Complications in
HEAD
and
NECK
SURGERY

Complications in
HEAD
and
NECK
SURGERY

Yosef P. Krespi, MD

Professor of Clinical Otolaryngology
Columbia University College of Physicians and Surgeons
Director, Department of Otolaryngology–Head and Neck Surgery
St. Luke's/Roosevelt Hospital Center
New York, NY

Robert H. Ossoff, DMD, MD

Guy M. Maness Professor and Chairman, Department of Otolaryngology
Vanderbilt University Medical Center
Attending Surgeon and Chairman, Department of Otolaryngology
Vanderbilt University Hospital
Nashville, TN

W. B. SAUNDERS COMPANY
Harcourt Brace Jovanovich, Inc.
Philadelphia   London   Toronto   Montreal   Sydney   Tokyo

W. B. SAUNDERS COMPANY
Harcourt Brace Jovanovich, Inc.

The Curtis Center
Independence Square West
Philadelphia, Pennsylvania 19106

Library of Congress Cataloging-in-Publication Data

Complications in head & neck surgery / [edited by]
Yosef P. Krespi, Robert H. Ossoff.
    p.   cm.

ISBN 0–7216–2980–6

1. Head—Surgery—Complications and sequelae.   2. Neck—
   Surgery—Complications and sequelae.   I. Krespi,
   Yosef P.   II. Ossoff, Robert H.   III. Title: Complications
   of head and neck surgery. [DNLM: 1. Head—surgery.
   2. Intraoperative Complications. 3. Neck—surgery.
   4. Postoperative Complications. WE 705 C7393]

RD521.C64 1993

617.5'101—dc20
DNLM/DLS   92–3580

Complications in Head and Neck Surgery   ISBN 0–7216–2980–6

Printed in the United States of America.

Last digit is the print number: 9   8   7   6   5   4   3   2   1

Contributors

———•———

ROBERT J. BACKER, MD
Staff Neurological Surgeon
St. John's Mercy Medical Center
St. Louis, MO
Neurotologic and Skull Base Surgery

SHAN R. BAKER, MD
Professor, Department of
    Otolaryngology
University of Michigan Medical
    School
Chief, Section of Facial Plastic and
    Reconstructive Surgery
Department of Otolaryngology
University of Michigan Medical
    Center
Ann Arbor, MI
*Tissue Transfer in Head and Neck
    Reconstruction: Skin Grafts, Skin
    Flaps, and Myocutaneous Flaps*
*Free Tissue Transfer in Head and Neck
    Reconstruction*

ANDREW BLITZER, MD, DDS
Professor of Clinical Otolaryngology
Department of Otolaryngology
Columbia University College of
    Physicians and Surgeons
Director, Division of Head and Neck
    Surgery
Columbia–Presbyterian Medical
    Center
New York, NY
Dysphagia and Aspiration

IOANA G. CARABIN, MD
Ear, Nose, Throat, Head and Neck,
    and Facial Plastic Surgeon

Satilla Regional Health Services
Waycross, GA
Paranasal Sinus Surgery

A. PHILIPPE CHAHINIAN, MD
Professor of Neoplastic Diseases
Mount Sinai School of Medicine
Senior Attending, Department of
    Neoplastic Disease
Mount Sinai Hospital
New York, NY
Complications of Chemotherapy

FRANCISCO J. CIVANTOS, MD
Assistant Professor, Department of
    Otolaryngology
University of Miami Medical School
Miami, FL
Carotid Artery Ligation

JACK A. COLEMAN, Jr., MD
Instructor, Department of
    Otolaryngology
Vanderbilt University Medical Center
Chief of Otolaryngology
Nashville Metropolitan General
    Hospital
Nashville, TN
Rigid Endoscopic Procedures

ISAAC ELIACHAR, MD
Staff Member and Section Head,
    Laryngotracheal Reconstruction
Department of Otolaryngology and
    Communicative Disorders
The Cleveland Clinic Foundation
Cleveland, OH
Laryngotracheal Devices

RON D. GOTTLIEB, MD
Chief Resident, Department of
    Otolaryngology–Head and Neck
    Surgery
New York Eye and Ear Infirmary
New York, NY
Acquired Immunodeficiency Syndrome;
    Precautions for Health Care Workers

MOSHE HAIMOV, MD
Clinical Professor of Vascular Surgery
Mount Sinai School of Medicine
Chief, Division of Vascular Surgery
Mount Sinai Hospital
Beth Israel Hospital North
New York, NY
Blood Vessels

GADY HAR-EL, MD
Assistant Professor and Director of
    Residency Training, Department
    of Otolaryngology
State University of New York—
    Health Science Center at
    Brooklyn
Director, Department of
    Otolaryngology
Kings County Medical Center
Brooklyn, NY
Tonsillectomy and Adenoidectomy

ELIZABETH HARRINGTON, MD
Assistant Professor of Vascular
    Surgery
Mount Sinai School of Medicine
Assistant Attending, Department of
    Surgery
Mount Sinai Hospital
New York, NY
Blood Vessels

JONAS T. JOHNSON, MD
Professor, Departments of
    Otolaryngology and Radiation
    Oncology
University of Pittsburgh School of
    Medicine
Vice Chairman, Department of
    Otolaryngology
The Eye and Ear Institute of
    Pittsburgh and The University of
    Pittsburgh Medical Center
Pittsburgh, PA
Head and Neck Infection

GARY D. JOSEPHSON, MD
Resident, Department of Surgery
Beth Israel Medical Center
Department of Otolaryngology–Head
    and Neck Surgery
New York Eye and Ear Infirmary
New York, NY
Functional Endoscopic Sinus Surgery

JORDAN S. JOSEPHSON, MD
Assistant Professor, Department of
    Otolaryngology–Head and Neck
    Surgery
State University of New York—
    Health Science Center at
    Brooklyn
Brooklyn, NY
Clinical Consultant, National
    Institutes of Health
Bethesda, MD
Chief, Division of Otolaryngology–
    Head and Neck Surgery
Director, Nasal and Sinus Center
Maimonides Medical Center
Brooklyn, NY
Functional Endoscopic Sinus Surgery

JAY R. KAMBAM, MD
Professor of Anesthesiology
Vanderbilt University Medical Center
Director, Division of Cardiovascular
    Anesthesia
Vanderbilt University Hospital
Nashville, TN
Anesthesia

SCOTT L. KAY, MD
Chief Resident, Department of
    Otolaryngology
Columbia University College of
    Physicians and Surgeons
Clinical Fellow in Otolaryngology
Columbia–Presbyterian Medical
    Center
New York, NY
Facial Reanimation Surgery

MONTE S. KEEN, MD
Assistant Professor of Otolaryngology
Columbia University College of
    Physicians and Surgeons
Director, Division of Facial Plastic
    and Reconstructive Surgery

Columbia–Presbyterian Medical
  Center
New York, NY
Cleft Lip Surgery
Facial Reanimation Surgery

ROBERT M. KELLMAN, MD
Associate Professor, Department of
  Otolaryngology and Pediatrics
Director of Maxillofacial Trauma
  Surgery
State University of New York—
  Health Science Center at
  Syracuse
Attending Physician
State University Hospital
Syracuse, NY
Maxillofacial Trauma

UMANG KHETARPAL, MD
Fellow, Department of
  Otolaryngology
Massachusetts Eye and Ear Infirmary
Boston, MA
Laryngeal Surgery

G. ROBERT KLETZKER, MD
Clinical Instructor, Department of
  Otolaryngology–Head and Neck
  Surgery
Washington University School of
  Medicine
Attending Surgeon
The Center for Cranial Base Surgery
St. John's Mercy Medical Center
Senior Attending, Washington
  University Medical Center
St. Louis, MO
Neurotologic and Skull Base Surgery

YOSEF P. KRESPI, MD
Professor of Clinical Otolaryngology
Columbia University College of
  Physicians and Surgeons
Director, Department of
  Otolaryngology–Head and Neck
  Surgery
St. Luke's/Roosevelt Hospital Center
New York, NY
Pharyngocutaneous Fistula
Dysphagia and Aspiration
Laryngeal Surgery
Stomal Recurrence and Mediastinal
  Dissection

DANIEL B. KURILOFF, MD
Assistant Professor of Clinical
  Otolaryngology
Columbia University College of
  Physicians and Surgeons
Assistant Director, Department of
  Otolaryngology–Head and Neck
  Surgery
St. Luke's/Roosevelt Hospital Center
Staff Otolaryngologist
Columbia–Presbyterian Medical
  Center
New York, NY
Tissue Transfer in Head and Neck
  Reconstruction: Skin Grafts, Skin
  Flaps, and Myocutaneous Flaps
Free Tissue Transfer in Head and Neck
  Reconstruction

KIN LAM, MD
Assistant Attending, Department of
  Medicine, Oncology and
  Hematology Section
St. Vincent Hospital
New York, NY
Complications of Chemotherapy

WILLIAM LAWSON, MD, DDS
Professor of Otolaryngology
Mount Sinai School of Medicine
Senior Attending
Mount Sinai Hospital
Chief, Department of Otolaryngology
Bronx VA Hospital
New York, NY
Paranasal Sinus Surgery

JOHN P. LEONETTI, MD
Assistant Professor of Otology,
  Neurotology, and Skull Base
  Surgery
Department of Otolaryngology
Co-Director, Center for Cranial Base
  Surgery
Loyola University Medical Center
Foster G. McGaw Hospital
Maywood, IL
Neurotologic and Skull Base Surgery

PAUL A. LEVINE, MD
Professor, Department of
  Otolaryngology–Head and Neck
  Surgery

Vice Chairman, Department of
Otolaryngology–Head and Neck
Surgery
University of Virginia Health Sciences
Center
Charlottesville, VA
Salivary Gland Surgery

FRANK E. LUCENTE, MD
Professor and Chairman, Department
of Otolaryngology–Head and
Neck Surgery
State University of New York
Health Science Center at
Brooklyn
Chairman, Department of
Otolaryngology
Long Island College Hospital
Brooklyn, NY
*Acquired Immunodeficiency Syndrome;
Precautions for Health Care Workers*

JUAN F. MOSCOSO, MD
Assistant Professor of
Otolaryngology–Head and Neck
Surgery
Mount Sinai School of Medicine
Fellow, Microvascular Surgery
Mount Sinai Hospital
New York, NY
Cranial Nerve Complications

MICHAEL NASH, MD
Assistant Professor of Surgery
Department of Otolaryngology
State University of New York—
Health Science Center at Stony
Brook
Stony Brook, NY
Tonsillectomy and Adenoidectomy

JAMES L. NETTERVILLE, MD
Assistant Professor, Department of
Otolaryngology
Vanderbilt University Medical Center
Director, Department of
Otolaryngology–Head and Neck
Surgery
Vanderbilt University Hospital
Chief, Division of Otolaryngology
Nashville VA Hospital
Nashville, TN
Carotid Artery Ligation

ROBERT H. OSSOFF, DMD, MD
Guy M. Maness Professor and
Chairman, Department of
Otolaryngology
Vanderbilt University Medical Center
Attending Surgeon and Chairman,
Department of Otolaryngology
Vanderbilt University Hospital
Nashville, TN
Laser Surgery

FRANCIS A. PAPAY, MD
Fellow, Cranial Facial and Pediatric
Plastic and Reconstructive
Surgery
Primary Children's Medical Center
Salt Lake City, UT
Laryngotracheal Devices

STEVEN J. PEARLMAN, MD
Assistant Professor of
Otolaryngology–Head and Neck
Surgery
Columbia University College of
Physicians and Surgeons
Assistant Director, Department of
Otolaryngology–Head and Neck
Surgery
St. Luke's/Roosevelt Hospital Center
New York, NY
Cranial Nerve Complications

GUY J. PETRUZZELLI, MD, PhD
Instructor, Department of
Otolaryngology
University of Pittsburgh School of
Medicine
Instructor, Department of
Otolaryngology
The Eye and Ear Institute of
Pittsburgh and The University of
Pittsburgh Medical Center
Pittsburgh, PA
Head and Neck Infection

HAROLD C. PILLSBURY, III, MD
Thomas J. Dark Distinguished
Professor of Surgery
University of North Carolina at
Chapel Hill School of Medicine
Attending Physician and Chief,
Division of Otolaryngology–Head
and Neck Surgery

University of North Carolina
    Hospitals
Chapel Hill, NC
Skull Base Surgery Complications

MICHAEL F. PRATT, MD
Assistant Professor, Department of
    Otolaryngology–Head and Neck
    Surgery
Director, Residency Training
    Education
Eastern Virginia Medical School
Chief, Department of Otolaryngology
DePaul Medical Center
Norfolk, VA
Surgery of the Pharynx and Esophagus

VITO C. QUATELA, MD
Associate Professor of Facial Plastic
    Surgery
Division of Otolaryngology–Head
    and Neck Surgery
University of Rochester Medical
    Center
Attending Physician in
    Otolaryngology
Strong Memorial Hospital
Highland Hospital
Genesee Hospital
Rochester, NY
Aesthetic Facial Surgery

JAMES F. REIBEL, MD
Assistant Professor, Department of
    Otolaryngology–Head and Neck
    Surgery
Attending, Department of
    Otolaryngology–Head and Neck
    Surgery
University of Virginia Health Sciences
    Center
Charlottesville, VA
Salivary Gland Surgery

HUGH REILLY, MD
Chief Resident, Department of
    Otolaryngology
Yale New Haven Hospital
New Haven, CT
Tracheotomy Complications

DALE H. RICE, MD
Tiber/Alpert Professor and Chairman,
    Department of Otolaryngology–
    Head and Neck Surgery

University of Southern California at
    Los Angeles School of Medicine
Los Angeles, CA
Functional Endoscopic Sinus Surgery

W. RUSSELL RIES, MD
Assistant Professor, Department of
    Otolaryngology–Head and Neck
    Surgery
Vanderbilt University Medical Center
Attending Physician
Vanderbilt University Hospital
Nashville, TN
Aesthetic Facial Surgery

CLARENCE T. SASAKI, MD
OHSE Professor of Surgery
Chief, Section of Otolaryngology
Yale University School of Medicine
Attending, Yale New Haven Hospital
New Haven, CT
Tracheotomy Complications

GARY L. SCHECHTER, MD
Professor and Chairman, Department
    of Otolaryngology–Head and
    Neck Surgery
Eastern Virginia Medical School
Norfolk, VA
Surgery of the Pharynx and Esophagus

GARY Y. SHAW, MD
Assistant Professor, Department of
    Otolaryngology–Head and Neck
    Surgery
University of Kansas Medical Center
Kansas City, KS
Attending Surgeon
VA Medical Center
Kansas City, MO
Management of Scars

GREGORY J. SHYPULA, MD
Clinical Fellow, Division of
    Hematology and Oncology
Department of Medicine
St. Luke's/Roosevelt Hospital Center
New York, NY
Complications of Chemotherapy

GEORGE A. SISSON, MD
Professor and Chairman (Emeritus)
Department of Otolaryngology–Head
    and Neck Surgery

Northwestern University Medical
School
Chicago, IL
*Stomal Recurrence and Mediastinal
Dissection*

HOWARD W. SMITH, DMD, MD
Professor of Clinical Otolaryngology
(Emeritus)
Columbia University College of
Physicians and Surgeons
Attending Surgeon, Department of
Otolaryngology
Columbia–Presbyterian Medical
Center
New York, NY
Cleft Lip Surgery

PETER G. SMITH, MD, PhD
Clinical Associate Professor,
Department of Otolaryngology–
Head and Neck Surgery
Washington University School of
Medicine
Co-Director, The Center for Cranial
Base Surgery
St. John's Mercy Medical Center
St. Louis, MO
Neurotologic and Skull Base Surgery

J. GREGORY STAFFEL, MD
Assistant Professor, Department of
Surgery
University of Texas Health Science
Center at San Antonio
Attending Physician
Medical Center Hospital
San Antonio, TX
Skull Base Surgery Complications

FRED J. STUCKER, MD
Professor and Chairman, Department
of Otolaryngology–Head and
Neck Surgery
Louisiana State University School of
Medicine
Attending, Louisiana State University
Medical Center
Shreveport, LA
Management of Scars

GORDON W. SUMMERS, DMD, MD
Attending Staff, Otolaryngology–
Head and Neck Surgery
Providence Medical Center
Portland, OR
Thyroid and Parathyroid Surgery

BHADRASAIN VIKRAM, MD
Professor of Radiation Oncology
Mount Sinai School of Medicine
Director, The Bernice and Charles
Blitman Department of Radiation
Oncology
Beth Israel Medical Center
New York, NY
Complications of Radiation Therapy

EDWIN F. WILLIAMS, III, MD
Facial Plastic and Reconstructive
Surgery
Otolaryngology–Head and Neck
Surgery
Albany Memorial Hospital
Albany, NY
Maxillofacial Trauma

Foreword

———•———

Earlier diagnosis of conditions requiring surgery and remarkable advances in surgical technique have greatly reduced the serious complications and morbidity that have accompanied head and neck surgery for generations. However, even present-day surgeons who limit their practice to the management of head and neck tumors face the unexpected challenge of complications; although complications occur far less frequently than in the past, they present more subtly. A contemporary thesis on head and neck complications edited by two widely experienced, well-respected surgeons is a welcome reference for both the practitioner and the full-time academic head and neck surgeon. The updates on laser surgery, facial plastics, and skull base problems make this text invaluable. Combining their vast surgical experience and that of their contributors, Dr. Krespi and Dr. Ossoff will help less experienced surgeons predict occasional or rare complications. We hope that early recognition of significant complications will allow for prompt management of problems and their timely resolution.

GEORGE A. SISSON, MD
Chicago, IL

Preface

———————•———————

Fifteen years ago, Dr. John Conley published his best-selling book, *Complications of Head and Neck Surgery.* Head and neck surgery has undergone tremendous changes since then, with recent advances in medical technology, pharmacology, radiology, laser surgery, anesthesiology, and intensive care.

The specialty of head and neck surgery practiced in the 1990s is completely different from that practiced in the 1960s. One major area of change is reconstruction following cancer surgery. In the last 30 years, new developments in anesthesia techniques and monitoring have allowed us to extend our horizon to former "no man's lands" like the mediastinum and the skull base; specifically, surgeons can perform surgical dissection around critical areas in the skull base, cavernous sinus region, carotid artery, cranial nerves, and orbit.

Having trained with prominent surgeons in the field of head and neck surgery, both editors of this book have seen the variety of developments since the early 1970s. Developments within the past 5 to 8 years include free flaps, laser surgery, skull base surgery, and endoscopic sinus surgery. As more surgeons have become involved with these types of surgical techniques, new complications that require management have become more evident. We hope this new volume of *Complications in Head and Neck Surgery* provides assistance to head and neck surgeons in avoiding complications and in managing these complications if they do occur.

Certainly, many surgeons remember discussing specific complications with an older surgical master and being answered with the following famous quotation, "Son, if you haven't seen this complication, it means that you have not done enough cases."

YOSEF P. KRESPI, MD
New York, NY

ROBERT H. OSSOFF, DMD, MD
Nashville, TN

Contents

———•———

CHAPTER 1

Anesthesia

JAY R. KAMBAM, MD

The scope of head and neck surgery may vary from a simple procedure like myringotomy and tube placement that lasts about 10 minutes in a patient with a normal airway to a complicated procedure that lasts several hours in a patient with a compromised airway. Head and neck surgery infrequently poses a challenge for the anesthesiologist. The surgery patients often have a compromised airway before operation, because of edema, infection, or altered anatomy as a result of benign or malignant growths from the structures of the airway. An understanding of the anatomy and pathophysiology of the airway, a thorough preoperative evaluation of the patient, familiarity with the surgical procedure, and last but not least a discussion with the surgeon about the perioperative management of the patient are essential to face this challenge and to manage these patients safely. It is absolutely necessary to adhere to sound airway management principles in conducting smooth and safe anesthesia for head and neck surgery. The surgeon's cooperation is often sought when the airway is either inaccessible or must be shared by both surgeon and anesthesiologist.

In addition to the airway problems from compromised airways, patients undergoing head and neck surgery are prone to certain complications: air embolism, pulmonary aspiration, cranial nerve reflexes leading to all types of arrhythmias, local anesthetic toxicity, and laser burns. Many patients are over 60 years of age and are vulnerable to the adverse effects of anesthesia because of their reduced margins of safety. An increased incidence of myocardial infarction (MI) associated with laser surgery is an example. The use of epinephrine and cocaine by the surgeon, and administration of nitrous oxide (N_2O) by the anesthesiologist during surgery, sometimes can cause serious problems. Many of these complications are discussed in this chapter; the complications related to laser surgery can be found in Chapter 30.

COMPLICATIONS RELATED TO AIRWAY MANAGEMENT [1-9]

The larynx, a boxlike structure, lies anterior to the bodies of the 4th, 5th, and 6th cervical vertebrae. The major skeleton of the larynx is formed anteriorly by the thyroid cartilage and posteriorly by the arytenoid and cricoid cartilages. The glottic opening is the narrowest part of the laryngeal cavity in adults. In children less than about 10 years of age, the narrowest part of the larynx is usually at the cricoid cartilage. The larynx is composed of nine cartilages—three paired (arytenoid, corniculate, and cuneiform) and three unpaired (thyroid, cricoid, and epiglottis).

Cricoid cartilage articulates with both thyroid and arytenoid cartilages. This is shaped like a signet ring, with the base lying posteriorly. This is the only structure that has a complete ring of cartilage, which lies anterior to the esophagus. Anesthesiologists frequently apply cricoid pressure to occlude the esophagus for prevention of regurgitation and aspiration of gastric contents. Arytenoid cartilage articulates with the cricoid cartilage to form a synovial joint. In rheumatoid arthritis there may be a significant narrowing of the airway because of the involvement of the cricoarytenoid joint. For this reason, blind insertion of an endotracheal tube in patients with rheumatoid arthritis is not recommended.

The epiglottis is a watchdog of the larynx. Thyroid cartilage is the largest cartilage of the larynx. Corniculate and cuneiform cartilages are of little importance in the structure of the larynx. The laryngeal muscles are voluntary and striated. The extrinsic muscles connect the larynx to the surrounding structures, and the intrinsic muscles lie within the larynx.

The vocal ligaments form the framework of the vocal cords. They are attached to the angles of the thyroid cartilage anteriorly and the arytenoid cartilage posteriorly.

Nerve Supply. The nerve supply to the larynx and trachea consists of the external and internal branches of the superior laryngeal nerve and the recurrent laryngeal nerve (both are branches of the vagus nerve or cranial nerve X), and branches from the glossopharyngeal nerve or cranial nerve IX. In addition, the pharynx, larynx, and trachea are supplied by the sympathetic nerves originating from the cervical sympathetic plexus.

Superior Laryngeal Nerve (External and Internal Branches). The external branch is a motor branch that supplies the cricothyroid muscle. The internal branch is sensory and pierces the posterior portion of the hyothyroid membrane above the superior laryngeal vessels at the greater cornu of the hyoid cartilage. The sensory branch divides into three sub-branches to supply (1) both surfaces of the epiglottis, (2) the aryepiglottic fold, and (3) the mucosa over the back of the larynx.

Recurrent Laryngeal Nerve (External and Internal Branches). The external branch is a motor branch that supplies all the intrinsic muscles of the larynx except the cricothyroid muscle, which is supplied by the external branch of the superior laryngeal nerve. The internal branch is a sensory branch that supplies the true vocal cords and the upper part of the tracheal mucosa. A few filaments communicate with the branches of the superior laryngeal nerve over the back of the tongue.

Stridor, Laryngeal Spasm, and Bronchospasm

The principal function of the larynx is to protect the tracheobronchial tree from aspiration of secretions and other foreign bodies. This is achieved by the glottic closure reflex of the adductor muscles of the larynx. This reflex is usually transient in nature and ends with removal of the stimulus. Two other important forms of laryngeal constriction are stridor and true laryngeal spasm.

Stridor is an incomplete form of glottic closure, usually caused by turbulent air flow through the larynx related to a tumor, edema, scarring, or nerve injury. Inspiratory stridor at rest indicates a severely compromised airway. To initiate general anesthesia before the airway is secured is a contraindication.

Laryngeal spasm is a form of complete glottic closure caused by a continued spasm of the false cords. Laryngeal spasm requires immediate therapy, which includes removal of the stimulus, gentle and sustained positive pressure breathing with 100 per cent oxygen, and sometimes administration of a rapidly acting muscle relaxant like succinylcholine (0.25 to 0.3 mg/kg, IV). Laryngeal spasm is frequently caused by painful stimuli anywhere in the body or stimulation of the airway under inadequate or light general anesthesia. Aspiration of gastric contents should always be suspected as another major cause of laryngeal spasm and bronchospasms.

Adequate oxygenation and ventilation of patients sometimes become difficult because of moderate-to-severe **bronchospasm** from airway stimulation. Bronchospasm is a frequent complication especially in patients with pre-existing airway disease. Treatment of bronchospasm includes increasing the depth of anesthesia, removing the stimulus until an adequate level of general anesthesia is achieved, administration of 100 per cent oxygen, and judicious use of bronchodilators. Ideally, patients should be evaluated and treated with bronchodilator drugs preoperatively to minimize this complication perioperatively.

Airway Edema

Edema of the upper airway is sometimes a serious complication of head and neck surgery. Manipulation of the airway with many kinds of laryngeal scopes and bronchoscopes and application of laser to the airway sometimes result in edema and airway obstruction. Treatment for airway edema includes parenteral administration of steroids (4 to 8 mg of dexamethasone); administration of racemic epinephrine (a mixture containing 50 per cent levo and 50 per cent dextro epinephrine; 0.25 to 0.5 ml in 2.5 ml of normal saline, every 4 to 6 hours) via a nebulizer; and/or reintubation of the trachea, depending upon the severity of obstruction.

Recurrent Laryngeal Nerve Injury

Unilateral nerve injury is rarely associated with an obstructed airway. However, bilateral recurrent nerve injuries can cause an acute obstruction of the upper airway. Typically, a patient with bilateral recurrent laryngeal nerve paralysis breathes well through an endotracheal tube, but when the tube is removed, the patient suddenly experiences severe difficulty in taking a breath. Reintubation of the trachea for several days is essential for a patient with bilateral nerve paralysis.

Noncardiac Pulmonary Edema

An airway spasm can result in pulmonary edema even in a patient with no pre-existing cardiopulmonary disease. Pulmonary edema may result from vigorous attempts to breathe against an obstructed upper airway because of the generation of large negative intrathoracic pressures leading to high negative interstitial hydrostatic pressures. In addition, high negative pressures can increase permeability leading to edema by injuring pulmonary capillaries and possibly alveoli.

A careful history regarding airway problems is essential prior to the induction of general anesthesia. Even with no evidence of known structural abnormalities (acquired or congenital), sometimes the anesthesiologist faces a difficult or impossible intubation. Proper planning and adherence to sound airway principles are necessary and are at times life-saving for patients with compromised airways. An airway can be secured in patients with compromised airways either by an awake oro- or nasotracheal intubation (with or without intravenous sedation and/or with topical anesthesia or nerve blocks) or by intubating a patient with the aid of a fiberoptic scope. A cricothyroidotomy, emergency tracheostomy, or insertion of a needle through cricothyroid membrane and careful oxygenation and ventilation with a Venturi-type jet ventilator are at times necessary. An elective tracheostomy under local anesthesia is sometimes absolutely necessary before the initiation of general anesthesia in certain patients.

Complications from Tracheal Intubation and Ventilation

Table 1–1 lists the major complications of various types of tracheal intubation and ventilation.

TABLE 1–1. Intubation and Ventilation Complications

Complications Related to Oro- and Nasotracheal Intubation	Complications Related to Jet Ventilation
Orogastric intubation	Barotrauma: Tracheal rupture, pneumomediastinum, pneumothorax, pneumoperitoneum, and subcutaneous emphysema
Nasogastric intubation	Hypoxemia and hypercapnia
Nasocranial intubation	Pulmonary aspiration
Bleeding	Inadequate anesthesia and intraoperative awareness
Aspiration pneumonitis	
Tissue damage	**Complications Related to Tracheostomy**
Teeth extraction	Bleeding
Vocal cord paralysis	Infection
Airway stenosis	Stenosis
Infection	Granulations
Adenoidectomy	Tracheomalacia
Granulomatosis	Mucus plugs from lack of humidity
Airway spasm	
Hypercapnia	
Cardiac arrest	
Hypoxia and hypoxemia	
Elevation in blood pressure, intracranial pressure, intraocular pressure, and intragastric pressure	
Arrhythmias	

LOCAL ANESTHETIC TOXICITY[10–15]

Local anesthetics that are used today are the *ester type* and the *amide type.*

Ester-type local anesthetics are cocaine, procaine, tetracaine, and chloroprocaine. They are metabolized primarily by an enzyme produced in the liver, called plasma cholinesterase or pseudocholinesterase.

Amide-type local anesthetics are lidocaine, bupivacaine, mepivacaine, prilocaine, and dibucaine. They are metabolized primarily in the liver.

Complications from the Use of Local Anesthetics

The occurrence of complications depends not only on the absolute amount of local anesthetic but also on its site of placement. For example, 1 ml of local anesthetic is enough to produce central nervous system toxicity if it is accidentally injected into the vertebral or carotid artery. Cardiovascular and respiratory toxicities usually follow central nervous system toxicity. Premonitory symptoms do not necessarily occur at all times. Some premonitory symptoms are tingling and numbness around the mouth, metallic taste, tinnitus or ringing in the ears, facial twitches, and nystagmus. Cardiovascular symptoms include bradycardia, hypotension, ventricular tachycardia, ventricular fibrillation, conduction blockade, and cardiac collapse. Respiratory arrest can occur from medullary ischemia, central depression, or both. Bupivacaine and cocaine are more cardiotoxic than the other local anesthetics.

Central Nervous System Toxicity

Therapy includes maintenance of the airway, oxygenation and ventilation, administration of thiopental sodium or a benzodiazepine (diazepam) and/or succinylcholine to treat seizures.

Cardiovascular System Toxicity

Cardiovascular support or cardiopulmonary resuscitation (CPR) or both may be necessary, depending on the severity of toxicity.

Anaphylactic Reactions

Anaphylactic reactions are very rare with the amide type of local anesthetic; if one occurs, it is usually from the preservative methylparaben. Anaphylactic reactions are also rare with the ester type of local anesthetic; when this occurs, it is usually from para-aminobenzoic acid, a metabolite of the ester. The same principles that apply to any drug-induced anaphylactic reaction also apply to the treatment of local anesthetic–induced anaphylactic reaction. In general, the treatment includes administration of epinephrine, histamine blockers, and corticosteroids; proper airway management; and fluid administration.

COCAINE TOXICITY [16–23]

Cocaine is an alkaloid derived from the South American shrub *Erythroxylon coca*, which has been extensively cultivated in the mountainous regions of Peru and Bolivia since at least the 7th century A.D. Cocaine is an ester type of local anesthetic and is primarily metabolized by an enzyme called pseudocholinesterase or plasma cholinesterase, which is produced in the liver. Unlike most of the other local anesthetics, cocaine produces vasoconstriction and shrinkage of the mucous membrane when applied topically. The anesthesiologist uses cocaine in patients primarily to attain topical analgesia of the nasal passages and to prevent bleeding from nasotracheal intubation. Head and neck surgeons use cocaine for shrinking nasal mucous membranes and to prevent bleeding, both of which produce a relatively dry surgical field.

Certain toxic effects of cocaine are of concern to both the anesthesiologist and the surgeon. If used in more than recommended doses, it can produce central nervous system toxicity, cardiorespiratory toxicity, and hypertensive crisis. Patients with hypertension, absent or abnormal pseudocholinesterase, and coronary artery disease are particularly prone to some of these cocaine-induced toxic reactions. The signs and symptoms of central nervous system toxicity include agitation, hallucinosis, headache, delirium, hyperthermia and diaphoresis, convulsions, and coma. Cocaine's major pharmacologic effect on the cardiovascular system is from its inhibition of the reuptake of norepinephrine at the synaptic clefts of sympathetic neurons. Because reuptake is a major route for elimination of neurotransmitter from its active receptor sites, the result is a potentiation of the response of sympathetically innervated organs to infused catecholamines, as well as to direct sympathetic stimulation. In addition, experimental evidence shows that cocaine may produce direct alpha-adrenergic stimulation through release of norepinephrine stored in peripheral sympathetic nerve terminals. Activation of postjunctional alpha-receptors is the major determinant of coronary and peripheral vascular resistance. It has been shown that cocaine, in fact, can cause coronary vasoconstriction and reduction of coronary blood flow, leading to ischemic syndromes.

Careful selection of patients, adherence to recommended doses (3 mg/kg), multiple applications rather than a single application of the entire recommended dose, and careful monitoring are absolutely essential to prevent some of the serious outcomes from cocaine toxicity. Combined use of a beta-blocker, nitrate, and a calcium channel blocker is a logical therapeutic choice if and when the toxic signs and symptoms of cocaine toxicity occur. Administration of a beta-blocker alone is not recommended as this may sometimes result in paradoxic hypertension.

EPINEPHRINE TOXICITY [24, 25]

Epinephrine is sometimes used by head and neck surgeons to produce vasoconstriction and to prevent bleeding in certain procedures, such as microsurgery of the ear and intranasal surgery. Administration of epinephrine is not without complications. The interaction with cocaine has already been discussed. Epinephrine frequently causes tachycardia, hypertension, and cardiac arrhythmias by itself. In addition, it produces marked cardiac arrhythmias when used with inhaled anesthetics. One should remember that concentrations of epinephrine greater than 1:50,000 do not provide further vasoconstrictive effect. The doses known to produce arrhythmias in 50 per cent of patients are (1) halothane (epinephrine injected in saline), 2.1 μg/kg, (2) halothane (epinephrine injected with 0.5 per cent lidocaine), 3.7 μg/kg; (3) isoflurane (epinephrine injected in saline), 6.7 μg/kg; and (4) enflurane (epinephrine in saline), 10.9 μg/kg. Suggested maximal single doses of epinephrine for submucosal injections are 1.5 μg/kg, 4.5 μg/kg, and 5 μg/kg when using halothane, isoflurane, and enflurane, respectively. One should not repeat these doses in less than 30-minute periods.

NITROUS OXIDE[26-28]

Nitrous oxide (N_2O) is an odorless to sweet smelling gas of low potency. It is most commonly administered in combination with other potent inhalation or intravenous anesthetics to produce general anesthesia. Although N_2O is a nonflammable gas, it will support combustion. For this reason either it is not used with the laser or if used will be discontinued a few minutes before applying laser near the airway. Even though N_2O is considered a relatively insoluble anesthetic, it is about 34 times more soluble in the blood than is nitrogen. In other words, N_2O can enter an air-filled cavity like the middle ear more rapidly than nitrogen can leave, resulting in a marked elevation of pressure in the middle ear. Under normal circumstances, this increase in middle ear pressure is passively vented via the eustachian tube into the nasopharynx. However, when the eustachian tube has narrowed because of inflammation, edema, or scarring, one can expect a tremendous elevation of middle ear pressure within a few minutes after N_2O administration. Tympanic membrane rupture, disruption of previous middle ear reconstructive

surgery, and tympanic membrane graft displacement are some of the adverse effects sometimes seen with the improper use of N_2O.

It is recommended that if N_2O is used during tympanoplasty, one should limit the concentration to 50 per cent, with gradual discontinuance at least 15 minutes prior to placement of the graft. Because of its solubility, discontinuation of N_2O can produce marked negative pressure in the middle ear, sometimes manifest as serous otitis media or transient postoperative hearing loss. The role of N_2O in air embolization is discussed in the next section.

AIR EMBOLISM[29-35]

Whenever an incision site is higher than right heart level, venous air embolism is a distinct possibility. Air embolism has been known as an intraoperative complication since 1818. A patient was undergoing operation in the seated position; a hissing sound was heard from within the incision and the patient lost consciousness and died within a few minutes. Autopsy revealed air in the right heart and pulmonary artery. The fact that a cut in a vein could act on the Venturi principle to entrain room air was well known by 1837. The position of the venous laceration in relation to the right heart and its size usually determine how much and how rapidly air can enter the circulation. If entrainment of air occurs steadily as small bubbles, these air bubbles travel to the lungs where normally they are rapidly absorbed by blood. On the other hand, rapid entrainment of air may produce right ventricular outflow tract obstruction, leading to cardiac arrest. In seated patients, however, air lock would be located not in the right heart but instead in the main pulmonary arteries.

Some patients undergoing major head and neck surgery are particularly prone to air embolization since the surgical field is usually elevated 15 to 20°, thereby creating a gravitationally induced negative pressure on the venous system and bony sinuses in the surgical field. The importance to the heart of the head position was first demonstrated by Senn in 1885 when he opened the superior sagittal sinus of horses and showed that air would enter with a hissing sound whenever the head was held elevated. Senn also demonstrated that lowering the head promptly stopped air entrainment. Systemic air embolism occurs only when a cardiac defect allows air bubbles to enter from the right heart to the left heart. Even though twenty-five per cent of the general population is said to have a patent foramen ovale, there should be a notable increase in right atrial pressure exceeding that of left atrial pressure before systemic arterial embolism can occur.

The constituents of the inspired gas mixture may have profound effects on the size of the air bubbles once they enter the circulation. Investigators found that continuous usage of nitrous oxide (N_2O) in animals at the time of air embolization is associated with grave effects on the outcome. Munson has shown that only one third the volume of air embolism is needed to kill rabbits breathing 70 per cent N_2O compared with breathing one hundred per cent oxygen. It is well known that N_2O, being about 34 times more soluble in blood than nitrogen, would expand the air bubbles two to four times, depending on the N_2O concentration used. However, prompt recognition of air embolism and discontinuation of N_2O would eliminate the problem of air bubble expansion.

Monitoring for air embolism is one of the most essential parts of perioperative management of patients undergoing head and neck surgery who are prone to have this complication. In many hospitals it is now standard practice to monitor such patients with one or more devices: (1) Doppler ultrasound, (2) end-tidal carbon dioxide tension ($P_{ET}CO_2$) or nitrogen tension with mass spectrometry or other means, (3) auscultation for murmurs with a precordial or esophageal stethoscope, (4) central venous pressure monitoring with a single or multipore catheter, and (5) pulmonary artery pressure monitoring with a Swan-Ganz catheter. A central venous or a Swan-Ganz catheter is indicated in high-risk patients as this not only aids in the diagnosis

but also helps in the treatment of air embolism. The advantages versus the disadvantages of one method of monitoring over another have been well reviewed elsewhere.

With the advent of improved monitoring and immediate diagnosis of air embolism, the perception of this condition has changed from that of a rare but catastrophic occurrence characterized by cardiovascular collapse to that of a frequent incidental finding that most often can be stopped with a plug of bone wax, tamponading the venous tear with a saline-soaked sponge, or application of an electrocautery device. In addition to lowering the incision site to a level below that of the right heart (head down or Trendelenburg position) and tilting the table to the left side (left lateral decubitus position to prevent air entering the right ventricular outflow tract and pulmonary artery), aspiration of air through a central venous catheter or a pulmonary artery catheter may be necessary at times.

PULMONARY ASPIRATION SYNDROME[36-45]

Anacreon, a Greek poet, died after inhaling grape seed in 475 B.C. Godwin of Wessex, proclaiming his innocence in the murder of Alfred the Etheling, said, "If I am guilty, may this bread choke me," whereupon he ate the bread, fell in a fit, and died. Humphrey Gilbert, an English poet, in 1583 aspirated a piece of mutton and died. Even poets and noblemen are not exempt from aspiration.

John Hunter in 1781 provided the first scientific observation of aspiration while testifying at a murder trial. Hunter said that it is in the mouth of everyone that a little brandy will kill a cat; it kills the cat by getting into its lungs, not its stomach. Curtis Mendelson in 1946 reported 66 cases of aspiration in obstetric patients undergoing general anesthesia for vaginal delivery. This classic report was so descriptive and complete that the acid pulmonary aspiration syndrome is now known as Mendelson syndrome. Mendelson also studied the clinical picture of aspiration syndrome in rabbits.

Pulmonary aspiration is a leading cause of anesthesia-related morbidity and mortality, accounting for about 10 per cent of anesthesia-related deaths. Available data from prospective studies indicate that the incidence of silent (unrecognized) aspiration of gastric contents occurring in patients undergoing general anesthesia is about 20 per cent. Patients undergoing head and neck surgery are frequently outpatients, and often they are apprehensive; often they do not have enough time to adjust to the strange hospital environment and are also suffering from their airway problems. In one study, adult outpatients had larger gastric volumes than inpatients. In addition, more outpatients had a gastric pH of less than 2.5. These patients are more vulnerable to regurgitation and subsequent aspiration of gastric and pharyngeal contents because of a difficult airway, loss of airway reflexes either from nerve damage or from topical anesthesia, or use of a small and incompletely sealed airway or no endotracheal tube at all in certain procedures.

Pulmonary aspiration frequently involves a liquid aspirate (over 90 per cent) and occasionally a solid aspirate. Aspiration of large, undigested particles of solid food leads to an acute airway problem by mechanically obstructing the major airway paths. This condition frequently requires rigid bronchoscopy and removal of foreign bodies.

Aspirated liquid material is either acidic (pH less than 2.5) or nonacidic or neutral (pH greater than 2.5). Nonacidic or neutral liquid aspirate can be subdivided into clear liquid and particulate aspirates. Both types of liquid aspirates usually produce acute hemorrhagic pulmonary edema leading to hypoxemia, acidosis, and hypotension if a large enough volume is aspirated. However, nonacidic liquid aspirates produce less severe lesions than do acidic aspirates. It is well established that the severity of the pulmonary damage depends on the acidity and volume of the liquid that is aspirated. The mortality rate appears to be lower for patients who aspirate nonacidic liquid material compared with acidic liquid material. The critical volume of the aspirate is considered to be around 25 ml (0.3 to 0.4 ml/kg). Aspiration

of blood or blood clots, other than causing mechanical obstruction of the airway, usually poses no high risk for pneumonitis. Signs and symptoms of severe acid aspiration include cyanosis; wheezing; tachycardia or bradycardia; acidosis; pink, frothy transudate, often in copious amounts; and hypotension.

Prevention of aspiration of gastric contents requires an appropriate number of hours of fasting before the planned operation, proper planning, and pharmacologic therapy. An intubation while the patient is awake or a rapid-sequence induction of anesthesia and endotracheal intubation with a cuffed tube and application of external cricoid pressure (Sellick maneuver) are sometimes necessary to prevent aspiration. However, frequently the nature of the operation necessitates no endotracheal intubation, which leaves the anesthesiologist to depend mainly on prophylactic pharmacologic therapy. This therapy includes an antacid (preferably a nonparticulate antacid), an H_2-antagonist (cimetidine, ranitidine, or famotidine), and a drug that empties stomach contents rapidly (metoclopramide).

Despite all preventive measures, pulmonary aspiration can still occur. Depending on the type and severity of aspiration, bronchoscopy, mechanical ventilation and application of positive end-expiratory pressure (PEEP), or continuous positive airway pressure (CPAP) for 24 to 48 hours may be necessary. Aggressive intravenous fluid replacement also may be required to treat the hypovolemia that occurs from the fluid shift caused by aspirate. The routine administration of corticosteroids and prophylactic antibiotic therapy are not recommended.

MYOCARDIAL INFARCTION[46-49]

Myocardial infarction (MI) is a potential complication of anesthesia and operation. The risk of sustaining an MI following anesthesia and surgery in a patient with no prior history of an MI is approximately 0.15 per cent (1 in 700 patients), with a mortality rate

TABLE 1–2. ASA Classification of Physical Status

Class 1:	No organic, physiologic, biochemical, or psychiatric disturbance
Class 2:	Mild-to-moderate systemic disturbance that may or may not be related to the reason for surgery
Class 3:	Severe systemic disturbance that may or may not be related to the reason for surgery
Class 4:	Severe systemic disturbance that is life threatening with or without surgery
Class 5:	Moribund patient who has little chance of survival but is submitted to surgery as a last resort (resuscitative effort)
Emergency (E):	Any patient in whom an emergency operation is required

Data from American Society of Anesthesiologists: New classification of physical status. Anesthesiology 24:111, 1963.)

of about 0.075 per cent (1 in 1400 patients). In patients with a previous MI, the incidence of fresh reinfarction is much greater and is related to the time elapsed since the previous MI. If the MI occurred more than 6 months previously, risk of reinfarction is about 6 per cent. If the MI is 0 to 3 months old, the risk of reinfarction is about 35 per cent (1 in 3 patients), and the risk decreases to about 15 per cent (1 in 7 patients) if the MI occurred between 4 and 6 months prior to anesthesia and operation. The mortality from such a perioperative reinfarction is between 50 and 70 per cent, much higher than that seen following a repeat MI not complicated by surgery. The site of the surgery, age (especially 70 years or more), the duration of the operation (more than 4 hours), preoperative congestive heart failure, ventricular aneurysm or ventricular dysfunction, left main coronary artery disease, and associated valvular heart disease (especially aortic stenosis) are some of the factors associated with a statistically significant increased risk for a perioperative MI. One should also note that the incidence of periprocedural myocardial ischemia and infarction is higher in patients undergoing laser airway procedures. Dumon and Vourc'h[46, 47] reported a mortality rate due to MI of about 0.6 per cent (1 in 160) in patients undergoing laser procedures, compared with 0.075 per cent (1 in 1400) due to MI in other procedures. The increased incidence of mortality was attributed to the age of the patients and preoperative cardiopulmonary disease.

Frequently occurring bronchospasm, laryngeal spasm, tachycardia, hypertension, hypercapnia, and hypoxemia are some of the other factors that may be responsible for increased mortality in MI patients undergoing airway surgery. A thorough evaluation of patients for cardiopulmonary disease and assuring that they reach the operating room in reasonably optimal shape are essential to reduce the perioperative mortality rate in these patients. Postponing surgery for at least 6 months after an MI will reduce the mortality rate significantly, as reported by several investigators.[48, 49]

CARDIAC ARREST[50–52]

The American Society of Anesthesiologists has grouped patients into five classes based on their physical status (Table 1–2). This classification is not intended to represent an estimate of anesthesia risk; however, intraoperative cardiac arrest is more common in the poor physical status classification, especially if emergency operation is performed.

Some causes of cardiac arrest under anesthesia are unrecognized hypoxemia, acidosis, hypovolemia, and an absolute or relative overdose of an anesthetic leading to cardiac depression and arrest. Another cause is the potential inability to intubate the trachea and ventilate the patient once general anesthesia is induced. Airway problems account for about 15 per cent of cardiac arrests in one recent report, compared with 44 per cent in another.[51]

MALIGNANT HYPERTHERMIA SYNDROME[53, 54]

Malignant hyperthermia (MH) is a hypermetabolic syndrome that can occur spontaneously in association with physical exercise, but it usually occurs with the use of halogenated inhalation anesthetics or succinylcholine. The incidence of MH has been reported to vary from 1 in 5000 to 1 in 50,000 surgical patients. MH may occur at any age but is most common in children, it is seen in decreasing frequency in those past age 40 years.

MH is an inherited disorder and follows an autosomal pattern in many families. It usually becomes manifest immediately following the induction of anesthesia but can occur at any point during anesthesia or in the first 24 hours following operation. Muscle rigidity (especially of the involuntary jaw muscles) is seen about 50 per cent of the time following the administration of succinylcholine in patients who eventually develop full-blown MH. Other early signs of MH include tachycardia, tachypnea, and rapid elevation of end-tidal P_{CO_2}. An elevation in temperature usually follows these early signs.

Blood gas tension determinations usually reveal a mixed respiratory and metabolic acidosis. Electrolyte determinations usually show hyperkalemia and hypocalcemia early in the course, followed by hypokalemia or normokalemia later. An increase in the CPK enzyme level (more than 20,000 U) when the level is measured every 6 hours for 48 hours will usually support the diagnosis. A muscle biopsy for the halothane-caffeine contracture test is presently recommended by many anesthesiologists in doubtful cases and for the family members of a patient who develops MH.

Treatment

In patients with a prior history of MH, all known triggering agents should be avoided. Dantrolene sodium, a muscle relaxant known to abort this syndrome, has been used for prophylactic therapy for several years; however, at present it is not routinely used for this purpose. The triggering agent is discontinued; vigorous hyperventilation with 100 per cent oxygen is begun; dantrolene sodium is administered intravenously immediately; cooling measures (ice packs, cool intravenous fluids, cooling blanket, air conditioning) are applied; and the operation is terminated as soon as possible. Cardiac arrhythmias are usually treated with intravenous procainamide, since use of lidocaine at this time is controversial.

With early diagnosis and prompt administration of dantrolene, the mortality rate should be near zero. If MH is not recognized early so that treatment with dantrolene can be initiated quickly, a 70 to 100 per cent mortality rate can be expected.

References

1. DeWeese DD, Saunders WH (eds): Textbook of Otolaryngology. 5th ed. St. Louis, CV Mosby, 1977, pp 89–101.
2. Fink BR: The Human Larynx; A Functional Study. New York, Raven Press, 1975, p 100.
3. Saunders WH: The Larynx. CIBA Found Symp 16:67–99, 1964.
4. Maze A, Block E: Stridor in pediatric patients. Anesthesiology 50:132–145, 1979.
5. Bryce DP, Briant TDR, Pearson FG: Laryngeal and tracheal complications of intubation. Ann Otol Rhinol Laryngol 77:442, 1968.
6. Keane WM, Rowe LD, Denneny JC, Atkins JP: Complications of intubation. Ann Otol Rhinol Laryngol 91:584–587, 1982.
7. Rex MAE: A review of the structural and functional basis of laryngospasm; Nerve pathways and clinical significance. Br J Anaesth 42:891–899, 1970.
8. McGonagle M, Kennedy TL: Laryngospasm-induced pulmonary edema. Laryngoscope 94:1583–1585, 1984.
9. Donlon JV: Anesthetic management of compromised airways. Anesth Rev 7:22–31, 1980.
10. Tucker GT, Mather LE: Clinical pharmacokinetics of local anesthetics. Clin Pharmacokinet 4:241–278, 1979.
11. Mather LE, Cousins MJ: Local anesthetics and their current clinical use. Drugs 18:185–204, 1979.
12. Liu P, Feldman HS, Covino BM, et al: Acute cardiovascular toxicity of intravenous amide local anesthetics in anesthetized ventilated dogs. Anesth Analg 61:317–322, 1982.
13. Kotelko DM, Shnider SM, Dailey PA, et al: Bupivacaine-induced cardiac arrhythmias in sheep. Anesthesiology. 60:10–18, 1984.
14. Voulgaropoulos DS, Johnson MD, Covino BG: Local anesthetic toxicity. Semin Anesth 9:8–15, 1990.
15. Tazelaar HD, Karch SB, Stephens BG, Billingham ME: Cocaine and the heart. Hum Pathol 18:195–199, 1987.

16. Digregorio GJ: Cocaine update: Abuse and therapy. Am Fam Physician 41:247–250, 1990.
17. Gawin FH, Ellinwood EH: Cocaine and other stimulants. Actions, abuse, and treatment. N Engl J Med 318:1173–1182, 1988.
18. Jatlow P: Cocaine: Analysis, pharmacokinetics, and metabolic disposition. Yale J Biol Med 61:105–113, 1988.
19. Gradman AH: Cardiac effects of cocaine: A review. Yale J Biol Med 61:137–147, 1988.
20. Gay GR: Clinical management of acute and chronic cocaine poisoning. Ann Emerg Med 11:562–572, 1982.
21. Rappolt RT, Gay GR, Inaba DS: Propranolol. A specific antagonist to cocaine. Clin Toxicol 10:265–271, 1977.
22. Ramoska E, Sachhetti AD: Propranolol-induced hypertension in treatment of cocaine intoxication. Ann Emerg Med 14:1112–1113, 1985.
23. Billman GE, Hoskins RS: Cocaine-induced ventricular fibrillation: Protection afforded by the calcium antagonist verapamil. FASEB J 2:2990–2995, 1988.
24. Johnston RR, Eger EI II, Wilson C: A comparative interaction of epinephrine with enflurane, isoflurane, and halothane in man. Anesth Analg (Cleve) 55:709–712, 1976.
25. Munson ES, Tucker WK: Doses of epinephrine causing arrhythmia during enflurane, methoxyflurane, and halothane anesthesia in dogs. Can Anaesth Soc J 22:495–501, 1975.
26. Munson SE: Transfer of nitrous oxide into body airway cavities. Br J Anaesth 46:202–209, 1974.
27. Patterson ME, Bartlett PG: Hearing impairment caused by intratympanic pressure changes during general anesthesia. Laryngoscope 86:399–404, 1976.
28. Owens WD, Gustave F, Scarloff A: Tympanic membrane rupture with nitrous oxide anesthesia. Anesth Analg 57:283–286, 1978.
29. Lesky E: Notes on the history of air embolism. German Med Monthly 6:159–161, 1961.
30. Durant TM, Long J, Oppenheimer MJ: Pulmonary (venous) air embolism. Am Heart J 33:269–281, 1947.
31. Senn N: An experimental and clinical study of air-embolism. Ann Surg 3:197–302, 1885.
32. Munson ES: Effect of nitrous oxide on venous air embolism. Anesth Analg 50:785–792, 1971.
33. Hybels RL: Venous air embolism in head and neck surgery. Laryngoscope 90:946–954, 1980.
34. Bedford RF: Venous air embolism: A historical perspective. Semin Anesth 2:169–176, 1983.
35. Brechner VL, Bethune RWM: Recent advances in monitoring pulmonary embolism. Anesth Analg 50:255–261, 1971.
36. Ong BY, Palahniuk RJ, Cumming M: Gastric volume and pH in outpatients. Can Anesth Soc J 25:36–39, 1978.
37. Simpson JY: The alleged case of death from the action of chloroform. Lancet 1:175, 1848.
38. Mendelson CL: The aspiration of stomach contents into the lungs during obstetric anesthesia. Am J Obstet Gynecol 52:191, 1946.
39. Pierce EC: Historical perspectives. Int Anesth Clin 22:1–16, 1984.
40. Blitt CD, Gutman HL, Cohen DD, et al: Silent regurgitation and aspiration during general anesthesia. Anesth Analg 49:707, 1970.
41. Sellick BA: Cricoid pressure to control regurgitation of stomach contents during induction of anesthesia. Lancet 2:404, 1961.
42. Manchikanti L, Colliver JA, Marerro TC, Roush JR: Ranitidine and metoclopramide for prophylaxis of aspiration pneumonitis in elective surgery. Anesth Analg 63:903–910, 1984.
43. Manchikanti L, Marerro TC, Roush JR: Preanesthetic cimetidine and metoclopramide for acid aspiration prophylaxis in elective surgery. Anesth Analg 61:48–54, 1984.
44. Gibbs CP, Scwartz DJ, Wynne JW, et al: Antacid pulmonary aspiration in the dog. Anesthesiology 51:380–385, 1979.
45. Chapman RL, Modell JH, Ruiz BC, et al: Effect of continuous positive pressure ventilation and steroids on aspiration of hydrochloric acid in dogs. Anesth Analg 53:556, 1974.
46. Dumon JF, Shapshay S, Bourcerean J, et al: Principles for safety in application of Neodymium-YAG laser in bronchoscopy. Chest 86:163–168, 1984.
47. Vourch'h G, Fischler M, Personne C, et al: Anesthetic management during Nd-YAG laser resection for major tracheobronchial obstructing tumors. Anesthesiology 61:63–67, 1984.
48. Tinker JH, Noback CR, Vlietstra RE, Frye RL: Managements of patients with heart disease for noncardiac surgery. JAMA 246:1348–1350, 1981.
49. Strong MS, Vaughan CW, Mahler DL, et al: Cardiac complications of microsurgery of the larynx: Etiology, incidence and prevention. Laryngoscope 84:908–920, 1974.
50. American Society of Anesthesiologists: New classification of physical status. Anesthesiology 24:111, 1963.
51. Keenan RL, Boyan CP: Cardiac arrest due to anesthesia. JAMA 23:2373–2377, 1985.
52. Harrison GG: Death attributable to anaesthesia: A ten year survey. Br J Anaesth 50:1041, 1979.
53. Gronert GA: Malignant hyperthermia. Anesthesiology 53:395–423, 1980.
54. Denborough MA: Malignant hyperpyrexia. Clin Anesthesiol 2:669–675, 1984.

CHAPTER 2

Blood Vessels

MOSHE HAIMOV, MD
ELIZABETH HARRINGTON, MD

The successful outcome of major head and neck surgery depends greatly on the prevention of the two major causes of intraoperative and postoperative morbidity and mortality—hemorrhage and airway obstruction. Frequently these two are interrelated. As with all surgical complications, prevention is better than treatment. Prevention of hemorrhage depends on meticulous surgical technique, thorough knowledge of head and neck anatomy, and proper preoperative evaluation of the coagulation factors essential for proper hemostasis. If hemorrhagic complications are anticipated and prevented, most major bleeding complications can be avoided.

Careful questioning will reveal a history of excessive bruising, previous hemorrhages, or underlying liver disease that may impair the coagulation mechanism. In obtaining a careful history, it is important to inquire about drug use, especially anti-inflammatory agents such as aspirin or aspirin-containing compounds, since many of these agents affect platelet aggregation and may cause excessive bleeding at the time of operation. If the tumor to be resected is clinically sus-

pected to involve major vessels, a computed tomography scan and arteriography should be considered to define the extent of carotid artery involvement. If these diagnostic studies confirm or are highly suspicious of major arterial involvement, the risk of carotid ligation or bypass should be discussed with the patient, and a vascular surgeon should be consulted and asked to be available at the time of operation for possible vascular reconstruction to prevent ischemic brain damage.

At operation, blood loss can be minimized by elevating the head 15 to 30 degrees, carefully monitoring vital signs. This elevation reduces venous congestion and also reduces small vessel oozing. Operating in the head and neck region requires knowledge of the anatomy of all major vessels and careful ligation of them. Inadvertent injury of major vessels occurs usually to the internal jugular vein or the common carotid artery and its major branches, i.e., the internal or external carotid arteries. Successful management of these injuries is to minimize blood loss, obtain proper exposure, and carry out the appropriate repair or ligature. Both venous and arterial bleeding can be temporarily controlled with pressure, allowing for proper proximal and distal dissection and exposure of the injured vessel. Haste and blind application of clamps not only increases the extent of the injury, making it less amenable to local pressure control, but also causes hypotension and shock, which greatly aggravate an ischemic injury. In addition, "blind" clamp application greatly increases the risk of major nerve injury with serious long-term consequences.

If a vein has been completely transected, by applying local pressure the ends of the vein can be identified and twisted with a hemostat, which will stop the bleeding and permit proper suture ligature application. If the vein has been only partially lacerated, the lacerated end can be grasped with an Allis clamp, which controls the bleeding and allows careful suturing of the laceration with monofilament vascular sutures. If the external carotid artery has been lacerated, it can be safely ligated without serious consequences. On the other hand, ligation of the internal or common carotid artery may result in severe, permanent neurologic damage or death and should be avoided if at all possible. Common carotid lacerations usually can be repaired with a lateral suture. If the internal carotid artery has been lacerated, lateral sutures may cause stenosis and predispose the patient to postoperative thrombosis, which may cause severe neurologic damage. This type of injury should be repaired with a vein patch.

The expertise of the vascular surgeon, if one is available, will greatly increase the success of these more complicated arterial repairs. Injuries that are close to the carotid bifurcation in elderly patients may require endarterectomy for repair; again, the help of an experienced vascular surgeon is required for successful outcome. If no such surgeon is available, it is safer to ligate the carotid artery rather than to proceed with a less than ideal repair, since postoperative thrombosis will put the patient at greater risk than will intraoperative ligation combined with postoperative anticoagulation. Although the duration of carotid clamping may be critical in a minority of cases, the use of temporary shunts by an inexperienced operator is inadvisable and should be avoided. The normotensive patient usually tolerates temporary carotid clamping better than poor arterial repair or traumatic shunting.

During extensive neck dissections, the subclavian artery may be injured, causing massive hemorrhage that may be difficult to control. The subclavian arteries are very friable vessels, and application of nonvascular clamps may cause further and frequently irreparable damage. If injury does take place, control should be obtained with local pressure, and proximal and distal control of the vessel should be obtained. Disarticulation or transection of the clavicle may be required on occasions to achieve proper control. Balloon catheters also can be used for temporary vascular control to allow for repair of the injured vessels. If difficult or impossible to repair, the subclavian artery can be ligated; this will seldom cause severe, acute ischemia, although arterial repair in the future may be required if severe functional impairment is noted.

POSTOPERATIVE BLEEDING

Postoperative bleeding is a serious complication in head and neck surgery. Excessive bleeding in the immediate postoperative period is usually caused either by technical mishaps or coagulopathy. When the bleeding is sudden, usually an untied vessel has reopened or the ligature of a major vessel has slipped. The major arteries that may cause this bleeding are usually the external carotid artery or its branches, most commonly the superior thyroid artery or the thyrocervical trunk in the lower portion of the neck. Venous structures that may be involved in acute bleeding include the internal jugular vein, the veins of the pterygoid and pharyngeal plexus, and the facial and external jugular veins. If suturing of the bleeding vessel is impractical, such as at the base of the skull or in the temporal bone region, tamponade with surgical gauze, Gelfoam, or muscle flaps may prove to be life saving. Surgicel, oxidized cellulose, has a specific applicability to bleeding in areas that are inaccessible from a technical point of view. Control of hemorrhage is life saving and should be done expeditiously. Adequate blood replacement should be given and special attention paid to maintain an adequate airway, either by endotracheal intubation or tracheostomy.

Acquired coagulopathy may also account for postoperative bleeding. Some of these complications may be caused by malnutrition, which diminishes the levels of vitamin K–dependent coagulation factors. Patients who have had radiotherapy and combination chemotherapy may have defective platelet function, which will cause generalized oozing and continuous postoperative blood loss. In addition, coagulopathy may be caused by failure to administer fresh-frozen plasma and platelets if only packed erythrocytes were used to replace extensive blood loss during operation.

Regardless of cause, the immediate effects of postoperative bleeding after head and neck surgery are usually obvious. If the drainage system is functioning properly, large amounts of blood are drained into the collection system; if the system is not functioning, hematoma forms under the skin flaps, which may cause severe respiratory distress. Once the bleeding complication is recognized—and one should always be alert and looking for it—supportive therapy in the form of fluid and blood replacement should be given immediately. All bleeding patients should be urgently returned to the operating room for re-exploration.

Delayed Postoperative Bleeding

Principal complications causing delayed postoperative bleeding relate to wound infection, fistula formation, and radiation necrosis. They may occur from 1 to 6 weeks following operation. The most common vessel associated with delayed postoperative bleeding is the carotid artery. This is one of the most catastrophic postoperative complications of head and neck surgery. Rupture of the carotid artery is an uncommon entity, occurring in 3 to 7 per cent of head and neck dissections. It has been reported to have a mortality of 50 per cent, and there are some reports that neurologic sequelae have occurred in excess of 60 per cent. An association of this complication with previous radiation is strong. Marchetta and Sakok documented a 7 per cent carotid artery rupture in 56 patients treated with radiation, as opposed to no rupture in those patients who had never received radiation.[1] Stell reported a 3 per cent carotid artery rupture rate in 280 patients undergoing head and neck surgery.[2] The risk of rupture in this group was also directly related to previous radiation. Other significant factors that are known to increase the risk of carotid rupture are the development of postoperative orocutaneous or pharyngocutaneous fistulas. The great majority of these fistulas appear during the first 2 weeks postoperatively, and they are almost always secondary to leakage of saliva at the pharyngeal closure. Five of ten patients reported by Coleman[3] and 43 of 60 reported by Heller and Strong[4] had these factors as predisposing cause. A large fistula positioned in the lateral portion of the neck in the proximity of the carotid artery should alert the surgeon to expect this complication.

Wound infections after breakdown of the pharyngeal closure predispose to carotid blowout. These wounds are often contaminated by *Staphylococcus aureus* as well as anaerobic flora of the mouth. The avoidance of flap incisions that parallel the carotid bulb is important. Many surgeons recommend use of the MacFee flap with horizontal incisions along the clavicle and submandibular fold to minimize carotid exposure in the event of skin breakdown. Placement of the suction drains over a previously radiated carotid artery should be avoided. Conley has stated that there are systemic factors that predispose to this complication: anemia, diabetes, and severe cardiovascular or chronic obstructive pulmonary disease.[5] A decreased ideal body weight of 10 to 50 per cent and hypoproteinemia also have been reported to predispose to rupture.

The etiology of carotid rupture has been

well delineated. Microscopic examination of the tissues has demonstrated premature atherosclerosis and fibrosis with obstruction of the vasa vasorum. Swain and colleagues have developed an experimental model of this in dogs and showed that an intact vasa vasorum prevented carotid artery rupture even when a pharyngocutaneous fistula with infection was present.[6]

Appropriate measures should be taken at operation to protect the vasa vasorum and the adventitia of the carotid artery. As noted, the placement of the flap incision is crucial to protect the artery should skin necrosis develop in cases in which there was a high risk of carotid artery rupture. In 1963 Corso and colleagues reported on the use of buried dermis for protecting carotid arteries.[7] Others have reported good results with this method. However, Smithdeal and associates in a 10-year review found no advantage to this coverage.[8] Coleman reported that the dermal graft has been shown to be ineffective.[3] Because the radiated neck is at risk for contamination by oral contents and the recipient bed is inadequate to receive a skin graft with the possibility of loss of the dermal graft and subsequent infection, this method of protection is no longer widely used. The musculocutaneous flap has been shown to be more resistant to infection and therefore more reliable in preventing complication. It is of major advantage to use such flaps as the pectoralis major or the latissimus dorsi, whose blood supply is outside the field of radiation. The regional neck flaps, such as the levator scapula flap and the trapezius muscle, have fallen into disfavor. They receive their blood supply from the transverse cervical artery, which may be affected by the radiation.

The pectoral and latissimus flaps provide muscle and tissue bulk above the vasculature and make them less prone to kinking and vascular compromise. However, they too have their problems. Care must be taken to avoid compression of the flap or its blood supply—that is, the thorocoacromial or thoracodorsal vessel. Adequate tunneling must be provided for these grafts. When the carotid artery is exposed to bacterial contamination, the vasa vasorum may not be able to withstand the insult. Emergency coverage of the artery must be provided. All necrotic tissue should be debrided and a musculocutaneous flap placed. If there is any evidence of necrosis of the carotid artery itself, it should be ligated proximally and distally to healthy arterial wall and the necrotic area excised. Failure to remove the unhealthy arterial wall completely may result in bleeding at a later date and act as a source of persistent infection.

The site of acute rupture is usually the common carotid artery, followed by the internal carotid artery and the carotid bulb. The external carotid artery is rarely the site of rupture. Cerebral complications occur within the first 24 hours postoperatively and include contralateral hemiplegia, hemianesthesia, aphasia, dysarthria, atrophy of the optic nerve, or monoplegia.[6] It has been suggested that these complications may be prevented to a certain extent by low-dose heparin. Massive hemorrhage should be controlled by manual pressure until intravascular volume can be restored and blood crossmatched. The airway should be controlled either by utilizing the previous tracheostomy or by placement of an endotracheal tube. Adequate blood pressure should be maintained. The patient should not be operated upon until stable. The incidence of neurologic complications decreases when operation is performed on a normotensive patient. The carotid artery should be treated as an infected foreign body when hemorrhage occurs. Vascular control should be obtained above and below the necrotic area through separate skin incisions. The involved arteries are suture-ligated and the stumps buried after coverage with vascularized muscle. This will decrease the chances of subsequent infection, septic emboli, and repeated hemorrhage.

CAROTID ARTERY RESECTION AND BYPASS FOR NECK CARCINOMA

The patient with recurrent neck cancer who has had prior radiation and operation is usually considered incurable when the tumor is fixed or surrounds the carotid artery either by metastasis or by direct extension. Resection of the carotid artery to eradicate this type of disease has significant morbidity and mortality. Recently, however, surgical excision with replacement of the artery has been shown to provide a chance of cure in these patients. With improved methods of vascular replacement, wound coverage, and control of infection, the morbidity and mortality can be reduced to an acceptable level, thus offering the chance of cure for a disease that is otherwise universally fatal.

Biller and colleagues reported a total of 28 carotid artery replacements in 26 patients.[9] This was achieved with a neurologic sequelae of 7 per cent and a postoperative mortality of 15 per cent. This is a significant improvement compared with previous results. Conley in 1953 and 1957 reported carotid artery replacement in 17 patients with 7 operative and 5 postoperative deaths.[10, 11] Lore and Boulos in 1981 reported 9 cases with a postoperative mortality rate of 22 per cent and a 30 per cent incidence of cerebral ischemia.[12] The diminished morbidity in the Biller series is attributed to the decreased duration of cerebral ischemia by using the subclavian artery for the proximal anastomosis in reconstructing the cerebral circulation. The subclavian artery is located at a distance from the pharynx and, accordingly, is better protected should an infection develop. It is outside the center field of radiation and is a healthier vessel for anastomosis. Furthermore, since the anastomosis is more lateral, the graft may be rerouted posteriorly at a greater distance from the area of recurrence. By using the subclavian artery, the duration of carotid flow interruption can be reduced an average of 4 minutes. Additionally, the use of myocutaneous flaps to replace compromised or resected neck skin and the creation of a pharyngostoma added to the success of this operation. The results in this series show that the patient with only neck disease has a better chance of cure compared with the patient with a primary lesion that has not been resected previously. Four of five patients with only neck disease in Biller's series survived 12 or more months without evidence of recurrence.

In summary, although the long-term prognosis of patients with primary or secondary malignancy involving the carotid arteries remains poor, radical excision with carotid replacement does offer a chance for cure or palliation with acceptable morbidity and mortality.

VASCULAR COMPLICATIONS OF HEAD AND NECK TRAUMA

The treatment of penetrating injuries in the head and neck region is still controversial. Some surgeons recommend mandatory neck exploration in all patients with penetrating injury deeper to the platysma muscle, while others show equally good results obtained with selective exploration based on defined indications. Almost all, however, agree that four-vessel angiography is indicated for all patients with penetrating neck trauma who are otherwise stable.

In a recent review of 85 penetrating injuries, Weaver and associates advocate arterial reconstructions in all patients with carotid artery trauma.[13] Their experience has shown that the presence of a neurologic deficit did not contraindicate arterial reconstruction; following this policy, all their patients improved and none developed the dreaded complication of revascularization in the presence of neurologic deficit, i.e., hemorrhagic infarction. If the internal carotid artery is injured at the base of the skull and cannot be repaired simply, ligation is advocated. The researchers conclude that the major determinant of morbidity and mortality in carotid artery injury is the ischemic insult and not the reperfusion hemorrhage.

Vertebral artery injury is uncommon and may be initially unrecognized.[14] Vertebral artery injuries may result in arteriovenous fistulas and pseudoaneurysms that may appear weeks or months following the injury. Surgical angiography used in the routine evaluation of patients with penetrating neck trauma readily demonstrates vertebral artery injury. Neurologic deficits are not usually caused by isolated vertebral artery injuries, since circulation to the basilar system may be adequately supplied by a single vertebral artery. The treatment consists of proximal and distal ligation of the vertebral artery. Ligation should be done, however, only when a patent contralateral vertebral artery is demonstrated and the arteriogram does not show that the spinal cord receives a substantial blood supply from the extracranial vertebral artery—which is rare but does occur in about 3 per cent of the population. If the contralateral vertebral artery is hypoplastic or if it significantly contributes to the blood supply of the spinal cord, an attempt should be made to restore vertebral artery flow using an interposition graft.

References

1. Marchetta FA, Sakok MW: Complications after radical head and neck surgery—performed through previously irradiated tissues. Am J Surg 114:835, 1967.
2. Stell PK: Catastrophic hemorrhage after major head and neck surgery. Br J Surg 56:525, 1969.
3. Coleman JJ: Complications in head and neck surgery. Surg Clin North Am 66:149–169, 1986.
4. Heller KS, Strong EW: Carotid artery hemorrhage after radical head and neck surgery. Am J Surg 138:607–610, 1979.
5. Conley JJ: Blood vessel complications. In Conley JJ: Complications of Head and Neck Surgery. Philadelphia, WB Saunders, 1979, pp 81–85.
6. Swain RE, Biller HF, Ogura JH: An experimental analysis of causative factors and protective methods in carotid cut rupture. Arch Otolaryngol 99:235, 1974.
7. Corso PF, Gerald PF, Frazell EL: The rapid closure of large salivary fistulas by an accelerated shoulder flap technique. Am J Surg 106:691, 1963.
8. Smithdeal CD, Corso PF, Strong EW: Dermis grafts for carotid artery protection: Yes or no? A ten year experience. Am J Surg 128:484–489, 1974.
9. Biller FW, Urken M, Lawson W, Haimov M: Carotid artery resection and bypass for neck carcinoma. Laryngoscope 94:181–183, 1988.
10. Conley J: Free autogenous vein graft to the internal and external carotid arteries in the treatment of tumors of the neck. Ann Surg 137:205–214, 1953.
11. Conley J: Carotid artery surgery in the treatment of tumors of the neck. Arch Otolaryngol 65:437–446, 1957.
12. Lore JM, Boulos EJ: Resection and reconstruction of the carotid artery in metastatic squamous cell carcinoma. Am J Surg 142:437–442, 1981.
13. Weaver FA, Yellin EA, Wagner WH, et al: The role of arterial reconstruction in penetrating carotid injuries. Arch Surg 123:1106–1110, 1988.
14. Meier DE, Brink EB, Fry TW: Vertebral artery trauma. Acute recognition and treatment. Arch Surg 116:236–239, 1981.

CHAPTER 3

Carotid Artery Ligation

FRANCISCO J. CIVANTOS, MD
JAMES L. NETTERVILLE, MD

The management of the compromised carotid artery is one of the most difficult problems in head and neck surgery. Most structures external to the deep cervical fascia can be summarily sacrificed for oncologic reasons. The internal and common carotid arteries, however, can be electively ligated only after careful evaluation of the adequacy of the collateral cerebral circulation, in order to avoid cerebral hypoperfusion and stroke. On the other hand, efforts to avoid ligation of the artery can predispose the patient to spontaneous rupture of the artery, requiring emergency resuscitation and carotid ligation.[1, 2]

Carotid ligation may be necessary for a variety of reasons. It can be electively performed in patients with cancer involving the carotid artery. More urgent ligation may be indicated in patients with postoperative fistulas or open wounds, often previously irradiated, who are at high risk for spontaneous rupture of an exposed carotid. Emergency ligation may prove necessary in the event of spontaneous carotid rupture. We will review the management of each of these three situations.

ELECTIVE CAROTID RESECTION FOR TUMOR

Indications

The internal carotid artery can be involved by tumors both in the neck and in the skull base. In the skull base, reconstruction of the artery is generally difficult due to limitations of exposure. Decisions regarding the potential benefits of carotid resection in skull base surgery vary with tumor histology and are beyond the scope of this chapter. When the artery is involved by carcinoma in the neck, management is controversial. Some surgeons argue that carotid resection secondary to involvement by cervical metastasis is not justified because of poor disease control and high complication rates.[3, 4] Others, however, indicate that long-term survival can be obtained by carotid resection in about 20 per cent of such cases, with few complications. Further palliative benefits also may obtained by controlling the tumors locally.[5-7] The differences between these two outlooks are probably due to patient selection. At our

19

institution, the philosophy is this: If a patient has massive disease adherent to the carotid but also with questionable resectability in other areas (i.e., skull base, mediastinum, and so on), we do not attempt carotid resection and treat the patient palliatively by non-surgical means. However, in patients with moderately advanced cervical metastases who are otherwise resectable but have carotid involvement, we support carotid resection. These cases are uncommon, though several are likely to occur in a major referral center each year. Carotid ligation can be contemplated in these cases, though carotid resection and reconstruction is also an option that shall be discussed.

Evaluation

Early involvement of the carotid artery by cervical metastases from head and neck squamous cell carcinoma is uncommon, probably occurring in fewer than 1 per cent of cases.[8] Carotid involvement is suspected when a neck mass is fixed to movement in the superoinferior plane.

The goal in evaluating such a patient is to determine whether the collateral flow through the circle of Willis will sufficiently perfuse the brain. Increased age, a history of symptoms suggesting cerebral ischemia, a history of ischemia of other organ systems secondary to atherosclerosis, and the presence of cervical bruits are all important points that can indicate the likelihood of a poor outcome from carotid ligation. Most surgeons advocate four-vessel cerebral arteriography as the first diagnostic test prior to carotid ligation.[7, 9] This will evaluate the patency and displacement of all the vessels contributing to the circle of Willis. Arteriography has about a 1 per cent risk of death or major complication in a population with known atherosclerosis, and this is probably lower in a population of patients with tumors.[10] In some situations, less invasive techniques such as computed tomography (CT) with digital subtraction and magnetic resonance (MR) angiography may be sufficient.[11] Certainly in patients with advanced tumors, CT

or MR imaging will provide additional information regarding the relationship of the tumor to the carotid artery. Duplex ultrasonography has not been useful in evaluating artery involvement by tumor, but it is useful in assessing flow through the involved and contralateral artery.[12]

Though simple angiography may indicate an anatomically adequate collateral circulation, it does not necessarily predict which patients will tolerate carotid ligation, even if collateral filling occurs with ipsilateral carotid compression. A variety of tests have been devised to provide such a prediction, both intraoperatively and preoperatively, with varying success. In reviewing the literature on this subject, the viewpoint of the various articles must be considered. Much has been written regarding the prediction of the patient's ability to tolerate temporary carotid occlusion during carotid endarterectomy without shunting. This is entirely separate from the patient's ability to withstand permanent carotid ligation. In fact, many have described experiences with patients who tolerated carotid ligation initially only to develop delayed neurologic sequelae at varying intervals postoperatively. Konno and associates have shown that 25 per cent of cerebrovascular accidents after carotid ligation occur 48 or more hours postoperatively.[13] Although some are caused by thrombosis,[14] others are due to marginal cerebral perfusion that may not be detected during a short period of trial occlusion.

For the intraoperative evaluation of candidates for carotid ligation, the measurement of distal internal carotid stump pressures is the best technique. Ehrenfeld and colleagues showed that intraoperatively measured carotid stump pressures greater than 70 mm Hg predicted the safety of carotid ligation.[14] Thirteen of twenty-five patients fell into this category. The remaining 11 patients had pressures of between 50 and 70 mm Hg, and 6 of these had postoperative cerebrovascular accidents. This represented a great advance in that a group of patients was identified in whom ligation could be performed fairly safely.[14] Enzmann and associates subsequently developed a method for measuring carotid back pressure angiographically.[15] However, Steed and colleagues, in a larger series, showed that while there is a correlation between cerebral blood flow and carotid stump pressures, the correlation is not exact. Their data indicate that stump pressures are not absolute indicators of the safety of carotid ligation.[16] At our institution, a patient with adequate carotid stump pressures experienced a fatal stroke 72 hours postoperatively.

One of the earliest methods for the preoperative estimation of the ability to tolerate internal carotid occlusion was oculoplethysmography. This technique involves the assessment of ophthalmic artery pressure by pressure measurements on the cornea. Martinez and associates used this technique in conjunction with carotid compression to assess collateral blood flow. They found a good correlation with intraoperative carotid stump pressures and used this technique to predict accurately the safety of ligation in four patients.[17] This technique presumed the ability to compress the carotid, which may prove difficult with neck tumors. In addition, one is measuring retinal artery pressure, which usually, but not always, correlates with carotid pressures. False-negatives can occur when collateral channels to the retinal artery exist. One might expect a higher failure rate using this technique on greater numbers of patients.

More recent tests have been based on a preoperative trial of internal carotid artery occlusion in the awake patient. This has been performed both angiographically and surgically under local anesthesia. Some researchers have recommended anticoagulation during this procedure. During the trial occlusion, the patient can be evaluated through a variety of methods. One of the simplest is to observe for neurologic signs and symptoms. This reasonably assesses a patient's ability to withstand temporary carotid occlusion when undergoing carotid replacement without shunting.[18] However, given the previously mentioned high incidence of delayed neurologic sequelae after carotid ligation, it obviously would be risky as the sole means of evaluating patients for carotid ligation.

Electroencephalography (EEG) has been added as a more sensitive means of detecting the patient with marginal cerebral blood flow after carotid occlusion. The use of intraoperative electroencephalographic monitoring during carotid endarterectomy has been well described in numerous reports, and characteristic EEG findings associated with ischemia have been described.[19-21] Andrews and colleagues successfully used this method to evaluate 24 patients requiring internal carotid ligation for skull base resections.[22]

Most recently, xenon computed tomographic cerebral blood flow mapping, in conjunction with carotid occlusion, has been shown to predict accurately the safety of carotid ligation in 22 of 23 patients.[16] This technique involves the inhalation of 32 per cent xenon as a radiodense tracer of blood flow, followed by computed tomography. This appears to be a very sensitive technique to predict the safety of carotid ligation, though like all the techniques mentioned, it is not foolproof.

Carotid Ligation—Operative and Perioperative Management

When resecting a tumor involving the carotid artery, the extent of the resection is dictated by the extent of disease. The portion of the tumor involving the artery should be dealt with last, after achieving proximal and distal control of the artery. Whenever possible the resection should be performed above the carotid bifurcation, thereby preserving the external carotid system with its potential collaterals to the cerebral circulation. Konno and colleagues showed a significantly lower incidence of neurologic complications with a preserved external carotid system.[13]

The actual technique of arterial occlusion has been discussed little in the literature. Konno and colleagues discussed gradual carotid occlusion over several days; they believed that neurologic complications were decreased if the carotid occlusion was performed gradually over greater than 13 days. How this was performed was not discussed, though apparently wounds were left open and clamps slowly tightened over this period. Permanent arteriographic balloon occlusion has been reported to be useful to skull base resections and in the control of acute or anticipated carotid hemorrhage.[16, 22, 23]

Surgical techniques for carotid ligation vary. In general, the artery should be doubly ligated with a secure, permanent suture such as 0 or 00 silk, and the end of the artery should be oversewn with a fine monofilament, nonreactive vascular suture. In the contaminated or radiated neck, the stumps of the arteries should be protected, either using local tissue (i.e., paraspinal muscles) or a myocutaneous flap.[24] During the ligation the anesthetist should seek to maintain a higher blood pressure and to avoid blood pressure swings. Arterial Po_2 and Pco_2 levels should be maintained in the normal range.[25]

The role of anticoagulation perioperatively in these cases is unclear. It is common practice to give a single dose of 5000 units of heparin intravenously when opening the carotid artery. Ehrenfeld and associates, in a population of patients undergoing urgent carotid ligation and not major resection, advocated 1 to 2 weeks of postoperative heparinization in all cases with stump pressures of less than 70 mm Hg.[14] Their population consisted largely of patients with vascular disease; those who died of stroke had demonstrated thrombus extending from the internal carotid artery to the middle cerebral artery. Some surgeons have advocated the use of subcutaneous heparin, 5000 units every 8 hours.[6] Most surgeons are opposed to full anticoagulation in a patient who has undergone a major resection, and in general stump thrombus has not represented a major problem. We routinely provide anticoagulation with heparin just before carotid clamping and partially reverse it with protamine sulfate if oozing continues during closure of the skin flaps.

Alternatives to Carotid Ligation

Despite advances in preoperative patient evaluation, cerebrovascular accidents are always a risk in resection of the carotid artery.

Postoperative carotid rupture is also a concern. Therefore, alternative ways of managing these cases have been sought. If the patient with a fixed neck mass has not received irradiation, many would support primary irradiation to be followed by neck dissection, in the hope that this would allow removal of the tumor from the artery without compromising the resection margins. However, often these patients have already received irradiation, or the carotid is extensively involved, so that primary irradiation is unlikely to salvage the carotid and is more likely to increase the complication rate. In such cases, the artery can be dealt with only surgically.

A surgical option supported by some is the so-called palliative peel, in which the tumor is dissected off the artery in a subadventitial plane. Some surgeons have argued that the carotid sheath represents a barrier to invasion by cancer cells in most cases.[26, 27] However, Huvos and associates reported malignant invasion of the adventitia and external elastic membrane in 27 of 64 resected carotid arteries (42 per cent).[28] If the tumor can be removed from the carotid cleanly, dissecting in a normal subadventitial plane, then this is certainly a reasonable course of action. However, peeling through an artificial plane and leaving a vessel wall with a highly abnormal appearance probably represents an incomplete tumor resection. To prevent tumor recurrence, postoperative radiation may be used if this is still an option.

Martinez and associates dealt with this problem by placing radioactive iodine seeds on the involved areas of the carotid after peeling the mass off the artery in 15 patients.[29] The data are difficult to interpret in relation to carotid disease as the patients with carotid involvement are not separated from a larger group of 48 patients treated with ^{125}I implants to other areas of questionable resectability. Only 18 patients with carotid involvement were considered to be in this group. The procedure was safe, however, as few complications and no carotid ruptures occurred. Its efficacy as a curative means of treating the carotid invaded by malignancy is questionable, and more information is needed. The researchers state that they do not believe this technique is a substitute for adequate surgical excision when this is possible.

A second alternative to carotid ligation is carotid resection followed by reconstruction of the artery. It has been clearly shown that this can be performed safely in noninfected and nonirradiated fields.[30] However, early reports of carotid reconstruction in irradiated or saliva-contaminated fields indicated a mortality rate of 41 per cent, owing to graft thrombus and, less frequently, fatal carotid hemorrhage.[31] Unfortunately, the majority of candidates for carotid resection are previously irradiated or contaminated cases or both. Recent advances, however, have made carotid reconstruction feasible in these patients. In particular, the major advance has been the use of myocutaneous flaps to cover the reconstructed artery. In addition, most surgeons prefer the use of saphenous vein interposition grafts rather that prosthetic materials, after several complications were noted with the use of Gore-tex grafts.

Studies have shown that in-line bypass grafting using saphenous vein can be performed safely in irradiated or contaminated cases.[6, 7, 18, 30] In the data of McCready and colleagues[7] and Biller and colleagues,[5] a total of 39 patients underwent carotid reconstruction with saphenous bypass and pectoralis major flap coverage. There were six postoperative strokes (15 per cent), of which two resolved completely. Two deaths resulted from stroke, and three deaths resulted from other causes (13 per cent mortality). One carotid blowout occurred. Biller and colleagues advocated the creation of a pharyngostoma in all cases with pharyngeal entry. They did this in all their patients except the one who suffered carotid blowout. This patient was salvaged by carotid ligation without sequelae.

Given the fact that the patients in both series were not selected for their ability to withstand carotid occlusion, these numbers are low in relation to the expected rate of neurologic sequelae after carotid resection without reconstruction. In addition, nine patients were without recurrence at a greater than 1 year follow-up; several additional patients lacked sufficiently lengthy follow-up periods to evaluate cure rate.

At our own institution, we have been performing carotid resection followed by saphenous vein reconstruction and myocutaneous flap coverage since 1987.[32] To date, we have assembled a series of 12 patients. Although it is too early to completely assess our series, our early data indicate that the procedure can be performed safely. In all 12 patients, the tumor was adherent to the carotid, and tumor invasion of the artery was subsequently shown histologically. The tumors were otherwise resectable. Seven patients had received preoperative radiation therapy. The majority of these cases involved saliva-contaminated wounds. There were no neurologic sequelae in any of these cases, with follow-up of from 5 to 52 months. No carotid ruptures have occurred. Four of the twelve patients developed wound infections. In two of these the myocutaneous flap prevented exposure of the arterial graft. In two cases the graft became exposed and was covered with a second myocutaneous flap without further sequelae. Four patients are alive without recurrence at a greater than 18 months' follow-up. Two have died of metastases without local recurrence. Two have died of other causes (one of pneumonia, one hemorrhaged from his gastrostomy site). One was lost to follow-up after 3 months without recurrence. The remaining three patients have had a very short follow-up at present. We feel that the key to success in these cases is meticulous, complete coverage of the reconstructed carotid with a muscle flap. We have used pectoralis or trapezius myocutaneous flaps for this purpose. We are encouraged by these early results and hope to gain further information. It is our feeling that in many cases carotid reconstruction may prove safer than carotid resection in patients with malignant invasion of the carotid artery. Carotid ligation can then be reserved for the treatment of skull base neoplasms and impending carotid rupture.

PREVENTION OF CAROTID RUPTURE

The risk factors for carotid rupture are well known. Radiation therapy and postoperative wound breakdown with infection, fistula formation, tissue necrosis, and vessel exposure are key predisposing conditions. There have been reports of spontaneous carotid rupture in well-healed patients many years after head and neck surgery and radiation, or after radiation alone.[33, 34] Similarly, rare carotid ruptures have occurred because of infections in patients without tumors.[35-37] However, such cases are extremely rare. In general, the patient at risk for carotid blowout is a previously irradiated patient, who has recently undergone major head and neck surgery and has now developed a major wound complication which is not improving. Nearly all patients who suffer carotid rupture have received both surgery and irradiation.[38, 39] Patients who have received primary radiation therapy for cure followed by salvage surgery for failure are particularly at risk.[40] In a series by Heller and Strong, major postoperative complications preceded carotid artery rupture in 92 per cent of patients.[2] Only 8 per cent did not have obvious fistulas or necrosis, and these were felt to have undetected wound sepsis or mucosal defects under intact skin.

Since the patient at risk for carotid rupture usually can be identified, preventive measures are often indicated. The literature clearly indicates that planned carotid ligation has a much lower morbidity and mortality than emergency ligation for spontaneous rupture. Moore and associates reported mortality rates of 17 per cent with elective ligation versus 38 per cent with emergency ligation.[41] Stroke occurred in 23 per cent of planned ligations, versus 50 per cent of emergency ligations. These data were obtained at a time when techniques for evaluating the adequacy of collateral cerebral circulation were not yet developed. The primary reason for the difference is related to the presence of acute blood loss and hypotension in the group that had emergency ligation. The researchers did not comment on the postoperative course of the electively ligated patients, but they imply that no difficulties with blowout of the carotid stumps were encountered.

Thus in the patient at risk for carotid rupture, preventive measures are prudent.

These patients can be divided into two groups. In patients with severe wound breakdown and early carotid exposure, but without evidence of bleeding, meticulous wound care should be performed, followed by carotid coverage. Patients who have exhibited vessel necrosis, characterized by dry, dark areas or crusted areas on the vessel surface, and patients who exhibit herald bleeding or oozing, should undergo urgent ligation.[38, 43]

The efficacy of various means of protecting the carotid artery has been greatly debated. Both the levator scapula flap and dermal grafts have been advocated for carotid protection at the time of neck dissection in high-risk patients.[44-47] Animal studies have lent some support to this concept,[47] but several clinical studies have found no clear benefit from these procedures. Since the underlying problem in these patients is poorly vascularized, irradiated tissue, it is not surprising that the use of nonvascularized tissue or tissue from the irradiated field affords little protection. Myocutaneous flaps from unirradiated areas offer more promise as a means of carotid protection. There have been no controlled experiments evaluating protection with vascularized muscle flaps, probably because most surgeons feel the benefits are so clear clinically that high-risk patients should not be denied it. As previously mentioned, all recent series discussing carotid resection have used vascularized flaps for coverage. The flap is most likely to provide benefit at the time of the initial resection. The problem that may be encountered in the infected wound with carotid exposure is that the necrotic, infected bed does not provide an adequate recipient site for a flap to adhere to, and the flap may simply detach from the wound. In this situation, carotid ligation may be the only alternative. A recent promising animal study yielded dramatic results using cyanoacrylate adhesive as a temporary means of carotid protection while allowing a wound to granulate and heal. More information is needed on this technique.[48]

If one decides that carotid ligation must be performed to prevent spontaneous carotid rupture, then, if possible, it should be performed through separate incisions in an uninfected area of the neck. If not possible, the stumps should be buried in uninfected tissue or covered with a flap. Concerns regarding the possibility of stump blowout with carotid ligation in an infected field have led some to perform permanent balloon occlusion with multiple balloons, including proximal occlusion near the origin of the carotid artery. Extensive data are not available on this approach, but it proved useful in at least one difficult case.[49]

In summary, protection of the carotid artery with a myocutaneous flap is probably indicated in patients at high risk for carotid rupture, and it may provide carotid protection in some cases after wound breakdown. If this fails and the artery shows signs of necrosis, or if herald bleeding occurs, urgent preventive ligation is indicated.

Finally, an additional group of patients at high risk for carotid rupture present surgeons with serious ethical and social considerations. These are the end-stage patients who have failed previous therapy and now show massive, uncontrolled tumor eroding the carotid artery. They often present with herald bleeding, and the family may be fearful of caring for the patient at home. These patients are not salvageable, and most head and neck surgeons would agree that surgical attempts to prolong their survival are generally not justified except in unusual circumstances at the request of the patient and family. If carotid rupture appears imminent, a hospital admission may provide a more comfortable setting for the patient and family in which to confront this experience.

MANAGEMENT OF SPONTANEOUS CAROTID ARTERY RUPTURE

Carotid artery rupture occurs in 3 per cent to 12 per cent of patients who have been treated with radiation and surgery.[17, 50] Because of its infrequency, appropriate management may be delayed by physicians and nurses unaccustomed to this problem. Porto and colleagues reviewed this topic in detail.[42] In their series of 22 patients experiencing

spontaneous carotid rupture, the mortality was lower than usual at 9 per cent. Another 9 per cent of patients experienced strokes with permanent hemiplegia. Patients who died at home were not included.

Several measures can increase success in salvaging patients after carotid rupture. Multiple units of blood should be readily available for any patient who is at risk. When rupture occurs, the patient should be packed immediately, and pressure should be held as needed to control bleeding as much as possible. Attempts at vessel ligation, however, should be deferred unless the vessel is immediately visible in an open wound and easily clamped. Otherwise, fluid resuscitation and replacement of blood volume should precede attempts to control hemorrhage, to minimize neurologic damage and decrease intraoperative mortality. A central catheter should be placed early to assist in assessment of appropriate fluid resuscitation. Four large-bore peripheral intravenous lines also should be inserted. Crystalloid and blood should be infused until the systolic blood pressure is stabilized at greater then 110 mm Hg. The airway must be controlled immediately and a PO_2 greater than 70 mm Hg must be maintained with ventilation if necessary. An operative procedure is delayed until these steps are taken.

When the patient has been appropriately prepared, he or she may be taken to surgery. The operation may be performed under local anesthesia if the risk of general anesthesia is too high. The procedure is performed in a manner similar to that described for planned preventive ligation. Porto and associates emphasized the importance of ligating the carotid artery proximally and distally through separate incisions, to avoid placing the stump in an infected field.[42] To achieve this, they state that one incision must occasionally be placed below the clavicle and the clavicle resected.

Postoperatively, the patients require placement in an acute care setting. They are often elderly and may be debilitated by cancer. Underlying pulmonary disease is often present. They have received large amounts of fluids and blood products and are at risk for stroke. Swan-Ganz catheter placement is commonly needed to manage fluids appropriately. Prolonged ventilator support also may prove necessary. Blood pressure should be maintained in the high-normal range to maximize cerebral effusion. A patient who survives may remain in guarded condition for several days after the event.

CONCLUSIONS

Despite the difficulties inherent in managing the compromised carotid artery in head and neck surgery, progress has been made in this area in the last 20 years. Better means of assessing the adequacy of cerebral circulation prior to elective resection are now available when needed. Better means of carotid protection are available than in the past, and guidelines for the appropriate management of spontaneous rupture are better defined. The frontiers lie in the areas of carotid reconstruction as well as in innovative techniques to avoid carotid resection, such as the use of radioactive seeds or synthetic means of carotid protection. Further work in these areas may provide greater advances in the future.

References

1. Moore OS, Baker HW: Carotid artery ligation in surgery of the head and neck. Cancer 8:712–718, 1955.
2. Heller KS, Strong E: Carotid artery hemorrhage after radical head and neck surgery. Am J Surg 138:607–610, 1979.
3. Kennedy JT, Krause LJ, Loevy S: The importance of tumor attachment to the carotid artery. Arch Otolaryngol 103:70, 1977.
4. Santos VB, Strong S, Vaughan CW Jr, et al: Role of surgery in head and neck cancer with fixed nodes. Arch Otolaryngol 101:645–648, 1975.
5. Biller HF, Urken A, Lawson W, et al: Carotid artery resection and bypass for neck carcinoma. Laryngoscope 98:181–183, 1988.
6. Atkinson DP, Jacobs LA, Weaver AW: Elective carotid resection for squamous cell carcinoma of the head and neck. Am J Surg 148:483–488, 1984.
7. McCready RA, Miller SK, et al: What is the role of carotid arterial resection in the management of advanced cervical cancer? J Vasc Surg 10:274–280, 1989.
8. Hiranandani LH: The management of cervical metastasis in head and neck cancers. J Laryngol Otol 85:1097, 1971.
9. Hibbert J: The compromised carotid artery. In Cummings CW, Fredrickson JM, Harker LA: Otolaryngology-Head & Neck Surgery (eds): Update I, 1989, pp 325–339.
10. Hass WK, Fields WS, North RR, et al: Joint study of extracranial arterial occlusion. JAMA 203:961–968, 1968.
11. McDonald KM, Gee W, Kamp HA, et al: Screening for significant carotid stenosis by ocular pneumoplethysmography. Am J Surg 137:244–249, 1979.
12. Baatenburg de Jong RJ, Rongen RJ, De Jong PC, et al: Screening for lymph nodes in the neck with ultrasound. Clin Otolaryngol, 1987.
13. Konno A, Togawa K, Iizuka K: Analysis of factors affecting complications of carotid ligation. Ann Otol Rhinol Laryngol 90:222–226, 1981.
14. Ehrenfeld WK, Stoney RJ, Wylie E: Relation of carotid stump pressure to safety of carotid artery ligation. Surgery 93:229, 1983.
15. Enzmann DR, Miller DC, Olcott C, et al: Carotid back pressures in conjunction with cerebral angiography. Radiology 134:415, 1980.
16. Steed DL, Webster MW, DeVries EJ, et al: Clinical observations on the effect of carotid artery occlusion on cerebral blood flow mapped by xenon computed tomography and its correlation with carotid artery back pressure. J Vasc Surg 11:38–44, 1990.
17. Martinez SA, Oller DW, Gee W, et al: Elective carotid artery resection. Arch Otolaryngol 101:744–747, 1975.
18. Olcott L, Fee WE, Enzmann DR, et al: Planned approach to the management of malignant invasion of the carotid artery. Am J Surg 142:123, 1981.
19. Artru AA, Strandnes DE Jr: Delayed carotid shunt occlusion detected by electroencephalographic monitoring. J Clin Monit 5:119–122, 1989.
20. McFarland HR, Pinkerton JAJ, Frye D: Continuous electroencephalographic monitoring during carotid endarterectomy. J Cardiovasc Surg (Torino) 29:12–18, 1988.
21. Collice M, Arena O, Fontana RA, et al: Role of EEG monitoring and cross-clamping duration in carotid endarterectomy. J Neurosurg 65:815–819, 1986.
22. Andrews JC, Valavanis A, Fisch U: Management of the internal carotid artery in surgery of the skull base. Laryngoscope 99:1224–1229, 1989.
23. Khoo CT, Molyneux AJ, Rayment R, et al: The control of carotid arterial haemorrhage in head and neck surgery by balloon catheter tamponade and detachable balloon embolisation. Br J Plast Surg 39:72–75, 1986.
24. Everts EC: Surgical Complications. Otolaryngology-Head & Neck Surgery. In Cummings CW, Fredrickson JM, Harker LA, et al (eds): 1986, pp 1411–1428.
25. Aki BF, Blakeley WR, Lewis CE, et al: Carotid endarterectomy: Is a shunt necessary? Am J Surg 130:760, 1975.
26. Ketchum AS, Haye RC: Spontaneous carotid artery hemorrhage after head and neck surgery. Am J Surg 110:649–655, 1965.
27. Dibbel DG, Gowen GF, Shedd DP et al: Observations on postoperative carotid hemorrhage. Am J Surg 109:765–770, 1965.
28. Huvos AG, Leaming RH, Moore OS: Clinicopathologic study of the resected carotid artery. Am J Surg 126:570–574, 1973.

29. Martinez A, Gossinet DR, Fee W, et al: Iodine implants as an adjuvant to surgery and external beam radiotherapy in the management of locally advanced head and neck cancer. Cancer 51:973–979, 1983.

30. Conley J: Free autogenous vein graft to the internal and common carotid arteries in the treatment of tumors of the neck. Ann Surg 137:205–214, 1953.

31. Conley JJ: Carotid artery surgery in the treatment of tumors of the neck. Arch Otolaryngol 65:437–446, 1957.

32. Reilly MK, Perry MD, Netterville JL, et al: Carotid artery replacement in conjunction with resection of squamous cell carcinoma of the neck. Presented at the 54th Annual meeting of the Society for Vascular Surgery, Boston, June 4–5, 1991.

33. Sobol SM, Rigual N, Jacocks MA: Successful angioplasty after delayed spontaneous rupture of the common carotid artery after head and neck surgery. Otolaryngeal Head Neck Surg 93:817–821, 1985.

34. Iannuzzi R, Metson R, Lofgren R: Carotid artery rupture after twice-a-day radiation therapy. Otolaryngol Head Neck Surg 100:621–622, 1989.

35. Blum DJ, McCaffrey TV: Septic necrosis of the internal carotid artery: A complication of peritonsillar abscess. Otolaryngol Head Neck Surg 91:114, 1983.

36. Endicott JN, Nelson RJ, Saraceno CA: Diagnosis and management decisions in infections of the deep fascial spaces of the head and neck, utilizing computerized tomography. Laryngoscope 92:630–633, 1982.

37. Wills PI, Vernon RP: Complications of space infections of the head and neck. Laryngoscope 91:1129, 1981.

38. Maran AGD, Amin M, Wilson JA: Radical neck dissection: A 19-year experience. J Laryngol Otol 103:760–764, 1989.

39. McCoy G, Barsocchini LM: Experiences in carotid artery occlusion. Laryngoscope 78:1195, 1968.

40. Joseph D, Shumrick D: Risks of head and neck surgery in previously irradiated patients. Arch Otolaryngol 97:381, 1973.

41. Moore OS, Karlan M, Sigler L: Factors influencing the safety of carotid ligation. Am J Surg 118:666–668, 1969.

42. Porto DP, Adams G, Foster C: Emergency management of carotid artery rupture. Am J Otolaryngol 7:213–217, 1986.

43. Grady ED, Robinson JS, White JB, et al: Technical suggestions for cancer of the tongue and floor of the mouth. N C Med J 17:466–470, 1956.

44. Staley JC: A muscle cover for the carotid artery after radical neck dissection. Am J Surg 102:815–817, 1961.

45. Corso PF, Gerold FP: Use of autogenous dermis for protection of the carotid artery and the pharyngeal suture lines in radical head and neck surgery. Surg Gynecol Obstet 117:37–40, 1963.

46. Schweitzer RJ: Use of muscle flaps for protection of carotid artery after radical neck dissection. Ann Surg 156:811, 1962.

47. Swain RE, Biller HF, Ogura JH: An experimental analysis of causative factors and protective methods in carotid artery rupture. Arch Otolaryngol 99:235–241, 1974.

48. Costantino DD, Atiyah RA, Mico AS, et al: The prevention of carotid artery rupture with isobutyl-2-cyanoacrylate. Laryngoscope 98:377–381, 1988.

49. Sanders EM, Davis KR, Whelan CS, et al: Threatened carotid artery rupture: a complication of radical neck surgery. J Surg Oncol 33:190–193, 1986.

50. Shumrick D: Carotid artery rupture. Laryngoscope 83:1051, 1973.

CHAPTER 4

Pharyngocutaneous Fistula

YOSEF P. KRESPI, MD

Pharyngocutaneous fistula can occur in the hands of the most senior and technically competent surgeons. The incidence of this complication can be kept low by good management of the surgical wound. A surgeon who performs head and neck surgery should be ready for pharyngocutaneous fistula and treat this complication in a competent manner. This complication is managed according to the surgeon's experience and the specific needs of the individual head and neck patient. The nursing staff, the patient, the family, and the house staff must be directly involved in the management and care; generally, patients require intensive wound care around the clock.

Pharyngocutaneous fistula requires special attention in head and neck surgery for prevention, early recognition, and management. The etiologic factors of pharyngocutaneous fistula must be understood and handled preoperatively. Most head and neck cancer patients are emaciated and require nutritional support prior to the cancer surgery. In addition to restoration of proper nitrogen balance and correction of albumin, levels of certain metallic elements, such as zinc and magne-

sium, and vitamins must be sufficient. Anemia must be corrected prior to operation to prevent major wound complications. Patients with severe arteriosclerosis and diabetes are considered at high risk for the development of pharyngocutaneous fistula. Diabetes must be controlled and cardiopulmonary status stabilized.

One of the major reasons for development of pharyngocutaneous fistula is residual microscopic or gross tumor at the surgical site or at the resection margins. This leads to disturbances in wound healing, early dehiscence, and the appearance of fistulization.

Technical errors in reconstruction of the surgical site also cause these fistulas, such as tension on the mucosal closure line, inability to invert the mucosal edges, kinking of the suture line, and reduced vascular supply of the suture line. The surgical technique in closing mucosa to mucosa or mucosa to skin flap must be meticulous, using full surgical skills. Every attempt must be made to obtain at least two layers of closure. A Connell suture using permanent suture material inverts the mucosal edges. This suture line can be supported with interrupted sutures to further strengthen the first layer. Ideally, a third layer of muscle closure further seals the suture line. Muscle can be harvested locally or can be rotated from a distant area. If one uses a flap, this flap must be secured to relieve suture line tension, either through the prevertebral fascia or through digastric muscles. These suspension sutures prevent gravity from pulling the flap away from the suture line. Extreme attention to technical detail is essential.

Another important factor in the development of fistulas is preoperative radiation therapy.[1] A radiation dose of more than 5000 rads administered within 6 months prior to surgery has the potential for surgical complications involving the pharyngeal closure and the survival of skin flaps. If the radiation dose exceeds 7000 rads, these complications can be even more hazardous due to the extreme risk of losing skin, muscle, and mucosal tissues in the surgical field.

The incidence of pharyngocutaneous fistula varies from 10 per cent to 50 per cent, and this depends directly upon the dose of radiation therapy. A small fistula will close with proper wound management and time. Meticulous care of wound edges, administration of antibiotics, and local debridement of the necrotic tissue are recommended in the immediate management.

PREVENTION

The main goal in the management of pharyngocutaneous fistula is prevention. The operating surgeon's technical expertise and surgical technique are essential in the prevention of this complication. Good hemostasis usually alleviates hematomas and the dead space that is necessary in the surgical technique. The handling of tissue edges with gentle surgical technique is mandatory. Prophylactic intravenous antibiotics should be started prior to operation and continued for 2 days after the procedure. Every surgical wound in a patient who has had preoperative radiation therapy carries an inherent secondary complication of potential carotid artery exposure and rupture. To cover the exposed and radiated carotid artery, muscle flaps from the levator scapula, digastric and mylohyoid muscles, or prevertebral fascia can be used for local coverage. Although these muscles have decreased vascularity due to local radiation, their use may provide additional safety in protecting the carotid artery. A dermal graft can be used to resurface the carotid bulb area. Muscle flaps from areas distant from the irradiated field, such as the pectoralis or trapezius muscles, can be rotated and used to cover the entire carotid system and support the pharyngeal closure as a third layer.

Surgeons must consider creating a controlled pharyngostoma in a potentially hazardous wound that was heavily radiated. A controlled pharyngostoma can be beneficial in protecting the remaining suture line and skin flaps. Before performing a pharyngostomy, one must be sure that the blood supply of the mucosa and the skin edges is adequate and will tolerate the suture tension (Table 4–1). Also, a suction catheter can be introduced

TABLE 4–1. Cutaneous Blood Supply of the Neck

Skin over	Supplied by
Submental triangle	—facial artery via submental branch
Submaxillary triangle	—facial artery via direct branches
Carotid triangle	—superior thyroid artery via intrahyoid and sternomastoid branches
Anterior (muscular) triangle	—superior thyroid artery
	—inferior thyroid artery via very small musculocutaneous perforators
Occipital triangle	—occipital artery via descending branches
Supraclavicular triangle	—transverse cervical artery via direct branches, supraclavicular artery

through the pharyngostoma to divert saliva away from the suture line. A controlled pharyngostoma can keep the flaps in place and usually eliminates dead space along the neck flaps.

Head and neck surgeons must plan the pharyngostoma preoperatively and place the neck incisions accordingly. In a patient undergoing laryngopharyngectomy, total laryngectomy, or partial pharyngectomy, a midline incision from the tracheostoma upward toward the hyoid area, which is slightly curved to one or the other side of the neck, can provide adequate exposure of the neck for limited neck dissection, excision of the primary tumor, and creation of a controlled pharyngostoma in the midline. Midline-controlled pharyngostomas along the pharynx or the tongue base are away from the great vessels, which provides ideal protection.

EARLY RECOGNITION

The successful management of pharyngocutaneous fistula requires early recognition. Swelling, erythema, and pain, with high temperature spikes, are the usual presenting signs of developing fistulas. In addition, an experienced head and neck surgeon looks for oral or wound odor. The sensitive nose of a senior surgeon can detect an early fistula even before local signs develop. Myocutaneous flaps may conceal the evidence of swelling and erythema around the wound edges. House staff and nursing staff must be alerted to the presence of the myocutaneous flap and its pedicle immediately after the procedure, so that neck swelling and erythema will not be mistaken for hematoma or abscess formation.

A pharyngocutaneous fistula usually begins to develop on the sixth to seventh day after operations. If a malodorous wound associated with a temperature spike occurs, the surgeon must open the wound along the pharyngeal closure in order to identify the fistula. It is essential that the wound be opened as far away from the carotid artery and tracheostoma as possible. Ideally, once

the fistula is identified, it should be diverted toward the midline and high up superiorly. An open fistula immediately above the tracheostoma may cause aspiration of the infected secretions directly into the airway. Suction drains must be placed into the opened pharyngocutaneous fistula to divert the salivary flow; once the salivary flow is reduced, a 25 per cent acetic acid solution is used to pack the fistula site, using gauze packing. A large fistula may require opening the wound further and partially creating a controlled fistula when the local wound infection is stabilized. This can be accomplished by placing three or four stabilizing sutures to invert the neck skin edge into the mucosal edge (Fig. 4–1).

MANAGEMENT

Culture and sensitivity studies of the wound and pharyngeal drainage must be obtained. Usually gram-negative bacteria are found, which require intravenous antibiotics.

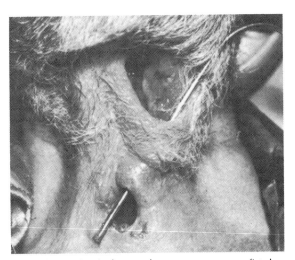

FIGURE 4–1. A large pharyngocutaneous fistula communicating with the tracheostome. The original attempt at closure of the pharynx was carried out with a minimum of mucous membrane closed under tension. This wound contracted and stabilized and was closed with regional tissue in 3 months. (From Conley J: Complications of Head and Neck Surgery. Philadelphia, WB Saunders, 1979.)

The neck drains must be directed toward the fistula, and an additional suction drain is placed in the pharyngostoma to divert the salivary output. The drains must be kept in place until the amount of discharge is minimal. This may take 10 to 12 days. Occasionally, a small fistula can be handled with the suction drain and an additional opening on the skin to divert the salivary flow to the midline. This should be away from the carotid artery, even if the carotid artery is protected, and also away from the tracheostoma, to prevent aspiration. A cuffed tracheostomy tube should be inserted upon the identification of a pharyngocutaneous fistula and remain in place until closure. Debridement of necrotic tissue, especially in a patient who received heavy preoperative radiation, is mandatory. This will keep the wound clean and healthy, and the surgical bed is thereby prepared for future flap reconstruction. An odorous pharyngocutaneous fistula is treated locally with acetic acid solution or Dakin solution. These solutions may be administered orally, 10 to 15 ml every 4 hours, to acidify the upper digestive tract. Also, the packing is saturated with the acetic acid solution and used as appropriate to cover the wound.

As the fistula site matures following control of the infection (usually 7 to 10 days), the fistula can be lightly packed with iodine-soaked gauze to decrease drainage and stimulate granulation. Most fistulas will start decreasing in size after the infection is controlled. Fistulas under 2 cm usually close spontaneously with proper wound care within 2 to 4 weeks. Mature fistulas or controlled pharyngostomas can be plugged with gauze to allow the patient to eat. Oral feedings of the patient with pharyngocutaneous fistula and an infection can be devastating; this can complicate the infection and promote mucosal and skin necrosis. Only small, mature pharyngostomas (3 to 4 weeks old) can be plugged so the patient may be fed orally.

Postoperative radiation therapy can be started with an open, mature pharyngostoma. If the fistula closure is anticipated within weeks, radiation therapy can be delayed until the pharyngostoma has closed.

Prior to postoperative radiation therapy, all exposed and infected hardware for mandibular reconstruction must be removed.

The surgical closure of a pharyngeal fistula depends on the size and the location of the pharyngostoma and the presence of irradiated tissue. Nonirradiated local tissue is used to close small (up 2 cm) fistulas. The surgical technique consists of turning the skin tissue around the pharyngostoma. A circumferential incision is made around the fistula at a distance equal to the width of the fistula; the surrounding tissue is undermined halfway in order not to interrupt the blood supply of the skin flaps. The skin flaps are turned in and sutured with single-layer interrupted inverting sutures, using nonabsorbable material. A second layer can be used for support of the suture line with a local muscle, if available. The skin around the pharyngostoma can be slightly undermined, or a rotation skin flap can be used to provide cutaneous closure. Skin grafts or dermal grafts are not sufficient to cover the suture line adequately.

This surgical closure is not recommended with irradiated tissue, owing to the diminished blood supply of the neck skin. A controlled pharyngostoma or a mature pharyngocutaneous fistula of an irradiated patient should be closed with an additional regional cutaneous flap or myocutaneous flap. Cervical skin can be turned in locally and a cutaneous flap used to cover the suture line. An exposed carotid artery is covered with a myocutaneous flap. Cervical skin viability must be assessed before rotating the myocutaneous flap. To prepare a viable surgical recipient site for the myocutaneous flap, the necrotic skin edges and other nonviable tissue must be debrided prior to swinging the flap. With a small pharyngeal defect, the myocutaneous flap (usually the pectoralis major) can be skin-grafted over the muscle, and this part can be used to close the pharyngeal defect. This creates a three-layer closure, with use of skin, subcutaneous tissue, and muscle. With large pharyngeal defects, in selected cases the myocutaneous flap skin can be turned in, in order to cover the pharyngeal defect, and a skin graft can be placed over the muscle to cover the cutaneous neck defect. The development of a pectoralis major myocutaneous flap in 1979 added major advantages in the management of the pharyngocutaneous fistula. This flap is versatile, tolerates major trauma, and provides an ample supply of nonirradiated tissue with a viable muscle pedicle that can support and protect the important structures in the neck and upper mediastinum (Fig. 4–2).

NECK INCISIONS AND CAROTID RUPTURE

The carotid artery is at greatest risk for exposure and subsequent rupture when radical neck dissection is combined with resection of a primary lesion involving any portion of the tongue, pharynx, and cervical esophagus. This is especially true following previous radiotherapy. Rupture of the carotid

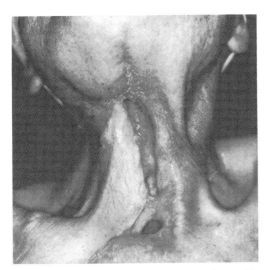

FIGURE 4–2. Maximal precautions have been taken in this heavily irradiated radical ablation of the lateral neck, thyroid, larynx, and associated skin by creating a large controlled pharyngostome and resurfacing the lateral neck with a thoracoacromial flap. This wound healed per primam. All features of this type of conservative and precautionary management give the best opportunity for healing. The stroma was closed in an interval of 6 weeks by undermining and direct approximation. (From Conley J: Complications of Head and Neck Surgery. Philadelphia, WB Saunders, 1979.)

artery is rare otherwise but can occur following any type of cervical skin necrosis and wound breakdown over the major vessels. Carotid artery blowout occurs most commonly at the bifurcation but may occur anywhere along the course of the common or the internal carotid arteries. Preoperative radiotherapy plays a major role in fistula formation and infection. Radiation therapy causes endarteritis and fibrosis of the skin and underlying tissue, which decreases perfusion in virtually all areas.

Skin incisions that are parallel to or lie directly over the carotid vessels are likely to expose these vessels when the skin edge sloughs. Carotid blowout is unavoidable when salivary contamination and infection accompany skin slough.

Another cause for carotid artery blowout, when associated with a fistula or infection, is direct injury to the blood vessel wall from suction catheters, tracheostomy tubes, or other prosthetic devices. Large vessel blowout may occur without skin slough under an intact skin flap. This may happen when the skin is not in direct contact with blood vessels and is associated with dead space and infection. The dead space may be the result of postoperative fistula associated with the contamination of the vessel wall and devitalization of the vessel adventitia.[5, 6]

PREVENTION OF CAROTID ARTERY BLOWOUT

Patients with poor oral hygiene may benefit from an antibacterial mouthwash using 1 per cent clindamycin or 1 per cent neomycin 48 hours prior to the procedure. Preoperative antibiotics may be necessary.

Skin incisions in the neck should be placed away from the great vessels and never cross them. Some surgeons popularized the use of horizontal incisions (MacFee) as the solution to this problem.[4] However, skin slough may occur directly over the great vessels due to injury from excessive retraction of the skin flaps during operation to obtain adequate exposure. Other types of skin flaps that avoid linear incisions over the vessels may include an inverted-Y incision or modifications of the apron flap.

Subplatysmal dissection of the skin flap should be done with great care to avoid damage to the blood supply. One must always include the cervical platysma in the flap unless there is a question of involvement of the platysma or skin by the neoplasm. In this situation, full-thickness excision is essential to provide adequate oncologic margins. One must avoid possible trauma to the skin flap from clamps resting on and lying over the flaps during the operative procedure. Flaps must be protected with warm irrigation and moist laparotomy pads during the entire procedure. One must also trim the edges of the flap at least 1 cm when viability is questionable.

Special precautions should be taken to preserve skin perfusion in the case of prior chemotherapy or radiation therapy. Suction drains are preferred to decrease dead space and allow proper apposition of the skin flaps. Drains should not cross the base of the skin flap, which could compromise perfusion. Drains should be secured with absorbable sutures and placement confirmed with neck mobility. When electrodissection is used to raise skin flaps, excessive heat must be avoided. The lowest possible current setting should be used to prevent thermal injury. Extreme care must be given to creating a watertight closure of defects in the upper aerodigestive tract (e.g., using suture techniques that invert mucosa).

The surgeon must carefully inspect the closure for leaks after repair. Also, the tissue that is used for closure must be viable, with adequate blood supply. The suture line must be free of tension, and the surgeon must prevent dead space under the oral cavity by using muscle flaps from the neck, a myocutaneous flap, or other transposed viable tissue.

When a pharyngocutaneous fistula is anticipated, a planned pharyngostoma may be appropriate. The pharyngostoma must be positioned away from the carotid sheath, ideally in the midline. In addition, a suction catheter may be placed into this pharyngostoma to divert pharyngeal secretions and minimize the amount of drainage and soiling of the skin incisions.

Prosthetic vascular grafts should not be used if infection is present or when there is likelihood of a postoperative pharyngocutaneous fistula. One can create a controlled pharyngostoma in these instances to avoid this serious complication.

It has been documented that the vasa vasorum of the carotid artery is crucial in determining the viability of the carotid artery and of the dermal graft placed over the carotid.[7-9]

References

1. Ellis M: Surgical techniques following irradiation of the neck. J Laryngol 77:872, 1963.
2. Babcock W, Conley J: Neck incisions in block dissection. Arch Otolaryngol 84:108, 1966.
3. Schobinger R: The use of a long anterior skin flap in radical neck dissection. Ann Surg 146:221, 1957.
4. MacFee W: Transverse incisions for neck dissection. Ann Surg 151:279, 1960.
5. Freeland AP, Rogers JH: The vascular supply of the cervical skin with reference to incision planning. Laryngoscope 85:714, 1975.
6. Rabson JA, Hurwitz DJ, Futrell JW: The cutaneous blood supply of the neck: Relevance to incision planning and surgical reconstruction. Br J Plast Surg 38:208–219, 1985.
7. Heller KJ, Strong EW: Carotid artery hemorrhage after radical head and neck surgery. Am J Surg 138:607–610, 1979.
8. Porto DP, Adams G, Foster C: Emergency management of carotid artery rupture. Am J Otolaryngol 7:213–217, 1986.
9. Swain RE, Biller HF, Ogura JH: An experimental analysis of causative factors and protective methods in carotid artery rupture. Arch Otolaryngol 99:235–241, 1974.

CHAPTER 5

Head and Neck Infection

JONAS T. JOHNSON, MD
GUY J. PETRUZZELLI, MD, PhD

Wound infection is the leading cause of morbidity in postoperative patients. The incidence of postoperative wound infection following clean-contaminated head and neck surgery ranges from 4 per cent to 25 per cent.[10, 12] In one study of patients undergoing major contaminated head and neck surgical procedures, the development of postoperative wound infection resulted in prolongation of hospitalization from an average of 17 days (encountered in patients with no evidence of infection) to an average of 34 days.[16] The economic impact of wound infection based on hospital charges alone (1985 dollars) was estimated to be greater than $10,000 per patient. These data clearly do not address the cost of prolonged hospitalization in terms of pain and suffering or its domestic economic impact.

It is apparent from these data that postoperative head and neck infection must be a major concern to every head and neck surgeon. This chapter will examine prevention, recognition, treatment, and complications of head and neck wound infection.

PREVENTION

Preoperative Care

The prevention of postoperative wound infection begins preoperatively. Efforts must be made to maximize the patient's opportunity to have complication-free surgery. This, in turn, requires that the patient be carefully evaluated so that abnormalities, both potential and real, can be identified and brought under optimal control prior to elective surgery.

The patient should be carefully queried regarding prior hospitalizations, tobacco and alcohol use, medications, and current health status. Preoperative tobacco use compromises pulmonary function. Avoidance of tobacco for even a few days prior to a general anesthetic may result in reduced postoperative pulmonary complications.[24] Similarly, excessive alcohol use (abuse) should be identified. Patients with a history of alcoholic withdrawal or those who report daily heavy consumption of alcoholic beverages should be either withdrawn from alcohol preoperatively or managed prophylactically during the operative and postoperative period to prevent acute postoperative alcoholic withdrawal. Occasionally patients will be encountered who abuse other drugs alone or in combination with alcohol. Table 5–1 lists drugs commonly misused/abused by patients with head and neck cancer. Also identified are the withdrawal periods for each agent.

Metabolic conditions must be optimized, including the management of fluid and electrolyte imbalance, titration of cardiac drugs, and optimization of pulmonary status. The preoperative laboratory investigations include a chest radiograph, electrocardiogram, complete blood count with quantitative platelets, serum electrolytes, blood glucose, and urea nitrogen and creatinine levels. Partial thromboplastin and prothrombin times and serum protein and albumin levels are also obtained. These studies rarely alter the preoperative management of our patients but serve as useful baseline data should complications arise in the postoperative period.

Particular attention is paid to the pulmonary status of patients undergoing conservation laryngeal surgery.[24] All these individuals undergo complete pulmonary function testing (spirometry and flow volume loops) to determine the extent of their pulmonary reserve. Room air arterial blood gas determinations are used to assess the degree of hypoxia present.

Patients with known cardiovascular or renal disease are evaluated by a medical consultant familiar with the nuances of the head and neck cancer population. Potential anesthetic risks are reviewed prior to operation with the anesthesia team.

The widespread availability of over-the-counter of salicylates and nonsteroidal anti-inflammatory drugs is of great concern to the surgeon. The anticoagulant effect of these medications requires that patients be carefully queried regarding their use so that disastrous side effects can be avoided. As much as 2 weeks may be required for the patient to recover from the antiplatelet effect of salicylates. A lesser and variable effect of the other nonsteroidal, noninflammatory drugs has important implications as well.

An assessment of the patient's nutritional status and correction of malnutrition must be made prior to any surgical intervention.[5, 17, 18, 25] Traditional methods of determining the adequacy of a patient's nutritional status have included height/weight ratios, anthropomorphic measurements, serum protein levels, total lymphocyte count, and delayed hypersensitivity responses. Reilly has divided these indices of nutritional status into "static" and "functional" parameters.[20] Static measurement defines the nutrition of the patient at a single time point and includes data such as weight, height, and levels of albumin, transferrin, retinol-binding proteins, and prealbumin. Functional measurements indicate the impact of malnutrition on the basic processes of growth, metabolism, and immune function.

TABLE 5–1. Drug Withdrawal Phenomena

	Symptoms Appear (*hours*)	Most Severe (*hours*)	Duration (*days*)
Alcohol	6–12	36–72	5–7
Barbiturates (pentobarbital, secobarbital)	8–24	36–72	5–7
Benzodiazepines (diazepam, chlordiazepoxide, temazepam, flurazepam, oxazepam)	72–96	120–192	10–14
Nicotine	24	36–48	5–21
Opiates (heroin, morphine, methadone, meperidine)	12–14	48–72	7–10

(Data from Jaffe JH: Drug addiction and drug abuse. In Goodman LS, Gilman A (eds): The Pharmacological Basis of Therapeutics. 5th ed. New York, Macmillan, 1975; and Khantzian EJ, McKenna GJ: Acute toxic and withdrawal reactions associated with drug use and abuse. Ann Intern Med 90:361–372, 1979.)

In an attempt to establish a quantitative relationship between nutritional status and surgical outcome, investigators at the University of Pennsylvania developed the Prognostic Nutritional Index (PNI).[8] Their equation considers the following parameters: thickness of the triceps skin fold, serum albumin, serum transferrin, and reactivity to delayed hypersensitivity testing. Patients with a PNI greater than .25 require aggressive nutritional support prior to operation. When the PNI is greater than .40, the surgeon is well advised to delay elective surgery until the nutritional deficiencies can be resolved. The PNI has been shown to be an accurate indicator of morbidity in the head and neck surgical population.

Most surgeons today concur that enteral feeding should be employed whenever possible.[23] Advanced head and neck lesions often cause significant dysphagia and trismus and prohibit adequate oral intake. In these cases nasogastric tube feeding is preferred. Successful prolonged enteral feedings can be provided via percutaneously placed gastrostomy or jejunostomy tubes. A small number of patients may require total parenteral nutrition (TPN) via a central venous catheter. We have used TPN in patients who are severely malnourished, those with obstructing hypopharyngeal or esophageal lesions, or who have ileus due to an operative procedure or chemotherapy.

The duration of preoperative nutritional therapy is individualized based on the patient's general physical examination and the degree of improvement in biochemical parameters. Generally 2 to 3 days in which a patient tolerates an enteral diet without complications of cramping or diarrhea should be considered the minimum prior to major ablative reconstructive surgery.

Lastly, coexisting infections should be treated. The oral cavity and the lungs are the two most common sources of infection associated with head and neck neoplasms.

The dentition represents a potential source for infection following head and neck surgery. The sequelae of radiation therapy in the presence of advanced periodontal disease and the need for dental hygiene are well recognized.[15] Osteoradionecrosis, caries, periapical abscesses, and alterations in the oral microflora have all been demonstrated following external beam radiation.[1, 3, 4] Aggressive dental therapy in conjunction with the radiotherapy has been shown to reduce the incidence and severity of these complications. We apply these same principles prior to ablative oncologic procedures. Preoperatively, patients receive a careful dental examination and, if necessary, active dental intervention. Hypererupted teeth, teeth that cannot be restored, or those with advanced sepsis are extracted. Every effort is made to preserve dentition to facilitate prosthetic rehabilitation. We feel that by reducing local contamination the healing of intraoral mucosal suture lines can proceed efficiently.

Aspiration and chronic pulmonary contamination may be caused by large tumors of the upper aerodigestive tract, including the glottis and hypopharynx. Initial nonsurgical measures to improve bronchopulmonary hygiene include incentive spirometry, antibiotics, bronchodilators, and intermittent positive-pressure breathing (IPPB). In some circumstances, these infections cannot be fully eradicated because of continued life-threatening bronchopulmonary contamination. In the face of persistent aspiration due to these neoplasms, the surgeon may be forced to proceed with aerodigestive separation (laryngectomy) with the patient in less than optimal medical condition.[6]

Intraoperative Care

The importance of operative technique cannot be overlooked in the prevention of postoperative healing complications.[2] This includes the gentle handling of tissue, avoidance of foreign bodies, and careful debridement of nonviable or necrotic tissue. Wounds must be carefully approximated, sutures accurately placed, and internal suture lines placed in a watertight fashion. Copious saline irrigation is appropriate at the end of every surgical case. The intraoperative use of antibiotic irrigation is an appealing, but unproved, addition to the armamentarium of the head and neck surgeon.

The administration of perioperative antibiotic prophylaxis will be considered, in this discussion, as an intraoperative issue. It has been clearly demonstrated that antibiotic prophylaxis is maximally effective when instituted at the time of, or just prior to, contamination of the wound. We recommend that the antibiotic be instituted either on call to the operating room or by the anesthesiologist during induction of anesthesia. The intravenous route is the most reliable and convenient.

Multiple prospective randomized trials have demonstrated a comparable efficacy of a number of antibiotic agents or combination of agents (Table 5–2). The presence of fungi and the enteric gram-negative organisms, such as *Escherichia coli, Serratia,* or *Proteus,* in cultures obtained from patients with postoperative head and neck wound infections properly reflects colonization rather than pathogenicity.[14] Routine administration of antibiotics effective against these organisms seems unnecessary. The antibiotic chosen should be effective against oral flora. This includes the aerobic streptococci and staphylococci as well as the oral anaerobic bacteria.

Various investigators have evaluated populations of patients undergoing major head and neck surgical procedures in an attempt to identify the optimal duration of antibiotic administration to maximize the efficacy of antibiotic prophylaxis.[7, 11, 19] No information exists to support the administration of antibiotics for greater than 24 hours postoperatively. In a prospectively designed, randomized multi-institutional trial, 109 patients scheduled for major head and neck surgical procedures using pectoralis major myocutaneous flaps were randomly assigned to receive antibiotics for either 1 day or 5 days postoperatively.[12] In every case, the antibiotic was administered intravenously and begun prior to operation. Fifty-three patients were randomized to receive 1 day of antibiotic prophylaxis. Infection was encountered in 10 patients (18.9 per cent). Fifty-six patients were randomly assigned to receive 5 days of antibiotic prophylaxis. Infection was encountered in 14 patients (25 per cent). These data support the observation that prolonged administration of antibiotics does not improve efficacy or does not reduce the incidence of infections observed.

At the completion of the procedure, the wound should be copiously irrigated to remove foreign particulate matter, bacteria, necrotic debris, and clot. Suction drains should be strategically placed in the wound in adequate numbers to properly evacuate serum or blood that may develop. Following isolated radical neck dissection, we routinely employ two drainage tubes; we ordinarily employ four drainage tubes in patients undergoing laryngectomy with neck dissection or composite resection.

The wound should be closed meticulously. Special attention must be paid to achieving a watertight mucosal closure. Poor judgment intraoperatively resulting in tension on the suture line may result in separation of the mucosal suture line postoperatively and cause postoperative wound infection. Similarly, repair of major soft tissue defects with inadequately vascularized or poorly planned flaps may cause postoperative necrosis, wound separation, and infection. It is abundantly clear that these so-called "technical" aspects of surgical care are critical to the successful outcome of a procedure.

At the completion of the operation, we immediately hook the suction drains to the suction apparatus, and a compressive cer-

TABLE 5–2. Incidence of Infection Encountered with Various 1-Day Antibiotic Regimens

Antibiotic Employed	Patients	Number Infected (%)
Cefazolin (500 mg)	21	7 (33)
Cefazolin (1 gm)	57	16 (2)
Cefazolin (2 gm)	59	5 (8.5)
Carbenicillin	72	10 (14)
Moxalactam (2 gm)	75	3 (4)
Clindamycin (600 mg)	52	2 (3.8)
Clindamycin-gentamicin	81	4 (5)
Cefoperazone (2 gm)	39	4 (10)
Cefotaxime (2 gm)	32	3 (9)

(Modified from Johnson JT: The use of antibiotics in head and neck surgery. In Myers EN, Suen JY (eds): Cancer of the Head and Neck. 2nd ed. New York, Churchill Livingstone, 1989.)

vical dressing is placed on most patients. The drains remain for an average of 4 to 5 days and are removed when the total drainage for 24 hours is less than 10 ml. The total amount of fluid collected in the drains is between 250 and 300 ml in the absence of mucocutaneous fistula or wound infection. In patients with bilateral neck dissection, compressive dressings are not used. Similarly, in patients with pedicle flaps compressive dressings are not used because of the potential for vascular compromise. In routine cases closed primarily, compressive dressings may aid in co-apting the cervical flaps to the deep tissues, may reduce the risk of hematoma, and further reduce the problem with postoperative serum collection.

Postoperative Care

Postoperatively, patients must be maintained nutritionally. This requires introduction of enteric feedings given through a nasogastric tube as soon as the bowel regains its motility. Caution should be used, however, in instituting these feedings: premature bolus feeding may result in emesis which, in turn, may cause disruption of the mucosal suture lines, which inevitably results in major postoperative infection. It is apparent, therefore, that every stage of surgical care requires good judgment.

Similarly, fluid and electrolyte balance must be maintained. This requires intermittent measurement of hematocrit and electrolytes and monitoring of urinary output.

Postoperative nursing care is critical to successful outcome. Nurses monitor drainage from the cervical catheters. These catheters are aspirated during every shift (every 8 hours) to assure patency and to prevent obstruction with particulate debris or clot. Aspiration is undertaken employing sterile technique.

Dressings are maintained until the drainage catheters are removed. Dressings are not routinely changed on a daily basis unless they become soiled or otherwise disrupted.

The postoperative program of oral hygiene includes careful brushing of teeth to reduce caries, flossing to remove interproximal debris, and the topical application of fluoride-containing compounds.

RECOGNITION AND TREATMENT OF POSTOPERATIVE WOUND INFECTION

The sine qua non of postoperative wound infection in the head and neck patient is development of a purulent collection under the cervical skin flap. Other factors such as fever or leukocytosis are less reliable and must be correlated with evaluation of the wound.

If the cervical drains are observed to contain purulent debris, a wound problem is apparent. Similarly, the observation of saliva in the Hemovac drain should be considered an indication that the mucosal suture line has been disrupted. Under these circumstances, the Hemovac drains must be maintained to effect drainage of the contaminated or infected material. Premature removal of the drains under these circumstances necessarily results in the development of a collection that may, in turn, compromise further the mucosal closure or skin flap, resulting in fistula formation.

If a subcutaneous collection is identified, then drainage must be instituted. Placement of the drain should be selected so that it allows nursing care and does not compromise the tracheotomy with aspiration of drainage material. Accordingly, it should be placed laterally rather than in the midline. It is apparent from this discussion that it is far better to have the Hemovac drains in place to evacuate a small wound infection or mucosa leak when a wound problem is identified rather than to re-establish drainage at some later date after a collection has developed.

The administration of antibiotics to patients with either a diagnosed wound infection or purulent debris or saliva in the drains is a matter of contention. Clearly, the most important factor in management of wound infection or compromise of the internal suture line is drainage. The administration of antibiotics is advocated to reduce cellulitis and prevent the development of systemic sepsis, reduce fever, avoid endocarditis, and so on. The chosen antibiotic should be effective against a broad spectrum of bacteria, especially the streptococcus, the staphylococcus, and the anaerobic bacteria.

The bacteriology of postoperative head and neck wound infections has been reported by numerous authors.[11, 14, 22] Most postoperative wound infections in the head and neck are polymicrobial in nature. Cultures commonly demonstrate multiple organisms, some of which are pathogenic while others may be only colonizing the cervical wound. From a practical point of view, it is often impossible to distinguish between truly pathogenic organisms and those that are only colonizing the wound. This requires, therefore, that blood cultures be made in patients who evidence sepsis, such as high fever, so that the specific offending organism may be identified.

When a mucocutaneous fistula develops, polymicrobial contamination invariably occurs. Administration of broad-spectrum antibiotics can be expected to affect the pattern of colonization, and long-term management of patients with fistulas invariably results in colonization with resistant organisms. Accordingly, patients must be closely monitored. Blood cultures should be obtained when patients develop high fever. When the condition of the wound worsens rather than improves, such as might be determined by increasing erythema, cellulitis, and induration, efforts to identify the offending organism must be intensified.

Complications

The most commonly encountered complication in postoperative wound infection is the development of mucocutaneous fistula. Fistula is more commonly encountered in patients who have had prior treatment with irradiation therapy. In a study of patients undergoing major head and neck surgical procedures in whom reconstruction had been undertaken with a pectoralis major myocutaneous flap, 100 per cent of patients who developed postoperative infection following prior treatment with irradiation therapy subsequently developed fistula.[9] This is in contrast to only 66 per cent of patients who developed fistula with wound infection with no prior radiation therapy.

Care of the patient with a postoperative fistula requires intensive nursing support. Efforts must be made to divert the salivary stream so that it does not contaminate the tracheotomy or bronchopulmonary tract. Techniques employed include dressings, packing, and use of cuffed tracheotomy tubes. Most patients with small mucocutaneous fistulas heal in 10 days to 2 weeks. However, it is apparent that this should be viewed strictly as a general estimate. In one study evaluating postoperative hospitalization in patients who develop wound infection, the average length of hospitalization was 34 days for those who developed wound infection and fistula following surgery alone, whereas hospitalization averaged 64 days in patients who had radiation therapy prior to surgery.[9] This increased hospitalization reflects the effect of radiation therapy on wound healing and the frequent need for subsequent procedures to control fistula in patients who had prior radiation therapy.

Large (more than 3 cm) mucocutaneous fistulas that develop postoperatively, especially in patients with prior irradiation therapy, frequently require secondary procedures to effect closure. Attempts to use local tissue such as rotation and turn-in flaps are frequently frustrated. We currently advocate use of either pedicled tissue, such as pectoralis major or trapezius myocutaneous flap, or we use free tissue transfers employing microvascular techniques. These techniques afford the surgeon well-vascularized healthy tissue to effect closure in contaminated and frequently irradiated surgical fields.

Exposure of the carotid artery in a postoperatively infected wound represents a potentially life-threatening complication. Patient care should be intensified, and dressings employing gauze moistened with an antibacterial solution should be applied and carefully tended. Efforts should be directed at returning the patient to the operating room at the earliest available time to cover the carotid artery with vascularized tissue. Appropriate techniques include the use of a pectoralis muscle or myocutaneous flap or some other similarly designed flap to cover the carotid artery.

If the carotid artery is allowed to become desiccated, carotid rupture or blowout may occur. Arterial bleeding from an infected postoperative wound must be considered a sentinel bleed indicative of a carotid artery injury. Patients must be managed on an emergency basis. When circumstances allow, evaluation with arteriography to determine the exact site of carotid erosion is appropriate. Under some circumstances, the erosion involves the external carotid artery, which then may allow the surgeon to ligate the external carotid artery electively. Unfortunately, more often the common or internal carotid artery is involved. This requires elective carotid ligation. Failure to undertake ligation electively frequently results in catastrophic hemorrhage.

Postoperative wound breakdown resulting in exposure of the mandible frequently results in osteomyelitis and sequestration. Efforts should be directed at intensified wound care. Debridement may be required.

SUMMARY

Prevention of infectious complications in head and neck surgery begins preoperatively. A careful assessment of the health of the patient, with particular attention to pre-existing pulmonary, cardiac, and renal diseases, is made. Treatment of coexisting infections and nutritional deficiencies is initiated prior to surgery. Appropriate perioperative antimicrobial chemoprophylaxis is instituted and continued at least 24 hours postoperatively.

Intraoperatively, meticulous surgical technique prevents tissue strangulation with resulting ischemia and necrosis. Watertight mucosal closures prevent postoperative salivary contamination, and closed suction drains prevent subcutaneous fluid collections.

Specialized nursing, including care of the drains and tracheotomy, is important to the prevention of postoperative infections.

In cases of postoperative wound infection, early recognition and prompt intervention may reduce the severity of the complications. Local wound care, debridement of nonviable tissue, coverage with healthy tissues, and systemic antibiotics may prevent fistula formation or carotid rupture.

The cornerstone in reducing the incidence and severity of infectious complications following head and neck surgery is the team approach. Frequent communication between the head and neck surgeon, nurse specialists, nutritionist, and medical consultants is integral to safe and successful surgery.

References

1. Beumer J, Harrison R, Sanders B, Kurrasch M: Preradiation dental extractions and the incidence of bone necrosis. Head Neck Surg 5:514–521, 1983.
2. Brown BM, Johnson JT, Wagner RL: Etiologic factors in head and neck wound infections. Laryngoscope 97:587–590, 1987.
3. Carl W: Dental management and prosthetic rehabilitation of patients with head and neck cancer. Head Neck Surg 3:27–42, 1980.
4. Casey D, Carl W: Dental considerations in oral cancer surgery. In Carl W, Sako K (eds): Cancer of the Oral Cavity. Chicago, Quintessence Publishing, 1986.
5. Chandra RK: Of nutritional status and disease outcome: Immunocompetence assessment. Ill Med J 172:111–113, 1987.
6. Eisele DW, Yarington CT, Lindeman RC: Indications for the tracheoesophageal diversion procedure and the laryngotracheal separation procedure. Ann Otol Rhinol Laryngol 97:471–475, 1988.
7. Fee WR Jr, Glenn M, Handen C, Hopp ML: One day vs two days of prophylactic antibiotics in patients undergoing major head and neck surgery. Laryngoscope 94:612, 1984.
8. Goodwin WJ, Torres J: The value of the Prognostic Nutritional Index in the management of patients with advanced carcinoma of the head and neck. Head Neck Surg 6:932, 1984.
9. Johnson JT, Bloomer WD: Effect of prior radiotherapy on postsurgical wound infection. Head Neck 11:132–136, 1989.
10. Johnson JT, Myers EN: Management of complications of therapeutic intervention. In Myers EN, Suen JY (eds): Cancer of the Head and Neck. 2nd ed. New York, Churchill Livingstone, 1989, pp 953–978.
11. Johnson JT, Myers EN, Thearle PB, et al: Antimicro-

bial prophylaxis for contaminated head and neck surgery. Laryngoscope 94:46–51, 1984.

12. Johnson JT, Schuller DE, Silver F, et al: Antibiotic prophylaxis in high-risk head and neck surgery: One-day vs. five-day therapy. Otolaryngol Head Neck Surg 95:554–557, 1986.

13. Johnson JT, Yu VL: Antibiotic use during major head and neck surgery. Ann Surg 207:108–111, 1988.

14. Johnson JT, Yu V, Myers EN, Wagner RL: An assessment of the need for gram-negative coverage in antibiotic prophylaxis for oncological head and neck surgery. J Infect Dis 115:331–333, 1987.

15. Keene HJ, Fleming TJ: Prevalence of caries-associated microflora after radiotherapy in patients with cancer of the head and neck. Oral Surg Oral Med Oral Pathol 64:421–426, 1987.

16. Mandel-Brown M, Johnson JT, Wagner RL: Cost-effectiveness of prophylactic antibiotics in head and neck surgery. Otolaryngol Head Neck Surg 92:520–523, 1984.

17. Mullen JL, Buzby GP, Waldman TG, et al: Predication of operative morbidity and mortality by preoperative nutrition assessment. Surg Forum 30:80, 1979.

18. Murray DP, Tunell WP, Whang R: Nutrition. In Papper S, Coussons RT, Williams GR (eds): Manual of Medical Care of the Surgical Patient. Boston, Little Brown, 1985, pp 169–184.

19. Piccart M, Dor P, Klastersky J: Antimicrobial prophylaxis of infections in head and neck cancer surgery. Scand J Infect Dis (Suppl) 39:92–96, 1983.

20. Reilly JJ: Nutritional management of patients with head and neck cancer. In Myers EN, Suen JY (eds): Cancer of the Head and Neck. 2nd ed. New York, Churchill Livingstone, 1989, pp 131–144.

21. Rodgers GK, Johnson JT, Petruzzelli GJ: Lipid and volume analysis of neck drainage in patients undergoing neck dissection. Otol Head Neck Surg, in press.

22. Rubin J, Johnson JT, Wagner RL, Yu VL: Bacteriologic analysis of wound infection following major head and neck surgery. Arch Otolaryngol Head Neck Surg 114:969–972, 1988.

23. Shike M, Berner YN, Gerdes H, et al: Percutaneous endoscopic gastrostomy and jejunostomy for long-term feeding in patients with cancer of the head and neck. Otolaryngol Head Neck Surg 101:549–554, 1989.

24. Tisi GM: Preoperative identification and evaluation of the patient with lung disease. Med Clin North Am 71:399–411, 1987.

25. Weiss SM: Nutritional aspects of preoperative management. Med Clin North Am 71:369–375, 1987.

Dysphagia and Aspiration

ANDREW BLITZER, MD, DDS
YOSEF P. KRESPI, MD

Aspiration and dysphagia are caused by a mechanical or neuromuscular disability creating a functional deficit. Alterations in the oral cavity, pharynx, larynx, or esophagus may cause significant problems with the swallowing effort, sometimes allowing pulmonary contamination with swallowed material. Most cases of postoperative dysphagia and aspiration are in patients with head and neck tumors. These are usually not complications but rather an expected morbidity of the disease and the treatment modalities. The disability will be related to the part surgically altered (e.g., tongue, pharynx, hypopharynx) or the cranial nerves sacrificed with resultant neuromuscular deficit or sensory loss (needed for coordination of motion and initiation of reflex events). Therefore, if the functional deficit can be anticipated, the treatment plan should include a means for compensating for the disability.[1]

NEUROLOGIC DYSFUNCTION

Both disease (including infection, trauma, and tumors) and the treatment of disease can cause neurologic impairment of the functions of the head and neck. Cranial nerves V, IX, X, and XII are all important in the production of swallowing disorders and aspiration. Most patients tolerate slow, gradual onset of neurologic impairment better than a sudden, complete nerve loss.

Failure of cranial nerve V may produce a swallowing disorder through a loss of sensation within the oral cavity and tongue and will interfere with the motor innervation of the masticatory muscles. Cranial nerve IX provides sensation to the tonsil, palate, posterior tongue, and pharynx, and motor function to the stylopharyngeus muscle, part of the soft palate, and part of the constrictor muscles. Classically, there is a loss of the gag reflex and a deviation of the uvula. Dysfunction of the tenth nerve causes the worst disabilities of swallowing and aspiration. Peripherally, the motor function to the larynx is provided by the recurrent and superior laryngeal nerves. Injury to the superior laryngeal nerve will also alter the sensation of the supraglottic larynx. The combination of motor disability and sensory impairment makes aspiration more likely. As the vagal lesion moves more centrally, the disability worsens. A section of the vagus at the skull base will disable the constrictors and the larynx and eliminate sensation of much of the larynx and pharynx. This is often impossible to overcome. Cranial nerve XII gives motor innervation to the tongue. A unilateral hypoglossal nerve paralysis usually is asymptomatic, but a bilateral hypoglossal paralysis can be devastating.[1–3]

Both diseases and surgical procedures that cause intracranial changes can also affect swallowing and allow for aspiration. Diffuse brain lesions can cause increased intracranial pressure that may produce stupor or coma. These diffuse lesions include neoplasia, hematoma, abscess, massive infarction; meningitis, encephalitis, cerebritis; excess ingestion of alcohol, narcotics, or barbiturates; or increased or decreased serum calcium, sodium, or glucose.[2]

SWALLOWING

Swallowing is a mixed voluntary and involuntary activity in which there is a synchronized, coordinated system of muscle contractions and relaxation. In the oral phase of swallowing (voluntary), the tongue prepares the food with saliva and sorts out the big particles that need to be chewed again before the swallow. The tongue then compresses the bolus against the palate, shaping it and coating it with mucus, and then squeezing it into the oropharynx. The soft palate is elevated to seal off the nasopharynx from the oropharynx, preventing nasal reflux. As the bolus passes the faucial pillars and reaches the vallecula epiglottica, the larynx is elevated and the involuntary portion or the pharyngeal phase of the swallow begins. Respiration is inhibited during this involuntary phase of swallowing.[1, 4]

In the pharyngeal phase, the tongue base first moves posteriorly, tipping the epiglottis posteroinferiorly. Simultaneously, the larynx is raised by the supraglottic musculature. The position of the epiglottis diverts the bolus posterolaterally, away from the airway. The collapse of the aryepiglottic folds and false cords, and the simultaneous closure of the vocal cords, protects the airway as the bolus descends into the hypopharynx.[1, 4–8]

When the bolus passes through the upper esophageal sphincter, the esophageal phase begins.[8] If the upper esophageal sphincter, the cricopharyngeus muscle, fails to open, swallowing will be impaired. This also will occur if the esophagus fails to contract or contracts dyssynchronously. The tonic contraction of the cricopharyngeus muscle is mediated by vagal fibers that provide tonic stimulation for contraction via lower motor activity.[9, 10] The tonic cricopharyngeal contraction is neurogenic, whereas central inhibition is responsible for the relaxation during swallowing.[11] The cricopharyngeus normally exerts a pharyngeal pressure of 15 to 23 mm Hg and must be overcome by the hypopharynx to induce the opening of the upper esophageal sphincter. Conditions that damage vagal fibers and interfere with the relaxation of the cricopharyngeus may cause cricopharyngeal achalasia, dysphasia, and aspiration.

The result of normal swallowing muscular activity is the movement of a bolus of material in the oral cavity into the pharynx, bypassing the laryngeal inlet, and into the esophagus. A dyscoordinated effort will allow aspiration, choking, nasal reflux, or regurgitation.[8]

ASPIRATION

Aspiration, or soiling of the tracheobronchial tree, can produce life-threatening pulmonary disease. Disordered oral, pharyngeal, or esophageal phases of swallowing or laryngeal dysfunction may allow pulmonary contamination with swallowed material. In some cases the aspiration is caused by a combination of laryngeal and swallowing dysfunction.[1] Intermittent or persistent aspiration may cause symptoms including cough, intermittent fever, recurrent tracheobronchitis, atelectases, pneumonia, and/or empyema. The pulmonary disease produced by aspiration may be associated with weight loss, cachexia, and dehydration. The quantity and frequency of aspiration increases with mechanical impairment of the larynx and pharynx, neurologic impairment, and decreasing levels of consciousness.[12–18]

Preoperative Management

Avoiding damage to the neural and muscular structures that are necessary for swallowing and protection of the airway is obvious. Treatment planning should include identifying the possibility of postoperative disorders of swallowing or aspiration or both. If aspiration is anticipated, a tracheostomy at the time of operation will help separate the airway from the pharynx temporarily and allow for adequate tracheal suctioning of airway contaminants and assisted ventilation when necessary.

The tracheostomy, however, should not be used as the sole method of management of aspiration. With use of a cuffed tracheostomy tube, an independent external airway port can be established. Secretions or food material that may pass through the larynx will be kept above the cuff on the tracheostomy tube. When the cuff is periodically deflated to prevent irreparable injury to the tracheal mucosa, the material will contaminate the airway unless meticulous suctioning has cleared it prior to cuff deflation. If the cuff is kept overinflated or is used for an extended period of time, the pressure will cause tracheomalacia. This will prevent an adequate seal around the tracheostomy tube and will allow airway soilage. Therefore, other solutions for continued use of tracheostomy should be employed.[1, 19, 20]

In some patients, neural or mechanical disability of the soft palate may produce velopharyngeal insufficiency, which allows for rhinolalia and nasal reflux. Treatment can consist of creating a prosthetic appliance to be inserted at operation to elevate the soft palate, soft palate or posterior pharyngeal wall augmentation, or pharyngeal flaps.[21] Other patients who have oral phase defects also can benefit from some types of obturators or guide-bar dental prostheses that can be used to guide food away from nonfunctional areas of the mouth, allowing the more functional areas to deal with the ingested food material.[22]

Surgical procedures that will disrupt the functional relationship of the tongue base, pharynx, and larynx often may produce aspiration. If a contemplated resection is likely to impair laryngeal elevation, the larynx can be suspended to alter the direction of the laryngeal inlet. Edgerton and Duncan,[23] Calcaterra,[24] and Goode[25] have described a midline, anteriorly based laryngeal suspension to decrease the likelihood of aspiration. These techniques utilize a suture from the mandible or other anterior structure to the upper edge of the thyroid lamina of the larynx. This tilts the larynx anteriorly and raises the larynx under the base of the tongue to avoid airway contamination. A modification of this concept was described by Hillel and Goode in 1983, in which the larynx was suspended laterally to increase the pharyngeal opening and change the direction of the laryngeal inlet.[26]

If parts of the larynx are either removed or disabled, augmentation or reconstructive procedures can be employed at operation to try to rehabilitate the functions of the larynx and allow swallowing without aspiration. Cricopharyngeal myotomy also may be useful in patients in whom part or all of the pharynx has been disabled.[27–30] In addition, a partial cricoid resection will allow for a larger opening at the upper esophageal sphincter, making swallowing more efficient with decreased resistance.[31] An alternative to this theme was described by Biller and Urken[78] for patients who have continued aspiration after supraglottic laryngectomy. Vertical cuts are made in half of the cricoid cartilage, allowing for a collapse of the hemilarynx and thereby decreasing the space available for airway soilage. Some patients continue to have a functional airway.

If a protracted swallowing disability is anticipated, occasionally a soft nasogastric tube or temporary feeding gastrostomy will allow for proper alimentation without risking aspiration.

Postoperative Management

Immediately after operation, most patients who have major head and neck surgical procedures will have some degree of swallowing disability or aspiration or both owing to swelling, pain, muscle spasm, and so on. If these disabilities continue, however, further investigation will be necessary. A review of the preoperative plan and operative procedure will sort out what is disabled. A fiberoptic direct laryngoscopic view of the larynx and pharynx during swallowing can identify any defects in the larynx or laryngeal motion, pooling of the hypopharynx, poor contractility of the pharynx, obstruction from a flap or other transposed tissue, and any mass lesions that may be causing obstruction. Laryngeal and pharyngeal electromyography also may help in determining a mechanical or neural disability.[32]

Using a radiologic examination termed a modified barium swallow or "cookie swallow," a video tape is made so that the study can be replayed at various speeds to identify subtle changes within the phases of the swallow. Small amounts of barium of different consistencies are given to the patient, who is kept in a natural upright position, to best assess the oral and pharyngeal phases of the swallow. The swallowing effort can be analyzed for adynamic areas, relative or true obstructions, and dyssynchrony. The patient's position can be changed to see in which position swallowing is the best. Aspiration also can be assessed in regard to consistency of the bolus, the position of the patient, and any other associated dysfunction.[3, 8]

Ultrasonography has been found useful in studying the oral phase of swallowing but cannot be used for the pharyngeal or esophageal phases because of interference of the cervical spine. This study is non-invasive and safe and can be repeated at regular intervals without harm to the patient.[33, 34] Radionuclide scans also have been found useful in evaluation of patients who have dysphagia and aspirate. A radioactive bolus, usually composed of ^{99}Tc sulfur colloid, is fed to the patient. The swallow is recorded with the gamma scintillation camera as the bolus passes from the oropharynx to the esophagus. The pharyngeal transit time, clearance rate, and degree of aspiration can easily be quantified.[34]

Manometry, utilizing an apparatus that measures pressures in the pharynx, cricopharyngeus, and esophagus, is a useful way of identifying subtle failures of pressure generation or hyperfunction of the sphincter. However, manometry does not yield any information about aspiration. Therefore, manometry and videofluoroscopy have been used together, as reported by McConnel, for the accurate evaluation of dysphagia and aspiration.[35]

Treatment of the swallowing disorders found is to correct or compensate for the underlying defect. Swallowing therapy can be of benefit in some of these individuals. Swallowing therapy should be individualized, based on observations during swallowing efforts, and the swallowing effort should be recorded on a videotaped barium swallow. The consistency, head and neck position, method of food introduction, the quantity of food, and other parameters of swallowing can be assessed and modified for each patient, to allow the maximum swallowing situation for that patient.[8] In patients who still cannot swallow, gavage feeding can be taught that will bypass the oral phase. In patients who do not improve with these techniques, nasogastric or pharyngotomy tube feedings may be useful. Some patients with nasogastric tubes continue to aspirate a reflux of material around the tube. These patients may need a gastrostomy, a tracheostomy, and/or other laryngeal and pharyngeal procedures to prevent life-threatening aspiration.[1, 3, 8, 36]

In patients who are found to have either

true or relative cricopharyngeal achalasia, a cricopharyngeal myotomy may help correct the associated dysphagia and aspiration. Cricopharyngeal myotomy is the treatment for true or relative cricopharyngeal achalasia, not for patients who have difficulty in all phases of swallowing from generalized mechanical failure, as some investigators suggest.[27–30, 37–40]

In some patients who develop esophageal motility disorders, pharmacologic agents can alter dysfunction. Most of the esophageal motility research has addressed increasing the pressure of the lower esophageal sphincter for the treatment of gastroesophageal reflux. Two agents commonly used to increase contractility of the esophagus are bethanechol (which increases esophageal contractility, but also increases the production of gastric acid) and metoclopramide (a potent antiemetic that has been found additionally to increase contractility without increasing gastric acidity).[39, 41, 42] The effect of these or other agents on the upper esophagus and upper esophageal sphincter is still not known precisely. In patients who have diffuse esophageal spasm, the use of histamine blockers in conjunction with calcium channel blockers such as nifedipine or diltiazem (although not FDA-approved for this purpose) has been shown to be effective in some cases.[43]

Alteration of laryngeal neural or mechanical function also may cause aspiration. Unilateral sensory stimulation of the normal larynx should produce a reflex adduction of the vocal cords. The sensory signal for this reflex closure is carried via the superior laryngeal nerve, and the bilateral motor response is carried via the recurrent laryngeal nerve. If there is a decreased or absent sensory signal, foreign material in the supraglottis and glottis may fail to trigger laryngeal adduction, allowing swallowed material to spill through the glottis until it is detected by sensory fibers of the subglottis, which are carried in the recurrent laryngeal nerve. If the vagal sensory fibers are also disabled, a cough may not be initiated, and the foreign material will descend into the tracheobronchial tree until it provokes a cough response produced by the vagal tracheal fibers, which have considerable crossover.[1, 19]

The unilaterally impaired vocal cord also may imperil a patient's airway if it is produced in conjunction with a swallowing dishability. In addition to the soiling of the airway owing to the incompetent vocal cord, the patient's cough is also diminished. It becomes much harder to build up an adequate amount of subglottic pressure when there is a unilateral paresis or paralysis, without blowing the paralyzed cord open. The treatment plan for an incompetent larynx should be based on the patient's underlying disease, the likelihood for recovery, general medical status, quality of life issues, and severity of the aspiration and laryngeal incompetence. Vocal cord paralysis can occur during thyroid operations, surgical procedures for Zenker diverticula, mediastinoscopy, and intrathoracic procedures, as well as other procedures that may imperil the recurrent laryngeal nerve. A tracheostomy, as discussed, may give a temporary benefit from the separation of the airway and food passage. The airway can be secured by means of a tracheostomy tube with a cuff. The cuff will keep secretions or food substances from entering the airway, and the tracheostomy will also provide access for good pulmonary toilet. Meticulous suctioning of secretions above the cuff is necessary to prevent soilage of the airway when the cuff is deflated. Tracheotomy is only a short-term solution, however, since with time cuff pressures produce tracheomalacia, and the inability to obtain an effective seal will allow continued airway soilage. Therefore, other solutions are necessary for long-term disability.[44–47]

In some patients, particularly those with a known permanent paralysis because of anatomic defect of a vocal cord, vocal cord augmentation may provide a return of good function. Bruning reported moving a paralyzed vocal cord toward the midline using paraffin injection.[48] However, paraffin was found to be inflammatory to the laryngeal tissues, producing granulomas. Other materials were tested, including glycerin, cartilage, bone dust, and tantalum. Tantalum and glycerin and then Teflon and glycerin were first used by Arnold in 1962.[49] Since then, Lewy, Rontal and colleagues, and Schramm and colleagues have separately reported successful treatment of vocal cord paralysis using Teflon or Gelfoam injection.[50–52] Teflon is injected into the larynx during a direct laryngoscopy, using local anesthesia so that the airway and voice can be assessed constantly. Vocal cord injection also can be performed in selected patients percutaneously via the cricothyroid membrane, as recently reported by Ward and colleagues.[53] Teflon injection also has been reported via an indirect technique with a right angle injecting apparatus. In addition to medialization, use of Teflon, Gelfoam, and collagen has been reported for augmentation of vocal cord contour.[50–52]

Teflon within the vocalis muscle may produce fibrosis and a "stiff cord" that changes or abolishes the mucosal wave and changes the resonant characteristics of the vocal cord. Teflon use, therefore, should be judicious since it is reactive and can cause granulomas and fibrosis. Teflon is also very difficult to remove from the larynx once injected.[54]

Some patients with brain stem stroke or neural trauma who suffer from aspiration have a reasonable chance for partial or full functional return. In these patients, vocal cord medialization can be accomplished with a Gelfoam injection.[52] This will medialize the vocal cord for 3 to 4 months until all the material is resorbed, allowing patients to have a functional benefit while awaiting functional return. If no return occurs and the patient again becomes symptomatic, a permanent method of vocal cord medialization can be used.

Meurmann in 1952 described a technique for augmenting large glottic incompetencies using autologous cartilage.[55] The cartilage implants were placed submucosally via a midline thyrotomy. The technique has been modified and refined by others.[56–59]

Within the past several years, Isshiki and others have introduced a series of surgical techniques to alter vocal cord position and function by altering the laryngeal framework.[60–62] Their Type I procedure (vocal cord medialization) is accomplished via a window in the ipsilateral thyroid ala and placement of a Silastic block to medialize the cord. The Isshiki arytenoid adduction procedure is useful in cases of significant incompetence in the posterior glottis. In this procedure the cricoarytenoid joint is dislocated, and a suture is placed through the lateral cricoarytenoid muscle attachment. The suture is then brought out through the ipsilateral thyroid lamina anteriorly and tied. This rotates the cord and vocalis process medially. Both the Type I and adductor procedures can be used together when there is cord atrophy and a posterior glottis opening. Others, including Koufman,[63] have confirmed superb results for correction of the voice and mild aspiration utilizing laryngeal framework surgery.

GLOTTIC PROSTHESES

Through the years some researchers have conceptualized management of severe aspiration with a tracheostomy for the airway and a glottic prosthesis as a "cork in a bottle" technique. These prostheses were often rigid and either prefabricated or custom made. They were placed endoscopically and usually held in place with transcutaneous sutures. Although these techniques diminished aspiration, patients continued to leak fluids around the prostheses.[64] A new hollow prosthesis made of soft silicone has been designed by Eliachar and colleagues.[65] This tube produces a more favorable seal and has a slit in the upper end allowing phonation while maintaining a glottic closure. This tube is inserted via the tracheostomy site.

GLOTTIC AND SUPRAGLOTTIC CLOSURE

In cases of intermediate to severe recurrent or persistent aspiration, several procedures for glottic or supraglottic closure have been described.

A glottic closure procedure was described by Montgomery in 1975.[66] His procedure was performed through a median thyrotomy. The mucosa of the vocal cords is stripped bilaterally, and a figure-of-eight suture closes the glottis and allows the vocal cords to produce a fibrous union. This technique achieves separation of the air and food passages with a permanent tracheotomy. However, the patient cannot phonate. In addition, if the vocal cords are functional preoperatively, the seal may pull apart before healing and allow aspiration of material through a posterior opening. The procedure is described as reversible, but laryngeal webs are often difficult to correct, leaving vocal cords with significant scarring and poor phonation.

Creation of a supraglottic laryngeal closure is an alternative to a closure of the larynx at the glottic level. This has the advantage of not causing any scarring in the area of the vocal cords. Habal and Murray in 1972 described a two-layered horizontal closure of the supraglottis via a pharyngotomy.[67] The epiglottis, aryepiglottic folds, arytenoids, and interarytenoid area are then incised and the tip of the epiglottis is then folded over the arytenoids and sutured in place. Patients cannot phonate and breath through a tracheotomy tube. Strome and Fried in 1983 reported the procedure to be reversible.[68] In some cases recurrent aspiration occurs, perhaps owing to the suture line opening posteriorly from the spring of the epiglottic cartilage. A vertical supraglottic closure was created to avoid the posterior opening and leave a small opening at the top by Biller and associates in 1983.[69] With an opening at the level of the tip of the epiglottis, aspiration does not occur, but phonation is possible in some patients. We have used this closure successfully in several patients with intractable aspiration, with excellent results. Patients often can again eat, and some can speak.[1]

LARYNGEAL DIVERSION

In 1975, Lindeman described a procedure that would separate the air and food passages.[70] This procedure is potentially reversible and could be performed without damage to the laryngeal structures. The trachea is first separated at the third or fourth tracheal ring, with the distal portion brought out and sewn to the neck skin. Next, the proximal tracheal stump and larynx are sewn to a small opening in the esophagus, allowing all material entering the larynx to exit into the esophagus, with a complete separation of the airway. Phonation does not occur following this treatment unless the patient recovers function and the procedure is reversed. Yarington and Lindeman reported two such reversals of his procedure.[71] We have used this technique many times with success. Lindeman[70] and Baron and Dedo[72] reported a modification of this technique in which a blind end-pouch of the proximal trachea is created. Another approach to the patient with a very high preliminary tracheostomy was described by Krespi and colleagues, who saved the mucosal lining to use as a superiorly based mucosal flap and performed cartilage resection from the cricoid cartilage and the first and second tracheal rings.[73] An esophagotomy is made at the level of the first tracheal ring, and the tracheal mucosal flap is sutured to the esophagotomy. An alternative diversion technique was described by Tucker, in which both the proximal and distal tracheal stumps are diverted to the anterior cervical skin, thereby creating a double-barreled tracheostoma.[74] The proximal trachea is brought out to the skin through a split in the sternocleidomastoid muscle; this maneuver supposedly compresses the trachea, minimizing leakage of aspirated material to the skin. This procedure has the obvious disadvantage of draining corrosive substances to the cervical skin.

LARYNGECTOMY

The oldest treatment for life-threatening aspiration is a total laryngectomy. Total laryngectomy provides a permanent cutaneous tracheostoma and a permanent separation of the airway and food passage, but it eliminates phonation, or the possibility of reversal in patients who might recover some or all of their function.[75] Some suggest that laryngectomy, particularly a narrow-field laryngectomy, is still indicated in patients with poor prognoses or associated medical problems.[76, 77]

FUTURE DIRECTIONS

The future of rehabilitation of patients with neural and mechanical disabilities creating problems with aspiration and swallowing is the reinnervation of denervated muscles and the transfer of neuromuscular pedicles. Electrical pacing of denervated muscles also may help allow contracture of denervated muscle, enhancing function. With the advent of these techniques, radical but life-saving techniques previously described may be unnecessary, and patients may well have better function.[79–86]

References

1. Blitzer A, Krespi YP: Pathophysiology, evaluation, and management of chronic aspiration. In Johnson JT, Blitzer A, Ossoff R, Thomas JR (eds): Instructional Courses—American Academy of Otolaryngology–Head and Neck Surgery. Vol 2. St. Louis, CV Mosby, 1989, pp 53–67.
2. Brin MF, Younger D: Neurologic disorders and aspiration. Otolaryngol Clin North Am 21:691–701, 1988.
3. Logemann JA, Bytell DE: Swallowing disorders in three types of head and neck surgical patients. Cancer 44:1095–1105, 1979.
4. Didio LJA, Anderson MC: The "Sphincters" of the Digestive System. Baltimore, Williams & Wilkins, 1968.
5. Ardan GM, Kemp FH: The protection of laryngeal airway during swallowing. Br J Radiol 25:406, 1952.
6. Atkinson M, Kramer P, Wyman SM, Ingelfinger FJ: The dynamics of swallowing. I. Normal pharyngeal mechanisms. J Clin Invest 36:581, 1957.
7. Negus JE: The second stage of swallowing. Acta Otolaryngol Suppl (Stockh) 78:78–82, 1949.
8. Logemann J: Evaluation and Treatment of Swallowing Disorders. San Diego, College Hill Press, 1983.
9. Van Overbeek JJ, Betlem HC: Cricopharyngeal myotomy in pharyngeal paralysis; Cineradiographic and manometric indications. Ann Otol Rhinol Laryngol 88:596–602, 1979.
10. Yoshida Y: Localization of efferent neurons innervating the pharyngeal constrictor muscles and the

11. Christenson J: Innervation and function of the esophagus. In Stipa S, Belsey RHR, Moraldi A (eds): Medical and Surgical Problems of the Esophagus. London, Academic Press, 1981, pp 14–16.
12. Bonano PC: Swallowing dysfunction after tracheostomy. Ann Surg 174:29, 1970.
13. Nahum AM, Harris JP, Davidson TM: The patient who aspirates—diagnosis and management. J Otolaryngol 10:10–16, 1981.
14. Bartlett JG, Gorbach SL: The triple threat of aspiration pneumonia. Chest 68:560–566, 1975.
15. Huxley EJ, Viroslav J, Gray WR, Pierce AK: Pharyngeal aspiration in normal adults and patients with depressed consciousness. Am J Med 64:564, 1978.
16. Mendelson CL: Aspiration of stomach contents into lungs during obstetrical anesthesia. Am J Obstet Gynecol 52:191, 1946.
17. Hawkins DB: Noninfectious disorders of the lower respiratory tract. In Bluestone CD, Stool SE (eds): Pediatric Otolaryngology. Philadelphia, WB Saunders, 1983, pp 1265–1269.
18. Awe WC, Fletcher WS, Jacob SW: The pathophysiology of aspiration pneumonitis. Surgery 60:232–239, 1966.
19. Blitzer A: Evaluation and management of chronic aspiration. N Y State J Med 87:154–160, 1987.
20. Cameron JL, Reynolds J, Zuidema GD: Aspiration in patients with tracheostomies. Surg Gynecol Obstet 136:68–70, 1973.
21. Wurster CF, Krespi YP, Davis JW: Combined functional oral rehabilitation after radical cancer surgery. Arch Otolaryngol 111:530–533, 1985.
22. Chalian VA, Drane JB, Standish SM: Maxillofacial Prosthetics: Multidisciplinary Approach. Baltimore, Williams & Wilkins, 1971.
23. Edgerton MT, Duncan MM: Reconstruction with loss of the hyomandibular complex in excision of large cancers. Arch Surg 78:425–436, 1959.
24. Calcaterra T: Laryngeal suspension after supraglottic laryngectomy. Arch Otolaryngol 94:306–309, 1971.
25. Goode RL: Laryngeal suspension in head and neck surgery. Laryngoscope 86:349–355, 1976.
26. Hillel AD, Goode RL: Lateral laryngeal suspension: A new procedure to minimize swallowing disorders following tongue base resection. Laryngoscope 93:26–31, 1983.
27. Stevens KM, Newell RC: Cricopharyngeal myotomy in dysphagia. Laryngoscope 81:1616–1620, 1971.
28. Calcaterra TC, Kadell BM, Ward PH: Dysphagia secondary to cricopharyngeal muscle dysfunction: Surgical management. Arch Otolaryngol 101:726–729, 1975.
29. Wilkins SA: Indications for the section of the cricopharyngeus muscle. Am J Surg 108:533, 1964.
30. Ross ER, Green R, Auslander MD, Biller HF: Cricopharyngeal myotomy: Management of cervical dysphagia. Otolaryngol Head Neck Surg 90:434–441, 1982.
31. Krespi Y, Sisson G: Management of chronic aspiration by subtotal and submucosal cricoid resection. Ann Otol Rhinol Laryngol 94:580, 1985.
32. Blitzer A, Lovelace RE, Brin MF, et al: Electromyographic findings in focal laryngeal dystonia (spastic

dysphonia). Ann Otol Rhinol Laryngol 94:591–594, 1985.

33. Shawker T, Sonies B, Stone M: Real-time ultrasound visualization of tongue movement during swallowing. J Clin Ultrasound 11:485, 1983.

34. Sonies BC, Baum BJ: Evaluation of swallowing pathophysiology. Otolaryngol Clin North Am 21:637–648, 1988.

35. McConnel FMS: Analysis of pressure generation and bolus transit during pharyngeal swallowing. Laryngoscope 98:71–78, 1988.

36. Shedd DP, Scatliff JA, Kirchner JA: A cineradiographic study of post-resectional alterations in oropharyngeal physiology. Surg Gynecol Obstet 110:69–89, 1960.

37. Mills CP: Dysphagia in pharyngeal paralysis treated by cricopharyngeal sphincterotomy. Lancet 1:455–457, 1973.

38. Lebo CP, Sang K, Norris FH: Cricopharyngeal myotomy in amyotrophic lateral sclerosis. Laryngoscope 86:862–868, 1976.

39. Schulze-Delrieu K: Esophageal Pharmacology. In Cohen S, Soloway RD (eds): Diseases of the Esophagus. New York, Churchill-Livingstone, 1982, pp 35–49.

40. Asherson N: Achalasia of the cricopharyngeal sphincter. J Laryngol Otol 64:747–758, 1950.

41. Reference deleted.

42. Diamant NE: Normal esophageal physiology. In Cohen S, Soloway RD (eds): Diseases of the Esophagus. New York, Churchill-Livingstone, 1982, pp 1–33.

43. Buchin PJ: Swallowing disorders: Diagnosis and medical treatment. Otolaryngol Clin North Am 21:663–667, 1988.

44. Bryant LR, Tinkle JK, Dubiler L: Tracheal damage from cuffed tracheostomy tubes. JAMA 215:625, 1971.

45. Thilenius OG, Vial CB: Chronic tracheotomy in dogs. J Appl Physiol 18:439–440, 1963.

46. Fee WE, Ward PA: Permanent tracheostomy: A new surgical technique. Ann Otolaryngol 86:635–638, 1977.

47. Fearon B, McDonald RE, Smith C: Airway problems in children following prolonged endotracheal intubation. Ann Otol Rhinol Laryngol 75:975, 1966.

48. Bruning W: Über eine neue Behandlungsmethode. Verh Dtsch Laryngol 18:151, 1911.

49. Arnold GE: Vocal rehabilitation of paralytic dysphonia. Arch Otolaryngol 76:358–368, 1962.

50. Lewy RB: Glottic rehabilitation with Teflon injection—the return of voice, cough, and laughter. Acta Otolaryngol 58:214, 1964.

51. Rontal E, Rontal M, Morse G, Brown EM: Vocal cord injection in the treatment of acute and chronic aspiration. Laryngoscope 86:625–634, 1976.

52. Schramm VL, May M, Lavorato AS: Gelfoam paste injection for vocal cord paralysis: Temporary rehabilitation of glottic competence. Laryngoscope 88:1268, 1978.

52a. Ford CN, Bless DM: Clinical experience with injectable collagen for vocal cord augmentation. Laryngoscope 96:863, 1986.

53. Ward PH, Hanson DG, Abemayor E: Transcutaneous Teflon injection of the paralyzed vocal cord: A new technique. Laryngoscope 95:644–649, 1985.

54. Rubin HJ: Misadventures with injectable polytef (Teflon). Arch Otolaryngol 101:114, 1975.

55. Meurmann Y: Operative mediofixation of the vocal cord in complete unilateral paralysis. Arch Otolaryngol 55:554, 1952.

56. Opheim O: Unilateral paralysis of the vocal cord. Acta Otolaryngol 45:226, 1955.

57. Waltner JG: Surgical rehabilitation of voice following laryngofissure. Arch Otolaryngol 67:99, 1958.

58. Levine HL, Tucker HM: Surgical management of the paralyzed larynx. In Bailey B, Biller HF (eds): Surgery of the Larynx. Philadelphia, WB Saunders, 1985, pp 117–147.

59. Smith GW: Aphonia due to vocal cord paralysis corrected by medial positioning of the affected vocal cord with a cartilage autograft. Can J Otolaryngol 1:295–298, 1972.

60. Isshiki N: Recent advances in phonosurgery. Folia Phoniatr (Basel) 32:119–154, 1980.

61. Isshiki N, Okamura H, Ishikawa T: Thyroplasty type I (lateral compression) for dysphonia due to vocal cord paralysis or atrophy. Acta Otolaryngol 80:465–473, 1975.

62. Isshiki N: Phonosurgery: Theory and Practice. Tokyo, Springer-Verlag, 1989.

63. Koufman JA: Laryngoplastic phonosurgery. In Johnson JT, Blitzer A, Ossoff R, Thomas JR (eds): Instructional Courses—American Academy of Otolaryngology–Head and Neck Surgery. St. Louis, CV Mosby, 1988, pp 339–352.

64. Weisberger EC, Huebsch SA: Endoscopic treatment of aspiration using a laryngeal stent. Otolaryngol Head Neck Surg 90:215–222, 1982.

65. Eliachar I, Roberts JK, Hayes JD, Tucker HM: A vented laryngeal stent with phonatory and pressure relief capability. Laryngoscope 97:1264–1268, 1987.

66. Montgomery WW: Surgical laryngeal closure to eliminate chronic aspiration. N Engl J Med 292:1390–1391, 1975.

67. Habal MB, Murray JE: Surgical treatment of life-endangering chronic aspiration pneumonia. Plast Reconstr Surg 49:305–311, 1972.

68. Strome M, Fried MP: Rehabilitative surgery for aspiration. Arch Otolaryngol 109:809–811, 1983.

69. Biller HF, Lawson W, Baek S-M: Total glossectomy: A technique of reconstruction eliminating laryngectomy. Arch Otolaryngol 109:69–73, 1983.

70. Lindeman RC: Diverting the paralyzed larynx: A reversible procedure for intractable aspiration. Laryngoscope 85:157–180, 1975.

71. Yarington CT, Lindeman RC, Sutton D: Clinical experience with the tracheoesophageal anastomosis for intractable aspiration. Ann Otol Rhinol Laryngol 85:609–612, 1976.

72. Baron BS, Dedo HH: Separation of the larynx and trachea for intractable aspiration. Laryngoscope 90:1927–1932, 1980.

73. Krespi YP, Quatela VC, Sisson GA, Som ML: Modified tracheo-esophageal diversion for chronic aspiration. Laryngoscope 94:1298–1301, 1984.

74. Tucker HM: Management of the patient with an incompetent larynx. Am J Otolaryngol 1:47–56, 1979.

75. Montgomery WW: Total laryngectomy. In Montgomery WW (ed): Surgery of the Upper Respiratory System. Philadelphia, Lea & Febiger, 1973, pp 484–496.

76. Cannon CR, McLean WC: Laryngectomy for chronic aspiration. Am J Otolaryngol 3:145–149, 1982.

77. Krespi YP, Blitzer A: Laryngectomy for aspiration: Narrow field technique. Laryngoscope, in press.

78. Biller HF, Urken M: Cricoid collapse, a new tech-

nique for the management of glottic incompetence. Arch Otolaryngol 111:740–741, 1985.

79. Blitzer A: Swallowing disorders and aspiration in the elderly. In Goldstein J, Kashima HK, Koopman CF (eds): Geriatric Otolaryngology. Toronto, BC Decker, 1989, pp 124–134.

80. Crumley R: Phrenic nerve graft for bilateral vocal cord paralysis. Laryngoscope 93:425–428, 1983.

81. Rice D: Laryngeal reinnervation with the ansa cervicalis. Arch Otolaryngol 109:480–481, 1983.

82. Tucker HM: Selective reinnervation of paralyzed facial muscles by the neuro-muscular island pedicle technique: New concepts in rehabilitation of the longstanding facial paralysis. In Fisch UJ (ed): Facial Nerve Surgery. Birmingham, AL, Aesculapius, 1977, pp 251–283.

83. Tucker HM: Neurologic disorders. In Tucker HM (ed): The Larynx. Stuttgart, Thieme Medical Publishers, 1987, pp 235–259.

84. May M: Muscle transposition for facial reanimation: Indications and results. Arch Otol Head Neck Surg 110:184–189, 1984.

85. Broniatowski M, Ilyes LA, Jacobs GB, et al: Artificial reflex arc: A potential solution for chronic aspiration. A canine study based on a laryngeal prosthesis. Laryngoscope 98:235–237, 1988.

86. Broniatowski M, Ilyes LA, Jacobs GB, et al: Artificial reflex arc: A potential solution for chronic aspiration. I. Neck skin stimulation triggering strap muscle contraction in the canine. Laryngoscope 97:331–333, 1987.

CHAPTER 7

Cranial Nerve Complications

STEVEN J. PEARLMAN, MD
JUAN F. MOSCOSO, MD

Modern surgical techniques have enhanced our ability to extirpate head and neck tumors once thought to be inoperable. With these enhanced surgical methods comes an increase in postoperative patient morbidity, affecting deglutition, respiration, cosmesis, and shoulder function. Prior to the era of surgical intervention, many syndromes that affected the cranial nerves of the skull base were described. Trauma, tumors, and infections were implicated in Vernet syndrome, marked by paralysis of the cranial nerves of the jugular foramen (the glossopharyngeal, vagus, and accessory).[1] Villaret syndrome added the sympathetic trunk, and Collet-Sicard syndrome involved cranial nerves IX through XII. Similar neurologic sequelae result from surgical intervention. Complications from these operations are discussed in this chapter, along with relevant anatomy, patient management, and rehabilitation.

THE OLFACTORY NERVE (I)

ANATOMY

The olfactory nerve (I) contains special fibers concerned with odor identification (ol-

faction). Fine, nonmyelinated axons arise from bipolar nerve cells within the olfactory epithelium, located on the roof of the nasal cavity and extending over the upper third of the septum and most of the superior concha. These nerve fibers gather into approximately 20 filaments that traverse the cribriform plate of the ethmoid bone and the meninges to synapse with the secondary olfactory neurons in the olfactory bulbs. The central projection of these neurons forms the olfactory tract.[2, 3] In addition to the neural inputs from the olfactory epithelium, inputs from cranial nerves V, IX, and X may be involved in odor identification.[4] Henkin and coworkers believe the vapor-sensitive mucosa served by the aforementioned cranial nerves acts as an accessory olfactory area.[5, 6]

OLFACTORY NERVE COMPLICATIONS

Loss of olfaction is not to be considered a minor inconvenience. Apart from the pleasure loss from inability to enjoy fragrances, being unable to smell food or gas is a serious handicap that could lead to unnecessary accidental deaths. Injury to the olfactory system can occur directly or indirectly. Any operation upon the ethmoids may result in direct injury to olfactory mucosal nerves. The bone of the cribriform plate is thin, and removal of tissue from this area can result in dural tears and olfactory nerve injury. Nonetheless, loss of olfaction is rarely reported as a complication of surgery upon the ethmoids. Anosmia was noted in one patient out of 1000 undergoing ethmoidectomies at the Mayo Clinic.[7] Maniglia has reported another case after intranasal ethmoidectomy.[8, 9] Friedman and Katsantonis did not report anosmia as a consequence of intranasal ethmoidectomy in over 1160 patients,[10] and it is yet to be reported as a complication of endoscopic sinus surgery.[11–13] Anosmia following exenterative surgery for chronic infection of the ethmoid or frontal sinuses is rarely encountered. Hardy and Montgomery reported only one case in 250 patients undergoing frontal osteoplastic sinusotomy.[14] Loss of olfaction following external frontoethmoidectomy or lateral rhinotomy has not been reported.

The techniques of craniofacial surgery developed by Dandy,[15] Ray and McLean,[16] and Smith and colleagues[17] and popularized by Ketcham and colleagues[18] have allowed the modern otolaryngologist–head and neck surgeon to pursue aggressively both benign and malignant disease of the anterior skull base, frontal sinus, or ethmoid sinuses previously thought unresectable. Resection of the cribriform plate during craniofacial procedures renders all these patients anosmic postoperatively.[19]

Following total laryngectomy, up to 95 per cent of patients reported altered or absent olfaction.[20] Henkin believes this is secondary to interrupted neural feedback from his postulated accessory olfactory areas (described earlier). However, no such anatomic neural pathways are known to exist. The most likely explanation for laryngectomy-induced hyposmia is the interruption in transport of odorant molecules to the olfactory epithelium from loss of nasal air flow.[5] With pulmonary assistance devices, the olfactory thresholds and odor identification scores of laryngectomees are similar to those of controls.[21] With this knowledge, strategies have been devel-

oped to rehabilitate the laryngectomized patient's sense of smell.[22]

THE OPTIC NERVE (II)

ANATOMY

The optic nerve (II) is formed within the retina by the confluence of the ganglion cell axons at the optic disk. These myelinated fibers pass posteromedially from the eyeball to exit from the orbit through the optic canal. This canal is located in the lesser wing of the sphenoid bone, in close proximity to the lateral wall of the sphenoid sinus and to the posterior group of ethmoid air cells. Being composed of the axons of secondary sensory cells, the optic nerve, like the olfactory nerve, is a tract of the central nervous system.[3] Its main blood supply is through the ophthalmic artery, a branch of the internal carotid artery. However, numerous communications occur with branches of the external carotid artery. Venous drainage is through the superior and inferior ophthalmic veins, to the cavernous sinus and pterygoid plexus of veins. The globe itself occupies the anterior third of the bony orbit, the posterior two thirds being occupied by the fat, muscles, vessels, and nerves that supply the globe.

OPTIC NERVE COMPLICATIONS

The globe sits within the bony orbit at the confluence of the middle and upper thirds of the face and is thus at risk from neoplasms in this area as well as from tumors originating within the surrounding sinuses, whose walls form the boundaries between the bony orbit and the sinuses. Orbital exenteration is required in 20 per cent to 45 per cent of sinus cancers and in most intraorbital neoplasms.[23] Less common, fortunately, is blindness secondary to the many operations for benign disease performed about the orbit. Blindness may follow anterior skull base surgery, surgical intervention about the ethmoid, maxillary, and sphenoid sinuses, or facial fracture reduction. The literature contains case reports of blindness occurring during or after malar fracture reduction,[24] zygomatic arch fracture reduction,[25] orbital floor reconstruction,[26] and decompression for thyroid orbitopathy.[27, 28]

Unilateral blindness secondary to intranasal, external, or endoscopic ethmoidectomy most likely follows transgression of the party wall between the sinus and orbit, with subsequent orbital hematoma formation.[9, 28] Treatment begins with recognition of increased intraorbital pressure. Repeated palpation of the orbit during surgery is advocated by Stankiewiecz.[29] Other signs of increased intraorbital pressure and intraorbital hemorrhage include proptosis, chemosis, ecchymosis, mydriasis, and ophthalmoplegia. Bradycardia may result from increased intraocular pressure and the activation of the ocular reflex. Initial management is medical and consists of eye massage and diuretics. Miotic eye drops and epinephrine can reduce intraocular pressure but interfere with the pupillary reflex. Decompression via lateral canthotomy or medial orbital wall decompression may become necessary if there is no response to these measures. Ophthalmologic consultation should be obtained immediately.[29] Direct optic nerve injury is much less common but can occur, given the close proximity of the optic nerve transection during endoscopic intranasal ethmoidectomy.[30] There is no treatment for loss of vision secondary to direct optic nerve trauma.

Blindness following bilateral radical neck dissection has been reported in five patients.[31] Pathologic study was available for one patient and revealed bilateral hemorrhagic intraorbital optic nerve infarction, which may have occurred secondary to systemic hypotension in combination with ophthalmic vein hypertension as a consequence of bilateral internal jugular vein ligation.

THE TRIGEMINAL NERVE (V)

ANATOMY

The trigeminal nerve, a compound nerve, is the largest of all cranial nerves. Its central role in the face is revealed by its many functions. It is responsible for the sense of taste for the anterior two thirds of the tongue; it is the major sensory nerve to the head, the face, and its mucosal membranes, and it provides motor innervation to the muscles of mastication. Four ganglia of the autonomic nervous system and their fibers are associated with the three divisions of the trigeminal nerve, distributing autonomic innervation to lacrimal, sweat, and salivary tissues of the head and neck. Sensory and motor roots, originating in the brain stem, as well as the gasserian ganglion, contribute to the three peripheral trunks of this nerve.[32]

TRIGEMINAL NERVE COMPLICATIONS

Because of its wide distribution, the trigeminal nerve is subject to injury from the multitude of surgical extirpative procedures performed upon the integuments of the head and neck and its cavities. The risk from surgery aimed at exenteration of malignant disease is obvious and will not be discussed at length here. The proclivity for squamous neoplasms to involve cutaneous nerves places the branches of the trigeminal nerve at risk for injury during resection for cutaneous carcinoma.[33] Similarly, because of the tendency for salivary gland tumors to invade perineural spaces (particularly adenoid cystic carcinoma), branches of the trigeminal nerve (the lingual nerve in particular) must frequently be sacrificed in the performance of an oncologically complete operation.[34] The large resections necessary to ablate oral cavity and sinus cancers frequently necessitate the sacrifice of regional branches of the trigeminal nerve. Loss of trigeminal function associated with these resections is generally not considered a complication of such surgical procedures. Rather, the inadvertent sacrifice of function that unexpectedly accompanies lesser operations in the region becomes a source of distress for the head and neck surgeon and of irritating disability for the patient.

The ophthalmic or first division of the trigeminal nerve is a purely sensory nerve supplying the globe, lacrimal gland, mucous lining of the orbit and nose, and skin and muscles of the eyebrow and forehead.[32] Its distal branches (frontal, supraorbital, supra-cochlear, lacrimal, and nasal nerves), particularly the first three, can be injured during operations upon the brow. Hardy and Montgomery, in reviewing 250 patients undergoing osteoplastic frontal sinusotomy, encountered 3 with persistent postoperative frontal neuralgias.[14] All patients with a brow incision, and most in whom a coronal incision was employed, complained of postoperative forehead numbness and paresthesias. In 65 per cent of cases the symptoms disappeared within 12 months; however, 35 per cent of patients developed persistent, albeit minor, sensory disturbances.[14] Similar deficits will result from external approaches to the ethmoid sinuses, such as the Lynch or Killian approach, or from supraorbital extension of a lateral rhinotomy incision. Sensory deficits are frequently unilateral, and patients have little trouble accommodating their existence.[35] For some surgeons these sensory disturbances do not merit inclusion in reviews of complications following frontal/ethmoid sinus surgery.[36, 37]

The superior maxillary nerve, or second division of the fifth cranial nerve, is also a sensory nerve. It enters the pterygomaxillary fossa through the foramen rotundum and passes forward into the infraorbital canal in the floor of the orbit, emerging at the infraorbital foramen. Branches of this nerve are distributed through the pterygomaxillary fossa (orbital, sphenopalatine, posterior dental), infraorbital canal (anterior dental), and on the face as the palpebral, nasal, and labial branches.[32] Injury to many of these branches is an expected sequela of operation for midfacial and sinus malignancies. However, operation for inflammatory sinus disease, transantral approaches to the orbit, and surgery of the pterygomaxillary fossa can endanger these nerves. Paresthesias of the upper lip, gums, and teeth are common after transantral procedures as a result of stretch of the infraorbital nerve or because of injury to the anterior dental nerve. These usually resolve after 3 to 6 months and are more common following revision surgery.[38, 39]

Transantral decompression of the orbit has become the favored surgical treatment of dysthyroid orbitopathy.[40] The reported incidence of postoperative facial, lip, or dental hypesthesia following this operation ranges from 20 per cent to 100 per cent, with up to 45 per cent of patients developing persistent sensory disturbance.[26, 27, 40, 41] Transantral approaches to the pterygomaxillary fossa, for the management of vasomotor rhinitis or for the control of posterior epistaxis, result in neurogenic injury to the fifth nerve branches in less than 3 per cent to 5 per cent of cases.[42–45] Trigeminal hypesthesias occur more commonly early in a surgeon's experience with this type of operation.[44]

The inferior maxillary nerve (lingual nerve, terminal branch) (Fig. 7–1) is the largest division of the trigeminal nerve. It consists of a large sensory root supplying branches to the lower teeth and gums and to the skin of the lower face, lip, and temple. A smaller, motor root innervates the muscles of mastication. In addition, taste fibers from the anterior two thirds of the tongue travel with the lingual branch of the third division.[32] Branches of the inferior maxillary nerve are most commonly sectioned during surgery for cancers of the oral cavity or of salivary gland origin, as noted. Any operation upon the submaxillary triangle and its contents places the lingual nerve at risk for injury. Milton and colleagues, in a review of morbidity associated with submandibular gland excision for benign disease, documented a 3 per cent incidence of permanent injury to the lingual nerve.[46] Although rarely reported, isolated mylohyoid nerve injury with resultant hypesthesia of the lateral lower lip and chin can also accompany submandibular gland excision.[47] Intraoral removal of ranulas and other benign lesions of the floor of the mouth also may be accompanied by lingual hypesthesia if care is not taken to identify and preserve the lingual nerve in the course of the dissection. No systematic evaluation of lingual nerve function following radical neck dissection exists in the English literature. In our experience, injury to the lingual nerve during radical lymphadenectomy is a rare occurrence in the absence of gross dis-

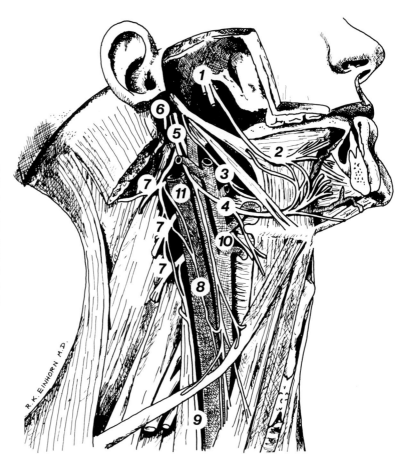

FIGURE 7–1. Cranial nerves in the skull base and neck. (1) Mandibular (V) nerve; (2) lingual nerve; (3) glossopharyngeal (IX) nerve; (4) hypoglossal (XII) nerve; (5) vagus (X) nerve; (6) accessory (XI) nerve; (7) cervical ventral rami; (8) ansa cervicalis; (9) phrenic nerve; (10) carotid artery; and (11) jugular vein.

ease within the submandibular triangle. Loss of taste to one side of the tongue is easily compensated for by the remaining normal side.

When possible, direct anastomosis or cable grafting of a resected mandibular nerve can lead to successful re-establishment of lower facial sensation.[48, 49] The free microvascular transfer of tissue for the reconstruction of postsurgical defects has become an established reconstructive modality in head and neck surgery. Urken and associates have reported the successful sensory reinnervation of free flaps used for mandibular reconstruction.[50] Two thirds of their patients in whom nerve grafts were used to reconnect the inferior alveolar nerve stump to a native flap nerve experienced return of sensation, as documented by the presence of discrimination to touch, pinprick, and temperature and improved subjective oral function.

THE GLOSSOPHARYNGEAL NERVE (IX)

ANATOMY (see Fig. 7–1)

The glossopharyngeal nerve (IX), as its name implies, is distributed to the pharynx and tongue. It carries special somatic sensory fibers from the mucous membranes of the pharynx, tonsillar pillars, posterior third of the tongue, external ear skin, and tympanic membranes. General small, visceral, afferent fibers emanate from the carotid body and sinus. Special sensory afferents for taste arise from the posterior one third of the tongue and vallate papillae. The motor function of nerve IX includes special visceral efferents to the stylopharyngeus muscle and general secretomotor fibers via the otic ganglion to the parotid gland.[3, 32, 33]

After emerging from the brain stem, nerve

IX gives off two branches within the skull: a tympanic branch to the middle ear and an auricular branch to the external ear. It exits from the skull base in the anteromedial part of the jugular foramen in a separate dural sheath, anterolateral to the vagus and the accessory nerves, medial to the internal carotid artery, and anteromedial to the jugular bulb. Upon its exit, nerve IX passes forward between the internal jugular vein and internal carotid artery, then descends between the internal and external carotid arteries deep to the stylopharyngeus muscle toward the pharynx, running between the superior and middle constrictor muscles, then forward deep to the hyoglossus muscle. Here it divides into the tonsillar, lingual, and pharyngeal branches. The carotid branch descends on the wall of the internal carotid artery, with the carotid branch of the vagus nerve, to the carotid sinus and carotid body.[3, 51]

Isolated nerve IX injuries rarely cause significant morbidity and will be discussed in the section on skull base surgery.

THE VAGUS NERVE (X)

ANATOMY (Figs. 7–1 and 7–2)

The vagus nerve (X) is the longest cranial nerve with the most extensive distribution, thereby making it more subject to injury than any other cranial nerve.[51] It carries visceral afferents for sensation from the larynx, trachea, and esophagus as well as from its thoracic and abdominal distribution. General somatic sensory afferents supply part of the external ear, external auditory canal, and external surface of the tympanic membrane and pharynx. Special visceral efferent motor innervation is carried to the striated muscle of the pharynx, palatoglossus muscle, and larynx. Smooth muscle and glands of the pharynx, larynx, and thoracic and abdominal viscera are supplied by general visceral efferent roots.[52]

The vagus nerve is formed from the convergence of several rootlets from the brain stem into a single nerve that exits from the skull via the jugular foramen, sharing its arachnoid and dural sheath with the accessory nerve. Its two sensory ganglia lie within the jugular fossa. In the superior ganglion, nerve X is joined by fibers of nerve IX and the sympathetic trunk. The inferior ganglion has contributions from nerve XII. After its exit from the skull base, nerve X runs anteriorly between the internal jugular vein and internal carotid artery, posterior to the styloid and its muscles.[3, 32, 51] Just below the inferior ganglion, in the neck, nerve X gives off the superior laryngeal nerve.

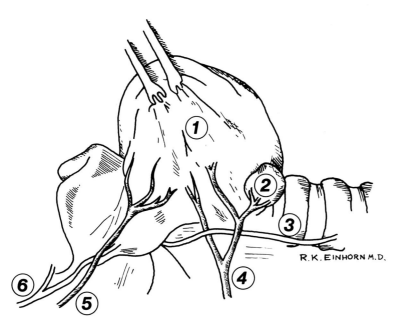

R.K. EINHORN M.D.

FIGURE 7–2. The thyroid gland. (1) Right lobe of thyroid; (2) inferior parathyroid; (3) recurrent laryngeal nerve; (4) inferior thyroid artery; (5) superior thyroid artery; and (6) superior laryngeal nerve.

The superior laryngeal nerve courses posterior then medial to the internal and external carotid arteries before dividing into external and internal branches. The external branch descends on the lateral surface of the inferior constrictor muscle, ending on the cricothyroid muscle, which it innervates. The internal branch travels on the thyrohyoid membrane with the superior laryngeal artery, pierces that membrane, and branches to provide sensation to the hypopharynx, vallecula, epiglottis, false vocal cords, ventricle, and piriform recesses. It also anastomoses with nerve IX in forming the pharyngeal plexus. A branch of this nerve may supply or contribute to the nerve supply of the transverse arytenoid muscle.[32, 53]

The recurrent branch of nerve X, or the recurrent laryngeal nerve, continues its descent in the carotid sheath, occupying a variable position between the internal jugular vein and common carotid artery. The right recurrent laryngeal nerve curves around the subclavian artery in an anterior-to-posterior direction and ascends in the tracheoesophageal groove to the larynx. The left recurrent laryngeal nerve hooks around the aortic arch to ascend in the left tracheoesophageal groove, often coursing farther from the trachea than the right recurrent nerve does. The right recurrent nerve is less reliably found in the tracheoesophageal groove, thereby making it more likely to be injured during surgery.[54, 55] Other anatomic variations of the recurrent laryngeal nerve include a nonrecurrent laryngeal nerve in association with an abnormal subclavian artery.[56] This was found in 0.52 per cent of over 6000 cases, of which only 2 of 33 were left sided.[57]

From the tracheoesophageal groove, the recurrent nerve ascends in close relationship to the posterior border of the thyroid gland, passing either over or under the inferior thyroid artery, and under the lower border of the inferior constrictor muscle to enter the larynx behind the cricothyroid joint.[58] Within the larynx, the recurrent nerve divides into anterior and posterior branches supplying all the intrinsic muscles of the larynx, excluding the cricothyroid muscle. Branching prior to entering the larynx may further expose the nerve to injury.[59] The recurrent laryngeal nerve also contains afferent fibers for sensation and stretch receptors below the vocal cords.

VAGUS NERVE COMPLICATIONS

Cranial nerve sequelae from thyroid, parathyroid, and other neck procedures follow. Injuries that involve other cranial nerves are discussed in the section on skull base surgery later in this chapter.

Surgery of the Thyroid and Parathyroid (Figs. 7–2 and 7–3)

Traditionally, surgical procedures for thyroid and parathyroid disease are centered on avoidance of neurologic and endocrine complications. Because of these concerns, the incidence of cranial nerve complications is generally low when the surgeon is well trained in the anatomy of the neck and its neurovascular structures. Cranial nerve injury becomes significant when an operation is performed for malignant disease due to preoperative cranial nerve invasion and for purposeful sacrifice. The complication rate also increases when secondary surgical exploration is necessary owing to scarring and distorted anatomy.

The incidence of recurrent laryngeal nerve injuries following partial thyroidectomy has a wide range and does not increase significantly when performed bilaterally. Beahrs and associates reported a 1.3 per cent incidence of recurrent laryngeal injuries in 1022 patients undergoing unilateral operation.[58] Mountain and associates found a 1.2 per cent temporary and a 0.14 per cent permanent incidence of vocal cord paralysis in 2101 patients.[59] They stressed the importance of identifying the recurrent laryngeal nerve—they found a three- to fourfold increase in vocal cord paralysis when the recurrent laryngeal nerve was not identified. Most reports range from 0.3 per cent to 5 per cent,[60] but a figure as high as 13 per cent has been reported.[61] The incidence of recurrent laryngeal nerve paralysis rose only slightly when reported for total thyroidectomy. Beahrs and

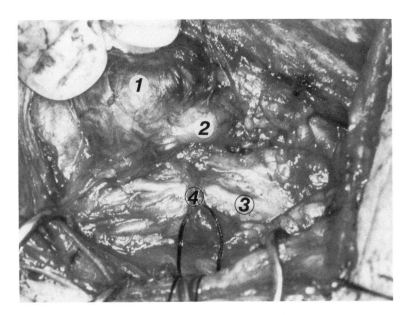

FIGURE 7–3. Specimen showing the first four structures depicted in Figure 7–2. (1) Right lobe of thyroid; (2) inferior parathyroid; (3) recurrent laryngeal nerve; and (4) inferior thyroid artery.

Paternak reported a 1 per cent incidence of recurrent nerve paralysis.[62] Fowler[63] found a 2 per cent incidence in benign disease, which ranged up to 7 per cent for Perzik and Catz,[64] who included cases of nerve sacrifice for malignant disease. Operations for malignant thyroid tumors had a higher incidence of nerve injury, but not as high as that for surgical re-explorations. Chonkich and colleagues found that the incidence of recurrent laryngeal nerve injury doubled from 0.6 per cent for benign disease to 1.5 per cent for malignant disease in 540 thyroid operations.[65] Recurrent laryngeal nerve complications increased to 9.2 per cent in 548 thyroid operations performed by Beahrs and Vandertoli in patients who had had two or more procedures; when considering cancer cases only, this number increased to 17 per cent.[66]

Review of parathyroid explorations and their complications demonstrated results similar to those of thyroid surgery. Recurrent laryngeal nerve complications were reported by Katz and Hopp[67] and Satava and group[68] in 1.7 per cent and 2.8 per cent of patients, respectively. Patow and colleagues, more recently, found 1.3 per cent recurrent laryngeal nerve complications for primary parathyroid explorations, which increased to 6.6 per cent for surgical re-explorations.[69] The literature on secondary operations of the parathyroid ranges from 0 of 19 patients with permanent

paralysis for Van Heerden and associates[70] to 2.7 per cent for Wang[71] and 9 per cent in Billings and Milroy's series.[72] Variability in reported results may be increased by the nonuniformity of reporting temporary versus permanent complications and methods of selecting patients for postoperative examination.

The literature on thyroid surgery is replete with articles on methods, results, and complications; thorough knowledge of anatomy and a good sound surgical approach are stressed as key factors for avoiding cranial nerve complications. Iatrogenic injury can be avoided by this knowledge, as well as by an understanding of the possible anatomic and pathologic variations that may exist. The recurrent laryngeal nerve should be identified along its entire length. Beahrs and colleagues used the inferior thyroid artery as a landmark, which is in direct relationship with but may run over or under the recurrent laryngeal nerve.[58] Wang traced the nerve from the inferior cornu of the thyroid cartilage.[71] Lore and colleagues favored identifying the recurrent laryngeal nerve in the tracheoesophageal groove and traced it up behind the posterior suspensory ligament of Berry.[61]

Injury to the superior branch of nerve X is less commonly addressed but not necessarily less frequently encountered.[73] Voice changes are usually subtle and may not be noticed unless the patient is a professional speaker or singer. Patients may report inability to reach high-pitched notes or easy voice fatigability. Aspiration is usually not a problem, since only the external branch of the superior laryngeal nerve is injured. Unilateral superior laryngeal nerve paralysis can be detected during laryngeal examination if the cord on the affected side appears shorter and more lax than on the normal side and if the affected side is lower than the normal side. The interior larynx tilts toward the normal side on phonation owing to unilateral contraction of the cricothyroid muscle. Bilateral superior laryngeal nerve paralysis may be missed, since the patients often remain asymptomatic. On examination, the epiglottis overhangs the anterior larynx, making viewing of the true vocal cords difficult. The vocal cords remain flaccid and bowed, failing to tense on phonation. Patients will have weak, breathy voices. Injury to the external branch of the superior laryngeal nerve can be avoided by careful dissection of the superior pole of the thyroid gland and identification of the superior thyroid artery prior to its ligation.

A thorough preoperation evaluation of the larynx, especially in patients with voice changes or prior neck operation, is essential for recognizing nerve injuries. Any vocal cord paresis should be noted, for this may indicate a possible malignancy. Awareness of prior vocal cord difficulties will also allow the surgeon to take precautions for potential airway compromise postoperatively, as well as providing the necessary medicolegal documentation. Most studies reviewed used voice changes as the only indication for postoperative evaluation of the larynx. This limited survey technique can alter postoperative reporting of cranial nerve complications.

Neurologic complications are not usually recognized until after operation,[74] when the patient complains of persistent voice changes. Management of these injuries should be addressed on a case-by-case basis. Known nerve transection at the time of surgery can be managed by primary anastomosis of the severed ends[74, 75] or treated with an immediate ansa hypoglossi–recurrent laryngeal nerve anastomosis. Permanent vocal cord paralysis will result from nerve transec-tion. Temporary nerve complications result from clamping, stretching, or pinching the nerve. Immediate re-exploration may be warranted to release suture ligatures that may have inadvertently been passed around the recurrent laryngeal nerve.[61, 75]

Delayed recognition of recurrent laryngeal nerve paralysis can be treated in a number of ways. Treatment by an irreversible method should be reserved until at least 12 months after operation in the event that the recurrent laryngeal nerve regenerates. If nerve transection was not purposely performed or noted during operation, the best initial treatment for unilateral paralysis is Gelfoam paste injection.[76] Gelfoam lasts from 4 to 8 weeks and repeated injections may be required before function returns. Permanent unilateral vocal cord rehabilitation is most simply accomplished by Teflon injection, when a known nerve section occurs, or after a delay of 12 months.[77] Teflon injection into the vocal cord may not be as effective when there are injuries to the central nerve X or recurrent laryngeal nerve simultaneously with the external branch of the superior laryngeal nerve, since the vocal cord is more flaccid and lies in a lower plane than the opposite side.

Better voice results are reportedly obtained via open thyroplasty. Isshiki described vocal cord rehabilitation performed surgically under local anesthesia with direct visual fiberoptic control.[78, 79] A Silastic implant, which can be modified for different tissue deficits along the length of the vocal cord, is used to medialize the paralyzed cord. Laryngeal reinnervation is a third type of vocal cord rehabilitation. Tucker first described the ansa hypoglossi nerve muscle pedicle for restoring vocal cord function.[80] This technique does not require recurrent laryngeal nerve interruption and adds muscle for tissue bulk. However, return of vocal cord mobility may take up to 6 months. Crumley advocates direct ansa hypoglossi to recurrent laryngeal nerve and anastomosis for laryngeal rehabilitation.[75] Neural reinnervation does not preclude temporary use of Gelfoam or thyroplasty, both of which are reversible. However, neural reinnervation does require a sacrifice or interruption of the recurrent laryngeal nerve.

Bilateral vocal cord paralysis requires more aggressive intervention. Initially, patients need to be reintubated. If the recurrent laryngeal nerves were preserved, steroids should be given and a tracheotomy performed if the patient fails extubation.[81] These patients may have strong voices immediately postoperatively, which will weaken with time with muscle atrophy and vocal cord lateralization. Reinnervation procedures can be attempted; however, no satisfactory reproducible method currently exists. Vocal cord lateralization is the next treatment of choice, most recently via laser arytenoidectomy.[82] Prior to introduction of the laser, Thornell performed an intralaryngeal arytenoidectomy.[83] Earlier surgical rehabilitation of bilateral vocal cord paralysis required open extralaryngeal arytenoidectomy, as described by King[84] and Woodman.[85]

Vagus Nerve Complications from Other Head and Neck Procedures

Carotid endarterectomy requires dissection in an area containing multiple cranial nerves. Among those at risk are nerve X, including superior and recurrent branches; nerve XII; and the marginal mandibular branch of nerve VII. In 1969, Ranson and associates found a 5.1 per cent incidence of nerve XII injuries, and a 1.4 per cent incidence of marginal mandibular nerve VII injuries.[86] DeWeese and group reported a 17.5 per cent incidence of nerve XII complications.[87] Matsumoto had an 8.5 per cent incidence of nerve XII injuries; 1.5 per cent, marginal nerve VII; and 2.3 per cent, nerve X.[88] More recent studies have seen an increase in reported complications, including 2.3 per cent to 5.4 per cent for nerve XII; 0 to 2.5 per cent for marginal nerve VII; and 3.9 per cent to 14 per cent for nerve X injuries, according to Hertzer and associates,[89] Evans and associates,[90] and Knight and associates.[91]

In a large prospective study by Weiss and colleagues, temporary injuries were distinguished from permanent complications.[92] There was an overall incidence of 14.4 per cent temporary and 6.6 per cent permanent

cranial nerve injuries. Of the 563 cases, 8.6 per cent had nerve XII injuries, of which 2.6 per cent were permanent. There were 6.2 per cent marginal nerve VII complications, of which 2.8 per cent were permanent, and 3.7 per cent nerve X pareses resulting in 0.6 per cent of permanent vocal cord changes. The actual incidence of these complications is difficult to compare among articles in the literature, since very few studies included full preoperative cranial nerve evaluation.

A number of explanations were given for the postoperative complications encountered. The first is anatomic variation in the course of the cranial nerves. Vigorous retraction is blamed for nerve injuries, especially those sustained by the marginal mandibular branch of nerve VII. High carotid bifurcation or high-lying carotid plaques can contribute to nerve XII complications. Mobilization of the superior thyroid artery puts the superior laryngeal nerve at risk. Postoperative dysfunction was evaluated only when patients complained of voice changes or dysphagia. Near-normal voices may not necessarily correlate with full cranial nerve function. Conversely, Aldoori and Baird found ten patients with postoperative voice changes, of whom only three had immobile vocal cords.[93] This may be due to other airway-induced changes by the endotracheal tube or to undetected and unreported superior laryngeal injuries. General recommendations were to perform careful dissections and avoid bilateral carotid endarterectomies or risk the rare complication of bilateral nerve XII or nerve X palsies and subsequent airway obstruction.

Any cervical procedure can cause cranial nerve injury, especially approaches to deep structures of the neck. Heeneman reviewed 85 anterior approaches to the cervical spine.[94] Surgical exposure is obtained by retracting the carotid sheath laterally and the thyroid gland and larynx medially. Nine (11 per cent) patients had postoperative voice changes. Six were temporary, and three were permanent injuries. Suspected causes of these complications were traumatic division (deemed unlikely), nerve pinching or stretching, and pressure from postoperative edema.

Many surgical procedures require endotracheal intubation, which has been implicated in vocal cord paralysis.[95] Direct compression of the anterior branch of the recurrent laryngeal nerve by the endotracheal tube cuff is the most likely mechanism. Another possible cause may be from hyperextension of the neck with subsequent stretching of nerve X. Nasogastric tubes, placed during many of the more extensive head and neck procedures, as well as with procedures performed elsewhere in the body, often elicit sequelae. Vocal cord paralysis with cricoid ulceration and edema has been attributed to their use.[96]

THE SPINAL ACCESSORY NERVE (XI)

ANATOMY

Cranial nerve XI is probably of dual—somatic and visceral—derivation, composed of bulbar and spinal contributions. The bulbar portion exits from the brain stem as 4 or 5 rootlets, which coalesce with the spinal portion at the jugular foramen. Just below the skull base, the bulbar portion leaves the nerve to join the vagus, eventually supplying striated, extrinsic laryngeal musculature and pharyngeal muscles. The spinal portion arises from cervical levels 2 through 5 and enters the brain through the foramen magnum to join with the bulbar portion. At the jugular foramen, the spinal portion emerges between the internal carotid artery and the internal jugular vein, passes posteroinferiorly either superficial or deep to the internal jugular vein, and pierces the deep aspect of the sternocleidomastoid muscle. Usually at this point the accessory nerve receives a sensory communicating branch from the second cervical central ramus.

The accessory nerve emerges from the posterior border of the sternocleidomastoid muscle at the junction of its upper and middle thirds and traverses the posterior triangle, where it is often joined by branches of the ventral rami of C3, C4, and C5. The nerve then passes beneath the anterior border of the trapezius muscle at the junction of its middle and lower thirds and continues inferiorly along the deep surface of the muscle to supply all three parts of it.[97]

The spinal accessory nerve classically has been thought of as the major motor innervation of the sternocleidomastoid and trapezius muscles.[1] The trapezius muscle provides primary supportive and rotatory actions on the shoulder girdle. Its three muscular divisions act in concert with other muscles attached to the scapula to steady and control the shoulder during movement and at rest.[32, 98] However, the observation by several researchers that surgical transection of the spinal accessory nerve does not uniformly lead to total loss of trapezius function implies the existence of an alternate motor supply.[99–101] For example, Love noted subjective symptoms in only 11 of 61 patients who underwent high division of the entire spinal accessory nerve during accessory-facial crossover surgery for facial paralysis.[102]

The results of extensive electrophysiologic and neural mapping experiments in both animals and humans suggest the existence of considerable exchange between the spinal accessory nerve and the cervical nerves at both motor and sensory levels.[103–109] Nonetheless, the most important motor supply to the sternocleidomastoid and trapezius muscles is via the spinal accessory nerve. Alternate motor pathways to the subtrapezius plexus, via the ventral roots of cervical nerves C2 through C5, are highly variable and minor in importance when compared with the motor supply provided by the accessory nerve.[97] Proprioceptive fibers from the trapezius muscle travel with the spinal accessory nerve. Pain fibers also course with the accessory nerve in its distal portion before entering the cervical plexus, and their disruption may account for the sensory disturbances occurring after surgical transection of this nerve.[110]

ACCESSORY NERVE COMPLICATIONS

Proximity of the spinal accessory lymphatic chain, subject to nodal enlargement of diverse causes, and its superficial location within the investing fascia of the posterior triangle make the spinal accessory nerve subject to injury during minor procedures of the posterior neck. Occasionally the nerve is inadvertently cut during diagnostic lymphadenectomy or excision of benign lesions of the posterior triangle.[111-113] Many surgeons have documented trapezius dysfunction after this type of surgical procedure.[113-117] Most spinal accessory injuries, however, occur during radical lymphadenectomy of the neck in the management of head and neck cancer. As advocated initially by Crile, the spinal accessory is included in the en bloc resection of the lymph-bearing structures of the neck during radical neck dissection.[118] Spinal accessory injury also can occur during mobilization of the sternocleidomastoid muscle to correct postparotidectomy facial depression or during neck exploration following penetrating trauma to the neck.[119] In these instances, the proximal portion of the nerve is at risk.

Sequelae from the loss of trapezius function are both subjective and objective. Patient complaints include pain, characteristically "dragging" in nature, shoulder droop, and an inability to carry weights on the affected side or to elevate loads above the head. Pain may occur at rest or only with attempts at motion[121] and is considered secondary to traction on the levator and rhomboid muscles, the brachial plexus, and the ligamentous supports of the shoulder joint.[97] As noted, there may also be a sensory component to the spinal accessory nerve, the loss of which component may contribute to the discomfort that follows this injury. Symptoms generally appear immediately after operation or develop when normal activities are resumed. Nahum and colleagues have described the following objective findings: (1) limitation of abduction at the shoulder, (2) loss of the rhythm of abduction, as the scapula now rotates abnormally, (3) winging of the scapula, and (4) loss of the sloping contour of the shoulder, which is replaced by a right angle appearance because of atrophy of muscle substance and loss of support.[121] A marked decrease in range of motion and muscle strength at the shoulder joint has been documented by Sobol and associates,[120] Remmler and group,[122] and Dewar and Harris.[123] Oncologic soundness notwithstanding, the

avoidance of this "shoulder syndrome" has led some surgeons to advocate nerve-sparing (modified) neck dissections in selected patients.[124-127]

Other factors may affect shoulder mobility adversely following the loss of the spinal accessory nerve, such as the degree to which the innervation of compensatory muscles (levator scapulae, rhomboids) has been preserved.[128] Postoperative radiotherapy or the use of ipsilateral pectoralis major muscle flaps also will limit shoulder mobility by up to 20 per cent.[129] Thus, neither patient complaints nor objective evidence of trapezius dysfunction is universally encountered after loss of the spinal accessory nerve. For example, Saunders and associates found that 67 per cent of their patients undergoing radical neck dissection volunteered mild subjective complaints in spite of the presence of profound muscle atrophy.[130] Similarly, in the series of Leipzig and associates, 40 per cent of patients undergoing classic radical neck dissection had mild shoulder dysfunction postoperatively.[131]

Many approaches exist to decrease the morbidity associated with loss of the spinal accessory nerve. Physical therapy, starting in the postoperative period under the direction of a physical therapist and continued at home, effectively addresses the shoulder syndrome and should be employed in all patients undergoing classic radical neck dissection.[132] Orthopedic reconstruction of the shoulder girdle is advocated by some.[123, 133] Modification of the technique of neck dissection to preserve the spinal accessory nerve has been mentioned. Prospective studies have shown that this technique results in the best average shoulder function upon subjective and objective evaluation.[97, 120, 130, 134] The abnormal shoulder function seen in a small percentage of patients undergoing this procedure is attributable to traction injury to the nerve and to devascularization during its dissection. Anecdotal evidence has shown that primary anastomosis of nerves transected during minor surgical procedures upon the posterior triangle results in a return of function in most cases.[112, 113, 135]

Cable grafting of a resected spinal accessory nerve was first described by Harris and

Dickey[136] and Ballantyne and Guinn.[128] They reported success based on clinical examination alone. Recent prospective studies employing electromyography as well as subjective and objective evaluation of shoulder function have proved the usefulness of cable grafting.[137] The average functional scores following cable grafting, although significantly better than those of patients undergoing classic radical neck dissection, fall below those of patients receiving nerve-sparing surgery.

THE HYPOGLOSSAL NERVE (XII)

ANATOMY (see Fig. 7–1)

The hypoglossal nerve (XII) carries general somatic motor fibers to all the intrinsic and extrinsic muscles of the tongue except the palatoglossus. It emerges from the skull via an individual canal in the posterior cranial fossa, the hypoglossal canal, located medial to the internal carotid artery and jugular foramen. Immediately upon its exit from the skull, it is in intimate association with all structures of the jugular foramen (internal jugular vein, nerves IX, X, XI), then passes inferolaterally behind the internal carotid artery close to the posterior surface of nerve X, deep to the posterior belly of the digastric muscle. After crossing lateral to the bifurcation of the common carotid artery, the nerve loops anteriorly above the greater cornu of the hyoid bone. It then runs medially on the hyoglossus muscle over the mylohyoid muscle to be distributed to the tongue musculature.[2, 31, 50]

Contributions are received from upper cervical branches, usually C1 or C2 or both at the skull base. These fibers pass into the descendens hypoglossi, forming the ansa cervicalis (also called the ansa hypoglossi) and form the nerves to the thyrohyoid and geniohyoid muscles. Hypoglossal fibers are distributed exclusively to the tongue musculature.[50]

Complications from hypoglossal nerve injuries will be discussed in the next section, on skull base surgery.

Skull Base Surgery

Surgical procedures for paragangliomas of the skull base have undergone a great number of recent advances.[138] Head and neck paragangliomas include glomus tympanicum, jugulare, and vagale, and carotid body tumors. Improved surgical techniques and constantly improving diagnostic methods, including computed tomography (CT), angiography, and magnetic resonance imaging (MRI), are now available. The treatment of choice for most paragangliomas is surgical excision. Earlier treatment of the disease favored limited surgery with adjunctive radiotherapy or radiotherapy alone.[139, 140] More recent comparative studies by Glasscock and colleagues,[141] Brachmann and colleagues,[142] and Jackson and group[143] showed the superiority of surgery with or without radiation therapy over radiation therapy alone. However, with these advanced methods and the aggressive resection of larger tumors, significant postoperative morbidity is encountered.

As early as 1914 Balfour and Wildner recognized that "a cure without permanent disability is rare."[144] The most common complication of skull base surgery is cranial nerve dysfunction, both temporary and permanent. In reviewing the Mayo Clinic experience with carotid body and cervical paragangliomas, Hallet and associates noted a significant decrease in the incidence of postoperative stroke and mortality rates after 1965, but no changes in the incidence of cranial nerve deficits.[145] The addition of preoperative embolization, which helps reduce intraoperative blood loss and operative time, did not affect neurologic sequelae.[146] Despite these surgical advances, cranial nerve preservation has not improved, which may be due to tumor adherence to the surrounding neurovascular structures.[145–148]

Surgical excision of paragangliomas confined to the middle ear, or glomus tympanicum, has a very low incidence of cranial nerve palsies, with only 1 of 45 patients sustaining hearing loss and 1 of 45 with a temporary nerve VII paralysis.[138] A much higher incidence of cranial nerve complications results from the skull base techniques

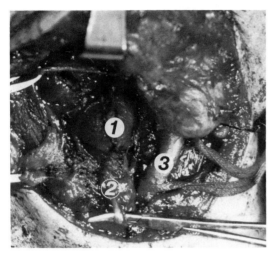

FIGURE 7–4. Surgical removal of glomus vagale tumor. (1) Tumor; (2) vagus (X) nerve; and (3) carotid artery.

required for complete surgical extirpation of glomus jugulare and vagale and carotid body tumors (Figs. 7–4 and 7–5).

The most common and serious complications of skull base surgery relate to cranial nerve deficits. The reported incidence of postoperative complications varies widely in the literature. In 1980, Spector and Sobel reported on 104 glomus tympanicum and jugulare tumors, of which 34 per cent presented with cranial nerve paresis.[149] Of 80 patients treated with surgery or surgery combined with radiation, only one had additional sensorineural hearing loss, and one sustained transient cranial nerve X palsy postoperatively. Fifteen patients developed postoperative permanent facial nerve palsy, of which seven were total and three were partial. Farrior preserved cranial nerve function in all but 2 patients with facial pareses and 1 with transient vocal cord (nerve X) pareses in 18 cases of large glomus jugulare tumors.[150*] Gardner and associates found 13 of 13 postoperative nerve VII pareses, of which 4 were permanent, with some dysfunction of nerve VI or nerves IX through XII in 9 patients, half of which were present preoperatively.[152]

In reviewing more recent series, Jackson and coworkers found a high percentage of cranial nerve palsies at operation in 91 glomus tumors.[138] Eighteen per cent of these patients had involvement of nerves IX through XII or pareses of nerve VII noted preoperatively. Cranial nerves IX through XII were injured or sacrificed in 23 of 46 (50 per cent) glomus vagale and jugulare tumors, and 22 patients (48 per cent) had nerve VII injuries. Cece and coworkers reported on 17 large glomus jugulare tumors.[148*] Seventeen of 17 patients had postoperative facial pareses, of which five were present preoperatively; function returned in all but three patients. A total of 15 patients had nerve X palsies, of which 8 were noted preoperatively and 10 were resected for tumor involvement. Ten patients had postoperative nerve XII palsies, of which six were present prior to operation.

In a report on preoperative embolization

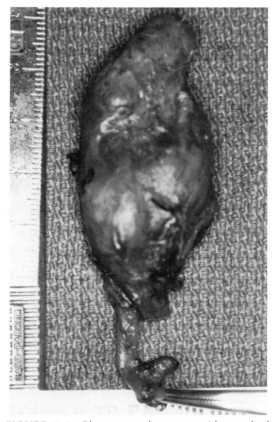

FIGURE 7–5. Glomus vagale tumor with attached vagus nerve.

---

*Class C or D in the classification of Jenkins and Fisch.[151]

of glomus jugulare tumors in 35 patients, Murphy found one nerve VII, 17 nerve IX, 13 nerve X, and 18 nerve XII deficits following operation.[146] Eighteen cases of glomus vagale tumors were reported by Biller and colleagues; one had preoperative and all 18 had postoperative nerve X loss.[153] Cranial nerve IX was affected in three cases preoperatively. Nerve XII dysfunction was present in 4 patients preoperatively and 12 patients postoperatively. In a large series of 153 carotid and cervical paragangliomas, Hallet and associates found postoperative injuries of cranial nerves VII and IX through XII, in 40 per cent of the patients, of which 48 per cent were permanent.[145] Leonetti and colleagues reported 154 skull base procedures for tumors of mixed histology.[154] Forty-six patients (30 per cent) suffered a new onset of at least transient cranial nerve pareses. The most frequent nerve affected was nerve VII (38 per cent), followed by nerve V (21 per cent) and nerves IX and X (18 per cent). The overall number of cranial nerve complications remained constant in their review of the literature.

A thorough knowledge of anatomy; good preoperative planning, including use of modern imaging techniques; and adequate surgical exposure are all necessary steps in reducing postoperative cranial nerve complications. Glomus vagale tumors by definition require sacrifice of the associated cranial nerve (see Fig. 7–1), in contrast to carotid body tumors from which cranial nerves may be peeled.[145] More extensive tumors may involve or encase cranial nerves of the jugular foramen and hypoglossal canal. Farrior reduced cranial nerve morbidity by preserving the medial wall of the jugular vein to protect cranial nerves IX through XII.[150]

The most commonly addressed cranial nerve injury in the literature is that of nerve VII,[155] since it results in the most visible disability. Surgical correction of facial nerve deficits is discussed elsewhere in this text. In summary, the principle of facial rehabilitation is to attempt primary reanastomosis without tension or to perform an interposition graft from the greater auricular or sural nerves. These procedures may require mobilization of the facial nerve from its canal. Recovery may take up to 18 months. Reinnervation or surgical reanimation is the next treatment of choice. In descending order of preference these procedures include a nerve XII to VII anastomosis, facial crossover, ipsilateral accessory (XI) nerve graft, and cervical nerve–muscle pedicle reinnervation.[156] Although a nerve XII to VII anastomosis is most desirable, it should not be performed in the presence of associated nerve IX or X paralysis, since this would add to swallowing difficulties and aspiration. Temporal muscle slings can restore resting tone and partial facial reanimation. Static slings can be performed using fascia lata.[157] Muscle or fascia procedures might better be applied to reanimation of the lower face by means of other operations, such as inserting a gold weight, unilateral brow lift, and lower lid shortening techniques for the ipsilateral eye.[158] Lastly, free flaps also can be used to rejuvenate the paralyzed face.[159]

Injuries to nerves IX and X often occur together and may result from neural traction, direct sectioning for tumor removal, or packing the inferior petrosal sinus orifice under the jugular bulb for hemostasis.[154] Isolated nerve IX injury has little more morbidity owing to overlap with nerve X. Nerve X injury alone causes vocal cord paralysis, dysphagia, and often aspiration, since these tend to be high nerve X injuries occurring prior to the takeoff of the superior laryngeal nerve. Patients with preoperative cranial nerve deficits have less aspiration and little or no dysphagia or voice changes postoperatively[148] because of accommodation to the gradual onset of cranial nerve dysfunction.

The lateral skull base approach to the medial skull base[160] often sacrifices cranial nerves V_3, VII, IX, and occasionally XII.[52] Resection of large tumors often results in dysphagia and aspiration from one of three causes: (1) resection of the anterior tonsillar pillar delaying food bolus transport by interruption of nerve IX and its feedback in the initiation of a swallow; (2) decreased tongue mobility secondary to reconstruction and loss of bolus control, exacerbated by hypoglossal nerve dysfunction; (3) decreased pharyngeal peristalsis with tongue interruption and re-construction with adynamic flaps.[52, 155] Cranial nerve involvement is usually found preoperatively; however, since this approach is more commonly used for highly malignant tumors, patient adaptation can occur by the gradual onset of cranial nerve involvement by tumor. If patient adaptation does not occur, surgical rehabilitation is necessary.

Diagnosis is best determined by physical examination and modified barium swallow. Radiographic evaluation often demonstrates failure of cricopharyngeal relaxation and hypopharyngeal pooling. Severe dysphagia is best treated initially by temporary nasogastric feeding and occasionally a tracheotomy.[155, 161] Most patients adapt with time and the tube can be removed. Swallowing and speech rehabilitation can be obtained by cricopharyngeal myotomy and staged Teflon injection into the vocal cords. Cece and colleagues[148] and Biller and colleagues[153] found that the improvement with cricopharyngeal myotomy merited its performance at the time of initial surgical resection with staged vocal cord augmentation. Their results were enhanced further when there were no preoperative vocal cord problems. This protocol effectively decreased postoperative dysphagia and aspiration.

Bilateral nerve X paralysis leads to severe dysfunction. Rehabilitation includes nasogastric tube feeding and tracheotomy, with eventual attempts at vocal cord lateralization or reanimation. The palate must also be rehabilitated, initially by obturator, and eventually it may require a pharyngeal flap.[155] High unilateral nerve X injuries prior to the takeoff of the superior laryngeal nerve may also complicate vocal rehabilitation. The paralyzed vocal cord will lie in a different plane from the normal side. Teflon injection may not restore vocal function fully. Other methods of rehabilitation are discussed elsewhere in this chapter.

Unilateral nerve XII paralysis is usually well tolerated. In the absence of other cranial nerve injuries, patients adapt quickly to the slight atrophy of the tongue and compensate with little speech changes. Bilateral nerve XII injury can be crippling, severely impairing both speech and swallowing. Airway obstruction may occur when the patient is supine. When bilateral nerve XII injury is coupled with deficits of nerves IX and X, antiaspiration procedures such as laryngeal diversion may be necessary.[155]

In the preoperative assessment, it is important to rule out the presence of synchronous occult lesions. There is a 10 per cent multicentricity rate in cervical paraganglioma.[162] Knowledge of another lesion may alter the surgical planning to avoid bilateral palsies of nerves X and XII. Patients with bilateral vagal body tumors should have surgical management of the larger tumor and radiation therapy for the smaller one[153] since bilateral nerve paralysis would result from surgery on both. A contralateral glomus jugulare should be treated surgically first. If there is no nerve X paralysis following the first procedure, the contralateral vagal tumor can be resected. If there is nerve injury, the second vagal tumor should be irradiated. Similarly, carotid body tumors should be resected prior to contralateral glomus vagale tumors.

Operation for these once inoperable tumors has become feasible. Advanced surgical techniques may cause a higher rate of cranial nerve deficits, especially facial paralysis, dysphagia, aspiration, and voice changes. Recognition of the potential for these complications and planning for patient rehabilitation, beginning before the operation, may reduce the postoperative burden from these cranial nerve complications.

References

1. Haymaker W, Kuhlenbeck H: Disorders of the brain stem and its cranial nerves. In Joynt RJ (ed): Clinical Neurology. Philadelphia, JB Lippincott, 1976.
2. Romanes GJ: Cunningham's Textbook of Anatomy. London, Oxford University Press, 1981.
3. Wilson-Powels L, Akesson EJ, Stewart PA: Cranial Nerves: Anatomy and Clinical Comments. Philadelphia, BC Decker Inc, 1988.
4. Alarie V: Sensory irritation by airborne chemical agents. CRC Crit Rev Toxicol 20:175, 1978.
5. Henkin RI, Royce RC, Ketcham AS, et al: Hyposmia following laryngectomy. Lancet 2:479, 1968.
6. Henkin RI, Larson AC: On mechanisms of hyposmia following laryngectomy in man. Laryngoscope 82:836, 1972.
7. Freedman HM, Kern EB: Complications of intra-

nasal ethmoidectomy: A review of 1,000 consecutive operations. Laryngoscope 89:421, 1979.

8. Maniglia AJ, Chandler JR, Goodwin WJ, Flynn J: Rare complications following ethmoidectomies: A report of eleven cases. Laryngoscope 91:1234, 1981.

9. Maniglia AJ: Fatal and major complications secondary to nasal and sinus surgery. Laryngoscope 99:276, 1989.

10. Friedman WH, Katsantonis GP: Intranasal and transantral ethmoidectomy: A twenty-year experience. Laryngoscope 100:343, 1990.

11. Stankiewicz JA: Complications in endoscopic intranasal ethmoidectamy: An update. Laryngoscope 99:686, 1990.

12. Schaefer SD, Manning S, Close LG: Endoscopic paranasal sinus surgery: Indications and considerations. Laryngoscope 99:1, 1990.

13. Stammberger H: Endoscopic endonasal surgery—concepts in treatment of recurrent rhinosinusitis. Part II: Surgical technique. Otolaryngol Head Neck Surg 94:147, 1986.

14. Hardy JM, Montgomery WW: Osteoplastic frontal sinusotomy. An analysis of 250 operations. Ann Otol Rhinol Laryngol 85:523, 1976.

15. Dandy WE: Orbital Tumors—Results Following the Transcranial Operative Attack. New York, Oskar Priest Publications, 1941.

16. Ray BS, McLean JM: Combined intracranial and orbital operation for retinoblastoma. Arch Ophthalmol 30:437, 1943.

17. Smith RR, Klopp CT, Williams JM: Surgical treatment of cancer of the frontal sinus and adjacent areas. Cancer 7:991, 1954.

18. Ketcham AS, Chretien PB, Van Buren JM, et al: The ethmoid sinuses: A re-evaluation of surgical resection. Am J Surg 126:469, 1973.

19. Hoye RC, Ketcham AS, Henkin RI: Hyposmia after paranasal sinus exenteration or laryngectomy. Am J Surg 120:485, 1970.

20. DeBeale G, Damste PH: Rehabilitation following laryngectomy; The result of a questionnaire. Br J Commun Dis 7:141, 1972.

21. Tatchell RH, Lerman JW, Watt J: Olfactory ability is a function of nasal air flow volume in laryngectomees. Am J Otolaryngol 6:426, 1985.

22. Damste PH: Extras in rehabilitation: Smelling, swimming and compensations for changes after laryngectomy. In Keith RL, Darly FL (eds): Laryngectomy Rehabilitation. Springfield, IL, Charles C Thomas, 1979.

23. Conley JJ: The risk to the orbit in head and neck cancer. Laryngoscope 95:515, 1985.

24. Gordon S, MacRae H: Monocular blindness as a complication of the treatment of a malar fracture. Plast Reconstr Surg 5:228, 1950.

25. Smith HW: Personal communication, 1991.

26. Scapini DA, Mathog RH: Repair of orbital floor fractures with Marlex mesh. Laryngoscope 99:607, 1989.

27. DeSanto LW: The total rehabilitation of Graves' ophthalmopathy. Laryngoscope 90:1652, 1980.

28. Calcaterra TC, Thompson JW: Antral-ethmoidal decompression of the orbit in Graves' disease: Ten-year experience. Laryngoscope 90:1941, 1980.

29. Stankiewicz JA: Blindness and intranasal endoscopic ethmoidectomy: Prevention and management. Otolaryngol Head Neck Surg 101:320, 1989.

30. Buus DR, Tse DT, Farris BK: Ophthalmic complications of sinus surgery. Ophthalmology 97:612, 1990.

31. Marks SC, Jaques DA, Hirata RM, Saunders JR: Blindness following bilateral radical neck dissection. Head Neck 12:342, 1990.

32. Gray H: Anatomy, Descriptive and Surgical. The Classics of Surgery Library, Gryphon Editions, Birmingham, 1984.

33. Mendenhall WM, Parsons JT, Mendenhall NP, et al: Carcinoma of the skin of the head and neck with perineural invasion. Head Neck 11:301, 1989.

34. Conley J, Myers E, Cole R: Analysis of 115 patients with tumors of the submandibular gland. Ann Otol 81:323, 1972.

35. Conley JJ (ed): Complications of Head and Neck Surgery. Philadelphia, WB Saunders, 1979, p 137.

36. Lillie HL: Postoperative complications of the radical external frontal sinus operations. Trans Am Laryngolog Assoc 53:136, 1931.

37. Friedman WH: Ethmoid sinus. In Blitzer A, Lawson W, Friedman WH (eds): Surgery of the Paranasal Sinuses. Philadelphia, WB Saunders, 1985, p 152.

38. Blitzer A: Surgery for infection and benign disease of the maxillary sinus. In Blitzer A, Lawson W, Friedman WH (eds): Surgery of the Paranasal Sinuses. Philadelphia, WB Saunders, 1985, p 187.

39. Goldman J, Blaugrund SM: Complications of surgery of the nasal cavity, sinuses and pharynx. In Conley JJ (ed): Complications of Head and Neck Surgery. Philadelphia, WB Saunders, 1979, p 178.

40. Ogura JH, Thawley SE: Orbital decompression for exophthalmos. Otolaryngol Clin North Am 13:29, 1980.

41. Warren JD, Spector JG, Burde R: Long-term follow-up and recent observations on 305 cases of orbital decompression for dysthyroid orbitopathy. Laryngoscope 99:35, 1989.

42. Goldin-Wood PH: Petrosal and vidian neurectomy in chronic vasomotor rhinitis. J Laryngol Otol 75:232, 1961.

43. Hiranadani NL Jr: Treatment of chronic vasomotor rhinitis with clinico-pathologic study of vidian nerve section in 150 cases. J Laryngol Otol 80:902, 1966.

44. Montgomery WW, Lofgren RH, Chasin WD: Analysis of pterygopalatine space surgery. Laryngoscope 80:1190, 1970.

45. Chasin WD, Lofgren RH: Vidian nerve section for vasomotor rhinitis. Arch Otolaryngol 86:129, 1967.

46. Milton CM, Thomas BM, Bickerton RC: Morbidity study of submandibular gland excision. Ann Coll Surg Engl 68:148, 1986.

47. Adjei SS, Hammersley N: Mylohyoid nerve damage due to excision of the submandibular salivary gland. Br J Oral Maxillofac Surg 27:209, 1989.

48. Hausamen JE, Schimidseder MS: Repair of mandibular nerve by means of autologous nerve grafting after resection of the lower jaw. J Maxillofac Surg 1:74, 1973.

49. Robinson PP: Observations of the recovery of sensation following inferior alveolar nerve injuries. Br J Oral Maxillofac Surg 26:177, 1988.

50. Urken M, Biller H, Weinberg H, et al: Oral mandibular reconstruction using musculocutaneous free-flaps: A review of 72 cases, and a new classification scheme for bone, soft tissue and neural defects. Presented at the Spring Meeting of the American Society of Head and Neck Surgery, May, 1990.

51. Hollinshead WH: Anatomy for Surgeons. Vol I: The Head and the Neck. Philadelphia, Harper and Row, 1982.

52. Tucker HM: Rehabilitation of patients with postoperative deficits; Cranial nerves VIII through XII. Otolaryngol Head Neck Surg 88:576, 1980.

53. Levine TM: Swallowing disorders following skull base surgery. Otolaryngol Clin North Am 21:571, 1988.

54. Hunt PS: A reappraisal of the surgical anatomy of the thyroid and parathyroid glands. Br J Surg 55:63, 1968.

55. Wang C: The use of the inferior cornu of the thyroid cartilage in identifying the recurrent nerve. Surg Gynecol Obstet 140:90, 1975.

56. Henry JF: Nonrecurring recurrent laryngeal nerve. Surgery 104:977, 1988.

57. Rustad WH: Revised anatomy of recurrent laryngeal nerves: Surgical importance based on the dissection of 100 cadavers. J Endocrinol Metab 14:87, 1954.

58. Beahrs OH, Ryan RF, White RA: Complications of thyroid surgery. J Clin Endocrinol Metab 16:1456, 1956.

59. Mountain JL, Stewart GR, Colcock BP: The recurrent laryngeal nerve in thyroid operations. Surg Gynecol Obstet 133:978, 1971.

60. Caldarelli DD, Hollinger LD. Complications and sequelae of thyroid surgery. Otolaryngol Clin North Am 13:85, 1980.

61. Lore JM, Kim DJ, Elias S: Preservation of the laryngeal nerves during total thyroid lobectomy. Ann Otol 86:777, 1977.

62. Beahrs EF, Paternak BM: Cancer of the thyroid gland. Curr Prob Surg (Dec):1, 1969.

63. Fowler EF: Preoperative and postoperative complications in patients with disease of the thyroid. Arch Surg 81:741, 1960.

64. Perzik SL, Catz B: The place of total thyroidectomies in the management of thyroid disease. Surgery 63:436, 1967.

65. Chonkich GD, Petti GH, Goral W: Total thyroidectomy in the treatment of thyroid disease. Laryngoscope 97:897, 1987.

66. Beahrs OH, Vandertoli DJ: Complications of secondary thyroidectomy. Surg Gynecol Obstet 117:535, 1960.

67. Katz AD, Hopp D: Parathyroidectomy: Review of 338 consecutive cases histology: location and reoperation. Am J Surg 57:557, 1977.

68. Satava RM, Beahrs OH, Scholz DA: Success rate of cervical explorations of hyperparathyroidism. Arch Surg 110:625, 1975.

69. Patow CA, Norton JA, Brenan MF: Vocal cord paralysis and reoperative parathyroidectomy. Ann Surg 144:411, 1982.

70. Van Heerden JA, Beahrs OH, Woolner JB: The pathology and surgical management of primary hyperparathyroidism. Surg Clin North Am 57:557, 1977.

71. Wang C: Parathyroid reexploration: A clinical and pathological study of 112 cases. Ann Surg 186:143, 1977.

72. Billings PJ, Milroy EJG: Reoperative parathyroid surgery. Br J Surg 70:542, 1983.

73. Ward PH, Berci G, Calcaterra TC: Superior laryngeal nerve paralysis: An often overlooked entity. Trans Am Acad Opth 85:78, 1977.

74. Green DC, Ward PH: The management of the divided recurrent laryngeal nerve. Laryngoscope 100:779, 1990.

75. Crumley R: Repair of the recurrent laryngeal nerve. Otolaryngol Clin North Am 23:553, 1990.

76. Schramm VL, May M, Lavorato AS: Gelfoam paste. Injection for vocal cord paralysis: Temporary rehabilitation of glottic incompetence. Laryngoscope 28:1268, 1978.

77. Arnold GE: Vocal rehabilitation of paralytic dysphonia. IX: Techniques of intracordal injection. Arch Otolaryngol 76:359, 1962.

78. Isshiki N, Morita H, Okamura H: Thyroplasty as a new phonosurgical technique. Arch Otolaryngol 78:451, 1974.

79. Isshiki N, Taira T, Kojima H, Shoji K: Recent modifications in thyroplasty type I. Ann Otol Rhinol Laryngol 98:777, 1989.

80. Tucker HM: Reinnervation of unilaterally paralyzed larynx. Ann Otol Rhinol Laryngol 86:789, 1977.

81. Netterville JL, Aly A, Ossoff RH: Evaluation and treatment of complications of thyroid and parathyroid surgery. Otolaryngol Clin North Am 23:529, 1990.

82. Ossoff RH, Sisson GA, Duncavage JA, et al: Endoscopic laser arytenoidectomy for the treatment of bilateral vocal cord paralysis. Laryngoscope 94:1293, 1984.

83. Thornell WL: Intralaryngeal approach for arytenoidectomy in bilateral abductor cord paralysis. Arch Otolaryngol 47:505, 1948.

84. King BT: A new and functional restoring operation for bilateral abductor cord paralysis. JAMA 112:814, 1979.

85. Woodman O: A modification of extralaryngeal approach to arytenoidectomy for bilateral abductor paralysis. Arch Otolaryngol 43:63, 1946.

86. Ranson JHC, Imparato AM, Claus RH, et al: Factors in the mortality and morbidity associated with surgical treatment of cerebrovascular insufficiency. Circulation (Suppl 1):269, 1969.

87. DeWeese JA, Rob CG, Satran R, et al: Results of carotid endarterectomies for transient ischemic attacks five years later. Ann Surg 178:258, 1973.

88. Matsumoto GH, Crossman D, Callow AD: Hazards and safeguards during carotid endarterectomy. Am J Surg 133:458, 1977.

89. Hertzer RN, Feldman BJ, Bevan EG, Tucker HM: A prospective study of the incidence of injury to the cranial nerves during carotid endarterectomy. Surg Gynecol Obstet 151:781, 1980.

90. Evans WE, Meldelowitz DS, Liapus Wolf V, Florence CL: Motor speech deficit following carotid endarterectomy. Ann Surg 196:529, 1982.

91. Knight FW, Yeager RH, Morris DM: Cranial nerve injuries during carotid endarterectomy. Ann Surg 154:529, 1987.

92. Weiss K, Kramar R, Fist P: Cranial nerve injuries: Local complications of carotid artery surgery. J Cardiovasc Surg 28:171, 1987.

93. Aldoori M, Baird RN: Local neurological complications during carotid endarterectomy. J Cardiovasc Surg 29:423, 1988.

94. Heeneman H: Vocal cord paralysis following approaches to the anterior cervical spine. Laryngoscope 83:17, 1973.

95. Cavo JW Jr: True vocal cord paralysis following intubation. Laryngoscope 90:1352, 1985.

96. Friedman M, Baim H, Shelton V, et al: Laryngeal injuries secondary to nasogastric tubes. Ann Otol Rhinol Laryngol 90:469, 1981.

97. Weissberger EC: The efferent supply of the trapezius muscle: A neuroanatomic basis for the preservation of shoulder function during neck dissection. Laryngoscope 97:435, 1987.

98. Hollinshead WH: Pectoral region, axilla and shoulder. In Anatomy for Surgeons: Back and Limbs. 2nd ed. Hagerstown, MD, Harper & Rowe, 1968.

99. Jones TA: A modified technique of radical neck dissection. Clin Otolaryngol 9:308, 1984.

100. Stell PM, Jones TA: Radical neck dissection. Preservation of function of the shoulder. J Laryngol Otol 8(Suppl):106, 1983.

101. Weitz JW, Weitz SL, McElhinney AJ: A technique for preservation of spinal accessory nerve function in radical neck dissection. Head Neck Surg 5:75, 1982.

102. Love JG: Nerve anastomosis in the treatment of facial paralysis. Arch Surg 62:379, 1951.

103. Fahrer H, Ludin HP, Mumenthaler M, et al: The innervation of the trapezius muscle—an electrophysiologic study. J Neurol 207:183, 1974.

104. Windle WF: The sensory components of the spinal nerve. J Comp Neurol 80:79, 1948.

105. Escolar J: The afferent connection of the 1st, 2nd, and 3rd cranial nerves in the cat during stimulation of the spinal accessory nerve. J Comp Neurol 89:79, 1948.

106. Holomanova AG, Benuska J, Durcovicova C, Cierny G: Localization of the motor cells after denervation of the sternocleidomastoid muscle in the cat. Folia Morphol (Praha) 21:335, 1973.

107. Rappoport S: Location of the sternocleidomastoid and trapezius motoneurons in the cat. Brain 156:339, 1978.

108. Vanner SJ, Rose PK: Dendritic distribution of motoneurons innervating the three heads of the trapezius muscle in the cat. J Comp Neurol 226:96, 1984.

109. Soo KC, Guiloff RJ, Oh A, et al: Innervation of the trapezius muscle: A study in patients undergoing neck dissections. Head & Neck 12:488, 1990.

110. Brown H, Burus S, Kaiser CW: The spinal accessory nerve plexus, the trapezius muscle, and shoulder stabilization after radical neck cancer surgery. Ann Surg 208:654, 1988.

111. Ferencsik M, Puikovics K, Bobynyl Z, Vargas G: Peripheral nerve injuries as a rare complication of cervical lymph node excision for diagnostic purposes. Orv Hetil 131:1465, 1990.

112. Autran JM, Hazan A, Senechaut JP, Peytral C: Postoperative iatrogenic lesions of the external branch of the accessory spinal nerve. Ann Otolaryngol Chir Cervicofac 105:339, 1988.

113. Woodhall B: Trapezius paralysis following minor surgical procedures in the posterior cervical triangle. Ann Surg 136:375, 1952.

114. Petrera JE, Trojabors W: Conduction studies along the accessory nerve and follow-up of patients with trapezius palsy. J Neurol Neurosurg Psychiatry 47:630, 1984.

115. Weidenbauer MM: An electromyographic study of the trapezius muscle. Am J Phys Med 31:365, 1952.

116. Sedel L, Abols Y: Iatrogenic lesions of the spinal accessory nerve. Microsurgical repair. Presse Med 12:1711, 1983.

117. Norden S: Peripheral injuries to the spinal accessory nerve. Acta Chir Scand 94:515, 1946.

118. Crile GW: Excision of cancer of the head and neck. JAMA 47:1780, 1906.

119. J.M.'s unpublished experience, 1991.

120. Sobol S, Jensen C, Sawyer W, et al: Objective comparison of physical dysfunction after neck dissection. Am J Surg 150:503, 1985.

121. Nahum AM, Mullally W, Marmor L: A syndrome resulting from neck dissection. Arch Otolaryngol 74:82, 1961.

122. Remmler D, Byers R, Scheetz J, et al: A prospective study of shoulder disability resulting from radical neck dissections. Head Neck 8:280, 1986.

123. Dewar FP, Harris RI: Restoration of function of the shoulder following paralysis of the trapezius by fascial sling fixation and transplantation of the levator scapulae. Ann Surg 132:1111, 1950.

124. Ward GE, Robben JO: A composite operation for radical neck dissection and removal of cancer of the mouth. Cancer 5:98, 1951.

125. Bocca E, Pignataro O: A conservation technique in radical neck dissection. Ann Otol Rhinol Laryngol 76:975, 1967.

126. Roy PH, Beahrs OH: Spinal accessory nerve in radical neck dissections. Am J Surg 118:800, 1969.

127. Jesse RH, Ballantyne AJ, Larson D: Radical or modified neck dissection: A therapeutic dilemma. Am J Surg 136:516, 1978.

128. Ballantyne AJ, Guinn GA: Reduction of shoulder disability after neck dissection. Am J Surg 112:662, 1965.

129. Nowak P, Parzuchowski J, Jacobs JR: The effects of combined modality therapy of head and neck carcinoma on shoulder and head mobility. J Surg Oncol 41:143, 1989.

130. Saunders JR, Hirata RM, Jaques DA: Considering the spinal accessory nerve in head and neck surgery. Am J Surg 150:491, 1985.

131. Leipzig B, Suen J, English JL, et al: Functional evaluation of the spinal accessory nerve after neck dissection. Am J Surg 148:526, 1984.

132. Gluckman JL, Myer CM, Aseff JN, Donegan JO: Rehabilitation following radical neck dissection. Laryngoscope 93:1083, 1983.

133. Hoaglund F, Duthie R: Surgical reconstruction for shoulder pain after radical neck dissection. Am J Surg 112:522, 1966.

134. Weisberger EC, Lingeman RE: Cable grafting of the spinal accessory nerve for rehabilitation of shoulder function after radical neck dissection. Laryngoscope 97:915, 1987.

135. Dunn WA: Trapezius paralysis after minor procedures in the posterior cervical triangle. South Med J 67:312, 1974.

136. Harris HH, Dickey JR: Nerve grafting to restore function of the trapezius muscle after radical neck dissection (a preliminary report). Ann Otol Rhinol Laryngol 74:880, 1965.

137. Anderson R, Flowers RS: Free grafts of the spinal accessory nerve during radical dissection. Am J Surg 118:796, 1969.

138. Jackson CG, Glasscock ME III, Nissen AJ, et al: Glomus tumor surgery: The approach, results, and problems. Otolaryngol Clin North Am 15:897, 1982.

139. McCabe BE, Fletcher M: Selection of therapy of glomus jugulare tumors. Arch Otolaryngol 89:156, 1969.

140. Rosenwasser H: Glomus jugulare tumors: Long-term tumors. Arch Otolaryngol 88:33, 1968.
141. Glasscock ME III, Jackson CG, Dickins JRE, Wiet RJ: The surgical management of glomus tumors. Laryngoscope 89:1640, 1979.
142. Brachmann DE, House WF, Terry R, Scanlan RL: Glomus jugulare tumors: Effect of irradiation. Trans Am Acad Ophthalmol Otolaryngol 76:1423, 1972.
143. Jackson SG, Glasscock ME III, Harris PF: Glomus tumors. Classification and management of large lesions. Arch Otolaryngol 108:401, 1982.
144. Balfour DC, Wildner F: The intercarotid paraganglion and its tumors. Surg Gynecol Obstet 18:203, 1914.
145. Hallet JN, Nora JD, Hollier LH, et al: Trends in neurovascular complications of surgical management for carotid body and cervical paragangliomas: A fifty-year experience with 153 tumors. J Vasc Surg 7:284, 1988.
146. Murphy TP, Brackman DE: The effect of preoperative embolization on glomus jugulare tumors. Laryngoscope 99:1244, 1989.
147. Shamlin WR, Remine WH, Sheps SG, Harrison EG Jr: Carotid body tumor (chemodectoma): Clinico-pathology and analysis of 90 cases. Am J Surg 122:732, 1971.
148. Cece JA, Lawson WL, Biller HF, et al: Complications in the management of large glomus jugulare tumors. Laryngoscope 97:152, 1987.
149. Spector GJ, Sobel S: Surgery for glomus tumors at the skull base. Otolaryngol Head Neck Surg 88:524, 1980.
150. Farrior JB: Intratemporal approach to the skull base for glomus tumors. Anatomic considerations. Ann Otol Rhinol Laryngol 93:616, 1984.
151. Jenkins MA, Fisch U: Glomus tumors of the temporal bone. Arch Otolaryngol 107:209, 1981.
152. Gardner G, Cocke EW Jr, Robertson JT, et al: Glomus jugulare tumors—Combined treatment: Part II. J Laryngol Otol 95:567, 1981.
153. Biller F, Lawson W, Som P, Rosefeld R: Glomus vagale tumors. Ann Otol Rhinol Laryngol 98:21, 1989.
154. Leonetti JP, Smith PG, Grubb RC: Management of neurovascular complications in extended skull base surgery. Laryngoscope 99:492, 1989.
155. Sataloff RT, Myers DL, Kremer FB: Management of cranial nerve injury following skull base surgery. Otolaryngol Clin North Am 17:577, 1984.
156. Tucker HM: Restoration of selective facial nerve function by neuro-muscular pedicle techniques. Clin Plast Surg 6:293, 1979.
157. Rubin LR: Entire temporalis muscle transposition. In Rubin LR (ed): Reanimation of the Paralyzed Face: New Approaches. St. Louis, CV Mosby, 1977, p 294.
158. Rubin LR: The anatomy of a smile: Its importance in the treatment of facial paralysis. Plast Reconstr Surg 53:384, 1973.
159. Hakelius L: Free muscle grafting. Clin Plast Surg 6:301, 1979.
160. Krespi YP, Sisson GA: Transmandibular exposure of the skull base. Am J Surg 148:534, 1984.
161. Mattox DE, Fisch U: Surgery of the skull base. In Johns ME: Complications of Head and Neck Surgery. Vol 2. Philadelphia, BC Decker Inc, 1986, p 307.
162. Zak FG, Lawson W: The Paraganglioma Chemoreceptor System: Physiology, Pathology, and Clinical Medicine. New York, Springer-Verlag, 1982, p 383.

CHAPTER 8

Neurotologic and Skull Base Surgery

G. ROBERT KLETZKER, MD
PETER G. SMITH, MD, PhD
ROBERT J. BACKER, MD
JOHN P. LEONETTI, MD

Surgeons embarking on cranial base surgery need to be acquainted with the complications occasionally encountered. Hemorrhage, cerebral edema, arterial or venous infarction, pneumocephalus, cerebrospinal fluid leak, infection, and acquired cranial nerve deficits may occur in any surgical procedure in which the dura is opened and the brain manipulated. Specific compartments of the cranial cavity have varying degrees of tolerance to operative alterations. For example, relatively small changes in the blood flow in the posterior fossa may severely alter the delicate functions of the brain stem.[21] Removal of lesions of the skull base may leave large intra/extracranial communications requiring complex reconstructive techniques for closure.

Minimization of complications begins with a comprehensive preoperative neuroradiographic assessment, including high-resolution computed tomography (HRCT), magnetic resonance imaging (MRI), and conventional or magnetic resonance angiography. Balloon occlusion test of the internal carotid artery estimates the patient's tolerance to carotid artery ligation. Anticipation of the limits of resection and of the neurovascular structures that may be involved is the cornerstone of the collaborative planning by a cranial base team to achieve a safe, oncologically sound resection.[33, 41, 49]

PERIOPERATIVE CONSIDERATIONS

In addition to the standard perioperative protocol established for a conventional neurosurgical procedure, the patient who undergoes a cranial base resection is evaluated by both a neuroanesthesiologist and an intraoperative electrophysiologist. Coordination with these members in positioning the patient and placement of critical monitoring leads requires cooperation and experience to minimize confusion or delay in the operating suite. Priority is given to the induction of general anesthesia in a manner that reduces the risk of increasing intracranial pressure. A preliminary tracheotomy is performed if entry into the upper aerodigestive tract is anticipated.[19] Once adequate airway control is obtained, an adjuvant arterial, intraventricular, or lumbar catheter is methodically inserted. A nasogastric tube, urinary catheter, and pneumatic stockings are secured prior to placement of the patient in three-point fixation (Fig. 8–1). Avoidance of excess neck flexion that may impair venous return is particularly important if major venous structures are obliterated or resected. Troublesome intracranial hypertension may occur if flow through the contralateral internal jugular vein is compromised. Monitoring leads are secured after the patient has been placed in the final operative position. Integrity of all electrophysiologic and hemodynamic monitors is confirmed prior to the isolation of the operative field.

Intracranial pressure is adjusted by removal of cerebrospinal fluid, hyperventilation, or osmotic diuresis by the neuroanesthesiologist at the request of the surgical team. Attainment of adequate oncologic exposure with minimal brain retraction is of paramount importance in these lengthy operations. Hypotensive anesthesia is often helpful in minimizing blood loss in the resection of vascular lesions. Caution must be exercised with this technique to prevent generalized cerebral hypoperfusion. As with any surgical procedure, communication between all members of the surgical team enhances the well-being of the patient and conduct of the operation.[52, 67]

MANAGEMENT OF INTRAOPERATIVE BLEEDING

Extirpation of extensive lesions of the cranial base entails long operations that fre-

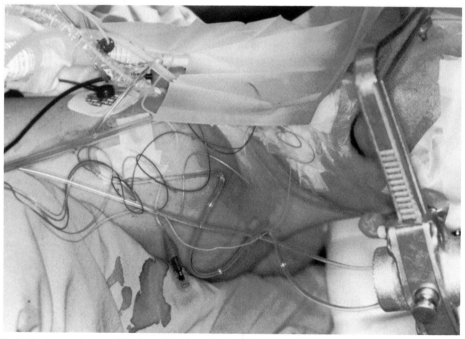

FIGURE 8–1. Perioperative positioning of patient in head holder, with cranial nerve monitoring electrodes secured to skin.

quently require a combination of surgical approaches.[1, 23, 56] A substantial portion of the operative time involves access to vascular structures of the cranial base. A working knowledge of intracranial and extracranial vascular anatomy and physiology, as well as techniques for the intraoperative control of bleeding from these structures, is a fundamental requisite for one who is involved with skull base surgery.[55, 75] Inadequate control of bleeding can hinder the effective removal of a tumor or lead to major, life-threatening complications.[66, 70]

Angiology of the Cranial Base

Venous System. Extracranial veins encountered during the course of lateral cranial base surgical procedures are tributaries of the retromandibular or external or internal jug-ular veins. Mastoid or occipital emissary veins also connect the dural sinus system with branches of occipital, postauricular, or retrofacial veins.[34] The pterygoid plexus of the subtemporal region is quite variable in its location and volume of return owing to an alteration of the angioarchitecture because of an underlying tumor (Fig. 8–2).

The dural sinuses serve as conduits for blood from the brain, meninges, and diploë of the skull. The sinuses are connected with the extracranial veins via emissary and other, larger venous channels, which are formed by the anatomic separation of the endosteal and meningeal layers of the dura mater. The transverse sinus serves as the drainage system for the outflow from the sagittal and straight sinuses. At approximately the occipitotemporal suture line, the transverse sinus empties into the sigmoid sinus, which takes a sinuous course through the mastoid portion of the temporal bone. The sigmoid sinus

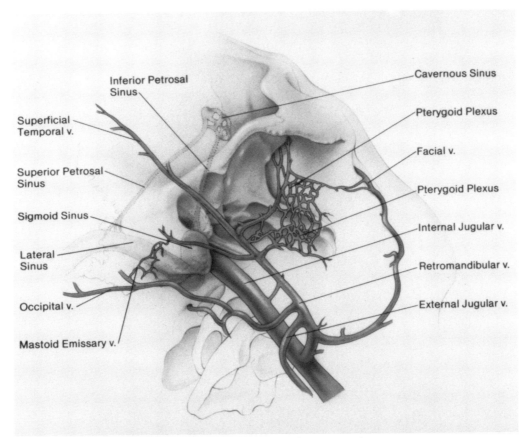

FIGURE 8–2. Infratemporal fossa exposure of extracranial venous anatomy.

drains into the internal jugular vein at the level of the jugular bulb. The superior petrosal sinus drains into the confluence of the transverse and sigmoid sinuses.[11] This conduit allows bidirectional flow of blood between the cavernous and transverse sinuses (Fig. 8–3). This smaller-caliber channel courses along the petrous bone within the dural layers of the tentorium and provides an alternate route of flow if the sigmoid sinus is obliterated.[51, 89] Venous outflow from the lateral cerebral cortex is through the inferior cerebral vein of Labbé that drains into the transverse sinus. Venous return from the lateral brain stem is through the petrosal vein that drains into the superior petrosal sinus.[2, 39, 45]

The cavernous sinus is a parasellar, trabeculated space that spans the gap between the petrous apex and the superior orbital fissure. It receives venous tributaries from the ophthalmic, cerebral, and retinal veins and the sphenoparietal sinus. The usual outflow tract from the cavernous sinus is to the transverse sinus by way of the superior petrosal sinus, the jugular bulb via the inferior petrosal sinus, and the pterygoid plexus through a complex of emissary veins. Contralateral flow is available through this midline venous cavern when normal pathways are altered by tumors or their surgical removal. Coursing through the thin-walled cavernous sinus are a number of cranial nerves and the cavernous portion of the internal carotid artery.[36] Management of lesions that involve the cavernous sinus has heretofore been a major surgical challenge. Fortunately, novel techniques have permitted an oncologic resection of this unique anatomic structure with preservation of integral neurologic structures.[83]

Arterial System. The extracranial blood supply to the scalp and neck is provided by the facial, superficial temporal, occipital, and

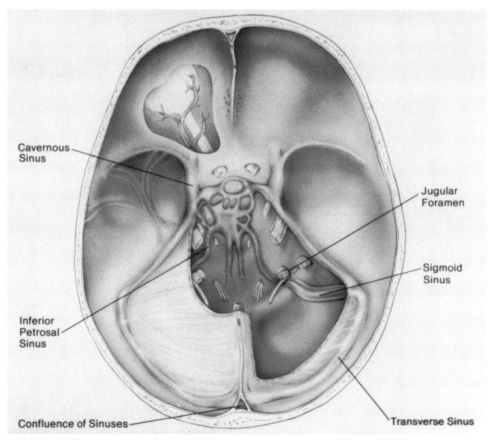

FIGURE 8–3. Intracranial anatomy of venous sinuses of the cranial base.

postauricular branches of the external carotid artery. The deep temporal and middle meningeal branches of the internal maxillary artery supply the base of the skull within the infratemporal fossa.[34] The ascending pharyngeal artery supplies structures of the anterior temporal bone through the inferior tympanic canaliculus (Fig. 8–4).

Major transcranial arterial structures are the internal carotid and vertebral systems. The cervical portion of the internal carotid artery ascends vertically from the carotid bifurcation and is located deep to the sternocleidomastoid, digastric, and stylohyoid muscles. It is in proximity to the superior constrictor, levator veli palatini, and medial scalene muscles along its posteromedial border. The carotid foramen lies anterior to the jugular foramen in the temporal bone, both of which are medial to the base of the styloid process at the vaginal plate of the tympanic ring.[81] The two foramina are separated by a thin partition of bone that widens medially and forms a valuable radiographic landmark known as the vascular crest or bony plate (Fig. 8–5). The petrous artery ascends vertically within the temporal bone and lies anterior to the cochlea.[4] The superior limit of the vertical portion of the petrous carotid artery is the junction of the bony and cartilaginous parts of the eustachian tube. The petrous carotid then courses horizontally along the axis of the eustachian tube. The greater petrosal nerve crosses the horizontal part of the petrous carotid artery. It is roofed by the ganglion and the mandibular and maxillary divisions of the trigeminal nerve as it enters the cavernous sinus[60] (Fig. 8–6). In its cavernous segment, the artery reaches its anterior limit. It then curves first cephalad then posteriorly in a 180° turn as it exits from the roof of the cavernous sinus. The main branching vessel proximal to the circle of Willis is the ophthalmic artery, which usually

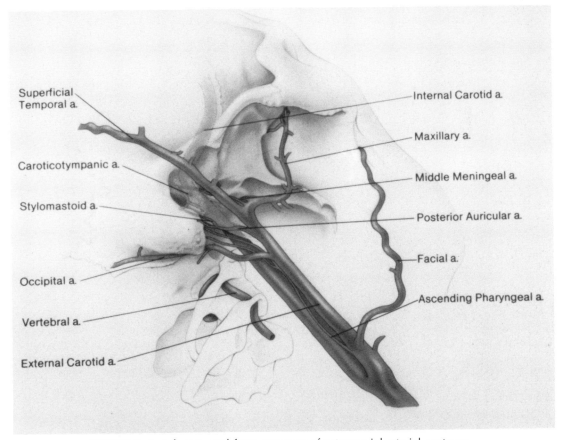

FIGURE 8–4. Infratemporal fossa exposure of extracranial arterial anatomy.

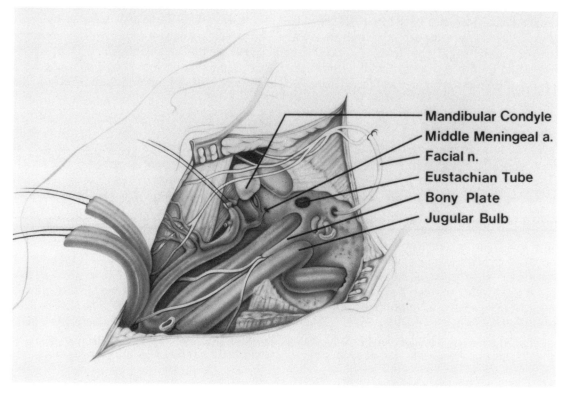

FIGURE 8–5. Lateral exposure of upper cervical neurovascular structures.

branches from the carotid within the cavernous sinus below the optic nerve.[85]

The vertebral artery enters the transverse process of the sixth cervical vertebra and ascends vertically. It exits from the foramen of the transverse process of the atlas (C1) and courses through the atlanto-occipital membrane into the intracranial cavity. The basilar artery, formed by the union of the vertebral arteries, provides the blood supply to elements of the posterior cranial fossa. Major branches of the basilar artery include

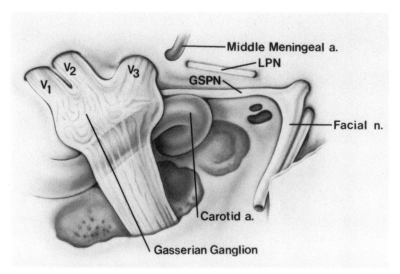

FIGURE 8–6. Middle cranial fossa exposure of the petrous portion of the internal carotid artery in relationship to anatomic landmarks. GSPN, greater superficial petrosal nerve; LPN, lesser petrosal nerve.

the posterior inferior cerebellar, anterior inferior cerebellar, superior cerebellar, and posterior cerebral arteries.

Management of Bleeding During Cranial Base Surgery

Nowhere is the surgical axiom that "bleeding is the enemy of the surgeon" more apropos than to cranial base surgery. Failure to control bleeding may result in a catastrophic outcome or, at the very minimum, obscure critical dissection. The approach used to obtain access to a particular lesion dictates the angiology that may be encountered.

BLEEDING FROM A DURAL SINUS

Any approach to the posterior fossa may require management of bleeding from one or more emissary veins that drain the transverse and sigmoid sinuses. Bone removal of the mastoid and occipital cortex is carried out with a rotary drill in sweeping motions with continuous suction irrigation. The blue coloration of the venous sinuses can be visualized under a thin shell of intact bone. Bleeding from emissary veins is controlled initially with bone wax impaction into their points of exposure. Thinning the bone between the site of bleeding and the emissary vein's point of exit from the sinus allows the greatest opportunity for complete coagulation. To avoid a tear at the emissary-sigmoid junction, bone should first be completely removed from the sinus, using a combination of cutting and polishing burs, a blunt dural elevator, and bone rongeurs. Bipolar electrocautery then can be used to ensure coagulation of the vein stump.[68]

Failure to identify the vein distal to the sinus can lead to troublesome bleeding if the vein is torn at its juncture with the sinus. The additional risk of air entry into the venous system exists if the head lies above the level of the right atrium of the heart. In the event of the inadvertent opening of the sinus—heralded by the brisk outflow of deoxygenated blood—the anesthesiologist should be alerted, so as to monitor for signs of air emboli. At the first sign of intravascular crepitation, hypotension, tachycardia, a decline in end-expiratory Pco_2, or other warnings of air emboli, treatment should be instituted. The patient should immediately be put in the Trendelenburg position, with the left side of the table rotated down to isolate any intravascular air into the right cardiac ventricle, where it may be aspirated through a central venous catheter. Discontinuance of nitrous oxide, administration of 100 per cent oxygen, positive-pressure ventilation, and vasopressors are provided while digital pressure is applied over the venous opening. Aggressive attendance to the earliest warning signs of intravascular air can prevent the major complications of air emboli.[15, 80]

Small dural tears can be controlled with bipolar cautery and placement of oxidized cellulose gauze (Surgicel), held in place for a short period under a cotton patty with the suction tip, to tamponade the bleeding. A simple or figure-of-eight 4-0 silk suture also can approximate the dural margins and hold the Surgicel in place over the vessel rent. Larger tears require some form of extraluminal or intraluminal packing with a large sheet of Surgicel. Placement of this packing in the presence of brisk venous bleeding can be performed in a controlled fashion as the surgical assistant compresses the proximal sinus with the firm placement of a Kirschner sponge. This frees the surgeon to use the suction tip both to keep the surgical field free of blood and to advance the packing within the vessel aperture until bleeding has ceased. Packing of a sinus in individuals with thin dura runs the risk of tearing the medial aspect of the vessel and bleeding within the posterior fossa. Gentle advancement of the packing within the lumen of the vessel will prevent this potential complication.

The planned resection of dural sinuses can be accomplished in the manner described. The sinus also may be ligated with 2-0 or 3-0 silk sutures passed circumferentially around the vessel through small stab incisions in the dura, several millimeters from the margin of the sinus.[24] Placement of a ligature or packing to occlude the sigmoid sinus should be performed in such a way as to maintain the transverse sinus' patency. High cervical ligation of the internal jugular vein is done in concordance with sigmoid sinus obliteration in cases of tumor removal around the region of the jugular bulb, such as in glomus tumor operations (Fig. 8–7). The internal carotid artery is isolated with vessel loops at the time of internal jugular vein exposure whenever the infratemporal approach is being utilized or when the petrous exposure of the carotid is anticipated.[29, 53]

Bleeding from the cavernous sinus can be brisk, with bright red blood that appears arterial owing to the pulsatile quality. Precautions to avoid air emboli are necessary, as with any major sinus opening. Controlling hemorrhage from the cavernous sinus is technically more difficult than obtaining hemostasis in the other venous sinuses. The exposure is usually more limited, and the vital neurovascular structures contained within the sinus cavity preclude injudicious pressure to tamponade the bleeding. The opening of the sinus should be covered with a cotton patty that is held in place with a medium-bore suction tip. Surgicel gauze is advanced

into the dural rent until the bleeding adequately slows to allow clot to form and seal the leak. Patience is required as firm but gentle pressure is held over the Surgicel with the cotton patty by the suction tip. Once bleeding is controlled, the Surgicel is trimmed with a few millimeters of excess gauze left over the outer surface of the torn dura. The button of excess gauze should be kept in sight whenever work is being done in that area of the operative field, to avoid the accidental dislodgement of the Surgicel from the sinus by suction or instruments that may snag the gauze and reinstitute bleeding. Using the minimum amount of Surgicel that can plug the hole in the sinus is best. Over-packing of the sinus with thrombotic gauze may result in pressure injury to cranial nerves III through VI or compression of the internal carotid.[82]

Obtaining access to the superior cervical vasculature, as routinely carried out in head and neck procedures, is a necessity in extended cranial base resections. In addition to isolating the great vessels for their proximal control, this exposure often allows access to arteries that may be contributing to the vas-

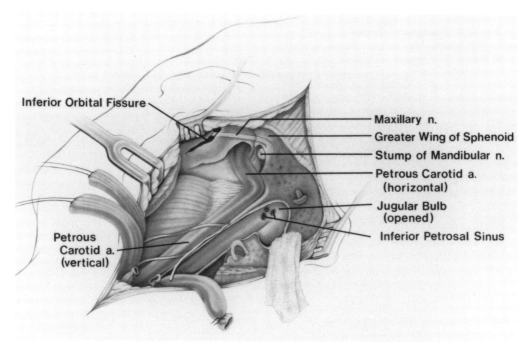

FIGURE 8–7. Lateral exposure of upper cervical neurovascular structures, with ligation of the internal jugular vein and sigmoid sinus obliteration.

cularity of the tumor. Ligation of feeding vessels can reduce operative blood loss immensely during tumor removal and improve the visibility during resection and thus the safety of the procedure. Guided by the preoperative angiogram, the ligation of select arteries is planned and carried out early in the procedure. Contrary to the occlusion of draining veins, the select intentional ligation of arteries has a more beneficial effect when there is a time lapse between arterial ligation and tumor removal. The longer the time between venous occlusion and tumor excision, however, the greater the potential for vascular congestion within the tumor and the more bothersome the operative bleeding. Tumors arising in the infratemporal fossa and upper aerodigestive tract often have contributing vascularity from the external carotid system. Preoperative angiogram-directed embolization of arterial feeders two days before resection is often helpful in hemostasis.[14] This has been used most successfully with paragangliomas, meningiomas, and angiofibromas. Ligation of the arteries as close to the tumor as possible offers significant vascular control, particularly when embolization has not been feasible. Gaining access to the tributaries of the internal maxillary artery can be accomplished after facial nerve and mandibular mobilization in the infratemporal fossa approach.[27] Mandibulotomy, when employed in combined lateral approaches, offers a similar advantage.

Specific vessels that require control to gain adequate tissue mobilization for tumor exposure vary with the approach. Care in electrocoagulation is warranted, keeping in mind adjacent structures that may be injured as hemostasis is obtained. The facial nerve, which is skeletonized or mobilized in posterior approaches, is vascularized by the stylomastoid artery in the vertical mastoid segment. Medial to the digastric ridge, this artery causes bleeding that requires coagulation. The facial nerve, because of its close proximity, may suffer irreversible electrothermal injury if it is included in the field of cautery.[12] Bipolar coagulation at a low setting, with concomitant irrigation, will minimize this risk. This technique is helpful in dissection of the peripheral portion of the facial nerve while controlling the venous and small arterial bleeding during parotidectomy. The superior occipital artery, the landmark of the superior limit in neck dissections, is also best controlled with bipolar coagulation or ligation, since vessel clamping or unipolar coagulation can cause injury to the underlying eleventh cranial nerve.

Control of the internal carotid artery is of paramount importance in most approaches to the cranial base. An awareness of its potential locations keeps the risk of inadvertent vessel injury to a minimum. This is particularly true of the anterior and inferior approaches, which provide access to the cranial base via the sphenoid sinus. The pterional and infratemporal fossa approaches are utilized whenever the carotid must be mobilized from its petrous encasement. Ideally, adequate proximal and distal exposure is obtained prior to any carotid mobilization. Pathology of the petroclival region may prohibit this degree of exposure.[40, 74] Intraluminal balloon occlusion affords available distal control in this situation. Preoperative balloon occlusion testing provides invaluable information concerning the collateral cerebral circulation and the capability of the patient to tolerate carotid resection without suffering irreversible neurologic sequelae.[22] Failure of the carotid occlusion trial warrants planning of bypassing the internal carotid artery with a vein graft if the histopathology dictates.[60, 84, 93] The petrous portion of the carotid can be reached safely and the artery gently mobilized when necessary. The caroticotympanic artery arises from the posterior aspect of the internal carotid, proximal to the genu at the bony-cartilaginous junction of the eustachian tube. This small-caliber vessel can bleed profusely if avulsed during carotid mobilization. Exposure of the petrous carotid is performed by thinning the bone with a diamond bur and then gently separating the "eggshell" fragments with a Freer elevator off the adventitia. Care is taken to remove bone away from the vessel, with contact to the artery itself kept to a minimum. With the bony surface of the superior aspect of the horizontal portion of the carotid removed, the artery can be cautiously retracted (Fig. 8–8). Inspection of the posteroinferior aspect of the vessel will allow identification of the tympanic branch, where it can be cauterized a few millimeters from the carotid's margin. With this vessel controlled, the dissection of the bone posterior to the carotid may proceed judiciously, with the process expedited by bone rongeurs.

Adjacent to the cochlea, at its superior aspect, the location of the geniculate ganglion should be determined. The greater superficial petrosal nerve typically is sharply sectioned while delineating the tensor tympani muscle along the medial margin of the eustachian tube. If the ganglion is exposed, care is taken not to traumatize the nerve bluntly or place traction on it while skeletonizing the genu of the carotid.[25] Procedures to preserve hearing[8] limit the amount of bone removal that can be performed around the carotid genu. In this instance the posterior margin of the carotid canal is removed through the protympanum and inferior tubal recess. The medial margin of the horizontal portion of the carotid, anterior to the cochlea, can be drilled out through the transtympanic approach to the petrous apex in combination with the exposure gained in the middle fossa extradurally.[77] In this latter, superiorly based approach, the bone anterior and inferior to the

genu is drilled away, allowing for complete removal of the carotid's bony encasement (Fig. 8–9). The superior aspect of the petrous carotid's surface is adjacent to the second and third divisions of the trigeminal nerve along the lateralmost margin of the cavernous sinus.

Separating the trigeminal nerve from the internal carotid is a thick dural fold that may be covered with a thin shell of bone or devoid of any hard tissue cover. The third and second branches of the trigeminal nerve may need to be sectioned at the foramen ovale and foramen rotundum respectively, to expose the sphenoid wing or infratemporal fossa adequately. This maneuver aids in the anterior mobilization of the carotid out of its canal by exposing the underlying floor of the middle cranial fossa and the bone adjacent to the carotid. Allowing adequate room to mobilize the carotid without compressing the vessel during retraction or kinking it at its genu is essential to prevent the potentially disastrous complication of vasospasm.[61]

Spasm of the carotid can occur with excess mechanical manipulation, temperature changes, drying of the adventitial surface, or prolonged exposure to blood. Gentle tissue handling and frequent irrigation of the carotid's surface with isothermal saline are the preventive measures taken whenever the

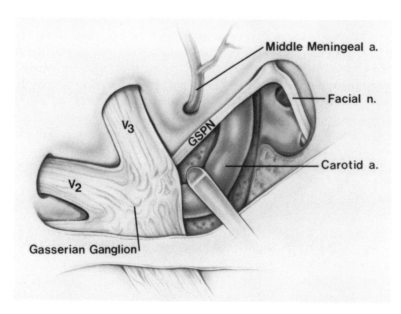

FIGURE 8–8. Middle cranial fossa exposure for mobilization of the petrous portion of the internal carotid artery.

Middle Meningeal a.

Facial n.

Carotid a.

V3

GSPN

V2

Gasserian Ganglion

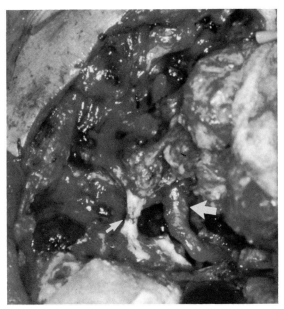

FIGURE 8–9. Intraoperative exposure of the internal carotid artery (*large arrow*) and facial nerve (*small arrow*) after removal of bony encasement.

vessel is uncovered. Despite these precautions, vasospasm may develop. The sequelae of this physiologic vascular activity vary with the severity and duration of the constriction. In our experience the most profound consequences occurred in the younger patients, whose vascular tonicity and reactivity were relatively hypersensitive.[87] Hemodilution and hypertensive therapy (utilized to treat vasospasm after subarachnoid hemorrhage) may be effective in preventing catastrophic infarction. At the earliest detection of segmental reduction of the vessel caliber, topical application of 10 per cent lidocaine, 1.5 per cent or 3 per cent papaverine, and 25 mg/ml of chlorpromazine has been shown to inhibit vascular smooth muscle contraction. These agents are effective spasmolytic agents that may be applied to the constricting vessel to counteract the myogenic response. The efficacy of calcium channel blockers such as nimodipine has not been proved in large-vessel spasm, though it is systemically administered in the management of medium-caliber cerebral artery spasm.

The sequelae of prolonged vasospasm are endothelial, intimal, and vessel media in-jury. Spasm unabated for as little as two hours can lead to irreversible injury and thrombosis. The darkened coloration of the vessel surface in the region of constriction is an ominous sign of significant vascular injury and impending thrombosis. Decreased vessel pulsations, distal to the site of constriction, may be detectable on visualization and palpation, thus warning of impaired perfusion.

Slowing of electroencephalographic waves has been seen during intraoperative monitoring when regional blood flow falls below 18 ml/100 gr/minute. Altered ventilation to elevate oxygen and carbon dioxide levels and maximizing of blood pressure are undertaken in an attempt to maintain cerebral perfusion.[63, 78] Anticoagulants are contraindicated at the time of operation but may be considered in the patient who has developed delayed thrombosis. The risk of delayed carotid spasm and decreased perfusion has been reported in both carotid mobilization and trauma. Declining neurologic status or increasing intracranial pressure in the postoperative period warrants evaluation by CT and angiography. Surgical dressings that may compress the carotid should be removed, and the wound should be explored to evacuate hematoma if carotid spasm is confirmed angiographically. Measures to decrease intracerebral pressure are concurrently undertaken.[61]

CEREBRAL EDEMA: EVALUATION AND MANAGEMENT

Tumors commonly incite edema in surrounding brain tissue.[16] Retraction or manipulation of brain also leads to varying degrees of cerebral swelling. The principles of treatment rely on the ability to alter the volume of brain, cerebrospinal fluid, or blood.[13, 38] Management of raised intracranial pressure begins with pharmaceutic, mechanical, and ventilatory measures. Computed tomography and magnetic resonance imaging provide the initial assessment of tumor volume, cerebral edema, mass effect, and midline shift. Ventricular size and shape allow one to estimate the volume of cerebrospinal fluid and the likelihood of hydrocephalus. The occurrence of cerebral edema after tumor resection is relatively common; clinical manifestations are usually present between 24 and 72 hours after operation. Clinically significant edema is most commonly heralded by evidence of increased intracranial pressure as measured by an intraventricular drainage catheter, a decline in the patient's mentation or level of alertness, or progressive focal neurologic deficits such as aphasia or limb weakness. Generalized edema that occurs as a result of brain manipulation or retraction or venous outflow obstruction becomes most pronounced several days after surgery.[26, 92] Depending on the degree of lethargy, the rapidity of the neurologic dysfunction, or the severity of the process, the first step in management is to obtain a CT head scan (Fig. 8–10). Expansile lesions, such as subdural hematoma and hydrocephalus, must be eliminated as a cause of the clinical decline prior to institution of pressure reduction maneuvers. Surgical exploration to evacuate intracerebral blood clots or subdural hematomas

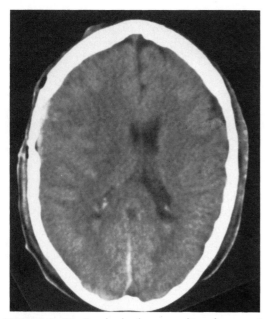

FIGURE 8–10. Cerebral edema resulting from postoperative hemorrhage, showing midline shift of ventricles.

that are compromising cerebral function is undertaken as early as these lesions are detected. Control of bleeding and removal of pressure-producing lesions often will arrest progression of neurologic injury and prevent irreversible sequelae if therapy is instituted efficaciously.

Postoperative cerebral edema occurring postoperatively that is diffuse and without a focal remediable cause should be addressed in an aggressive manner to prevent the neurologic injury subsequent to ischemia.[3, 6, 17] Placement of an intraventricular drain is useful for monitoring intracranial pressure, and regulating the volume of spinal fluid is a therapeutic measure. Epidural manometric measurements of intracranial pressure provide an alternative method of quantifying pressure changes and monitoring the response to therapy. This is preferable to the intraventricular drainage catheter when the ventricles are collapsed from cerebral edema or contraindications exist to removal of spinal fluid. Maintaining a reliable measurement with the epidural monitors may be difficult, making the intraventricular catheter the preferred device.[91]

Preoperative intravenous steroids (dexamethasone in 4- to 10-mg doses) are begun at least 12 hours preoperatively and continued every 6 hours for 3 days. The dose is tapered and discontinued over the ensuing 7 to 10 days, as the patient's recovery allows.[86] This regimen is used routinely to minimize edema associated with tumor removal, when significant dissection or retraction of brain is required.

Cerebrospinal fluid drainage through a temporary, closed sterile system is routinely employed to regulate the intracranial fluid volume and allow greater room for brain retraction. Lesions of the infratentorial compartment that have demonstrated obstruction of the aqueduct, as indicated by dilated ventricles, require intraventricular drainage catheter placement, as lumbar drainage techniques may lead to brain herniation. Lesions that transgress the intracranial compartments and may require dissection in the posterior fossa also require ventricular drains in the event of outflow obstruction near the aqueduct, resulting from edema due to manipulation.

Hyperventilation is a short-acting method of decreasing the intravascular blood volume, secondary to the effect of hypocapnia on the autoregulatory controls of the cerebral vasculature. The arterial PCO_2 should be maintained between 25 and 35 mm Hg, through hyperventilation.[78] This method of pressure control is most effective in the immediate perioperative period and loses efficacy as a pressure control modality after approximately 36 hours of continuous use. Controlled hypotension, hypothermia (30 to 32 degrees Centigrade), and barbiturate-induced coma are other perioperative modalities that may be employed adjunctively to hyperventilation, to minimize cerebral edema.

In addition to steroids, which are used prophylactically, hyperosmolar agents and diuretics are useful medications to reduce interstitial fluid volume. Their rapidity of action allows their use intraoperatively or to arrest acute edema. Mannitol is a hyperosmolar dehydrating agent that remains in the intravascular compartment and draws interstitial fluid into blood vessels by its osmotic gradient. Mannitol is given intravenously in doses of 0.5 to 2.0 mg/kg/body weight, infused over 20 minutes, every 6 to 12 hours. There is considerably less rebound effect than is seen with urea, which diffuses into intercellular spaces more readily. Furosemide (Lasix) is a frequently used diuretic that promotes the egress of interstitial edematous fluid by the renal excretion of excess water and electrolytes. This creates an osmotic gradient that, as occurs with mannitol, mobilizes excess fluid from the extracellular compartment. Furosemide is administered intravenously in doses of 20 to 60 mg every 4 to 6 hours. Care must be taken with its use to monitor serum potassium levels and replenish electrolytes.

POSTOPERATIVE STROKE: EVALUATION AND MANAGEMENT

The cause of the cerebrovascular accident may be embolic or thrombotic vascular occlu-sion, arterial spasm, venous infarction, or progressive intraluminal occlusion due to intimal dissection[59] (Fig. 8–11). The detection by CT of an area of a confined infarction or intracerebral hemorrhage may warrant only aggressive medical therapy, unless the hemorrhage is expansile or creating undue mass effect, as evidenced by ventricular compression. A focal intracranial accumulation of fluid or air most likely will create focal neurologic defects requiring emergency exploration and evacuation to relieve the pressure effect and prevent irreversible sequelae.[88, 94] The timing of the neurologic alteration may prove helpful in the initial clinical assessment, as cerebral edema is most apt to occur in the first few days, whereas postoperative stroke may occur in the immediate recovery period or remote from the operative session.

HEMORRHAGE

Prevention of bleeding around the dura is accomplished by meticulous hemostasis with bipolar coagulation, especially of the bridging veins to the sinuses. Dural tacking sutures

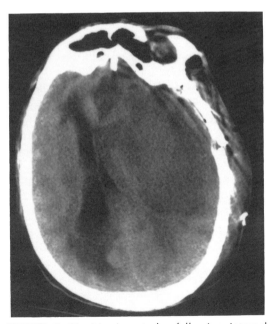

FIGURE 8–11. Massive stroke following internal carotid artery thrombosis in the postoperative period.

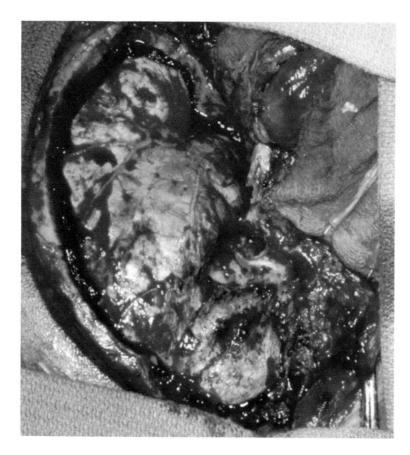

FIGURE 8–12. Coagulant material in the epidural space about the periphery of the craniotomy for hemostasis.

prevent blood from enlarging the epidural space. Coagulants, such as oxidized cellulose (Surgicel) or microfibrillary collagen (Avitene), are used to promote clot formation at the periphery of the craniotomy bone flap (Fig. 8–12). Subdural and epidural hemorrhages that are venous in origin arise from bridging veins between the brain, dura, and diploë. The tacking sutures should tamponade any bleeding from a venous source.[72] Branches of the middle meningeal artery, which supply the dura mater, must be coagulated adequately prior to wound closure to prevent hematoma formation. The presence of accumulating blood will by mass effect generate focal neurologic signs, such as hemiparesis or aphasia, or can first be detected after the onset of focal seizures. Hemiparalysis with obtundation, a fixed, dilated pupil, and respiratory distress are the hallmarks of rapidly increasing intracranial pressure with peduncular herniation. An urgent search for and treatment of a focal

hemorrhage is mandatory in attempting to reverse the neurologic decline.[54, 58] Carotid rupture, a rare complication, mandates immediate exploration to control bleeding and evacuate extravasated blood. The prognosis for recovery without devastating neurologic sequelae is extremely poor in the rare survivor of this complication (Fig. 8–13).

Postoperative hematomas can occur in the subdural or epidural space or within the excavation site of tumor removal. Application of warm saline, peroxide-soaked cotton, or freshly cut muscle plugs often will stop the seepage of blood from the surface of the brain at the tumor bed. Meticulous hemostasis is essential at the surface of brain tissue to prevent intraparenchymal hemorrhage. The risk of intraventricular hemorrhage is greater following removal of tumors around the cerebellar flocculus, in the cerebellopontine angle. Bipolar cauterization of the vascular choroid plexus, which is abundant in this region, will prevent blood accumulation

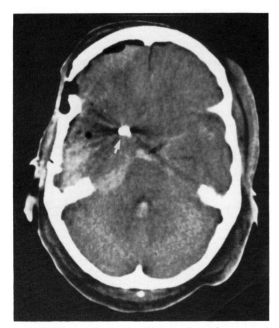

FIGURE 8–13. Intracerebral hemorrhage from a postoperative internal carotid artery rupture. The lucency (*arrow*) is the vascular clip applied to the petrous carotid for control of bleeding. The patient died 1 week later of irreversible cerebral edema following her subsequent stroke.

within the ventricular systems and reduce the risk of obstruction of the aqueduct with clot.

The rate at which focal neurologic signs develop varies with location and source. Arterial bleeding usually leads to the rapid collection of blood in the epidural space. Venous bleeders generally cause hematoma formation in the subdural space with a more gradual onset of symptoms and signs.[73] Identifying the location and size of the hematoma requires CT scanning. Rapid brain stem deterioration after posterior fossa surgery requires immediate wound exploration. Time should not be wasted on imaging. If a clot is not found, the wound can be irrigated and closed and the patient then transported for computed tomography.

BLOOD TRANSFUSIONS

The majority of cranial base operations require blood replacement, since losses often exceed 1 liter. The risk of transmission of infections such as acquired immunodeficiency syndrome (AIDS) and hepatitis is outweighed by the necessity of restoration of blood volume and hemostatic fluid balance. Excessive hemorrhage, often encountered in tumor extirpation from the lateral cranial base, poses additional potential complications with blood replacement. The incidence of direct transfusion reactions, acid-base derangements, coagulation defects, and cardiopulmonary complications increases proportionally to the number of required transfusions.[8]

Hypotension, bradycardia, and other cardiac arrythmias may be induced by the binding of citrate within preserved blood to the circulating ionized calcium. This relative hypocalcemia can be remedied by the administration of 1 gm of calcium chloride for every 2 units of transfused blood. Cardiac arrest can be induced as well by the administration of banked blood, which may have high levels of potassium. Massive transfusions should be a mix of fresh and stored whole blood to prevent induction of hyperkalemia. Lowered cardiac output or acid-base alterations may be induced by the rapid infusion of blood that has been refrigerated; transfusion of 3 to 5 units given over a 2-hour period may lower core temperature 4 degrees Centigrade. All transfusions must be warmed to body temperature prior to administration.

Coagulopathies resulting from dilutional thrombocytopenia or the clotting factor deficiencies of banked blood may increase the risk of hemorrhage and make the task of obtaining hemostasis excessively difficult. Hypocalcemia from the binding of citrate to ionized calcium may also induce aberrancies in the calcium-dependent clotting cascade, which compounds bleeding tendencies. Frequent intraoperative monitoring of prothrombin and partial thromboplastin times, serum calcium, and potassium, as well as platelet counts, is warranted during these lengthy procedures. One unit of fresh-frozen plasma and platelet packs should accompany the administration of each 4 to 5 units of banked whole blood or packed cells.[59]

Massive or rapid transfusion of blood products may precipitate acid-base derangements, coagulation defects, or cardiopulmonary complications, as previously summarized. The circulatory overload resulting from rapid volume replacement may lead to pulmonary edema and acute respiratory distress syndrome in the early postoperative period. Disseminated intravascular coagulation due to escape of fibrin and microaggregated cells from standard mesh filters may obstruct the pulmonary microvasculature and further impair oxygen diffusion. Pulmonary emboli may prove lethal, particularly in this compromised state, underlining the importance of careful attention to antithrombosis measures, use of micropore filters, and meticulous fluid balance.

PNEUMOCEPHALUS

Focal neurologic deficits can result from the accumulation of air in the cranial vault. Pressurized ventilation through a tracheostomy tube, in the setting of large, combined, intracranial and parapharyngeal resections, manufactures the situation at risk for air to be forced intracranially. Parapharyngeal tumors that after resection leave considerable dead space are most prone to this problem, owing to the surface area of pharyngeal lining which is reconstructed along with the close proximity of the intracranial cavity with the aerodigestive tract. Pneumocephalus is not uncommonly seen on postoperative CT. These small collections of air normally resorb within 7 to 10 days. Air accumulating under pressure, creating a tension pneumocephalus, is a potentially fatal complication.[64] "Ball valving" of soft tissues in the basicranial reconstruction after removal of bone, with forced inspired air entering the epidural space, can lead to mass effect and subsequent neurologic deterioration. Continuous lumbar catheter drainage may create a relative intracranial negative pressure as fluid is tapped from the subarachnoid space. This "vacuum" effect draws air into the intracranial space, through the perioperative tissue planes and the aerodigestive tract incision lines. Partic-

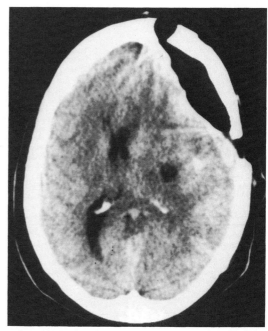

FIGURE 8–14. Tension pneumocephalus leading to midline shift of ventricles.

ular caution with lumbar drains is warranted in elderly patients whose relative laxity of brain increases the risk of pneumocephalus development.[71] Intracranial air is significant when tension develops, as indicated by signs of increased intracranial pressure or CT evidence of midline shift of the ventricles (Fig. 8–14).

A tension pneumocephalus must be rapidly decompressed, and the access of air sealed off with appropriate tissues of fascia or vascularized muscle or both. Clinically silent pockets of air, noted on scans, may need to be evacuated if their resolution is not evident on repeat scans. A search for associated cerebrospinal fluid leak is appropriate in the presence of a persistent pneumocephalus, as a concurrent cerebrospinal fluid leak has been found approximately one third of the time.

CEREBROSPINAL FLUID LEAKAGE

The development of a cerebrospinal fluid leak after skull base resection is one of the most common complications reported. Patients undergoing posterior fossa acoustic tumor removal have an average incidence of spinal fluid leakage nationwide of 10 per cent. Violation or resection of large segments of dura with extensive tumor removal has led to leaks of spinal fluid in a significant number of patients undergoing cranial base surgery through combined surgical approaches.[18, 28, 31, 42, 69, 88] The method of reconstruction seems to influence greatly the incidence of cerebrospinal fluid leakage. Whenever the continuity of the dura has been disrupted, there is a greater difficulty in re-establishing a watertight seal. Autologous grafts of fascia are used to reconstitute defects in the dura (Fig. 8–15). A watertight seal of the dura layer, although obtained whenever possible, is not essential for competent wound closure. Posterior fossa surgical defects, from a translabyrinthine approach, have been reconstructed successfully for years with autologous fat grafts. Skull base surgery, which exposes large areas of the basicranium, requires more sophisticated methods of reconstruction.[5, 43, 44, 47, 79] Free tissue transfer, with myogenous and myocutaneous grafts, has markedly decreased the incidence of postoperative cerebrospinal fluid leaks and subsequent wound infections.[47, 48]

Intraoperative lumbar drainage catheters are used to aid in the control of intracranial pressure and assist in relaxation of the brain, to minimize retraction. The catheter may be left in place in the recovery period, during which time the cerebrospinal fluid may be siphoned at a maximum rate of 300 ml/24 hours to prevent the development of a spinal fluid leak. The length of time that the drain is left in place varies with the amount of resection. On average, lumbar catheters are left in place for 5 days. The patient is kept on strict bed rest, with the head of the bed elevated between 15 and 30 degrees. A sterile mastoid style or Barton compression dressing is maintained over the wound to help with healing of the tissues. Prophylactic antibiotics are administered during the period of the catheter's occupation of the intrathecal space.[35, 65]

Reduction of cerebrospinal fluid production is aided by the use of acetazolamide sodium (Diamox Sustained-Release Tablets), administered orally in doses of 500 mg twice daily. This therapy is instituted when a persistent spinal fluid leak is apparent, adequate lumbar drainage is not completely successful, and an associated obstructive hydrocephalus is not present.

Cerebrospinal fluid leaks are one of the instigating factors in wound infections, fistula formation, and meningitis. Prevention has become more feasible with the advent of microvascular reconstructive techniques that

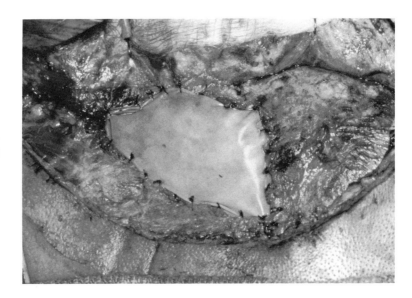

FIGURE 8–15. Dural graft reconstruction for a watertight closure.

allow closure of massive defects with well-vascularized tissues. Reconstituting the separation of the aerodigestive tract from the intracranial cavity, and preventing the egress of spinal fluid and inflow of contaminated saliva, depend upon the viability of the tissues used for reconstruction. In the event of a leak that fails to resolve after all the preventive measures mentioned, a re-exploration of the wound to replace a fascial graft may be necessary. Clear rhinorrhea or otorrhea, with a "halo sign" on a cotton sheet, alerts the clinician to the likelihood of a leak. If collectable, the fluid chemical analysis showing greater than 30 mg/ml of glucose concentration is felt confirmatory for cerebrospinal fluid, when found in the high-risk patient. Identification of beta-1 or beta-2 transferrin by immunoelectrophoresis is more specific for spinal fluid but is not a widely available test. Chloride concentration is higher in cerebrospinal fluid than in serum and is readily available in all hospitals. Documentation of a suspected leak in the nasopharynx by intrathecal instillation of radioactive isotopes and concomitant nucleotide scanning of cotton pledgets, which are left in the nasal cavity for 12 hours, is helpful when direct fluid collection is impossible. Contrast cisternography with CT imaging is available to confirm the presence of a leak and may be helpful in the localization of the site of origin.

INFECTIONS

The incidence of wound infections that can lead to complications of meningitis or peridural abscesses fortunately is not high following cranial base operations. The risk of wound infection rises with the extent of resection, length of surgery, potential dead space, and hematoma formation.[50] The development of a wound infection in the early postoperative period is highly significant, since numerous potentially life-threatening complications may ensue. The use of prophylactic antibiotics is warranted in intra- and extracranial resections owing to the in-

herent contamination of the upper aerodigestive tract bacterial flora. Antibiotics that attain high cerebrospinal fluid levels are not a primary consideration in the choice of prophylactic regimen. Vancomycin hydrochloride, 500 mg intravenously every 8 hours or 1 gram every 12 hours, provides adequate tissue levels when begun more than 6 hours preoperatively and continued for at least 24 hours after surgery. Skin pathogens, particularly the gram-positive organisms, are well covered, with minimal risk of ototoxicity or nephrotoxicity, provided the serum creatinine level is normal. Usage beyond the perioperative period should be monitored with serial creatinine and serum drug levels to ensure the adequacy of therapeutic levels. Prophylaxis against some gram-negative bacilli or anaerobic organisms when gross contamination with aerodigestive secretions is anticipated can be accomplished with ampicillin in doses of 500 to 1000 mg and metronidazole hydrochloride (Flagyl), 500 mg every 6 hours, intravenously. Gentamicin sulfate (80 mg every 8 hours) and clindamycin phosphate (300 to 600 mg every 8 hours) also make an effective prophylactic regimen, providing coverage against gram-positive and -negative organisms, as well as anaerobes. Precautions for nephro-ototoxicity are needed with the aminoglycosides, particularly when used with vancomycin.

Preparations of ampicillin sodium with sulbactam (Unasyn) offer single-regimen administration in doses of 1.5 to 3.0 gm every 6 hours, to provide broad-spectrum coverage against mixed flora, including beta-lactamase–producing gram-positive organisms and anaerobic bacteria. These can be used for perioperative prophylaxis in surgical fields contaminated by upper aerodigestive tract flora or therapeutically in the event of a documented infection. The newer generation of cephalosporins provides better gram-negative coverage, and these are indicated when contamination with *Pseudomonas* is likely. Ceftazidime, 1 to 2 gm intravenously every 8 hours, provides excellent anti-*Pseudomonas* coverage but is usually reserved for documented infections.

Wound infections are frequently associated

with problems resulting from inadequate or complicated reconstructions. Large defects that have been reconstructed with poorly vascularized tissues or autologous grafts are more prone to breakdown and resultant complications of spinal fluid leakage and fistula formation.[9, 10] The classic findings of skin erythema, swelling, tissue hyperemia, and drainage may be absent in the early stages of deep wound infection. Febrile episodes noted on routine vital sign records are often early warning signs of a postoperative infectious process. White blood cell counts with leukocyte differential, chest radiograph, urinalysis, and serial blood cultures are the immediate laboratory studies with which to search out a cause for the temperature elevations. A common cause of fever is pulmonary atelectasis. Alveoli are readily re-expanded by vigorous pulmonary toilet, incentive spirometry, or positive-pressure ventilation. A visible pulmonary infiltrate on chest radiograph is managed similarly while broad-spectrum antibiotic therapy is begun pending the identification of a specific pathogen by sputum culture. Indwelling urinary or central intravenous catheters in place for more than 5 days after surgery should be cultured, replaced, or discontinued if they are suspected as a nidus for infection by urinalysis or blood culture results. Meningitis should always be considered and lumbar puncture performed when a febrile source can not be found.[30] Consultation by infectious disease specialists can be of considerable benefit when an infection is not readily located but is suspected on clinical grounds. Rare causes of fever, such as medication reactions, deep venous thrombosis, pulmonary embolus, parotitis, or prostatis, can be identified more quickly when consultation is obtained.

The identification of a deep tissue infection is aided greatly by computed tomography or magnetic resonance imaging of the head and neck (Fig. 8–16). Areas of lucency adjacent to sites of the primary resection with contrast enhancement of the periphery are highly suspicious for an abscess. Computer-directed aspiration or, if accessible, direct drainage techniques will document the infection. Ad-

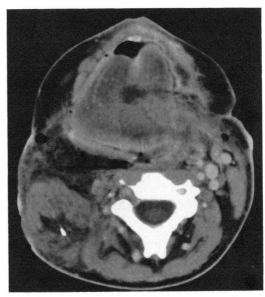

FIGURE 8–16. Deep tissue infection in parapharyngeal space following cranial base resection.

equate drainage and antibiotic therapy directed toward specific sensitive organisms is the required management. Subdural, epidural, and parapharyngeal abscesses mandate emergency open drainage and may require revision of the reconstruction with well-vascularized tissues, as afforded by pedicled myocutaneous or freely transferred myogenous grafts.[79] Reconstruction revisions occasionally are staged after the primary infection is controlled, to preclude loculating an abscess by a more competent technique in closure. The goal of obtaining separation of the intracranial cavity from the aerodigestive tract must be accomplished with the reconstruction to prevent the sequela of meningitis when a spinal fluid leak exists.

Antibiotic therapy is directed by the culture and organism sensitivity results, serum levels of the drugs, and advice from infectious disease consultants. Combinations of antibiotics are frequently necessary to clear the deep soft tissue infections that may occur following extensive skull base resections.[90] Vigilant monitoring to recognize potential adverse effects of therapy and to ensure eradication of the infection is paramount to the patient's eventual recovery.

CRANIAL NERVE INJURIES

Cranial nerves I through XII may be at risk for dysfunction postoperatively after cranial base resection, depending on the extent of dissection and location of the primary lesion (Fig. 8–17). The decision to resect specific nerves involved with tumor is dictated by the histologic process and the degree of function present before surgery.[76] When malignant lesions involve neural structures their removal is mandatory and a careful search must be made for microscopic neural involvement by frozen section examination at the time of operation. Squamous cell and adenoid cystic carcinomas have a great propensity for intra- and perineural growth, thus necessitating aggressive excision of nerves adjacent to tumor (Fig. 8–18). Benign lesions that cause compressive neuropathies, such as meningiomas and paragangliomas, may exhibit extensive involvement of the nerves

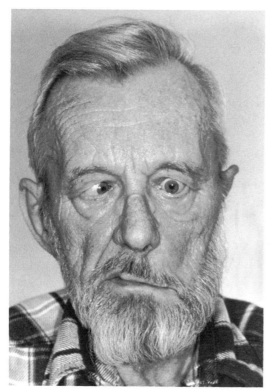

FIGURE 8–17. Paralysis of left abducens and facial nerves secondary to a temporal bone lesion involving the petrous apex.

exiting from the cranial base.[32] Their preservation may not be feasible. Microdissection techniques and electrophysiologic monitoring have evolved to enhance the preservation of cranial nerves during tumor resection.[37, 67] Attempts to control bleeding, particularly at the jugular foramen and cavernous sinus, may produce nerve paresis due to overzealous packing with oxidized cellulose. Prevention of this complication may be avoided by gentle surgical technique to obtain hemostasis with the least amount of packing possible. Locating the several inferior petrosal sinus openings into the medial jugular bulb, which may be packed with small pledgets of Surgicel, is helpful in the prevention of overpacking of the jugular fossa (see Fig. 8–7).

The management of the sequelae of cranial neuropathies following cranial base resection has evolved over the past decades to afford considerable remediation. The common problems associated with facial paralysis involve incompetent eye closure and exposure keratitis. Lacri-Lube ophthalmic ointment and a moisture chamber or lid taping at night, along with the application of artificial tears every 2 hours, will prevent drying of the eye in the immediate postoperative period. Ophthalmologic evaluation with corneal staining is advisable for a baseline examination to rule out any corneal abrasions. The placement of a gold weight or spring in the upper eyelid will restore competent lid closure on a temporary or permanent basis (Fig. 8–19). Canthoplasty of the lower eyelid is necessary in those individuals who develop significant ectropion or have extreme lower lid laxity that prevents complete corneal protection. Marked disfigurement of the face, with asymmetry and oral incompetence, may need to be corrected by muscle sling procedures using the temporalis or masseter muscle. Primary or crossed facial nerve grafting, or hypoglossal-to-facial nerve anastamosis, is useful in restoring tonus to the facial musculature, as are primary nerve grafts in suitable candidates.[7, 20] Electrical stimulation of the face, massages, and biofeedback exercises are directed by the physical therapists and are often helpful in maximizing the effects of the facial reanimation procedures.

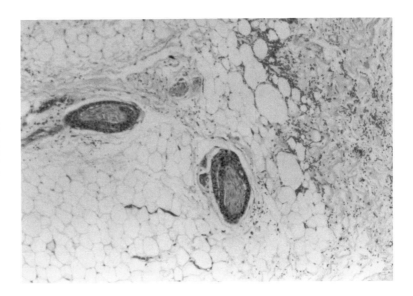

FIGURE 8–18. Perineural growth of an adenoid cystic carcinoma along peripheral nerves resected from the infratemporal fossa.

Problems with deglutition and phonation are not infrequent following skull base surgery, owing to the paresis or paralysis of the glossopharyngeal and vagus nerves. Perioperative pulmonary toilet through the tracheostomy helps prevent pneumonia. Decannulation of the tracheostomy is accomplished, along with assessment of the vocal cord function, by direct fiberoptic laryngos-copy, and swallowing evaluation by modified barium cineradiography. Persistent aspiration may require medialization of the vocal cord by endoscopic injection of Teflon or collagen or an external thyroplasty procedure. Pooling of secretions in the piriform sinus, resulting in aspiration, may be corrected by cricopharyngeal myotomy.[62] The latter problem may be particularly bother-

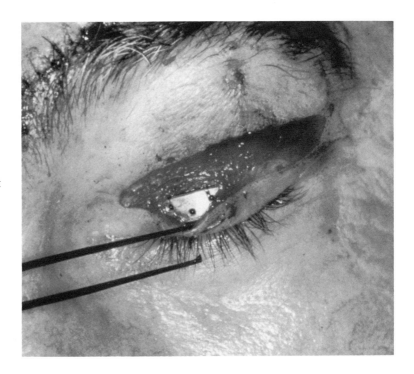

FIGURE 8–19. Gold weight implant in upper eyelid.

some and seems to be caused by the lack of pharyngeal sensation following glossopharyngeal nerve section. Swallowing training by a speech pathologist is often most beneficial to patients so afflicted.

SEIZURES

The occurrence of seizures in the postoperative period may signal the development of a hemorrhage, venous or arterial infarction, hematoma, or other complication leading to a mass effect and cerebral irritation. Manipulation, dissection, or resection of brain parenchyma can lead to an irritable focus of the cerebrum manifesting as focal seizures. Prophylactic anticonvulsant therapy with phenytoin (Dilantin) is advocated whenever considerable manipulation or resection of the brain has been required for tumor removal. The initial loading dose is 18 mg/kg intravenously followed by maintenance dosing of 300 mg per day. Clinical observation of persistent seizure activity, along with serial serum drug levels, guides adjustment of the dosing regimen.[38, 63]

References

1. Al-Mefty O: Supraorbital-pterional approach to skull base lesions. Neurosurgery 21:474–477, 1987.
2. Al-Mefty O, Fox JL, Smith RR: Petrosal approach for petroclival meningiomas. Neurosurgery 22:510–517, 1988.
3. Ames A, Wright RL, Masayoshi K, et al: Cerebral ischemia: The no-reflow phenomenon. Am J Pathol 52:437–447, 1987.
4. Ariyan S, Sasaki CT, Spencer D: Radical en bloc resection of the temporal bone. Am J Surg 142:443–447, 1981.
5. Bakamjian VY, Souther S: Use of temporal muscle flap for reconstruction after orbito-maxillary resections for cancer. Plast Reconstr Surg 56:171–177, 1975.
6. Bakay L, Lee JC: The effect of acute hypoxia and hypercapnia on the ultrastructure of the central nervous system. Brain 91:697–706, 1968.
7. Baker DC, Conley J: Facial nerve grafting: A 30 year retrospective review. Clin Plast Surg 6:343–351, 1979.
8. Baker RJ, Nyhus LM: Diagnosis and treatment of immediate transfusion reaction. Surg Gynecol Obstet 130:665–670, 1970.
9. Baker SR: Closure of large orbital-maxillary defects with free latissimus dorsi myocutaneous flaps. Head Neck 6:828–835, 1984.
10. Baker SR: Surgical reconstruction after extensive skull base surgery. Otolaryngol Clin North Am 17:591–599, 1984.
11. Balo J: The dural venous sinuses. Anat Rec 106:319–325, 1950.
12. Brackmann DE: The facial nerve in the infratemporal approach. Otolaryngol Head Neck Surg 97:15–17, 1987.
13. Brookes GB, Graham M: Benign intracranial hypertension complicating glomus jugulare tumor surgery. Am J Otol 5:350–354, 1984.
14. Brugge KG, Lasjaunias P, Chiu MC: Super-selective angiography and embolization of skull base tumors. Can J Neurol Sci 12:341–344, 1985.
15. Cece JA, Lawson W, Biller HF, et al: Complications in the management of large glomus jugulare tumors. Laryngoscope 97:152–157, 1987.
16. Challa VR, Moody DM, Marshall RB, et al: The vascular component in meningiomas associated with severe cerebral edema. Neurosurgery 7:363–368, 1980.
17. Chiang J, Masayoshi K, Ames A, et al: Cerebral ischemia: Vascular changes. Am J Pathol 52:455–465, 1968.
18. Close LG, Mickey BE, Samson DS, et al: Resection of upper aerodigestive tract tumors involving the middle cranial fossa. Laryngoscope 95:908–914, 1985.
19. Condon RE, Nyhus LM: Blood transfusion reactions. *In* Manual of Surgical Therapeutics. Boston, Little, Brown, 1975, pp 298–300.
20. Conley J, Baker DC: Hypoglossal-facial nerve anastomosis for reinnervation of the paralyzed face. Plast Reconstr Surg 63:63–72, 1979.
21. Dandy WE: The brain. In Lewis D (ed): Practice of Surgery. Vol 12. Hagerstown, MD, WF Prior Co, 1945, pp 1–671.
22. Devries EJ, Sekhar LN, Janecka IP, et al: Elective resection of the internal carotid artery without reconstruction. Laryngoscope 98:960–966, 1988.
23. Fisch U: Infratemporal fossa approach to tumors of the temporal bone and base of the skull. J Laryngol Otol 92:949–967, 1978.
24. Fisch U: Infratemporal fossa approach for glomus tumors of the temporal bone. Ann Otol Rhinol Laryngol 91:474–479, 1982.
25. Fisch U, Derald J, Senning A: Surgical therapy of internal carotid artery lesions of the skull base and temporal bone. Otolaryngol Head Neck Surg 88:548–554, 1980.
26. Fitz-Hugh GS, Robins RB, Craddock WD: Increased intracranial pressure complicating unilateral neck dissection. Laryngoscope 76:893–906, 1966.
27. Friedman WH, Katsantonis GP, Cooper MH, et al: Stylohamular dissection: A new method for en bloc resection of malignancies of the infratemporal fossa. Laryngoscope 91:1–11, 1981.
28. Gardner G, Robertson JH, Clark WC: Transtemporal approaches to the cranial cavity. Am Otol 6:114–120, 1985.
29. Gardner G, Cocke EW, Robertson JH, et al: Skull base surgery for glomus jugulare tumor. Am J Otol 6:126–134, 1985.
30. Garfield J: Intracranial abscess. In Symon L, Thomas D, Clark K (eds): Rob and Smith's Operative Surgery, Neurosurgery. 4th ed. London, Butterworth and Co, 1989, pp 83–93.

31. Glasscock ME, Dickins JRE: Complications of acoustic tumor surgery. Otolaryngol Clin North Am 15:883–895, 1982.
32. Glasscock ME, Jackson CG, Dickins JRE, Wiet RJ: Panel discussion: Glomus jugulare tumors of the temporal bone: The surgical management of glomus tumors. Laryngoscope 89:1640–1655, 1979.
33. Glasscock ME, Smith PG, Schwaber MK, Nissen AJ: Clinical aspects of the skull base. Laryngoscope 94:869–873, 1984.
34. Goldenberg RA: Surgeon's view of the skull base from the lateral approach. Laryngoscope 94:1–21, 1984.
35. Graf CJ, Gross CE, Beck DW: Complications of spinal drainage in the management of cerebrospinal fluid fistulae: Report of three cases. J Neurosurg 54:392–395, 1980.
36. Harris FS, Rhoton AL: Anatomy of the cavernous sinus. J Neurosurg 45:169, 1976.
37. Hitselberger WE, House WF: A combined approach to the cerebellopontine angle. Arch Otolaryngol 84:267–285, 1966.
38. Horwitz NH, Rizzoli HV: Postoperative Complications of Intracranial Neurological Surgery. Baltimore, Williams and Wilkins, 1982, pp 1–34.
39. Huang YP, Wolf BS: The veins of the posterior fossa—superior or galenic draining group. Am J Roentgenol 45:808–821, 1965.
40. Humphreys DH, Schwartz MR, Jenkins HA: Meningioma: A case of transcranial recurrence managed by base-of-skull technique and a review of the tumor. Otolaryngol Head Neck Surg 93:563–570, 1985.
41. Jackson CG, Glasscock ME, McKennan K, et al: The surgical treatment of skull-base tumors with intracranial extension. Otolaryngol Head Neck Surg 96:175–185, 1987.
42. Jackson CG, Glasscock ME, Nissen AJ, Schwaber MK: Glomus tumor surgery: The approach, results and problems. Otolaryngol Clin North Am 15:897–915, 1982.
43. Jackson IT: Advances in craniofacial tumor surgery. World J Surg 13:440–453, 1989.
44. Jackson IT, Adham MN, Marsh WR: The use of galeal frontalis flap in craniofacial surgery. Plast Reconstr Surg 76:905, 1986.
45. Johanson C: The central veins and deep dural sinuses of the brain. Acta Radiol Suppl 107, 1954.
46. Johns ME, Winn HR, McLean WF, Cantrell RW: Pericranial flap for the closure of defects of cranial resections. Laryngoscope 91:952–958, 1981.
47. Jones NF, Schramm VL, Sekhar LN: Reconstruction of the cranial base following tumour resection. Br J Plast Surg 40:155–162, 1987.
48. Jones NF, Sekhar LN, Schramm VL: Free rectus abdominis muscle flap reconstruction of the middle and posterior cranial base. Plast Reconstr Surg 78:471–479, 1986.
49. Kazan R: The neurosurgeon in skull base operations. Otolaryngol Clin North Am 4:925–938, 1982.
50. Ketchum AS, Hoye RC, Van Buren JM, Johnson RH: Complications of intracranial facial resection for tumors of the paranasal sinuses. Am J Surg 112:591–596, 1966.
51. Kinal ME: Hydrocephalus and the dural venous sinuses. J Neurosurg 19:195–201, 1962.
52. Kinney SE, Sebak BA: Rare tumors of the skull base and temporal bone. Am J Otol (Suppl), 1985, pp 135–142.
53. Krespi YP: Cancer surgery of the skull base. Clin Plast Surg 12:389–392, 1985.
54. Krespi YP, Sisson GA: Skull base surgery in composite resection. Arch Otolaryngol 108:681–684, 1982.
55. Kumar A, Valvassori G, Mafee M, Jafar J: Skull base lesions: A classification and surgical approaches. Laryngoscope 96:252–263, 1986.
56. Lambert PR, Johns ME, Winn RH: Infralabyrinthine approach to skull-base lesions. Otolaryngol Head Neck Surg 93:250–258, 1985.
57. Landolt AM, Millikan CH: Pathogenesis of cerebral infarction secondary to mechanical carotid artery occlusion. Stroke 1:52–62, 1970.
58. Leonetti JP, Smith PG, Grubb RL: Management of neurovascular complications in extended skull base surgery. Laryngoscope 99:492–496, 1989.
59. Leonetti JP, Smith PG, Grubb RL: Control of bleeding in extended skull base surgery. Am J Otol 11:254–259, 1990.
60. Leonetti JP, Smith PG, Grubb RL: The perioperative management of the petrous carotid artery in contemporary surgery of the skull base. Otolaryngol Head Neck Surg 103:446–451, 1990.
61. Leonetti JP, Smith PG, Linthicum F: The petrous carotid artery: Anatomic relationships in skull base surgery. Otolaryngol Head Neck Surg 102:3–12, 1990.
62. Levine TM: Swallowing disorders following skull base surgery. Otolaryngol Clin North Am 21:751–759, 1988.
63. Malis LI: Surgical resection of tumors of the skull base. In Wilkins RH, Rengachary SS (eds): Neurosurgery. New York, McGraw-Hill, 1985, pp 1011–1021.
64. Matsuba HW, Thawley SE, Smith PG: Tension pneumocephalus: A case following surgery. Am J Otol 7:208–209, 1986.
65. McCallum J, Maroon JC, Janetta PJ: Treatment of postoperative cerebrospinal fluid fistulas by subarachnoid drainage. J Neurosurg 42:434–437, 1975.
66. Mickey B, Close L, Schaefer S, Samson D: A combined frontotemporal and lateral infratemporal fossa approach to the skull base. J Neurosurg 68:678–683, 1988.
67. Moller AR: Electrophysiologic monitoring of cranial nerves in operations in the skull base. In Sekhar LN, Schramm VL (eds): Tumors of the Cranial Base—Diagnosis and Treatment. New York, Futura Publishing Co, 1987, pp 124–132.
68. Moloy PJ, Brackmann DE: Control of venous bleeding in otologic surgery. Laryngoscope 96:580–582, 1986.
69. Myers DL, Sataloff RT: Spinal fluid leakage after skull base surgical procedures. Otolaryngol Clin North Am 17:601–611, 1984.
70. Nager G, Heroy J, Hoeplinger M: Meningiomas invading the temporal bone with extension to the neck. Am J Otol 4:297–324, 1983.
71. Pitta LH, Wilson CB, Dedo HH, et al: Pneumocephalus following ventriculoperitoneal shunt: Case report. J Neurosurg 43:631–633, 1976.
72. Poppen JL: Prevention of postoperative extradural hematoma. Arch Neurol Psychiatry 34:1068–1069, 1935.
73. Rosen HM, Simeone FA: Spontaneous subdural hygromas: A complication following craniofacial surgery. Ann Plast Surg 18:245–247, 1987.

74. Samii J, Ammirati M, Mahran A, et al: Surgery of petroclival meningiomas: Report of 24 cases. Neurosurgery 24:12–17, 1989.
75. Sasarki C: Spectrum of exposures for skull base tumors. Clin Neurosurg 34:467–484, 1988.
76. Sataloff RT, Myers DL, Kremer FB: Management of cranial nerve injury following surgery of the skull base. Otolaryngol Clin North Am 17:577–589, 1984.
77. Sataloff RT, Myers DL, Lowry LD, Spiegel JR: Total temporal bone resection of squamous cell carcinoma. Otolaryngol Head Neck Surg 96:4–14, 1987.
78. Schettini A, Cook AW, Owre ES: Hyperventilation in craniotomy for brain tumor. Anesthesia 28:363–371, 1967.
79. Schuller DE: Latissimus dorsi myocutaneous flaps for massive facial defects. Arch Otolaryngol 108:414–417, 1982.
80. Schuller DE, Hart M, Goodman JH: The surgery of benign and malignant neoplasms adjacent to or involving the skull base. Am J Otolaryngol 10:305–313, 1989.
81. Sekhar LN, Janecka IP, Jones NF: Subtemporal-infratemporal and basal subfrontal approach to extensive cranial base tumors. Acta Neurochir (Wien) 92:83–92, 1988.
82. Sekhar LN, Moller AR: Operative management of tumors involving the cavernous sinus. J Neurosurg 64:879–889, 1986.
83. Sekhar LN, Sen CN, Jho HE, Janecka IP: Surgical treatment of intracavernous neoplasms: A four-year experience. Neurosurgery 24:18–30, 1989.
84. Sekhar LN, Schramm VL, Jones NF, et al: Operative exposure and management of the petrous and upper cervical internal carotid artery. Neurosurgery 19:967–982, 1986.
85. Sekhar LN, Schramm VL, Jones NF: Subtemporal-preauricular infratemporal fossa approach to large lateral and posterior cranial base neoplasms. J Neurosurg 67:488–499, 1987.
86. Smith HP, Challs VR, Moiody DM, et al: Biologic features of meningiomas that determine the production of cerebral edema. Neurosurgery 8:433–458, 1981.
87. Smith PG, Killeen TE: Carotid artery vasospasm complicating extensive skull base surgery: Cause, prevention and management. Otolaryngol Head Neck Surg 97:1–7, 1987.
88. Smith PG, Grubb RL, Kletzker GR, Leonetti JP: Combined pterional-anterolateral approaches to cranial base tumor. Otolaryngol Head Neck Surg 103:357–363, 1990.
89. Spector GJ, Sobol S: Surgery for glomus tumors at the skull base. Otolaryngol Head Neck Surg 88:524–530, 1980.
90. Strong AJ, Ingham HR: Surgical and microbiologic management of subdural and extradural abscesses. In Symon L, Thomas D, Clark K (eds): Rob and Smith's Operative Surgery, Neurosurgery. 4th ed. London, Butterworth and Co, 1989, pp 94–101.
91. Symon L: Control of intracranial tension. In Symon L, Thomas D, Clark K (eds): Rob and Smith's Operative Surgery, Neurosurgery. 4th ed. London, Butterworth and Co, 1989, pp 1–11.
92. Symonds CP: Hydrocephalic and focal cerebral symptoms in relation to thrombophlebitis of the dural sinuses and cerebral veins. Brain 60:531–550, 1937.
93. Urken ML, Biller HF, Haimov M: Intratemporal carotid artery bypass in resection of a base of skull tumor. Laryngoscope 95:1472–1477, 1985.
94. Weiss RM: Massive epidural hematoma complicating ventricular decompression: Report of a case with survival. J Neurosurg 21:235–236, 1968.

CHAPTER 9

Skull Base Surgery Complications

J. GREGORY STAFFEL, MD
HAROLD C. PILLSBURY, III, MD

Skull base surgical procedures encompass a broad anatomic area and multiple types of tumors. Each tumor requires a specifically tailored surgical approach. The skull base itself is composed of the frontal bone, encircling the posterior table of the frontal sinus; the floor of the anterior cranial fossa, which consists of the cribriform plate, the fovea ethmoidalis, and the roofs of the orbit; progressing posteriorly to sphenoid bone; and subsequently to the petrous apex and the rest of the temporal bone, ending in the occipital bone. The clivus is also considered part of the skull base.

The first decision to be made in the management of any patient with a tumor of the skull base is whether or not to operate. This decision is based on many factors, including overall health and age of the patient, type of tumor, life expectancy after resection, expected morbidity, and quality of life after resection. Although an unresectable tumor is an issue that must be discussed and individualized with each patient, in general certain factors predispose the physician to nonop-

erative treatment: involvement of the sphenoid sinus with a malignant process, involvement of both orbits or both optic nerves with a malignant process, invasion of the cavernous sinus, complete destruction of the clivus, involvement of the carotid artery near the sphenoid sinus or petrous apex, and distant metastasis. As always in medicine, these are only general guidelines, and few inviolable rules exist.

The delineation of the extent of the tumor has advanced logarithmically with the development of computed tomography (CT) and magnetic resonance imaging (MRI). These have assured the possibility of appropriate preoperative consultations as well as counseling of the patient. This was not always possible prior to these imaging modalities. Although this chapter focuses on the complications of skull base surgery, the postoperative deficits are more often expected sequelae of extirpative and curative tumor surgery rather than unexpected technical complications.

A partial listing of tumors that often involve the skull base includes esthesioneuro-blastoma, squamous and adenocarcinoma of the ethmoid and maxillary sinuses, sinonasal undifferentiated carcinoma, juvenile naso-pharyngeal angiofibroma, chordoma, glomus jugulare or vagale and carotid body tumors, acoustic neuroma, and petrous apex choles-teatoma and meningioma. What follows is a description of some of the complications of operation for these and other skull base neo-plasms.

CEREBROSPINAL FLUID LEAKS

Cerebrospinal fluid (CSF) leaks are a con-stant concern in any skull base operation. At best, they are annoying, and at worst, they lead to meningitis. They occur most com-monly when a large piece of dura must be resected. The larger the defect in the dura, the more likely a CSF leak. Thus, in resection of large acoustic neuromas via a translabyrin-thine approach in which a significant piece of the dura may be resected and reconstruc-tion is usually limited to placing strips of fat into the defect, the chance of a CSF leak is perhaps higher than in the case of a cranio-facial resection, in which good visualization of the dura can be had. If any dura is resected in a craniofacial resection, a repair can be accomplished in a multilayered fashion with suturing. As with any complication, the best way of treating it is to prevent it. Preventing CSF leak includes determining preopera-tively how much of the dura is involved. This often includes obtaining CT scans in both the axial and coronal planes and an MRI scan in consultation with a neurosurgeon.

If, during the operation, a tear in the dura is encountered, it is reapproximated, if pos-sible, with a watertight technique. This can be reinforced with pericranium temporalis fascia, cadaver dura, or fascia lata grafts. If the region is then to be exposed to the upper aerodigestive tract, a split-thickness skin graft may be applied. If a large piece of dura has to be resected because of involvement with a tumor, the reconstruction is done, once again, by creating a watertight seal with pericranium, temporalis fascia, fascia lata, or cadaver dura. Another possibility is a micro-vascular transfer of a free myofascial flap, and this is often the preferred method of reconstruction when the area being resected has received previous radiation therapy.

Johnson and associates have used tempo-ralis fascia covered with a rectus abdominis microvascular free flap with good success in large skull base tumors that invade the cra-nial cavity.[1] Reconstruction of the floor of the anterior cranial vault after craniofacial resec-tion classically has involved a pericranial flap rotated through the bottom of the craniotomy defect and sewn to the dura near the planum sphenoidale.[2] Certain surgeons have added bone or cartilage before placing the skin graft on the nasal side of the defect.[3] Nasal packing is generally used for 5 to 7 days until the skin graft has taken. More recently, Snyder-man and associates have determined not only that bone or cartilage is not necessary for adequate support, but also that the skin graft and nasal packing may not be needed.[4] They observed the appearance of good nasal sur-face mucosa with no increase in the incidence of meningitis or CSF leak. In the translaby-rinthine approach to an acoustic neuroma, the most common method of preventing CSF leaks is by using fat to obliterate the defect in the bone and the dura. It is also important to use bone wax to prevent the cerebrospinal fluid from leaking into the mastoid air cells and subsequently into the ear and nasophar-ynx. If this is not adequate, a middle fossa approach may be necessary in order to repair the dura as previously mentioned.

Another way of preventing CSF leaks is to check for them at the end of the procedure; thus, a Valsalva maneuver should be per-formed by the anesthesiologist, or, if possi-ble, the patient's head should be dropped lower than the heart to increase the CSF pressure at the possible site of leak. A lumbar drain should be left in place for 5 to 7 days after the operation if the possibility of a CSF leak is felt to be high.

CSF leaks may develop postoperatively de-spite all attempts at prevention. The symp-tom is usually clear fluid draining into the nasopharynx or out the ear. This fluid, if mixed with blood, may exhibit the classic ring sign if placed on any surface exposing the liquid to capillary action, such as filter paper or bed linens. This clear fluid, if it can be collected, also will reveal a significant amount of glucose if the patient does not have meningitis. Normal CSF contains approximately two thirds the glucose concentration of serum; normal nasal secretions do not contain glucose. CSF also contains about 124 mEq/l of chloride whereas nasal secretions do not contain chloride. Tau transferrin is another entity found only in CSF, and it may be detected by electrophoresis, immunofixation, and silver staining.[5, 6]

Once the diagnosis of CSF leak has been made, the surgeon usually has a pretty good idea of where it is coming from. Occasionally, however, the exact anatomic site of the leak may not be obvious. Attempts to localize the site of leak include injecting a dye into the CSF and watching for its appearance in either the wound, the nose, or the ear. Indigo carmine, methylene blue, and fluorescein all have been used; however, methylene blue has caused neurologic sequelae and should be avoided.[7] Fluorescein also can cause an arachnoiditis and should be used in low concentration.[8] Neuropatties are placed in the decongested nose after injection of the dyes, and direct visualization and staining of these neuropatties may lead to localization of the fistula. An ultraviolet light can be used to help look for the fluorescein both in the nose and on the neuropatties. Once the dye is in, the patient may be asked to perform the Valsalva maneuver, or the patient's head may be placed lower than the heart to encourage leakage of the dye. The same technique can be used with radioactive tracers such as technetium-99m DTPA and albumin labeled with ^{131}I; however, the localization in this particular case is less accurate and requires a gamma counter. An advantage of this technique is the minimal meningeal irritation. One disadvantage is the absorption of the isotope into the blood with subsequent secretion into the nasal secretions, causing a false-positive result.

In another method, contrast radiography using iodophendolate or metrizamide in-

trathecally can be used. After the contrast is injected into the intrathecal space, the patient is once again placed in the head down position and a CT scan is obtained to try to locate the leak. Iodophendolate is quite viscous and has a high incidence of meningeal irritation. Metrizamide is less viscous; however, it does not last as long so imaging must be done fairly quickly. There is a significant incidence of headache, nausea, and vomiting with metrizamide; valium or phenobarbital can be given to reduce the risk of seizure. As one might expect, large leaks are more easily visualized with contrast medium followed by CT scanning, whereas small leaks are perhaps best localized by dyes and radioactive tracers. If the metrizamide scan is negative but there is still significant suspicion of CSF leak, an overpressure metrizamide study can be obtained. In this study, the intrathecal pressure is raised to 40 to 50 cm H_2O for approximately 15 minutes utilizing a Harvard pump and artificial CSF (Elliot solution) to promote leakage and subsequent visualization. Radioactive tracers may be used at the same time.

Initial treatment of a CSF leak simply may involve placement of a lumbar drain and observation for several days. Coverage with antibiotic therapy is controversial, with views both supporting and opposing it.[9] In general, if the leak is into a contaminated area such as the nose, antibiotic coverage should be considered strongly. If, on the other hand, the leak is into a relatively sterile area such as the ear, antibiotic coverage may be withheld.

If the leak does not stop with an adequate trial of a lumbar drain, repair must be undertaken. The technique to be used depends upon the location of the leak. If the leak is near the cribriform plate, a septal mucoperichondrial flap may be used. If it is in the sphenoid sinus, a fascia graft followed by filling the sinus with fat may be used. If it is fairly large and in the anterior cranial base, the same techniques should be used as for intraoperative repair, including watertight closure with pericranium temporalis fascia, fascia lata, or cadaver dura. A regional myocutaneous or free myofascial flap also may be considered. The technique of repair is usually tailored to the site and size of the leak.[10] Success in operative repair of CSF leaks is not assured. Even experienced surgeons have a failure rate of approximately 20 per cent.[9]

MENINGITIS

Meningitis is a rare but serious complication of skull base surgery. Often the meninges are exposed directly to the upper aerodigestive tract during surgery and so are protected only by a pericranial flap and skin graft or some other relatively thin material. It is almost puzzling why meningitis does not occur more often in view of the extensive exposure of the meninges during operations such as craniofacial resection.

Many factors predispose to meningitis; probably the most significant is a residual CSF leak from the time of operation. Indeed, infection rates range from 9 per cent to 36 per cent when CSF leakage persists beyond two weeks.[11] Other factors that predispose to infection include procedures lasting several hours and with many people entering and leaving the operating room. Measures to reduce the chances of meningitis include standard surgical techniques that prevent infection, use of perioperative antibiotics, obliteration of dead space, meticulous hemostasis, debridement of any devitalized tissue, avoidance of any foreign material in the wound, and irrigating the wound with antibiotic solution.[12]

If meningitis develops, the clinical signs are usually headache, fever, and a stiff neck. Laboratory values show CSF leukocytosis with a preponderance of neutrophils, a glucose level that is usually less than one half of the simultaneous serum glucose, and an elevated CSF protein concentration. Culture and sensitivity study results should direct the antibiotic therapy. The advent of newer antibiotics with broad-spectrum gram-negative coverage combined with excellent CSF penetration (such as ceftriaxone) has helped prevent and treat these infections.

Another possibility includes aseptic meningitis in which the clinical picture is one of bacterial meningitis; however, no organisms are cultured from the CSF. Although not well understood, the etiology has been suggested to be the presence of blood breakdown products in the CSF. It is sometimes difficult to differentiate between aseptic meningitis and a partially treated bacterial meningitis, in which case the safest course is to treat the patient as if it initially were a case of bacterial meningitis.[12]

HEMORRHAGE

Hemorrhage is a frequent and serious complication of skull base surgical procedures for many reasons. Tumors that involve the skull base are often quite vascular, with predictable and multiple blood supplies, particularly the juvenile nasopharyngeal angiofibroma, as well as the carotid body, glomus jugulare, or glomus vagale tumor. Also, venous drainage often occurs through intradural venous sinuses. These cannot be tied off in the same manner as a peripheral vein, and back bleeding can be a problem. In addition, operation of the skull base often involves drilling away bone and exposing marrow, which can be a significant source of blood loss as well as a possible source of air embolism.

Aside from the standard surgical techniques of adequate exposure and vessel ligation, adjunctive measures have been taken to reduce bleeding during operation on some of these tumors. Specifically, in the juvenile nasopharyngeal angiofibroma, preoperative embolization of the vascular supply was first performed in the early 1970s by Dr. Roberson and his colleagues, Drs. Biller, Sessions, and Ogura.[13] Following this, in 1975, Pletcher and associates published their series of 7 embolized juvenile nasopharyngeal angiofibromas compared with 16 historical controls. These patients were embolized using Gelfoam and the surgeons noted that the average amount of blood lost in the embolized group was one half that of the control group.[14] Later followup series of juvenile nasopharyngeal angiofibroma resection cases by Economou and colleagues,[15] as well as the experience of Spector,[16] confirm that preoperative embolization decreased the amount of blood loss in these cases.

Once embolization of juvenile nasopharyngeal angiofibromas was shown to be effective, it was just a matter of time before radiologic technology progressed to the point at which superselective embolization could be performed. It was left, then, for Ward and associates to confirm the usefulness of superselective embolization in carotid body tumors[17] and for Young and group to confirm the usefulness of superselective embolization in glomus jugulare tumors.[18] Ward's series was composed of 17 cases of carotid body tumors. Eleven cases were resected without embolization, with an estimated blood loss of greater than 1000 ml per case. Six cases were operated with polyvinyl ethanol embolization, and the estimated blood loss averaged less than 400 ml. The operating time for the nonembolized cases was also two to three times as long as the operating time for the embolized cases. No cranial nerve injuries occurred in the embolized patients; however, numerous cranial injuries were sustained during the resection of the nonembolized group. The patients were heavily sedated when they were undergoing the embolization, and operative resection occurred within 24 hours of the embolization. In Young's series of glomus jugulare tumors, in ten cases without superselective embolization, the estimated blood loss averaged 2800 ml, and the average operating time was 9.6 hours. Three cases were done with superselective embolization: the average blood loss was only 750 ml and the average operating time was only 7.6 hours. Murphy and Brackmann noted a significant decrease in blood loss (2769 versus 1122 ml) and operative time (7.95 versus 7.04 hours) in 18 embolized patients compared with the 17 controls.[19]

Amid the enthusiasm for embolization and superselective embolization of vascular skull base tumors, some surgeons have not had such dramatic success with embolization. Indeed, Duvall and Moreano noted that the last five patients of their series had been embolized using Gelfoam. They did not notice a large decrease in bleeding and, indeed, the specimens failed to demonstrate the presence of Gelfoam or histologic tumor infarction on microscopic examination. This brings to light the fact that technique is important during embolization of skull base tumors. In general, the resection should occur within 24 hours of the embolization as collaterals open up quite quickly. Possible complications of embolization include stroke and cranial nerve palsies secondary either to tumor swelling or embolization of the vasa nervosa.[18, 21] The nerves affected are usually nerves IX through XII, which are supplied by the posterior neuromeningeal branch of the ascending pharyngeal artery.[22] Nerve VII also can be affected, and it is supplied by the middle meningeal, accessory meningeal, and stylomastoid arteries.[21] Also, the availability of an experienced neuroradiologist is certainly a positive factor in choosing preoperative embolization. These procedures are both complex and rare, and there is not an overabundance of neuroradiologists who are comfortable with doing this type of work.

Another method for decreasing the danger due to bleeding during resection of skull base tumors has been for the patient to donate autologous blood for transfusion. Fortunately, these tumors are not often resected emergently. Therefore, the patients generally have time to give up to 5 or 6 units of their own blood preoperatively. This minimizes any risk of transmissible disease and transfusion reaction associated with giving blood.

THE FACIAL NERVE

The facial nerve is most commonly involved with acoustic neuromas since it is confined in the internal auditory canal to the space immediately adjacent to the tumor. Although it is often found splayed out over the tumor, quite commonly the anatomic integrity of the nerve can be preserved during dissection of even fairly large acoustic neuromas. Glomus tumors also can involve the facial nerve in its course through the middle ear and as it exits the stylomastoid foramen. Other cerebellopontine angle tumors, as well as temporal bone lesions, also can involve the facial nerve. Another source of injury to the facial nerve at the skull base is trauma, including gunshot wounds and stab injuries. Squamous cell carcinoma also can involve the facial nerve at the base of the skull, as can adenoid cystic carcinoma of the parotid gland.

The facial nerve itself consists of approximately 10,000 fibers, 7000 of which are motor fibers to the mimetic facial musculature, the posterior belly of the digastric, and the stylohyoid and postauricular muscles. The nerve exits the midbrain in the form of two roots: a motor root and a mixed sensory and parasympathetic root known as the nervus intermedius, nerve of Wrisberg, or glossopalatine nerve. The nervus intermedius is a rather small filament lying between nerve VIII and the voluntary portion of nerve VII for a variable distance, often well into the internal acoustic meatus.[23] At the geniculate ganglion, the greater superficial petrosal nerve is given off. Distal to the ganglion, the branch to the stapedius comes off followed by the chorda tympani. After exiting from the stylomastoid foramen, the nerve courses through the parotid to the peripheral musculature. The branches to the postauricular muscles, the posterior belly of the digastric, and the stylohyoid muscle come off the nerve just as it exits from the stylomastoid foramen.

Principles of facial nerve management during skull base surgery follow a set hierarchy. If at all possible, the anatomic integrity of the nerve should be preserved. This is usually possible even in quite large acoustic neuromas and also in tumors that invade the temporal bone but do not invade the nerve itself. Sometimes, for better exposure, the nerve will have to be mobilized out of its bony canal in the temporal bone. This can generally be performed via a postauricular transmastoid approach. If the nerve must be cut, direct reanastomosis is the procedure of choice. This should be done under minimal tension, since tension is the biggest enemy of any neural anastomosis.[24] The nerve may be mobilized to gain approximately 1 cm of length if it is removed from its bony canal in the temporal bone. If direct reanastomosis is not possible, the procedure of choice is a nerve interposition graft. This is generally done with the greater auricular nerve since it is often in the field and approximately the correct diameter. However, if it is unavailable or not large enough, the sural nerve may be used. Before the anastomoses are made, the nerve ends should be cut cleanly, and the anastomosis may be made with 6-0 or 7-0 nylon stitches in the epineurium. Only enough stitches to hold the nerve in place are necessary, and, once again, tension is the biggest enemy of ultimate nerve function and should be strictly avoided at the anastomotic sites.

If the nerve has to be taken just as it exits from the midbrain or if several branches have to be taken quite distally, facial reanimation procedures are the only options. The most devastating complication from facial paralysis is blindness from corneal ulceration secondary to inability to close the eye. This is best prevented by patching the eye at night and using artificial tears during the day. Another recent innovation has been implantation of a small gold weight in the eyelid in order to aid with blinking. This has helped in preventing corneal desiccation; however, it is still difficult to make the blinking motion completely symmetric with only the use of a gold weight.[25] Another method of facial reanimation involves a nerve XII to VII transfer. This is used in resection of the nerve to the midbrain with preservation of a distal stump. It should be done before 1.5 to 2 years of denervation, because the motor end-plates on the facial musculature undergo complete degeneration at that time. The subsequent possibility of tongue hemiatrophy can be addressed with a tongue Z-plasty as described elsewhere in this chapter. Other facial reanimation procedures are available but are beyond the scope of this chapter.

The lack of taste on the anterior two thirds of the tongue is usually fairly well tolerated without any further therapy. The lack of parasympathetic innervation to the submandibular gland and glands of the nose does

not seem to create much functional disturbance, nor does the lack of a stapedial reflex.

One other area where the facial nerve can
be injured is during an infratemporal fossa
approach. This often may involve stretching
of the frontal branch of the facial nerve. This
branch is the least likely to recover if significantly injured or severed. However, the dysfunction caused by the lack of this branch is
not usually a major problem, especially in
patients who have had a skull base tumor
requiring the infratemporal fossa approach.

THE VESTIBULOCOCHLEAR NERVE

Cranial nerve VIII is most commonly
involved with an acoustic neuroma. Other
cerebellopontine angle tumors, such as meningiomas, petrous apex cholesteatomas,
cholesterol granulomas, eosinophilic granulomas, or various temporal bone lesions, can
affect this nerve.

Cranial nerve VIII is separated into the
vestibular and cochlear components fairly
easily as the nerve leaves the brain stem. The
cochlear component is the more anterior and
inferior part of the nerve, whereas the more
superior and posterior part of the nerve is
the vestibular section. Acoustic neuromas
most commonly arise from the superior vestibular nerve; however, both the vestibular
and cochlear components of nerve VIII usually must be sacrificed in removing acoustic
neuromas because of the size that they often
attain before presentation. However, there
has been an attempt at preserving functional
hearing. Many surgeons agree that tumor
size is inversely proportional to the chance
of saving hearing.[26-29] Thus, the smaller the
tumor, the better the chance of salvaging
hearing.

Glasscock and associates rate the possibility of a relationship between the normality
of the auditory brain stem response (ABR)
and the chance for successful hearing conservation.[29] Thus, the closer to normal the
ABR, the better the chance at successful hearing conservation. Even more intriguing is the
idea from Shelton and colleagues that an

abnormal electronystagmogram (ENG) is a
better prognostic indicator.[30] They base this
on the hypothesis that the caloric response
reflects only the superior vestibular nerve
function. If the calorics are not hypoactive,
the investigators are more inclined to suspect
an inferior vestibular nerve tumor as opposed
to a superior vestibular nerve tumor. If the
tumor lies on the inferior vestibular nerve,
the chance of successful hearing conservation
surgery is lower in their hands, probably
owing to trauma to the adjacent cochlear
nerve or interruption of cochlear blood supply.

Longer-term studies have become available
recently suggesting more definite prognostic
factors for hearing conservation.[31] Although
initially some surgeons felt that certain operative approaches would allow better hearing preservation, further studies have shown
that the actual size of the tumor is more
important than the operative approach.
Hearing is more likely to be preserved with
tumors of less than 1.5 cm. Furthermore,
preoperative speech receptor threshold (SRT)
scores of less than 30 dB and speech documentation in quiet (SDQ) scores of greater
than 70 per cent are good prognostic factors.[32]
A recent study by Kemink and colleagues
suggests that intraoperative loss of wave V
on the ABR correlates with profound hearing
loss.[31] A shift in wave V latency of less than
2 msec, however, still was associated with
hearing preservation. These workers suggest
monitoring wave V latency intraoperatively
as a guideline to hearing preservation. This
may be especially useful in cases of only one
hearing ear.[31]

The importance of attempting hearing
preservation has been underscored in a study
by Shelton and colleagues showing that hearing in the operative ear decreases more
quickly over time than hearing in the nonoperative side.[27] The loss of hearing due to
either sectioning of the cochlear nerve or
interruption of the blood supply to the cochlea or the cochlear nerve is not remediable.
Some patients who require the ability to
localize sound may be offered a CROS (contralateral routing of sound) hearing aid. If
they have a hearing loss on the contralateral
side, a BI-CROS aid may be indicated.[29, 30]

The symptom caused by sectioning the vestibular nerve is dizziness. This is caused by asymmetric peripheral vestibular input to the brain; however, this is rather quickly compensated for in the otherwise healthy patient. Generally, the peripheral vestibular function will be somewhat hypoactive for quite a while before the patient goes to surgery, as evidenced by the fact that most patients claim to be at least slightly unsteady for more than 6 months prior to their diagnosis.[27, 30, 33] Patients with a long history of deteriorating vestibular function have time to adjust to decreased unilateral input from their semicircular canals. Indeed, there may not be much function left and removing the tumor may not have a significant impact on their dizziness if the vestibular nerve was not functioning at all prior to surgery. It is important to remind these patients not to walk in the dark without a light until they are very well compensated.

THE VAGUS NERVE

The vagus nerve is quite commonly involved by tumors that erode the region of the skull base. Glomus vagale tumors involve the nerve by definition. Carotid body tumors and glomus jugulare tumors arise in such close proximity to the nerve that it is often the first cranial nerve to be involved with these tumors.

Nerve X passes through the anterior portion of the jugular foramen separate from nerve IX and closely paralleling the accessory nerve. As it passes through the foramen, it has a small superior ganglion from which arise the auricular and meningeal branches of the vagus. Just outside the jugular foramen, the vagus expands to form the large inferior or nodose ganglion. Initially, the vagus lies medial to both the internal jugular vein and the internal carotid artery, but as it descends the vessels shift slightly so that the vein comes to lie lateral to the artery; the vagus lies behind and somewhat between the two.[34] Just below the nodose ganglion the nerve gives off a pharyngeal branch that combines with the pharyngeal branch of nerve IX. The pharyngeal branch of nerve X is the chief motor supply to the pharynx. The vagus also contributes some fibers to the carotid nerve, although this is mostly a glossopharyngeal branch. The superior laryngeal nerve is the next branch to arise off the vagus. It picks up sympathetic innervation from the superior cervical ganglion and divides into the internal and external branches, with the internal branch supplying sensation to the supraglottic larynx and the external branch supplying motor innervation to the cricothyroid muscle and a small part of the inferior pharyngeal constrictor. The recurrent laryngeal nerves exit from the right vagus just distal to its crossing the subclavian and on the left side, just distal to the aorta, to loop back upward and supply innervation to all the muscles of the larynx with the exception of the cricothyroid.

Sectioning the vagus nerve leads to significant functional difficulty with swallowing because of the paralysis of the constrictor muscles. Patients also have problems with aspiration secondary to inability of the supraglottic larynx to detect the presence of food as well as inability of the vocal cord on the involved side to adduct. Often in skull base surgery, the nerve is taken above the takeoff of the superior laryngeal nerve; thus, even the cricothyroid muscle is not innervated on the involved side. This differs slightly from having only the recurrent nerve cut, as the cricothyroid muscle can help adduct the vocal cord. Along with the dysphagia and problems with aspiration, hoarseness is a third complication of dividing the vagus nerve.

Immediate treatment if the vagus nerve must be divided includes placement of a large nasogastric tube for gastric decompression and performing a tracheostomy at the time of surgery. The large nasogastric tube may be replaced by a softer, smaller-caliber feeding tube once the danger of gastric outlet obstruction has passed. The tracheostomy should remain with the cuff inflated until the danger of aspiration has passed. This may be done with compensation by the contralateral cord, a Teflon injection, or a thyroplasty operation.

If the vagus nerve is sectioned bilaterally, immediate treatment may also include a palatal obturator. Long-term treatment may include a pharyngeal flap.[35] Bilateral vocal cord paralysis is usually treated with a tracheostomy. If the superior laryngeal nerves are preserved, the voice may be quite good owing to the adduction provided by the cricothyroid muscles. If the nerves are divided above the superior laryngeal nerve takeoff, the voice may not be quite as good; however, the vocal cords actually come to lie at rest somewhat in adduction.[35]

Rehabilitation after sectioning the vagus nerve generally includes modifying the diet toward foods that are easy to swallow, such as semisolid foods. Swallowing rehabilitation therapy by a trained therapist can be helpful. Often these patients use the "supraglottic" swallow, in which they take a breath, double swallow, and then cough at the end of deglutition.[35] Vocal cord paralysis also can be treated with a Teflon injection. The patient with a high vagal lesion will not have as good a result from a Teflon injection of the paralyzed vocal cord as a patient with a simple recurrent nerve lesion because the level of the vocal cord is slightly different with denervation of the cricothyroid muscle. An adequate voice usually can be obtained with the injection, and aspiration can be significantly reduced.

Another option in rehabilitation of the larynx is the Isshiki thyroplasty operation, which involves excising a small strut of cartilage from the lateral ala of the thyroid cartilage and inserting this lateral to the true cord in such a fashion as to push the true cord medially.[36] The amount of medialization can be evaluated if the operation is done under local anesthesia and the patient is asked to talk during the procedure. Once the ideal location for the cartilage strut has been determined, it is secured into place. This operation has the advantage of being adjustable and reversible, whereas the Teflon injection is not. If the posterior glottic chink is quite wide or the level of the cords is quite disparate, an arytenoid adduction procedure may be added at the time of laryngoplasty.[37]

Although the Teflon injection and Isshiki operation have served well, neither is perfect for all cases. New methods of laryngeal rehabilitation are still being sought. Kuriloff and coworkers have used a canine model to evaluate vocal cord medialization using an implanted miniature tissue expander.[38] In theory, this would allow fine vocal adjustments to be made after implantation.

THE CAROTID ARTERY

The carotid artery is often involved by tumors of the skull base, specifically carotid body tumors, glomus jugulare tumors, and glomus vagale tumors. The carotid artery also can be involved high in the neck with squamous cell carcinoma. Attempts at resecting the carotid artery involved with squamous cell carcinoma in the neck have not led to increased survival.[39]

Whenever a benign skull base neoplasm involves the carotid artery, two decisions must be made preoperatively. The first is whether or not to resect the carotid artery, and the second is whether or not to attempt bypass of the carotid artery if resection is performed. Since 85 per cent of the cerebral blood flow is via the carotid and only 15 per cent is via the vertebral artery, resection of the carotid can lead to massive stroke. However, collateral circulation from the circle of Willis often will provide adequate perfusion to the cerebral hemispheres bilaterally. Historically, therefore, attempts have been made to determine which patients are most likely to suffer a stroke, compared with those patients who would have adequate cerebral perfusion in the face of carotid resection.

The earliest attempts at prediction included the Matas test. This involved carotid occlusion in the neck with subsequent neurologic examinations.[40] Angiography and measurement of carotid stump pressure were the next techniques to evolve. Indeed, carotid stump pressure has remained somewhat of a standard despite many attempts at new ways of evaluating patients, including ocular plethysmography, radioactive washout techniques, transcranial Doppler ultrasound, and monitoring of evoked potentials.[41–43]

Hays and coworkers believed that a carotid artery stump pressure of greater than 50 mm Hg indicated a safe level for occlusion.[42] Andrews felt that carotid artery back pressure of greater than 70 mm Hg was adequate, with a level of between 50 and 70 mm Hg being marginal and a level of less than 50 mm Hg being a contraindication to resection.[41] Another method, used by Andrews and associates, utilizes detachable balloon technology to make an empiric evaluation aided by electroencephalography (EEG). These workers transiently occlude the internal carotid for 15 minutes while monitoring the patient. If neurologic signs or symptoms develop or the EEG changes, the balloon is immediately deflated and the patient is not considered a candidate for carotid resection or occlusion. If the patient tolerates the procedure, a detachable balloon is used to occlude the internal carotid artery as close to the ophthalmic artery as possible. Resection is undertaken within 3 days. These workers had good results, but problems with this technique include false-negative and false-positive EEG changes.[41, 44]

The most exciting new breakthrough has recently come from de Vries and coworkers.[44, 45] These workers have developed a way of actually quantifying cerebral blood flow (not just pressure) during temporary balloon occlusion of the internal carotid artery. If patients tolerate 10 to 15 minutes of temporary balloon occlusion without neurologic deficit, they then breathe xenon gas until equilibrium results. A xenon CT scan is then performed, and cerebral blood flow (CBF) is calculated.[45] Xenon computed tomographic mapping of cerebral blood flow is an actual measure of cerebral blood flow. Normal cerebral blood flow to the brain is approximately 55 ml per 100 gm per minute. Patients usually do not develop neurologic symptoms until the cerebral blood flow has diminished to less than 20 ml per 100 gm per minute.[45] A permanent stroke occurs if cerebral blood flow is diminished to 10 to 15 ml per 100 gm per minute over a long period of time. De Vries and associates believed that the patient would tolerate permanent internal carotid artery occlusion if the CBF did not change after temporary balloon occlusion. The patient would tolerate temporary occlusion for a vein graft repair if the CBF decreased ipsilaterally during temporary balloon occlusion. Either nonoperative therapy or external/internal carotid bypass was indicated if neurologic deficit developed during xenon CT scan. Using these guidelines, 136 patients were studied using the xenon CT method. Eleven patients failed, and 96 patients were thought to be at minimal risk. Twenty-one of the 96 patients underwent either permanent occlusion or resection of the internal carotid artery with no neurologic sequelae. Of the 13 patients in the marginal blood flow category, one permanent and one temporary hemiparesis occurred. The investigators recommend temporary occlusion with a graft if operation is absolutely necessary on moderate-to-high-risk patients. If the patient develops neurologic symptoms during temporary balloon occlusion and operation is the only hope, an extracranial-intracranial bypass may be considered, but this has not been studied well.

If the decision is made to bypass the internal carotid artery, generally a saphenous vein graft or Dacron graft is used. Obviously, the higher the carotid artery is involved with the tumor, the more difficult any distal anastomosis will be. Vein grafts have a tendency to thrombose, and there is a risk of stroke by either thrombus propagation or distal embolization. If the nasopharynx is entered, antibiotics should be used and consideration should be given to the use of vascularized flaps to close any resected part of the upper aerodigestive tract.[47] In cases of wound infection with a graft, the risk of blowout and fatal hemorrhage is significantly increased.

Another decision which must at times be made intraoperatively is how to handle inadvertent injury to the carotid. In this case, reconstruction should be attempted. A small hole should be simply closed with direct suturing of the carotid artery wall during temporary arterial occlusion with clips. If a segment of the artery is significantly damaged or if the artery must be resected, consideration should be given to a vein graft. Some surgeons reconstruct with direct vein grafts in patients with benign tumors. In patients with malignant tumors and a short life expectancy or in those in whom the upper aerodigestive tract has been exposed, they prefer to occlude and excise the vessel in those who have tolerated a xenon CT cerebral perfusion test.[45] If the common carotid or the internal carotid artery is occluded low in the neck, a long thrombus may form within the internal carotid artery that can propagate distally into the middle cerebral artery or anterior communicating artery. Small emboli then can occlude distal branches of these vessels. This is less likely to occur if the internal carotid artery is occluded close to the ophthalmic or posterior communicating artery.[45]

The carotid artery also may be approached in the sphenoid sinus either during a craniofacial resection or during any of various procedures to resect tumors that may involve the sinus. The midline septum of the sphenoid always ends at one of the two carotid canals, owing to its embryologic derivation. The carotid artery runs just lateral to the sphenoid sinus and can be dehiscent within it. If the carotid artery is injured while the sphenoid sinus is being operated upon, massive life-threatening hemorrhage results. The treatment is to place a Foley catheter into the sphenoid sinus and inflate the balloon in order to tamponade the hemorrhage. A detachable balloon can then be floated into the carotid artery and used to block off the bleeding site. Obviously, this involves the possibility of a stroke; however, the only other option is exsanguination. This is also a technique for treating traumatic carotid cavernous fistulas.[48]

AIR EMBOLISM

Air embolism is a constant danger in skull base surgery because the patient can undergo cardiovascular decompensation within a matter of seconds after it happens. It occurs in skull base surgery because often the head is placed above the heart in positioning the patient to reduce venous bleeding. However,

this can lead to a situation in which the pressure in the right heart is less than the pressure at the level of the open vein. Although this no doubt happens quite frequently during standard operations in the neck, the collapsibility of the veins often prevents any entrance of air. The venous structures dealt with in skull base surgery, however, often consist of dural venous sinuses that do not collapse after being transected, as well as diploic bone that is also noncompressible and must be sealed with bone wax. Both of these venous structures can predispose to air embolism.

Once the air enters the vein, it proceeds to the right atrium and through the right ventricle into the pulmonary arterial circulation. If it is a very small amount of air, it will diffuse into the alveoli and be expelled during ventilation. If it is a larger amount of air, several things can occur. First, intensive pulmonary arterial vasoconstriction occurs, which can lead to cor pulmonale and pulmonary edema.[49] Larger amounts of air actually can lodge in the right atrium and ventricle, causing an air lock, with subsequent absence of any cardiac output. Severe hypotension and hypoxia then immediately occur. Also, in approximately 20 per cent of people, the foramen ovale, although generally closed with high left-sided heart pressures, can become functionally open to allow air to pass from the right atrium into the left atrium. This air can then embolize in the cerebral or coronary circulation with obvious disastrous effects.[50] Also, nitrous oxide is more soluble in blood than in air; thus, if a large air embolism occurs, a concentration gradient exists between the concentration of nitrous oxide in the blood and the concentration of nitrous oxide in the air. The nitrous oxide will diffuse into the air embolus, causing it to increase in size if nitrous oxide is being used for anesthesia at the time of the embolus.[51]

Clinically, the signs and symptoms of air embolus include an audible sucking sound at the site of entry of air into the venous system. If a chest Doppler is in place, it will immediately detect the presence of as little as 1 cc of air in the circulation,[52] although it can also miss certain episodes.[53] A "mill wheel" type of cardiac murmur may be heard, and any number of cardiac dysrhythmias may also occur. If a large air embolus is present and an air lock occurs in the right ventricle, sudden systemic hypotension will ensue. Also, since the lungs are not being perfused with blood, the end-expiratory CO_2 will drop. The central venous pressure will rise acutely, since the venous return to the heart has been cut off by the air lock in the right ventricle.

Treatment of an air embolism includes packing the wound immediately with saline-soaked sponges and occluding the open vein. The jugular veins should also be compressed bilaterally in the neck to prevent any further entrance of air. The air should be aspirated from a previously placed right atrial catheter, though this is sometimes difficult.[53] Ventilation should be switched immediately to 100 per cent oxygen, and any nitrous oxide should be discontinued. Vasopressors may be used in severe hypotension to help ensure adequate perfusion to vital organs. The patient should be placed in the left lateral Trendelenburg position to attempt to trap the air in the right side of the heart and prevent it from embolizing in the pulmonary arterial circulation. If for some reason a right atrial catheter has not been placed previously, a needle may be inserted into the right ventricle from a subxiphoid approach to aspirate the air.

The best way to treat an air embolism is to prevent it. This includes using great care during the operation to prevent having an open vein, an open dural venous sinus, or a large amount of diploic bone exposed without bone wax. Although it would be ideal to keep the patient's head below the level of the heart, this increases bleeding so much that it is not feasible. Also, in any skull base operation, a right atrial catheter should be in place, end-tidal CO_2 should be continuously monitored, and a chest Doppler should be used for the detection and treatment of any air embolism.

THE SPINAL ACCESSORY NERVE

Involvement of the spinal accessory nerve by tumors of the skull base is quite common. The nerve leaves the jugular foramen as the most posterior of the three nerves traversing this structure. Initially, it is medial to the jugular vein between the internal jugular and the internal carotid artery, and it usually passes between the vein and artery to cross the lateral surface of the vein. Embryologically, however, the vein forms a ring around the spinal accessory nerve and occasionally the lateral ring will persist instead of the medial ring. This leads to the spinal accessory nerve being medial to the jugular vein. Anatomic studies have given the incidence of this to be 20 to 30 per cent; however, clinically this appears to be a somewhat high estimate.[54]

The nerve then passes through, or occasionally deep to, the sternocleidomastoid muscle. It gives a branch to this muscle before traversing the posterior cervical triangle to enter the trapezius. It carries voluntary motor fibers to both the sternocleidomastoid muscle and the trapezius. Division of the spinal accessory nerve results in denervation of these muscles. Functionally, this results in difficulty in raising the shoulder and pulling it back, as in reaching into the back pocket for a wallet. There is also concomitant strain placed on supporting shoulder muscles, related to loss of the trapezius. This can lead to a chronic pain syndrome for which intensive physiotherapy regimens have been devised.

THE HYPOGLOSSAL NERVE

At the skull base, the hypoglossal nerve exits from the skull at the hypoglossal canal (anterior condyloid foramen). Normally a venous plexus accompanies the nerve through the canal that connects the marginal sinus with the vertebral vein. This plexus can be quite large when the occipital sinus is large.[55] The nerve as it exits is medial to the internal jugular vein and internal carotid artery. It then passes laterally and downward posterior to the vagus nerve and then runs outward between the jugular vein and the internal carotid artery. It courses under the sternocleidomastoid branch of the occipital artery and then proceeds medial to the posterior belly of the digastric toward the intrinsic muscles of the tongue.

Injury to nerve XII can occur during extensive dissections for skull base neoplasms. Glomus tumors can become sufficiently large so that sacrifice of nerve XII is unavoidable. The nerve also may be stretched in attempting to retract structures, which may be necessary to resect these tumors. Probably the most common reason for having to sacrifice nerve XII is direct involvement with a squamous cell carcinoma in the neck or involvement of the nerve with an adenoid cystic carcinoma of the submandibular gland. In these cases, the nerve is included in the en bloc resection. Sectioning the nerve inadvertently should be followed by an attempt at primary reanastomosis without tension. This is often impossible. Division of the nerve results in denervation of the ipsilateral intrinsic muscles of the tongue. The amount of tongue hemiatrophy with resultant dysarthria and dysphagia varies significantly from patient to patient. Conley noted that about 25 per cent of patients progress to marked atrophy, 53 per cent have moderate atrophy, and the remaining 22 per cent have little or no muscle degeneration.[56]

Rubin and colleagues were the first to show in animals, and subsequently in humans, that if innervated muscle was imbedded into the atrophic and denervated tongue, nerve fibers would grow from the innervated muscle into the denervated muscle and eventually would innervate the previously atrophied muscle.[57] After demonstrating this in a cat model, Rubin performed the midline tongue Z-plasty that transposes an innervated flap of tongue muscle from the functioning side into the denervated side of the tongue. Since the tongue is divided into right and left halves by a median fibrous septum that is fixed to the body of the hyoid bone, innervation does not occur without this surgical transfer of muscle. Within a few months after the Z-plasty procedure, patients generally have good muscle tone and symmetric muscle movement, as well as improvement in any dysarthria or dysphagia that they may have had.

If the hypoglossal nerve is involved in a skull base tumor, generally so are cranial nerves IX and X and possibly XI. Although most people do quite well with isolated unilateral sectioning of nerve XII, combining this with the sensory and motor deficits in the pharynx and the larynx due to loss of nerves IX and X can add significant difficulty. The Z-plasty, therefore, is a way of lessening the overall impact of the operation on the patient. Bilateral division of the hypoglossal nerves precludes use of the Z-plasty and is functionally devastating. Deglutition becomes impossible, and a gastrostomy or feeding jejunostomy should be placed. If cranial nerves IX and X have also been resected, consideration may need to be given to laryngeal division or an antiaspiration procedure.[35]

THE GLOSSOPHARYNGEAL NERVE

The glossopharyngeal nerve is often involved in skull base tumors but rarely to the exclusion of other neurovascular structures at the skull base. The glossopharyngeal nerve exits from the skull through the jugular foramen. It is the most anterior of the three nerves exiting from this foramen. The nerve usually lies in a groove in the anterior part of the jugular foramen and is separated from the other neurovascular structures in the foramen by a band of fibrous tissue. Occasionally, this fibrous tissue will ossify, creating a "pseudocanal" for the nerve. Just outside the jugular foramen, the inferior petrosal sinus, often the most anterior structure in the foramen, usually passes between nerves IX and X to enter the superior bulb of the internal jugular vein. This relationship, however, is variable.[58]

The glossopharyngeal nerve carries motor fibers to the stylopharyngeus muscle and preganglionic parasympathetic fibers arising from the inferior salivatory nucleus and going via the Jacobson nerve (nervus tympanicum) to anastomose in the otic ganglion to provide parasympathetic innervation to the parotid gland. The sensory fibers of nerve IX go to the middle ear, the eustachian tube, the lateral and posterior pharyngeal walls, and the posterior third of the tongue. A limited region of the external acoustic meatus and ear is also involved. As it emerges from the jugular foramen, the glossopharyngeal nerve lies anterolateral to the vagus and accessory nerves, medial to the internal carotid artery, and anteromedial to the jugular bulb.

Just after leaving the jugular foramen, it passes laterally between the jugular vein and the internal carotid artery and then forward between the internal and external carotid lying deep to the styloid process and its attached muscles. At this point, it is most easily located by looking on the medial border of the stylopharyngeus muscle. It curves around from the medial to the lateral aspect of the stylopharyngeus and then arborizes into a lingual and tonsillar branch as it enters the posterior aspect of the tongue medial to the hyoglossus. The glossopharyngeal nerve also has a branch that goes to the carotid sinus. This branch descends between the internal and external carotid and unites with the carotid branch of the vagus to supply the carotid body and carotid sinus.[58]

Care should be taken when working around these nerves, the carotid sinus, and the carotid body to avoid bradycardia and subsequent hypotension. If this occurs, a small amount of 1 per cent lidocaine without epinephrine can be injected into the carotid bulb to prevent reflex bradycardia. Although one would expect a large area of numbness in the pharynx due to isolated sectioning of nerve IX, as well as possible dysphagia from dysfunction of the stylopharyngeus, clinically these have not been a large problem when isolated division of the glossopharyngeal nerve is performed. However, when nerve IX is sectioned in conjunction with the vagus nerve, these problems can be more severe. The loss of the gag reflex is also associated more with sectioning of nerve X than of nerve IX, despite the theoretic loss of the afferent limb of this reflex after sectioning of nerve IX. Apparently, both nerves IX and X supply sensation to the pharynx, and their sensory distributions probably overlap somewhat.

THE CERVICAL SYMPATHETIC TRUNK

Occasionally, the cervical sympathetic trunk may be involved with skull base tumors. This trunk consists of two to four ganglia, generally referred to as superior, middle, vertebral, and inferior, with an interconnecting trunk. The fibers consist largely of ascending preganglionic sympathetic fibers that have emerged through the ventral roots of the upper thoracic nerves, entering the cervical sympathetic trunk via the white rami communicantes and passing upward to synapse in the higher ganglia. The superior cervical ganglion lies somewhat posteromedial to the first portion of the internal carotid artery and just anterior to the inferior (nodose) ganglion of the vagus. Postganglionic fibers leave the superior cervical ganglion to form the internal carotid plexus and course upward with the internal carotid artery to supply sympathetic innervation to the face, nose, and eye.[59] Interruption of the cervical sympathetic chain results in Horner syndrome, which includes ptosis due to lack of innervation of the Mueller muscle, which holds up the eyelid. Anhidrosis of the unilateral face results, since no sympathetic innervation goes to the sweat glands on the skin. Also, miosis is present as there is no sympathetic input to the pupil. To date, there is no good way to reverse these symptoms after sectioning of the cervical sympathetic plexus.

THE OLFACTORY NERVE

The olfactory nerve may sometimes be involved with or cut during the resection of several types of tumors involving the anterior skull base. These include esthesioneuroblastomas, sinonasal undifferentiated carcinomas, and squamous and adenocarcinomas of the paranasal sinuses. The olfactory nerves themselves lie just on top of the cribriform plate and have filaments that traverse the cribriform plate into the superior recess of the nose. The elevation of the contents of the anterior cranial fossa leads to transection of this connection between the olfactory nerve and the cribriform plate with resultant anosmia. Attempts to limit the dissection to one side may preserve the contralateral sense of smell; however, often both sides must be elevated. This creates a hole in the dura that should be repaired primarily and then reinforced with some type of facial graft.

Functionally, the loss of smell is bothersome to the patient. It greatly decreases, although does not completely eliminate, the sense of taste. There is no known method of rehabilitating the loss of the sense of smell at this point. Patients with anosmia need to be warned to check expiration dates on food and milk. Although noxious fumes are mediated through the trigeminal nerve, these patients also may be slow to smell smoke, so they should have working smoke alarms and fire extinguishers in their homes and places of work. They should use electric appliances as they cannot smell a gas leak.[36]

Dysosmia can result from drainage from or trauma to the olfactory system. If the site of the lesion is the olfactory tract, there is no treatment except to release any tension or impingement on the olfactory bulbs. This should be differentiated from uncinate fits, which are a seizure disorder that may respond to antiseizure mediators.[36]

OCULAR COMPLICATIONS

Although ocular complications are rare, they can be devastating when they occur. The most serious complication is blindness. This can occur in several ways. Orbital exenteration due to tumor extent is obvious. Previous indications for orbital exenteration are being re-evaluated in cases of sinus malignancy.[60] Trauma at the skull base can cause either an orbital hematoma or direct trauma to the optic nerve, resulting in visual loss. If the loss of vision does not respond to medical therapy, optic nerve decompression may be indicated.[61, 62] Damage to the ophthalmic division of the trigeminal nerve can lead to corneal anesthesia with possible ulceration, infection, and blindness. This may be significantly compounded by a facial nerve paralysis. A retrobulbar hematoma, such as may occur if an ethmoid artery retracts into the orbit or venous bleeding accumulates within the periorbita, also can cause blindness. The mechanism for this is not entirely clear, although high pressure causing venous outflow obstruction and subsequent hypoxia in the retina and optic nerve has been postulated.[63] Treatment includes ophthalmologic consultation if not already obtained, eye massage, 1 to 2 gm per kg of mannitol intravenously, and lateral canthotomy. If this does not relieve the pressure, a Lynch medial orbital decompression of the orbit with or without decompression of the optic nerve is indicated.[63] Sympathetic uveitis also may occur if an injured eye is not removed.[35]

Less devastating complications include enophthalmos, diplopia, and epiphora. Diplopia can occur if cranial nerve III, IV, or VI is involved with the tumor or in the resection. If the tumor involves the cavernous sinus, this is often the case. If the resection must involve the periorbita, resultant scarring and contraction of the extraocular muscles can occur, causing diplopia. Diplopia can also occur if the medial canthus is not reattached medially.[64, 65] This can be done with a transnasal wire secured to a medial canthal button or a permanent suture from the medial canthal tendon to the bony remnant of the medial orbit.[64] Epiphora also can occur if the lacrimal drainage system is interrupted; this is treated with a dacrocystorhinostomy. Enopthalmos may occur if the periorbita is resected and, as yet, there is no good treatment for this.

MISCELLANEOUS COMPLICATIONS

Miscellaneous complications include pain and dysfunction of the temporomandibular joint after disarticulation or retraction of the mandible during certain skull base approaches. This can be treated with physical therapy. It is interesting that this condition does not seem to develop frequently in patients in whom the condyle is actually resected.[66] Various nerve palsies can occur from patient positioning during very long skull base procedures, and care should be taken to prevent these in positioning the patient for the operation.

Neurosurgical complications are beyond the scope of this chapter; however, they merit mention and include, in addition to cerebrospinal fluid leaks and meningitis, subperiosteal abscess, major cerebral artery occlusion, intracerebral hematoma, subdural hematoma, epidural hematoma, pulsating exophthalmos, cerebral edema, intracranial hematoma, brain stem ischemia and infarction, pneumocephalus, and hydrocephalus.

References

1. Johnson GD, Jackson CG, Fisher J, et al: Management of large dural defects in skull base surgery: An update. Laryngoscope 100:200–202, 1990.
2. Johns ME, Winn HR, McLean WC, Cantrell RW: Pericranial flap for the closure of defects of craniofacial resections. Laryngoscope 91:952–959, 1981.
3. Baker SR: Surgical reconstruction after extensive skull base surgery. Otolaryngol Clin North Am 17:591–599, 1984.
4. Snyderman CH, Janecka IP, Sekhar LN, et al: Anterior cranial base reconstruction: Role of galeal and pericranial flaps. Laryngoscope 100:607–614, 1990.
5. Kinney SE: Trauma. In Cummings CW, Fredrickson JM, Harker LA, et al (eds): Otolaryngology–Head and Neck Surgery. Vol 4. St. Louis, Mosby-Yearbook, 1986, pp 3033–3045.
6. Yokoyama K, Hasegawa M, Shiba KS, et al: Diagnosis of CSF rhinorrhea: Detection of tau-transferrin in nasal discharge. Otolaryngol Head Neck Surg 98:328–332, 1988.
7. Wolman L: The neuropathological effects resulting from the intrathecal injection of chemical substances. Paraplegia 4:97–115, 1966.
8. Calcaterra TC: Extracranial surgical repair of cerebrospinal rhinorrhea. Ann Otol 89:108–116, 1980.
9. Myers DL, Sataloff RT: Spinal fluid leakage after skull base surgical procedures. Otolaryngol Clin North Am 17:601–612, 1984.
10. Kirchner JC, Sasaki CT: Reconstructive surgery of the sinuses. In Thawley SE, Panje WR (eds): Comprehensive Management of Head and Neck Tumors. Vol 1. Philadelphia, WB Saunders, 1987, pp 433–444.
11. Westmore GA, Whittam DE: Cerebral spinal fluid rhinorrhea and its management. Br J Surg 69:489, 1982.
12. Persing JA, Kassell NF, Jane JA: Neurosurgical perspectives of special perioperative consideration. In Cummings CW, et al (eds): Otolaryngology–Head

and Neck Surgery. St. Louis, CV Mosby, 1986, p 3383.
13. Roberson GH, Biller H, Sessions DG, Ogura JH: Presurgical internal maxillary artery embolization in juvenile angiofibroma. Laryngoscope 82:1524–1532, 1972.
14. Pletcher JD, Newton TH, Dedo HH, Norman D: Preoperative embolization of juvenile angiofibroma of the nasopharynx. Ann Otol 84:740–746, 1975.
15. Economou TS, Abemayor E, Ward PH: Juvenile nasopharyngeal angiofibroma: An update of the UCLA experience, 1960–1985. Laryngoscope 98:170–175, 1988.
16. Spector JG: Management of juvenile angiofibromata. Laryngoscope 98:1016–1026, 1988.
17. Ward PH, Liu C, Vinuela F, Bentson JR: Embolization: An adjunctive measure for removal of carotid body tumors. Laryngoscope 98:1287–1291, 1988.
18. Young NM, Wiet RJ, Russell EJ, Monsell EM: Superselective embolization of glomus jugulare tumors. Ann Otol Rhinol Laryngol 97:613–620, 1988.
19. Murphy TP, Brackmann DE: Effects of preoperative embolization on glomus jugulare tumors. Laryngoscope 99:1244–1254, 1989.
20. Duvall AJ, Moreano AE: Juvenile nasopharyngeal angiofibroma: Diagnosis and treatment. Otolaryngol Head Neck Surg 97:534–540, 1987.
21. Valavanis A: Preoperative embolization of the head and neck: Indications, patient selection, goals, and precautions. AJNR 7:943–952, 1986.
22. Davis KR: Embolization of epistaxis and juvenile nasopharyngeal angiofibromas. AJNR 7:953–962, 1986.
23. Hollinshead WH (ed): Anatomy for Surgeons. Vol 1: The Head and Neck. 3rd ed. Philadelphia, Harper & Row, 1982, p 81.
24. Gantz BJ: Intratemporal facial nerve surgery. In Cummings CW, et al (eds): Otolaryngology–Head and Neck Surgery. St. Louis, CV Mosby, 1986, p 3353.
25. Bojrab DI: Upper eyelid gold weight implantation in facial paralysis. Insights Otolaryngol 4:1–8, 1989.
26. Mangham CA: Complications of translabyrinthine vs. suboccipital approach for acoustic tumor surgery. Otolaryngol Head Neck Surg 99:396–400, 1988.
27. Shelton C, Hitselberger WE, House WF, Brackmann DE: Hearing preservation after acoustic tumor removal: Long-term results. Laryngoscope 100:115–120, 1990.
28. Shelton C, Brackmann DE, House WF, Hitselberger WE: Middle fossa acoustic tumor surgery: Results in 106 cases. Laryngoscope 99:405–408, 1989.
29. Glasscock ME, McKennan KX, Levine SC: Acoustic neuroma surgery: The results of hearing conservation surgery. Laryngoscope 97:785–789, 1987.
30. Shelton C, Brackmann DE, House WF, Hitselberger WE: Acoustic tumor surgery. Arch Otolaryngol Head Neck Surg 115:1213–1216, 1989.
31. Kemink JL, LaRouere MJ, Kileny PR, et al: Hearing preservation following suboccipital removal of acoustic neuromas. Laryngoscope 100:597–602, 1990.
32. Wade PJ, House W: Hearing preservation in patients with acoustic neuromas via the middle fossa approach. Otolaryngol Head Neck Surg 114:85–87, 1984.
33. Wiegand DA, Fickel V: Acoustic neuroma—the patient's perspective: Subjective assessment of symp-

toms, diagnosis, therapy, and outcome in 541 patients. Laryngoscope 99:179–187, 1989.

34. Hollinshead WH (ed): Anatomy for Surgeons. Vol 1: The Head and Neck. 3rd ed. Philadelphia, Harper & Row, 1982, p 495.

35. Sataloff RT, Myers DL, Kremer FB: Management of cranial nerve injury following surgery of the skull base. Otolaryngol Clin North Am 17:577–589, 1984.

36. Isshiki N, Morita H, Okamura H, Hiramoto M: Thyroplasty as a new phonosurgical technique. Acta Otolaryngol 78:451–457, 1974.

37. Isshiki N, Tanabe M, Sawada M: Arytenoid adduction for unilateral vocal cord paralysis. Arch Otolaryngol 104:555–558, 1978.

38. Kuriloff DB, Goldsher M, Blaugrund SM, Krespi YP: Controlled laryngoplasty for vocal cord medialization: A technique using tissue expansion. Laryngoscope 100:615–622, 1990.

39. Osguthorpe JD, Hungerford GD: Transarterial carotid occlusion: Case report and review of the literature. Arch Otolaryngol 110:694–696, 1984.

40. Matas R: Testing the efficiency of the collateral circulation. JAMA 63:1441–1447, 1914.

41. Andrews JC, Valavanis A, Fisch U: Management of the internal carotid artery in surgery of the skull base. Laryngoscope 99:1224–1229, 1989.

42. Hays RJ, Levinson SA, Wylie EJ: Intraoperative measurement of carotid back pressure as a guide to operative management for carotid endarterectomy. Surgery 72:953–960, 1972.

43. Ehrenfeld W, Stomy RJ, Wylie EJ: Relation of carotid stump pressure to safety of carotid artery ligation. Surgery 95:299–305, 1983.

44. de Vries EJ, Sekhar LN, Horton JA, et al: A new method to predict safe resection of the internal carotid artery. Laryngoscope 100:85–88, 1990.

45. de Vries EJ, Sekhar LN, Janecka IP, Eibling DE: Elective resection of the internal carotid artery without reconstruction. Laryngoscope 98:960–966, 1988.

46. Yonas H, Gur D, Goode BC, et al: Stable xenon CT blood flow mapping for evaluation of patients with extracranial/intercranial bypass surgery. J Neurosurg 62:333, 1985.

47. Sekhar LN, Schramm VL, Jones NF, et al: Operative exposure and management of the petrous and upper cervical internal carotid artery. Neurosurgery 19:967–982, 1986.

48. Debrun G, Lacour P, Vinuela F, et al: Treatment of 54 traumatic carotid-cavernous fistulas. J Neurosurg 55:678–692, 1981.

49. Munson ES, Paul WC, Perry JC, et al: Early detection of venous air embolism using a Swan-Ganz catheter. Anesthesiology 42:223–226, 1975.

50. Everts EC: Surgical complications. In Cummings CW, et al (eds): Otolaryngology–Head and Neck Surgery. St. Louis, CV Mosby, 1986, p 1411.

51. Marshall WK, Bedford RF: Use of a pulmonary-artery catheter for detection and treatment of venous air embolism: A prospective study in man. Anesthesiology 52:131–134, 1980.

52. Maroon JC, Goodman JM, Horner TG, Campbell RL: Detection of minute venous air emboli with ultrasound. Surg Gynecol Obstet 127:1236–1238, 1968.

53. Bedford RF, Marshall WK, Butler A, Welsh JE: Cardiac catheters for diagnosis and treatment of venous air embolism. A prospective study in man. J Neurosurg 55:610–614, 1981.

54. Hollinshead WH (ed): Anatomy for Surgeons. Vol 1: The Head and Neck. 3rd ed. Philadelphia, Harper & Row, 1982, p 497.

55. Hollinshead WH (ed): Anatomy for Surgeons. Vol 1: The Head and Neck. 3rd ed. Philadelphia, Harper & Row, 1982, p 85.

56. Conley J: Management of facial nerve paresis in malignant tumors of the parotid gland. In Rubin LR (ed): Reanimation of the Paralyzed Face: New Approaches. St. Louis, CV Mosby, 1977, p 230.

57. Rubin LR, Mishriki YY, Speace G: Reanimation of the hemiparalytic tongue. Plast Reconstr Surg 73:184–192, 1984.

58. Hollinshead WH (ed): Anatomy for Surgeons. Vol 1: The Head and Neck. 3rd ed. Philadelphia, Harper & Row, 1982, pp 78–79.

59. Hollinshead WH (ed): Anatomy for Surgeons. Vol 1: The Head and Neck. 3rd ed. Philadelphia, Harper & Row, 1982, pp 490–492.

60. Perry C, Levine PA, Williamson BR, Cantrell RW: Preservation of the eye in paranasal sinus cancer surgery. Arch Otolaryngol Head Neck Surg 114:632–634, 1988.

61. Knox BE, Gates GA, Berry SM: Optic nerve decompression via the lateral facial approach. Laryngoscope 100:458–462, 1990.

62. Sofferman RA: Sphenoethmoid approach to the optic nerve. Laryngoscope 91:184–196, 1981.

63. Stankiewicz JA: Blindness and intranasal endoscopic ethmoidectomy: Prevention and management. Otolaryngol Head Neck Surg 101:320–329, 1989.

64. Levine PA, Scher RL, Jane JA, et al: The craniofacial resection—eleven-year experience at the University of Virginia: Problems and solutions. Otolaryngol Head Neck Surg 101:665–669, 1989.

65. Schuller DE, Goodman JH, Miller CA: Reconstruction of the skull base. Laryngoscope 94:1359–1364, 1984.

66. Fisch U, Pillsbury HC: Infratemporal fossa approach to lesions in the temporal bone and base of the skull. Arch Otolaryngol 105:99–107, 1979.

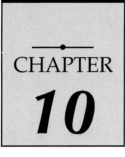

CHAPTER 10

Paranasal Sinus Surgery

WILLIAM LAWSON, MD, DDS
IOANA G. CARABIN, MD

The various surgical procedures performed on the paranasal sinuses carry a morbidity that is related to the operative route (e.g., intranasal, sublabial, transorbital, direct facial, combined cranial), the type and extent of the disease process, and factors that influence healing (e.g., systemic disease, prior radiation).

The paranasal sinuses are strategically located in relation to the orbit and skull base, from which they are separated by the lamellae of bone, placing vital organs at risk of serious injury. The range of complications varies from the cosmetic to the life-threatening.

FRONTAL SINUS SURGERY

TREPHINE

This procedure is designed to provide access into the frontal sinus by the creation of an opening in the medial aspect of its orbital wall. Its principal indication is for the drainage of pus in acute sinusitis and for the elevation of fractures of the anterior table.[1] The incision is made at the inferomedial aspect of the eyebrow. Placement more laterally may result in injury to the supratrochlear or supraorbital nerves with regional paresthesia or anesthesia of the adjacent eyebrow and forehead. Creating the trephine more laterally also may produce damage to the trochlea, with diplopia resulting from imbalance of the superior oblique muscle.[1] Failure to create the bony opening medially may result in the sinus cavity's being missed entirely and the catheter inserted intracranially.[1] If the opening is made in the anterior wall of the frontal sinus, a visible depression may result.

FRONTAL SEPTOPLASTY

This procedure entails removal of the intersinus septum (occasionally with the superior bony septum) to create a common opening into the nasal cavity. It is mainly of historical interest but may be performed when a patient's nasofrontal duct is injured

115

by ablative tumor surgery or trauma and the opposite duct is utilized to provide communal drainage.[2] It presently is not employed for cases of chronic unilateral infection secondary to duct obstruction, since it invites the risk of contralateral contamination and spread of disease. Its complications are the same as with the frontal trephine, along with potential injury to the olfactory groove. Another major limitation to its application is the development of stenosis.

EXTERNAL FRONTOETHMOIDECTOMY

The transorbital approach to the frontal sinus entails exenteration of the ethmoid labyrinth with enlargement of the nasofrontal duct and its marsupialization into the nasal cavity.[3] The extent to which the floor of the frontal sinus is removed depends on the amount and type of disease present (e.g., chronic inflammation, osteoma, mucocele) and the size of the sinus. The newly created duct is relined by a mucosal flap, stented with Silastic sheeting, or both. Closure of the neoduct is the limiting factor to the success of this procedure, with restenosis leading to chronic infection and mucocele formation. The failure rate has been reported to be from 20 per cent to 35 per cent.[4–6] The actual rate may be even higher, since many years often elapse before symptoms reappear and few long-term studies exist. This is exemplified by the report of Neel and associates in which an initial failure rate of 7 per cent at 3 years rose to 20 per cent after a 10-year follow-up.[7]

The procedure entails removal of the medial portion of the orbit and accordingly places regional structures at risk. Failed ligation of the anterior and posterior ethmoid arteries as they traverse the frontoethmoidal suture line may result in formation of an orbital hematoma. This is manifested by proptosis, chemosis, ophthalmoplegia, and progressive visual loss leading to blindness if not decompressed. A retrobulbar hemorrhage also may result from a torn ciliary vein caused by retraction of the globe. The mechanism of blindness is from direct pressure on the optic nerve, thrombosis of the retinal artery, and anterior ischemic optic neuropa-

thy. Visual loss also may result from direct injury to the optic nerve. The lacrimal sac may be traumatized, resulting in the development of dacryostenosis with recurrent infection and epiphora postoperatively. Injury to the trochlea or failure to reattach it produces diplopia and compensatory head tilt to compensate for the superior oblique muscle imbalance. Similarly, failure to coapt the periosteum and reattach the medial canthal ligament may cause pseudohypertelorism. The removal of bone above the frontoethmoidal suture line will violate the floor of the anterior cranial fossa and can produce a cerebrospinal fluid leak if the dura is penetrated. Hypertrophic scarring of the incision can cause an epicanthal-like fold.

In a series of 47 external ethmoidectomies reported by Kimmelman and colleagues, only 53 per cent of the patients were complication free.[8] The complications encountered consisted of facial edema (two), hemorrhage (four or five requiring transfusion), wound infection (three), hypertrophic scarring (two), temporary periorbital edema (eight), temporary supraorbital anesthesia (three), supraorbital hematoma (two), upper lid ptosis (one), and transient visual disturbances (two).

FRONTAL COLLAPSE

The collapse (Riedel) procedure represents an early attempt at controlling chronic disease of the frontal sinus by its obliteration; however, the resultant cosmetic deformity caused it to fall into disrepute. Nevertheless, it still holds an important place in the management of chronic osteomyelitis of the frontal sinus.[1]

Implicit in its proper performance is the creation of a significant cosmetic defect by removal of the supraorbital ridges as well as the anterior wall of the sinus to appose the forehead skin completely to the posterior table. In the management of chronic osteomyelitis, the removal of bone to where it is freely bleeding suggests that the nonviable portions have been removed but does not guarantee it. The recrudescence of infection with fistula or subgaleal abscess (Pott puffy tumor) formation may develop after an interval of months to years from a smouldering focus of osteomyelitis despite prolonged antibiotic therapy. This may occur at a distance from the original sinus cavity by extension of the infection through the diploë and may require a partial craniectomy for control. Equally important to adequate bone resection is total removal of the sinus mucosa to prevent mucocele formation. This is performed in the same fashion as with the osteoplastic flap in which all surfaces and recesses of the sinus are cleansed of any epithelial remnants by drilling.[1]

OSTEOPLASTIC FLAP

This procedure involves the creation of a hinged osteoperiosteal flap of the anterior wall of the frontal sinus for the removal of a lesion and the obliteration of the sinus cavity without cosmetic deformity. Although a variety of alloplastic and autogenous materials have been employed to achieve obliteration,[1] adipose tissue harvested from the abdominal wall is currently the material of choice. The success of the fat graft is predicated on its maintained viability by revascularization from the surrounding bone. Should this fail to take place, the resulting fibrosis and contraction of the autograft permits re-epithelialization of the sinus from the nasofrontal duct with the formation of a mucocele. Any retained mucosal remnant may produce a mucocele despite excellent graft viability. Mucosal tags may be present in a deep recess of the sinus (e.g., orbital extension) or along diploic veins, or they may arise from a supraorbital ethmoid air cell or from epithelial fragments adherent to dura in cases with posterior table erosion.

Another method of eliminating the sinus cavity relies upon auto-obliteration by osteoneogenesis.[9, 10] The paranasal sinuses have a tendency to fill with fibrous tissue and bone following removal of their epithelial lining; however, there is a degree of unpredictability in the extent and uniformity with which this occurs. Incomplete sinus obliteration leads to microcyst formation with recurrent infection or the development of a mucocele.

In cases of severe craniofrontal trauma with extreme comminution and loss of bone, some workers[11–13] remove the posterior sinus wall, permitting the brain and dura to herniate forward and fill the sinus, a process called cranialization. Again, retained mucosal remnants or proliferation of epithelium upward from a patent nasofrontal duct may lead to recurrent infection or mucocele formation.

Complications of the osteoplastic flap procedure are related to technical aspects of the operation, difficulties in healing, and failure to achieve sinus obliteration. These include bleeding (hematoma, seroma), infection (at the frontal and donor areas), difficulties with the bone flap (fracture, nonviability, embossment, migration) (Figs. 10–1 and 10–2), the creation of a bone cut beyond the sinus with dural penetration, graft failure (fat necrosis), neurologic disorders (supraorbital neuralgias and paresthesias), and cosmetic deformities (brow ptosis, frontalis contraction and paresis, incision scarring).

In a series of 250 cases reported by Hardy and Montgomery, complications developed in 47 patients (18 per cent).[14] These consisted of 6 frontal and 11 abdominal hematomas and seromas, 8 frontal and 2 abdominal abscesses, 8 bone cuts outside the sinus (7 with dural penetration), 2 forehead skin sloughs, 1 anosmia, 1 temporary eyelid ptosis, and 1 temporary frontalis paresis. The development of a frontal abscess is a serious complication: six of the eight cases of Hardy and Montgomery in whom it developed required revision surgery. These workers also reported 12 patients with persistent forehead pain refractory to medication. Surgical exploration was performed on four patients without any evidence of disease found. This underscores the principle that revision surgery should not be performed unless there is clinical or radiographic evidence of disease. This is especially true when using the direct brow approach in which the supraorbital nerves are sectioned, resulting in paresthesias, anesthesias, and neuralgias in a small number of patients. These workers also reported that 12 per cent of their patients had an unsatisfactory scar and 6 per cent had poor bone contour.

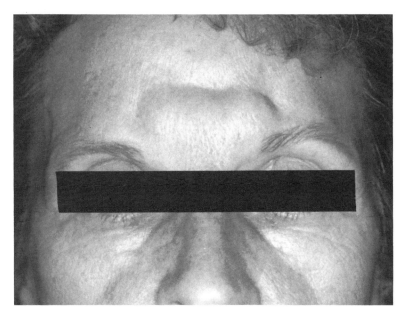

FIGURE 10–1. Embossment following frontal osteoplastic flap with fat obliteration. The contour irregularities represent new bone formation secondary to a reactive periostitis and areas of osseous resorption.

Although the coronal approach provides excellent scar camouflage and avoids injury to the supraorbital and supratrochlear nerves, it is associated with an increased blood loss. The direct brow (gullwing) incision used in patients with male pattern baldness should be made adjacent to the upper edge of the eyebrow, beveling the incision to provide protection to the hair follicles and achieve better scar camouflage. Nerve injuries are unavoidable by this approach, and the patient should be informed of the expected regional anesthesia and of the possibility of neuralgias. Irregularities in forehead contour result not only from hypertrophic bone changes by periosteal irritation (embossment) but also from areas of bone resorption along the line of the bone cut.

Construction and placement of the template used to create the bone flap is of vital importance. Care must be taken that it is prepared from a true Caldwell (posteroanterior projection) radiograph to minimize any magnification error and that at operation it is seated correctly over the supraorbital rims so as not to extend beyond the limits of the sinus. Similarly, beveling of the bone cut is important in preventing overshooting of the frontal sinus with intracranial entry.

In addition to these complications, we have seen the postoperative formation of an epidural abscess with an intact posterior table, presumably by extension of infection along a diploic vein.

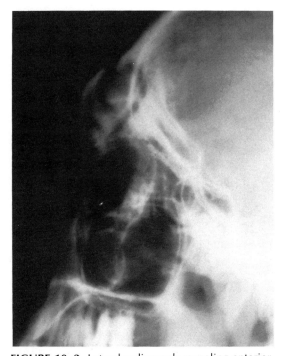

FIGURE 10–2. Lateral radiograph revealing anterior displacement of the bone flap following frontal osteoplastic flap procedure.

INTRANASAL
SPHENOETHMOIDECTOMY

The complications of intranasal sphenoeth-moidectomy may be subdivided into orbital, intracranial, sinonasal, and other.

ORBITAL

Entry into the orbit in performing an eth-moidectomy may be through the lacrimal bone anteriorly or the lamina papyracea of the ethmoid bone more posteriorly. The peri-osteum is closely adherent to the bone, and once the osseous boundary of the labyrinth is violated the periorbital fat is readily en-gaged. Instrumentation of the fat may result in the tearing of a ciliary vein with develop-ment of an orbital or retrobulbar hematoma. Significant orbital hemorrhage also may re-sult from injury to the anterior and posterior ethmoidal arteries, with the rapid develop-ment of a retrobulbar hematoma. Clinically, a superior orbital fissure syndrome (propto-sis, chemosis and ophthalmoplegia) appears (Fig. 10–3), which is associated with progres-sive visual loss. Management is related to the degree of bleeding present, which is reflected in the severity of the clinical find-ings. Relatively minor orbital bleeding may be managed by diuretics, mannitol, steroids, eye massage, and lateral canthotomy.[15, 16] However, with active intraorbital hemor-rhage, orbital decompression must be per-formed within 1 to 2 hours to reduce intra-ocular pressure and prevent the loss of visual acuity from becoming permanent.[17]

Another mechanism for the development of blindness is by direct injury to the optic nerve posterolaterally in the ethmoid laby-rinth or in the lateral wall of the sphenoid sinus. This is a less common cause of blind-ness and is generally complete and irrevers-ible. Clinically, the patient has a normal-appearing eye with a dilated pupil that fails to respond to light both directly and consen-sually.

Unrecognized injury into the orbit with continued instrumentation will cause dam-age to the extraocular muscles and their nerves, as well as to the fat and its vascula-

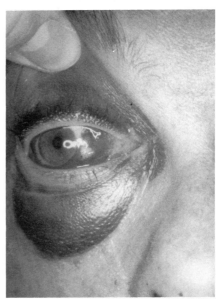

FIGURE 10–3. Retrobulbar hematoma following in-tranasal ethmoidectomy. Proptosis, ophthalmople-gia, and chemosis are present in addition to perior-bital ecchymosis.

ture. The medial rectus is most commonly injured;[18–20] however, a high orbital penetra-tion may damage the superior oblique muscle and infratrochlear nerve. Inferior rectus in-jury also has been reported following nasal polypectomy and antrostomy.[21] Damage to the muscle and its innervation results in impaired ocular mobility with diplopia. Im-mediate exploration and repair is under-taken, otherwise the resultant mass of mus-cle, nerve, scar, and fat immobilizes the eye.

The most minor orbital complication is the development of a fracture of the outer wall of the ethmoid labyrinth, with the extrava-sation of blood and the passage of air into the eyelids producing periorbital ecchymosis and subcutaneous emphysema. Patients who develop this complication are treated expec-tantly. They are hospitalized and observed to determine that more serious orbital bleed-ing does not develop. Prophylactic antibiotics are administered to prevent the development of an orbital cellulitis.

Regarding the incidence of these compli-cations, Maniglia and associates initially re-ported four cases of blindness (two from orbital hematoma with proptosis and two from optic nerve injury) among nine patients who developed major complications following ethmoidectomy.[20] In a later study, Maniglia described seven cases of blindness (one bilateral), in six of which an orbital hematoma was present following intranasal ethmoidectomy.[22] There were also two patients with intraocular muscle injuries and diplopia. Stankiewicz reported six cases of orbital hemorrhage following endoscopic ethmoidectomy, three of which resulted in permanent blindness.[16]

INTRACRANIAL

Violation of the floor of the anterior cranial fossa may result in a variety of complications that include cerebrospinal fluid (CSF) leak, pneumocephalus, meningitis, brain abscess, frontal lobe laceration, intracranial hemorrhage, and carotid–cavernous sinus fistula, all of which are serious and potentially lethal injuries. The development of a CSF leak is the most commonly encountered complication of intranasal ethmoidectomy. It most often occurs in the area of the cribriform plate (Fig. 10–4), fovea ethmoidalis, and superolateral to the sphenoid sinus. Kainz and Stammberger claimed that the anterior roof of the ethmoid labyrinth, where the anterior

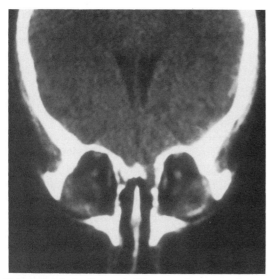

FIGURE 10–4. Coronal CT scan demonstrating a defect in the cribriform plate after intranasal sphenoethmoidectomy.

ethmoid artery passes across the olfactory groove to become intracranial, was also a point of vulnerability.[23] The dura is closely adherent to the bone, and osseous penetration or fracture generally produces a tear in the dura with CSF rhinorrhea. However, Wigand believed that CSF leaks could also occur from the stripping of diseased mucosa from the middle and superior turbinates and septum, which contain small branches of the fila olfactoria that communicate with the subarachnoid space.[24] Perforation or fracture of the posterior or superior wall of the sphenoid sinus also may result in a CSF leak.

If a CSF leak develops intraoperatively, it should be sealed immediately by fascial or dermal grafting (with or without a supplemental mucosal flap) through an endonasal approach. A leak that is detected in the immediate postoperative period is treated with bed rest, head elevation, and lumbar puncture with CSF drainage. If spontaneous closure is not achieved, or a delayed leak occurs, coverage of the defect is attempted through a rhinologic approach. A craniotomy is performed only after the failure of a primary nasal repair.

Despite intracranial entry, a CSF leak may not develop immediately from herniation of the brain downward into the defect but may manifest itself by the development of a suppurative complication days or weeks following surgery.[25] Management is by the administration of intravenous antibiotics for meningitis and cerebritis (Fig. 10–5) and craniotomy for drainage of abscesses.

Intracranial air (pneumocephalus) may develop with or without an accompanying CSF leak and also signals violation of the skull base (Fig. 10–6). Simple pneumocephalus is treated with intravenous antibiotics and computed tomographic monitoring to determine whether the defect has spontaneously sealed with the resorption of the intracranial air.

As with the orbit, continued instrumentation following unrecognized violation of the skull base may produce progressively more devastating injuries.[26] Laceration of the frontal lobes and the overlying branches of the anterior cerebral blood vessels may occur from penetration of the cribriform plate or

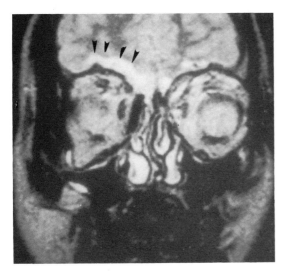

FIGURE 10–5. Coronal MRI revealing cerebritis of the frontal lobes *(arrows)* after intranasal ethmoidectomy.

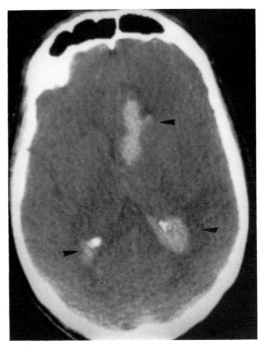

FIGURE 10–7. Axial CT scan showing multiple areas of intracranial hemorrhage *(arrows)* following intranasal sphenoethmoidectomy.

fovea ethmoidalis. Severe intracranial hemorrhage (Fig. 10–7) also may result from injury to the internal carotid artery with the formation of a pseudoaneurysm or carotid–cavernous sinus fistula. This most commonly occurs from instrumentation in the lateral recess of the sphenoid sinus where the bone

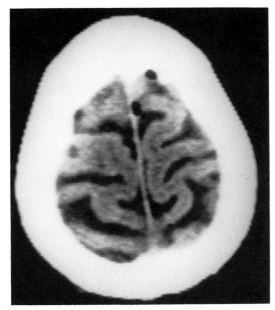

FIGURE 10–6. Axial CT scan of pneumocephalus secondary to intranasal sphenoethmoidectomy. The intracranial air outlines the cerebral gyri.

over the artery is dehiscent or has been perforated. Management of a major intracranial vascular injury is by nasal packing to tamponade the bleeding until an anterior craniotomy can be performed to repair or ligate the injured vessels and evacuate the hematoma.

The occurrence of these complications is documented in several reviews. Among nine patients with major complications following ethmoidectomy, Maniglia described three cases with a CSF leak accompanied by meningitis or epidural abscess, one case of carotid–cavernous sinus fistula, and one fatal instance of brain laceration.[20] In a later study, Maniglia reported six patients sustaining intracranial injuries following sinonasal surgery, two of which were fatal.[22] This consisted of four CSF leaks, two with meningitis; two intracranial hemorrhages; and one frontal lobe laceration. The two lethal cases consisted of massive intracranial hemorrhage from internal carotid artery injury in one patient, and an anterior cerebral artery laceration in another following endoscopic sphenoid sinus biopsy. Stankiewicz also described 7 instances of CSF leak among 700 endoscopic ethmoidectomies.[27]

SINONASAL

Scarring following instrumentation of the frontal recess may result in obstruction of the nasofrontal duct, with the development of acute or chronic frontal sinusitis or mucocele formation.[28] Injury to the nasolacrimal duct from carrying a middle or inferior meatus antrostomy too far anteriorly may produce stenosis with epiphora and dacryocystitis developing clinically. The nasolacrimal duct is also vulnerable to damage in cleaning out well-pneumatized agger nasi cells. The development of dacryostenosis requires endoscopic repair or dacryorhinocystostomy. Anosmia may result from removal of olfactory mucosa or fibrosis developing in the region of the cribriform plate. Wigand recommended that the superior portion of the middle turbinate be preserved to prevent the loss of mucosa that potentially contains olfactory elements.[29] The occurrence of atrophic rhinitis following resection of the middle turbinate as part of a complete sphenoethmoidectomy has been observed rarely.[29–31] We have not observed its development in over 1000 ethmoidectomies if a normal inferior turbinate was present.[32]

Closure of antrostomies made in both the middle and inferior meatus can occur no matter how wide they were created if circumferential enlargement is performed. Synechia formation results from adhesions forming between denuded mucosal surfaces present on the middle and inferior turbinate and the lateral nasal wall and septum from instrumentation. This most commonly occurs between inferior turbinate and septum and middle turbinate and lateral nasal wall. The former produces some degree of airway destruction. The latter may accompany endoscopic sinus surgery when the lateral surface of the middle turbinate has been removed and may result in middle meatus obstruction with recurrent infection.

Nasal hemorrhage results from injury to the sphenopalatine or ethmoid arteries and their branches and may have an immediate or delayed onset. Control of the bleeding may be achieved by electrocautery and light nasal anterior packing, or control may require posterior packing, arterial ligation, and blood transfusion.

OTHER COMPLICATIONS

Transient or persistent neuralgia of the face, lips, gingiva, teeth, and palate may arise from irritation of branches of the infraorbital, superior alveolar, and ethmoid nerves. Pain control may require analgesics and antineuralgic medications (phenytoin, carbamazepine).

Since extensive sinusitis and polyposis often develop in asthmatic patients, the precipitation of an acute attack intra- or postoperatively, under local or general anesthesia, may occur. Management may require administration of intravenous or inhalant steroids and bronchodilators.

A review of the large series reported of intranasal ethmoidectomies, whether performed conventionally,[28, 31, 33, 34] endoscopically,[29, 35–38] or microscopically,[39, 40] generally reveals a rate of serious complications of about 1 per cent to 3 per cent. Comparative evaluation does not reveal any one operative technique to be inherently safer, with the incidence of complications directly related to operator experience.

MAXILLARY SINUS SURGERY

CALDWELL-LUC PROCEDURE

Caldwell in 1893, Sprier in 1894, and Luc in 1897 described entry into the maxillary sinus via the canine fossa, also incorporating a nasoantral window for drainage.[41, 42] Although the Caldwell-Luc procedure was devised initially for the treatment of chronic maxillary sinusitis, subsequent applications include access to the ethmoid labyrinth and the orbital floor for the decompression of malignant endocrine exophthalmos; access to the pterygomaxillary space for the ligation of the internal maxillary artery; vidian neurectomy or sphenopalatine ganglionectomy; the repair of malar, orbital floor, and nasomaxillary fractures; and the removal of odontogenic and other benign sinonasal tumors.[43] After more than 90 years and numerous applications, the Caldwell-Luc procedure remains controversial for the treatment of chronic maxillary sinusitis because of the associated morbidity. The advent of endoscopic sinus surgery has reduced the number of Caldwell-Luc procedures performed; however, to what extent and with what efficiency it will eradicate chronic maxillary sinus inflammatory disease remains to be determined by longitudinal study.

The sublabial approach to the maxillary sinus through the canine fossa employs a mucoperiosteal incision and removal of the lateral antral wall. This disrupts both mucosal and osseous branches of the superior alveolar nerve. The anterior, middle, and posterior portions of this nerve extensively anastomose along the lateral wall of the maxilla to form the alveolar plexus.[44] Entry into the antrum entails disruption of the plexus, with the degree of nerve injury directly related to the extent of bone removal. Moreover, operative manipulation superiorly encroaches upon and may result in damage to the infraorbital nerve, directly or by retraction. Accordingly, the most common complication of this operation is paresthesia of the cheek, gingiva, and the teeth, which may persist for as long as 6 months. Direct damage to the nerve may produce persistent pain or neuroma formation. Prolonged and profound paresthesias and neuralgias are more commonly encountered following wide entry into the maxillary sinus for access to the pterygopalatine fossa or for orbital decompression. Retraction of the soft tissues over the anterolateral surface of the maxilla results in facial swelling secondary to edema, bleeding, periosteal reaction, lymphatic obstruction, and fibrosis. This may last days to weeks and in rare cases may be permanent.

The reported morbidity of the procedure ranges from 3 per cent to 40 per cent.[42, 45, 46] Yarington reported 8 complications (3 per cent) among 127 Caldwell-Luc procedures performed in 70 patients.[45] These included postoperative anesthesia (one), devitalized teeth (two), postoperative bleeding (one), postoperative ethmoiditis (two), acute otitis media (one), and pulmonary atelectasis (one). Murray described postoperative problems in 24 of 45 patients undergoing 60 Caldwell-Luc procedures.[46] These included recurrent sinusitis in ten, numbness persisting more than 6 months in eight, nasal synechiae in three, persisting facial swelling in two, and an abscessed tooth in one patient.

DeFreitas and Lucente reviewed 670 cases performed over a 10-year period at one institution, to better understand and classify the postoperative complications associated with this surgical procedure.[41] These were subdivided into immediate and long-term complications. The immediate complications included facial swelling in 89 per cent, cheek discomfort in 33 per cent, and epistaxis requiring repacking in 2.9 per cent of the cases. The long-term complications included recurrent sinusitis in 12 per cent, facial paresthesias in 9.1 per cent, recurrent polyps in 5.4 per cent, dacryocystitis in 2.6 per cent, gingivolabial fistula in 1.5 per cent, oroantral fistula in 1.1 per cent, and a devitalized tooth in 0.4 per cent. Overall, approximately 19 per cent of the cases manifested some operative complication.

Hutterbrink and Clemens reported that sensory disturbances following the Caldwell-Luc procedure could be significantly decreased by creating an osteoplastic flap of the anterior wall of the maxillary sinus.[47]

The radiologic changes that occur in the maxillary sinus following the Caldwell-Luc procedure include fibro-osseous proliferation, antral contraction, and compartmentalization.[48] These findings cause difficulties in distinguishing postoperative changes from recurrent disease on plain x-ray films. However, with the use of the CT scan this differentiation can be made in the majority of cases.[48]

We have also seen several cases of secondary mucocele formation (Fig. 10–8). They arise from subtotal removal of the lining mucosa, with circumferential fibrosis producing compartmentalization of the antrum; epithelial proliferation now leads to the development of a mucocele in the enclosed space.

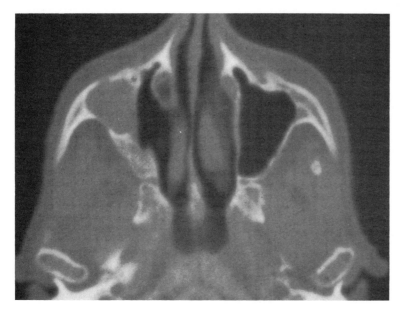

FIGURE 10–8. Axial CT scan revealing the formation of a secondary mucocele in the zygomatic recess of the maxillary sinus after the Caldwell-Luc procedure.

ANTROSTOMY

The creation of an intranasal antrostomy in the inferior meatus was first described by Mikulicz, in 1886, as an attempt to control infection of the maxillary sinus.[49] His procedure was later revised by Krause and Siebermann, who placed the opening in the middle meatus.[48] An antrostomy is presently employed not only for drainage but also for repeated irrigations and the removal of debris or foreign bodies from the maxillary sinus. Among the complications reported with this procedure are hemorrhage, formation of synechia, and closure of the window.[49] Closure of the antrostomy commonly occurs despite the creation of a wide aperture, if the margins have been denuded of mucosa circumferentially. It should also be noted that antrostomy patency does not guarantee control of chronic maxillary sinus disease. The creation of an antrostomy in both the middle and inferior meatus carries the risk of epiphora and dacryocystitis from nasolacrimal duct injury if bone removal is performed too far anteriorly. Excessive enlargement of the opening posteriorly in the inferior meatus may result in hemorrhage from injury to lateral branches of the sphenopalatine artery. Instrumentation of the maxillary sinus through an antrostomy can also result in paresthesias of the teeth and gingiva.

In small children, special consideration should be given to the presence of unerupted teeth when performing an antral irrigation or creating a nasoantral window. However, Tjellstrom and Sagne studied a group of children following antrostomy and antral irrigation over a 3-year period and found no significant effects on the formation and mineralization of the permanent dentition between the control group and the operated group.[50]

TRANSANTRAL ETHMOIDECTOMY

The transantral ethmoidectomy, which is indicated when extensive maxillary sinus disease as well as ethmoid pathology is present, carries the added potential morbidity of ethmoidectomy. Kimmelman and colleagues reported a 20 per cent complication rate in their series of 74 cases.[8] These included temporary facial edema (ten), facial pain (four), hemorrhage (three—two of which required transfusion), nasolacrimal duct injury (one), temporary lip and facial anesthesia (seven), persistent gingival anesthesia (three), and oroantral fistula (one). Friedman and Katsantonis described 2 major (one CSF leak, one epistaxis requiring arterial ligation) and 8 minor (seven postoperative pain and numbness, one epistaxis) complications among 137 transantral sphenoethmoidectomies.[30]

RHINOTOMY

The lateral rhinotomy provides access to the nasal cavity through its lateral wall for the removal of a variety of benign and malignant tumors. In itself it gives limited exposure of the anterior nasal cavity alone; however, it gains versatility by combining it with a medial maxillectomy or an external ethmoidectomy, or modifying it into a superior or total rhinotomy depending on the histology, location, and extent of the lesion to be resected.

Among the 162 rhinotomies performed in 148 patients by Bernard and group, 139 (86 per cent) were combined with another procedure.[51] This included a medial maxillectomy in 120 cases, a bifrontal craniotomy with craniofacial resection in 12 cases, a mandibulotomy in 3 patients, a partial maxillectomy in 2 patients, and a transpalatal and trans-sphenoid approach in 1 patient each.

A variety of complications have been described, the incidence and severity of which are related to the extent of the adjunctive procedure—that is, whether unilateral or bilateral osteotomies, a medial maxillectomy, or craniofacial resection is performed.

In a review of 13 cases of lateral rhinotomy combined with a medial maxillectomy, Myers and associates reported six patients developing epiphora, three having chronic dacryocystitis requiring dacryocystorhinostomy, and one with diplopia.[52]

In the series of 226 cases reported by Mertz and colleagues, there was an immediate complication rate of 2 per cent and a later postoperative complication rate of 15 per cent.[53] The immediate complications included meningitis (one), hemorrhage (two), and cardiac arrest (two). The late complications included the development of ectropion and epiphora in 14 patients, CSF leak in 3, and hematoma, frontal sinus mucocele, frontal duct obstruction, and facial neuralgia in 1 each. Other reported complications were poor cosmetic results in five patients, and synechia, nasal collapse, and septal perforation in another eight patients.

Among the ten cases of rhinotomy and medial maxillectomy published by Sessions and Larson, two patients developed epiphora.[54]

In the series of 162 rhinotomies reported by Bernard and group, 32 patients (21 per cent) developed complications.[51] Early complications occurred in 16 patients (11 per cent), with 4 having epiphora and intermittent dacryocystitis, 2 with diplopia, and 2 a CSF leak that resolved spontaneously. The majority (13 patients) developed transient blepharitis and eyelid edema.

Epiphora and dacryocystitis are relatively common postoperative complications, resulting either from edema or stenosis of the nasolacrimal duct. Although Sessions and Larson modified their resection to maintain the anatomic integrity of the nasolacrimal drainage system, this did not prevent its development.[54] Sessions and Humphrey later reported transecting the lacrimal sac and then stenting the opening with a polyethylene tube.[55] Bernard and group reported good results with just marsupialization of the cut end of the duct; however, the ducts of four patients subsequently stenosed and eventually required dacryocystorhinostomy.[51]

Transient diplopia results from detaching the trochlea from the superior aspect of the orbit. Simple reattachment of the orbital periosteum is generally sufficient for the patient to regain adequate support and function.

Nasal crusting generally can be anticipated with this procedure, but it tends to resolve within the first 6 months as re-epithelialization of the operative cavity occurs. Meticulous nasal hygiene, with frequent irrigation and periodic cauterization of granulations, hastens the healing process. Persistent crusting should be anticipated in patients who have received previous radiation therapy.

Telecanthus is another well-recognized complication of rhinotomy and medial maxillectomy. Sessions and Humphrey recommended wiring the medial canthal ligament to the frontal process of the maxilla.[55] However, good results were reported by Bernard and group simply with careful suture approximation of the medial canthal ligament to the periosteum.[51]

Transection of the nasofrontal duct carries the risk of stenosis and the possibility of

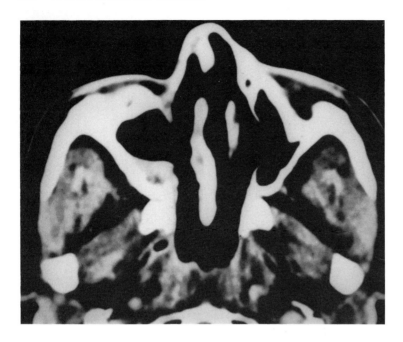

FIGURE 10–9. Axial CT scan demonstrating nasal collapse following lateral rhinotomy and medial maxillectomy.

development of a frontal sinus mucocele. This complication is fortunately rare; so far, only four cases have been reported.

Vestibular stenosis is principally a complication of total rhinotomy. It can be avoided by leaving a strip of skin between the alar and columella incisions and by carefully reapproximating these incisions, along with the placement of nasal packing.[51]

Nasocutaneous fistulas generally arise in irradiated patients undergoing medial maxillectomy. Two such cases occurred in Bernard and group's series, one of which closed spontaneously, with the other requiring repair with a nasolabial flap.[51]

Late cosmetic complications also occur with this procedure. Mertz and associates reported that 5 of their 226 patients had unacceptable scars.[53] Bernard and group reported a 10 per cent incidence of cosmetic complications.[51] Improper incision placement resulted in unacceptable scars in six patients. In one patient, the incision was placed too close to the medial canthus and webbing developed; another had depilation on the medial aspect of the eyebrow secondary to injury to the hair follicles from an unbeveled incision, and four had incisions placed too far laterally on the cheek. Ten other patients developed nasal collapse due to a combination of shift of the nasal pyramid, saddle deformity, columella collapse, and alar retraction (Fig. 10–9). It is noteworthy that eight of the ten patients with this complication had a medial maxillectomy, with six of the ten having undergone a total rhinotomy, demonstrating the importance of a strong, undisrupted nasal support, both laterally and centrally.

MAXILLECTOMY

Maxillectomy is generally performed for the extirpation of malignant tumors of the antrum; however, it may be required for the management of benign but destructive lesions (e.g., osteomyelitis, hemangiomas, giant cell tumors, ameloblastoma, aggressive fibromatosis). The extent and nature of the lesion determine the type of resection performed, which can vary from a partial (medial, infrastructure) maxillectomy to a total maxillectomy, with orbital preservation or exenteration, and even can be combined with a craniofacial resection when involvement of the anterior skull base is present. The operative and postoperative complications vary with the extent of the resection and whether the patient has received radiotherapy.

The total maxillectomy is among the oldest of the "monoblock" operations for cancer.[56] Although the surgical approach has remained relatively the same, the operative mortality and rehabilitation of the patient have improved. Nevertheless, a variety of functional and cosmetic complications are associated with maxillectomy because of its strategic relationship to the orbit, skull base, paranasal sinuses, and oral cavity. In addition to severe hemorrhage, serious orbital and intracranial complications are common.

Hemorrhage remains a major complication of maxillectomy. Intraoperatively, this results from inadequate exposure of the pterygomaxillary area, with poor control of the internal maxillary artery and its branches and damage to the pterygoid venous plexus and the anterior and posterior ethmoidal arteries. Postoperatively, epistaxis and hemorrhage can become uncontrollable, leading to death, as reported by La Vertu and associates.[57] Orbital hemorrhage is a rare but serious complication of maxillectomy due to inadequate control of the anterior or posterior ethmoid arteries.[58] Immediate medical and surgical intervention is necessary to reduce intraocular pressure and preserve vision in the affected eye.

Cerebrospinal fluid leaks occur when the dissection is carried along the cribriform plate and with a combined craniofacial resection. Gelfoam, dermis, muscle, and fascia can be used to cover the defect and seal off the leak. Meningitis may occur postoperatively but generally resolves with systemic antibiotic therapy. Nevertheless, death from meningitis has been reported by La Vertu and colleagues, who also mentioned the formation of subdural hematomas that required surgical drainage.[57] Suppuration within the maxillectomy cavity, which led to the development of a fatal brain abscess, was described by Bridger.[59]

In addition to the intracranial complications of craniofacial resection, osteomyelitis of the frontal bone flap requiring surgical debridement also has been reported. One death occurred from infection and brain herniation secondary to loss of the pericranial flap during radiation therapy.[56]

Larson and coworkers described ophthalmologic complications developing in 56 per cent of the patients in whom the orbital contents were preserved.[60] In this series, one patient developed an ipsilateral exposure keratitis and a contralateral optic atrophy, due to postoperative radiation, resulting in bilateral blindness.

In a review of 19 patients undergoing radical maxillectomy and followed 1 to 18 years, Smith and coworkers reported all to possess some degree of enophthalmos (100 per cent).[61] Cicatricial ectropion was present in 32 per cent; permanent diplopia in primary gaze position was evident in 11 per cent; early nasolacrimal duct obstruction was present in 32 per cent but rose to 63 per cent after 6 months. Also, transient diplopia was present in 37 per cent, and visual loss occurred in 16 per cent. These workers concluded that the cicatricial ectropion that developed from late contracture of the split-thickness skin graft used to line the maxillary cavity was the most difficult problem to correct.[61]

Although the cheek flap raised as part of the Weber-Ferguson incision is lined with a split-thickness skin graft to prevent flap contracture, the skin graft may slough, producing facial deformity. Ahmad reported a case of skin graft failure, which led to exposure and partial necrosis of the zygomatic arch.[62] When the malar bone is resected to achieve total maxillectomy for lesions with posterior antral extension, severe facial deformity is universally present.

In cases in which the orbital contents are preserved, reconstruction of the orbital floor is mandatory. Sobol and coworkers[63] reported good results using homologous lyophilized dura as did Larson and associates.[60] However, we favor the use of Marlex mesh, which provides rigid support. Despite this, the ocular complications of ptosis, diplopia, enophthalmos, ectropion, epiphora, and exposure keratitis are common (Fig. 10–10). The adjunctive use of radiation increases their incidence and severity and predisposes the patient also to cataract, optic atrophy,

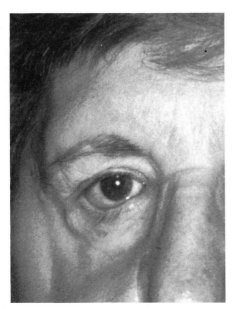

FIGURE 10–10. Facial deformity following total maxillectomy with orbital floor reconstruction. The lateral midfacial depression results from resection of the malar bone. Loss of the support of the infraorbital rim produces an ectropion.

and ophthalmitis. The ectropion that results following resection and reconstruction of the orbital floor generally cannot be corrected by skin grafting alone but requires the insertion of a cartilage graft to provide additional support to the tarsus.

When a lower eyelid incision is required for exposure, persistent postoperative edema may develop from interruption of the venous and lymphatic drainage. Eyelid edema is more pronounced and may even be permanent in patients having received radiotherapy. Ectropion has also been reported with this type of incision.[61] The standard horizontal eyelid incision meets that along the side of the nose to form an acute angle. The tip of the flap created has a tendency to slough, especially in irradiated cases, with the formation of a nasocutaneous fistula. To prevent this, Dr. Max Som modified the standard Weber-Ferguson incision by eliminating the eyelid component and carrying the nasal limb straight upward to the medial aspect of the eyebrow. Sobol and coworkers also reported success with this modification.[63]

A combined median mandibulotomy and

Weber-Ferguson maxillectomy approach has been devised for the management of advanced maxillary tumors involving the infratemporal fossa. The complications associated with the mandibulotomy include the development of nonunion (more commonly seen in diabetics) and orocutaneous fistulas. The latter generally respond to conservative management.[51]

References

1. Lawson W: The frontal sinus. In Blitzer A, Lawson W, Friedman AH (eds): Philadelphia, Surgery of the Paranasal Sinuses. WB Saunders, 1985, pp 120–144.
2. Goode RL, Strelzow V, Fee WE: Frontal sinus septectomy for chronic unilateral sinusitis. Otolaryngol Head Neck Surg 88:18, 1980.
3. Lawson W: The external frontoethmoidectomy. Goldman JL (ed): In The Principles and Practice of Rhinology. New York, John Wiley, 1987, pp 413–423.
4. Goodale RL: Some causes for failure in frontal sinus surgery. Ann Otol 51:648, 1942.
5. Harris HE: The use of tantalum tubes in frontal sinus surgery. Cleve Clin Q 15:129, 1948.
6. Williams HL, Holman CB: The causes and avoidance of failure in surgery, for chronic suppuration of the fronto-ethmosphenoid complex of sinuses: With a previous unreported anomaly which produces chronicity and recurrence, and the description of a surgical technique usually producing a cure of the disease. Laryngoscope 72:1179, 1962.
7. Neel HG, McDonald TJ, Facer GW: Modified Lynch procedure for chronic frontal sinusitis: Rationale, technique and long-term results. Laryngoscope 97:1274, 1987.
8. Kimmelman CP, Weisman RA, Osguthorpe JD, et al: The efficacy and safety of transantral ethmoidectomy. Laryngoscope 98:1178, 1988.
9. MacBeth RG: The osteoplastic operation for chronic infection of the frontal sinus. J Laryngol 68:465, 1954.
10. Bosley WA: Osteoplastic obliteration of the frontal sinuses: A review of 100 patients. Laryngoscope 82:1463, 1972.
11. Donald PJ, Bernstein L: Compound frontal sinus injuries with intracranial penetration. Laryngoscope 88:225, 1978.
12. Donald PJ: Frontal sinus ablation by cranialization. Report of 21 cases. Arch Otolaryngol 108:142, 1982.
13. Duvall AJ, Porto DP, Lyons D, Boies LR: Frontal sinus fractures. Analysis of treatment results. Arch Otolaryngol 113:933, 1987.
14. Hardy JM, Montgomery WW: Osteoplastic frontal sinusotomy. An analysis of 250 operations. Ann Otol 85:523, 1976.
15. Stankiewicz JA: Complications of endoscopic nasal surgery: Occurrence and treatment. Am J Rhinol 1:45, 1987.
16. Stankiewicz JA: Blindness and intranasal endoscopic ethmoidectomy: Prevention and management. Otolaryngol Head Neck Surg 101:320, 1989.

17. Sacks SH, Lawson W, Edelstein D, Green RP: Surgical treatment of blindness secondary to intraorbital hemorrhage. Arch Otolaryngol 114:801, 1988.
18. Mark LE, Kennerdell JS: Medial rectus injury from intranasal surgery. Arch Ophthalmol 97:459, 1979.
19. Flynn JT, Mitchell KB, Fuller OG, et al: Ocular motility complications following intranasal surgery. Arch Ophthalmol 97:453, 1979.
20. Maniglia A, Chandler J, Goodwin W, Flynn J: Rare complications following ethmoidectomies. A report of 11 cases. Laryngoscope 91:1239, 1981.
21. Rosenbaum AL, Astle WF: Superior oblique and inferior rectus muscle injury following frontal and intranasal sinus surgery. J Pediatr Ophthalmol Strabismus 22:194, 1985.
22. Maniglia AJ: Fatal and major complications secondary to nasal and sinus surgery. Laryngoscope 99:276, 1989.
23. Kainz J, Stammberger H: The roof of the anterior ethmoid: A place of least resistance in the skull base. Am J Rhinol 3:191, 1989.
24. Wigand ME: Transnasal ethmoidectomy under endoscopical control. Rhinology 19:7, 1981.
25. Sachdev V, Drapkin A, Hollin S, Malis L: Subarachnoid hemorrhage following intranasal procedures. Surg Neurol 8:122, 1977.
26. Forbes G, Bradley A: Fatality resulting from intranasal polypectomy. J Laryngol 73:445, 1959.
27. Stankiewicz JA: Cerebrospinal fluid leak and endoscopic sinus surgery. Presented at the Middle Section Meeting of The American Laryngological, Rhinological, and Otological Society, January, 1990.
28. Friedman WH, Katsantonis GP: The role of standard technique in modern sinus surgery. Otolaryngol Clin North Am 22:759, 1989.
29. Wigand ME: Endoscopic Surgery of the Paranasal Sinuses and Anterior Skull Base. New York, G. Thieme, 1990.
30. Friedman WH, Katsantonis GP: Intranasal and transantral ethmoidectomy: A 20-year experience. Laryngoscope 100:343, 1990.
31. Taylor JS, Crocker PV, Keebler JS: Intranasal ethmoidectomy and concurrent procedures. Laryngoscope 92:739, 1982.
32. Lawson W: The intranasal ethmoidectomy: An experience with 1077 procedures. Laryngoscope 101(4):367, 1991.
33. Freedman HM, Kern EB: Complications of intranasal ethmoidectomy: A review of 1000 consecutive operations. Laryngoscope 89:421, 1979.
34. Eichel BS: The intranasal ethmoidectomy: A 12-year perspective. Otolaryngol Head Neck Surg 90:540, 1982.
35. Schaefer SD: Endoscopic total sphenoethmoidectomy. Otolaryngol Clin North Am 22:727, 1989.
36. Levine HL: Functional endoscopic sinus surgery: Evaluation, surgery, and follow up of 250 patients. Laryngoscope 100:79, 1990.
37. Stankiewicz JA: Complications of endoscopic intranasal ethmoidectomy. Laryngoscope 97:1270, 1987.
38. Stankiewicz JA: Complications of endoscopic surgery. Otolaryngol Clin North Am 22:749, 1989.
39. Bagatella F, Mazzoni A: Microsurgery in nasal polyposis transnasal ethmoidectomy. Acta Otolaryngol (Suppl 431):1, 1986.
40. Silverstein H, McDaniel AB: Microsurgical sphenoethmoidectomy. In Goldman JL (ed): The Principles
and Practices of Rhinology. New York, John Wiley, 1987, pp 435–442.
41. DeFrietas J, Lucente F: The Caldwell-Luc procedure: Institutional review of 670 cases. Laryngoscope 98:1297, 1988.
42. MacBeth R: Caldwell-Luc operation 1956–1966. Arch Otolaryngol 87:630, 1968.
43. Blitzer A: Surgery for infection and benign diseases of the maxillary sinus. In Blitzer A, Lawson W, Friedman WH (eds): Surgery of the Paranasal Sinuses. Philadelphia, WB Saunders, 1985, p 187.
44. Harrison DH: The surgical anatomy of maxillary and ethmoid sinuses. A reappraisal. Laryngoscope 81:1658, 1971.
45. Yarington CT: The Caldwell-Luc operation revisited. Ann Otol 93:380, 1984.
46. Murray P: Complications after treatment of chronic maxillary sinus disease with Caldwell-Luc procedure. Laryngoscope 93:282, 1983.
47. Hutterbrink KB, Clemens S: Spatfolgen der Caldwell-Luc operation. Laryngol Rhinol Otol 65:69, 1986.
48. Som PM: The paranasal sinuses. In Bergeron RT, Osborn AG (eds): Head and Neck Surgery, Excluding the Brain. St. Louis, CV Mosby, 1989, pp 1–142.
49. Sogg J: Intranasal antrostomy—causes of failure. Laryngoscope 92:1038, 1982.
50. Tjellstrom A, Sagne S: Effects of intranasal antrostomy and antral lavage upon unerupted permanent teeth. J Laryngol Otol 93:883, 1979.
51. Bernard J, Lawson W, Biller HF, LeBenger J: Complications following rhinotomy. Ann Otol Rhinol Laryngol 98:684, 1989.
52. Myers EN, Schramm VL, Barnes FL: Management of inverting papilloma of the nose and paranasal sinuses. Laryngoscope 91:2021, 1981.
53. Mertz JS, Pearson BW, Kern EB: Lateral rhinotomy; Indications, technique and review of 226 cases. Arch Otolaryngol 109:236, 1985.
54. Sessions RB, Larson DL: En bloc ethmoidectomy and medial maxillectomy. Arch Otolaryngol 103:195, 1977.
55. Sessions RB, Humphrey DH: Technical modifications of the medial maxillectomy. Arch Otolaryngol 109:575, 1983.
56. Curtin JM: Malignant disease of the ethmoid and maxillary antrum. Br J Med Sci 6:488, 1957.
57. La Vertu P, Roberts JK, Kraus DH, et al: Squamous cell carcinoma of the paranasal sinuses: The Cleveland Clinic Experience 1974–1986. Laryngoscope 99:1130, 1989.
58. Thompson RF, Gluckman JL, Kulwin D, Savoury L: Orbital hemorrhage during ethmoid sinus surgery. Otolaryngol Head Neck Surg 102:45, 1990.
59. Bridger MW: Carcinoma of the paranasal sinuses: A review of 158 cases. J Otolaryngol 7:383, 1978.
60. Larson DL, Christ JE, Jesse RH: Preservation of the orbital contents in cancer of the maxillary sinus. Acta Otolaryngol 108:370, 1982.
61. Smith B, Lisman RD, Baker D: Eyelid and orbital treatment following radical maxillectomy. Ophthalmology 91:218, 1984.
62. Ahmad K: Squamous cell carcinoma of the maxillary sinus. Arch Otolaryngol 107:48, 1981.
63. Sobol SM, Wood B, Levine M: An approach to total maxillectomy with emphasis on orbital preservation. Plast Reconstr Surg 69:945, 1982.

CHAPTER
11

Functional Endoscopic Sinus Surgery

JORDAN S. JOSEPHSON, MD
DALE H. RICE, MD
GARY D. JOSEPHSON, MD

Functional endoscopic sinus surgery is a relatively new technique, recently introduced into the United States. The technique not only stresses precise surgical dissection but also and more importantly provides detailed diagnostic assessment and accurate postoperative care.[1-4] Functional endoscopic sinus surgery has been shown to be safe and effective in the hands of experienced surgeons; however, it still carries the risks and complications of traditional intranasal sinus surgery.

The functional endoscopic approach is based on the meticulous studies performed by Messerklinger on mucociliary clearance and on the pathophysiology of inflammatory sinus disease. Messerklinger further stressed atraumatic technique, restoration of the mucociliary clearance pathways, and operation tailored to the extent of disease, thus providing a functional result.[5, 6]

Mosher stated that "intranasal ethmoidectomy is one of the most dangerous and blindest of all surgical operations."[7] This certainly applies to functional endoscopic sinus surgery, which adds better visualization but does not provide binocular vision (depth perception). This combination may give the novice surgeon a false sense of security and lead to a subsequent disastrous complication. To minimize the chance of complications, it is recommended that the inexperienced surgeon obtain appropriate didactic training and multiple cadaver dissections, so that he or she may become familiar with the anatomy and the use of the instruments.

All sinus procedures, traditional and endoscopic, have advantages and disadvantages. The incidence and potential sites of complications seem to depend upon the particular procedure and on the experience of the surgeon with that procedure. The surgeon must clearly discuss the risks and benefits with the patient preoperatively and, based upon all factors, should choose the safest procedure that will provide the best result for the patient.

In general, the external approach to the ethmoid sinuses provides the safest and most familiar approach with the best control of potential bleeding sites. Intranasal techniques carry the highest risk of complication because of the limited access and potential for injury to the orbit and ethmoidal roof.[8] When combined with septal mobilization, turbinate resection, or the transantral approach, the intranasal technique provides good access to most areas.[9] However, a significant limitation to the intranasal approach, even when combined with microscopic magnification, is the inability to see the frontal recess area.

Performing intranasal ethmoidectomy under endoscopic control provides improved visualization and the ability to see into the frontal recess and sometimes into the frontal sinus, as well as visualize the maxillary and sphenoid sinuses, without additionally performing septal mobilization, turbinate removal, or a transantral approach. However, it is important that the surgeon be comfortable operating with monocular vision. Meticulous atraumatic tissue handling and precise hemostatic techniques become critical when using the endoscopic approach because blood on the tip of the endoscope may obstruct the surgeon's view. The functional endoscopic surgical approach stresses accurate endoscopic and tomographic preoperative assessment, meticulous intraoperative surgical technique, and precise postoperative cleaning.

COMPLICATION RATE

Many surgeons have discussed their complication rates. Although Stammberger and Messerklinger were able to perform over 2500 procedures without serious complications, significant complications still may occur in experienced hands, and the potential for complications is great.[9–11]

Vleming and de Vries report a 1.8 per cent minor complication rate with no major complications.[12] Stankiewicz, on the other hand, reports a 29 per cent complication rate, 8 per cent consisting of major complications.[13]

However, this report reviewed his first 90 patients undergoing endoscopic ethmoidectomy. He later brought his series up to date and reported an overall complication rate of 9.3 per cent on 300 ethmoidectomies in 180 patients.[14] His overall complication rate in his second 90 cases was reported at 2.2 per cent, which is comparable to complication rates published for intranasal ethmoidectomy. He further states that "the low complication rate in the second group of 90 patients (150 ethmoidectomies) indicates that safe ethmoidectomy surgery can be performed once experience is gained. However, this does not mean that the surgeon should 'let down his guard.' Constant attention to anatomic detail and location is paramount."[14]

MAJOR COMPLICATIONS

Hemorrhage

Sinus surgery need not be a bloody procedure despite the fact that the tissues of the nose and paranasal sinuses are well vascularized. However, severe bleeding from this area, necessitating blood replacement, would be subject to all the risks of receiving a transfusion. Bleeding during functional endoscopic sinus surgery also may interfere with visualization, and may even obligate the surgeon to conclude the surgery and finish later. Careful attention to detail usually will obviate this complication.

Preoperatively, potential bleeders must be identified by obtaining a complete history. Any medicines that may cause bleeding should be discontinued far enough in advance to permit reversal of their anticoagulant properties. Any coagulation disorders must be attended to thoroughly and treated appropriately before operation.

Whether the operation is performed under local or general anesthesia, careful application of topical and infiltrative vasoconstrictive agents is required. Adequate time must be allowed for the hemostatic effects to take place.

When dealing with significant polyposis, laser surgery performed to remove the polyps usually will provide adequate hemostasis during the procedure. The laser may also be used to remove a concha bullosa or to coagulate an area of bleeding to provide good hemostasis during the operation. As well, it is important to control the patient's blood pressure. Sedation or hypotensive anesthetic techniques should be used in addition.

Meticulous technique throughout the entire procedure allows for good hemostasis. When thickened sinus mucosa is present, removal may be preceded by direct application of vasoconstrictive agents to reduce bleeding.

Bleeding from the anterior or posterior ethmoid vessels or a branch is usually controlled with a topical vasoconstrictive cottonoid, as is most bleeding in the area. However, it is occasionally necessary to use oxidized cellulose, a gelatin sponge, or microfibrillar collagen for hemostasis. Oxidized cellulose also inhibits bacterial growth but may be irritating in large amounts because of its low pH. Microfibrillar collagen seems to be the most effective agent for hemostasis; however, it is more difficult to apply. Both the cellulose and the collagen may be difficult to remove.

The occurrence of bleeding from the ethmoid vessels should alert the surgeon of the close proximity to the skull base. In addition, any bleeding into the orbit from anterior or posterior ethmoid artery injury can result in visual disturbance. Intraorbital or periorbital bleeding is rare during this type of surgery but will be discussed in the blindness and visual disturbance section later.

During the sphenoid portion of the surgery, care must be taken to avoid the sphenopalatine artery and its major branches, which cross inferiorly on the face of the rostrum. Cavernous sinus bleeding, although profuse, usually responds well to light packing. Postoperatively these patients must be carefully monitored and evaluated by computed tomographic scan or magnetic resonance imaging for evidence of an intracranial bleed. In addition, the carotid arteries lie in the grooves of the lateral aspect of the sinus. Occasionally the carotid canal wall may be dehiscent or the canal may lie in the party wall between the sphenoid and the most posterior ethmoid cell. In any case, violation of the carotid artery can lead to disastrous bleeding, possible stroke, and death.

If the patient is bleeding significantly at the end of the procedure or if the surgeon is worried about bloody postnasal discharge causing bronchospasm in the asthmatic patient, a sponge may be placed lateral to the middle turbinate. A sponge also may be helpful in reducing scarring in the presence of tight anatomy or very reactive nasal mucosa. A Merocel sponge with a silk suture at one end is cut to size and coated with antibiotic ointment. The sponge is placed lateral to the middle turbinate under direct visualization and removed within 24 hours. If it is anticipated that leaving the sponge for a longer period of time may be desirable, the Merocel sponge is placed in an antibiotic-coated finger cot prior to insertion. The silk suture is taped to the patient's cheek for easy removal.

As a rule, epistaxis following endoscopic sinus surgery is easily controlled by topical vasoconstrictive and hemostatic agents but may occasionally require packing. Arterial ligation is rarely required but should be preoperatively evaluated with angiography. Radiologic embolization may be considered.

Cerebrospinal Fluid Leak

The chance of cerebrospinal fluid (CSF) leak may be minimized by several factors. Strong knowledge of the anatomy is certainly very important. Close study of the preoperative CT scan for possible anatomic variation and dehiscent areas, and utilization of this "roadmap" at the time of surgery, are paramount. True coronal plane sections are preferred as they provide the most information regarding the ethmoid roof/skull base. The roof may vary from being almost vertical to being almost horizontal. The difference in height between the cribriform plate and the roof may vary from 4 to 16 mm (Fig. 11–1).[15]

The primary sites for intracranial complication are the roof of the ethmoid sinus immediately posterior to the ethmoid dome and the posterior ethmoid superior to the

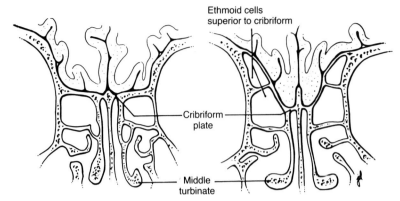

FIGURE 11–1. The anatomy of the ethmoidal sinuses varies widely. It is extremely important to review coronal views of this area prior to operation because these views delineate the difference in height between the skull base and the cribriform plate. The most common site of intracranial entry is where the roof slopes down to the middle turbinate. However, with this type of anatomy, dissection that does not proceed above the origin of the middle turbinate ultimately will leave a layer of ethmoidal cells behind. (From Kennedy DW: Surgery of the sinuses. *In* Johns ME: Complications in Otolaryngology–Head and Neck Surgery. Vol 2. Philadelphia, BC Decker Inc, 1986.)

sphenoid sinus (Fig. 11–2). If bleeding occurs during the dissection in the ethmoid dome, it should be assumed that the skull base has been reached unless proved otherwise. Posteriorly, the last ethmoid cell is usually lateral to the sphenoid sinus and is in close proximity to the optic nerve. In this case, if the surgeon tries to reach the sphenoid by going posterior to this lateral posterior ethmoid cell, undesirable intracranial encroachment will occur. The anterior sphenoid face usually lies more inferiorly than expected. The ostium is approximately 30° from the floor of the nose and measures approximately 7 cm from the nasal aperture in the adult. Finding the sphenoid ostium as a landmark is the safest way to enter the sphenoid.

Identifying the middle turbinate and only operating lateral to it enables the surgeon to avoid the cribriform plate. Identification of the anterior and posterior neurovascular bundles provides the surgeon with the superior limit—the skull base. The dome of the ethmoid, the frontal recess, the sphenoid rostrum, and the medial orbital wall further demarcate the operative field. In addition, in

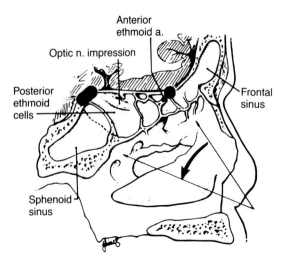

FIGURE 11–2. Sagittal section through the paranasal sinuses, revealing two areas for potential injury during intranasal ethmoidectomy *(blackened areas)*. The curved arrow shows the range of instrument rotation required to perform the dissection. The posterior-most ethmoid cell is seen wrapping around the lateral aspect of the sphenoid sinus *(dotted line)*. (From Kennedy DW: Surgery of the sinuses. *In* Johns ME: Complications in Otolaryngology–Head and Neck Surgery. Vol 2. Philadelphia, BC Decker Inc, 1986.)

surgical procedures under local anesthesia, both the skull base and the medial orbital wall show increased sensitivity to pain, and this should alert the surgeon to having encroached upon those areas.

The most frequent cause of CSF leakage during sinus surgery is intranasal ethmoidectomy or polypectomy. Dural exposure may occur as a result of a congenital defect, chronic disease, or previous sinus or neurosurgery and must be identified preoperatively, when possible. The surgeon must bear in mind that the CT scan may not be fully accurate and may in fact miss a small dehiscence. Any white or pulsatile mass or one occurring in an unusual area should be considered as a potential meningocele or encephalocele. Aspiration with a small-bore needle is recommended prior to resection.

In the sphenoid sinus, the primary concern when dural injury occurs is not the leak but rather the possibility of damage to the surrounding adjacent structures. Most sphenoid sinus leaks respond well to packing the sinus. After removing the sinus mucosa, fascia is placed against the opening, and the sinus is packed with fat. The anterior wall is reconstructed with fascia, and bone or cartilage may be used to reconstruct the opening. Occult CSF leak in the case of cavernous sinus bleeding must be considered.

CSF leaks may be noted intraoperatively or postoperatively. If noted intraoperatively, the leak should be identified by direct visualization. A blunt probe or instrument may be used to mark the site, and the point of injury may be documented radiographically with lateral skull films. This is important, since subsequent postoperative identification may be difficult. Most small leaks will probably close spontaneously; however, any leak large enough to be recognized should be closed immediately by utilizing a mucosal flap or free tissue graft. If the operation is terminated in the presence of a leak, the patient's nose should be lightly packed or not packed at all. Tight packing may increase the risk of meningitis and probably does not increase the chance of closure.

Neurosurgical consultation may provide additional assistance. Occasionally, placement of a lumbar drain at the time of surgery or serial lumbar punctures may allow the leak to close early and with minimal morbidity. Bed rest, refraining from the Valsalva maneuver, and neurologic monitoring are important.

The use of antibiotics is controversial. Some surgeons recommend antibiotic prophylaxis[16] and others cite no significant difference in the infection rate with prophylactic antibiotic administration.[17] However, together the otolaryngologist and neurosurgeon should decide whether their specific case requires antibiotics and administer them if necessary. In our practice, antibiotics are used for patients with CSF leaks who have been treated for chronic sinus infections or those who have an indwelling lumbar catheter.

Any patient with intraoperative leak should have an early postoperative CT scan to provide information about the possibility of intracranial hemorrhage or damage. A later CT scan may be indicated for follow-up or to check for infection.

CSF leaks that do not respond to closure from below or spinal drainage require neurosurgical exploration and closure from above. A transfrontal approach with subsequent fat obliteration of the sinus may be utilized; however, the technique of choice should be based on the experience of the surgeon.

Any CSF leaks that are recognized postoperatively need further evaluation. Endoscopy may be helpful in identifying the site of the leak, but identification may not always be possible.

Further studies may be helpful in identifying the leak if direct visualization fails. Intrathecal fluorescein and endoscopy with a blue light may be used in combination. Radioactive tagged albumin or water-soluble contrast agents (metrizamide) intrathecally injected with CT scan monitoring may localize the leak.

The patients usually complain of persistent clear nasal discharge or the feeling of fluid passing down the posterior pharynx. Low-pressure headaches (bifrontal headaches exacerbated by sitting up) and pneumocephalus are common. Meningitis frequently develops, particularly if the leak persists.

The initial treatment of a leak discovered postoperatively should be medical. The treatment consists of bed rest and diverting the CSF from the leak site to allow closure of the opening by normal wound contracture processes. Repeated lumbar puncture or indwelling percutaneous lumbar cistern drainage catheters have been used successfully to treat CSF leaks. The amount of CSF drainage varies with each case and is important to the success of stopping the leak. Simple elevation of the head just above the heart lessens intracranial CSF pressure and lessens the pressure gradient of the leak. On the other hand, overdrainage of the CSF fluid may lead to exacerbation of headache and may result in pneumocephalus and the development of subdural hematomas. If the CSF leak has not significantly decreased or stopped in 7 to 10 days, operative treatment is elected.

Blindness and Visual Disturbances

It is important preoperatively to uncover any pathologic conditions of the eye. As discussed in the section on hemorrhage, all risk factors for hemorrhage must be screened for preoperatively. It is necessary to obtain ophthalmologic consultation for amblyopia, glaucoma, anisocoria, or functional abnormalities such as retinal vascular disease or diabetic neuropathy. At a minimum, a careful history of eye disease along with gross vision testing should be performed on each patient before operation. It is important to realize that previous operations may have distorted the normal anatomy. This should be examined by reviewing the history for any change in vision before and after previous operations and by reviewing the CT scan for any dehiscence in the bone separating the sinus from the orbit.

The paranasal sinuses and the orbit are intimately related and are separated in these areas by thin bone. This bone may be paper thin, the lamina papyracea, and may on occasion be dehiscent. The dehiscence may be secondary to the disease process or pre-

vious operation, or it may be congenital. It may be noted in the medial or superior walls of the orbit in the areas of the lamina papyracea or posteriorly in the area of the optic nerve. The periorbita is very important; in the case of dehiscent bone, it is the only soft tissue barrier between the ethmoid sinus and the orbital contents. It is tough and fibrous but may be opened easily as it is thin.

The medial orbital wall, which is a crucial landmark used during the endoscopic technique, is formed from anterior to posterior by the frontal process of the maxilla, the lacrimal bone, the lamina papyracea of the ethmoid, and the sphenoid bone anteriorly only to the optic nerve foramen. The lacrimal sac rests in the lacrimal groove anteriorly. The anterior and posterior ethmoidal neurovascular bundles lie in the roof of the ethmoid sinus, and their foramina are located in the frontoethmoidal suture line. These bundles run from the orbit to the ethmoid sinus in a bony canal in the roof of the sinus. This bony canal travels medially to the septum. The globe of the eye occupies most of the space in the anterior orbit. Along with this lie the extraocular muscles, the trochlea, and the lacrimal sac apparatus.

The pathophysiology of blindness and visual disturbance varies. Direct injury to the optic nerve or its blood supply comprises one mechanism leading to visual disturbance. Cases of surgically severed optic nerves, causing immediate total blindness, have been reported. Chiasmatic or bilaterally severed optic nerves may lead to the devastating complication of bilateral blindness.

The optic nerve may become exposed posteriorly or may lie just adjacent to the lamina papyracea as the result of an air cell that is overly large and protrudes into the orbit. If the bony canal of the optic nerve is dehiscent, then the periorbita may be entered, and the optic nerve may be damaged during an ethmoidectomy.

Hemorrhage into the orbit from sinus surgery is most commonly secondary to periorbital encroachment. Ecchymosis, chemosis, and subconjunctival hemorrhage may occur secondary to entrance through the lamina papyracea alone; however, proptosis secondary to retrobulbar hemorrhage usually occurs slowly in this instance. The blood slowly extravasates into the orbital tissues. Various mechanisms may explain the visual disturbance. For one, the limitation of the bony confines of the orbit with a significant hemorrhage may cause an increase in the orbital pressure to the extent that there is impairment of the venous outflow facility and a rise in intraocular tension. Second, the hemorrhage also may cause an apparent paresis of the extraocular muscles, but this is reversible.

Also, there have been reports of visual disturbance secondary to overzealous globe retraction. Monopolar cautery also has been implicated but probably is not responsible unless being utilized adjacent to the optic nerve.

In optic nerve damage, both the direct and consensual pupillary reflex are affected, the afferent pupillary reflex is absent, and light does not stimulate the pupil to constrict. An afferent pupillary defect consisting of a diminished amplitude of pupillary light reaction, a lengthened latent period, and pupillary dilation with continuous light stimulation may be the first indication of optic nerve damage.

Proptosis may be caused by either hemorrhage or orbital emphysema. The onset of lid edema, lid ecchymosis, chemosis, mydriasis, and proptosis is the hallmark of retrobulbar hemorrhage. If the periorbita is entered, these changes may occur immediately. The mechanism of blindness may not be clear; however, it is clear that intervention must be immediate to offer the best chance to avoid ischemia and neural injury.

A dilated pupil with the presence of vision and pupillary reflexes probably reflects local anesthetic effects and is usually a temporary problem. When the operation is performed under local anesthesia, the vision should be constantly monitored. The vision and pupillary response also should be checked on the ipsilateral side before any operation on the contralateral sinus. When the patient is under deep general anesthesia, the pupillary response may be altered but should return as the anesthetic is lightened. The pupil should be checked throughout the operation.

The surgeon should know the narcotics given by the anesthesiologist because they also may alter the pupillary response. Whether the operation is performed under local or general anesthesia, the eye should be directly visualized by a member of the operating team for any movement during the procedure. If any movement is noted, the surgeon should consider that he or she is near the periorbita or into the orbit, until proved otherwise. Gentle palpation on the eyelid over the globe with endoscopic visualization of the sinus will allow identification of the lamina papyracea.

The surgeon must know how to provide adequate local anesthesia, and the patient must be able to tolerate it. A good local anesthesia is advantageous because it leads to a decrease in bleeding, increases the awareness of the surgeon to increased patient discomfort at the skull base and periorbita, and facilitates gross visual testing during the operation. Visual disturbance may occur secondary to injection of local anesthetic/ vasoconstrictive agents, although this is rare.

The surgeon may perform the procedure under general anesthesia; however, the surgeon must be constantly aware of anatomic location without the aid of an awake patient to alert her or him of being in danger areas.

The surgeon also should be aware that the infundibular incision may lead into the lacrimal sac or orbit. Damage to the trochlear or medial rectus may cause diplopia. Should periorbital fat be visualized, it should not be removed. Instead, dissection may be continued around it, leaving it in place. This should be noted in the operative report. The patient should be informed that if any further sinus surgery is performed, the next surgeon should be alerted to the fact that there is a break in the periorbita. Also, packing should be avoided, if possible, as the packing may contribute to increasing the intraorbital pressure. The patient should be observed for signs of orbital hematoma. In most cases, orbital changes will not progress beyond lid edema and ecchymosis.

Postoperative visual loss, pupillary change, or evidence of orbital bleeding requires immediate ophthalmologic or neuro-ophthalmologic consultation and re-exploration. Although injury to the optic nerve may not be reversible, it may be difficult to differentiate from retrobulbar hematoma. Therefore, both the otolaryngologist and the ophthalmologist must work closely to treat this complication. As soon as signs of retrobulbar hematoma appear (ecchymosis, lid edema, chemosis, pupil dilation, or proptosis), management requires immediate mannitol administration, 1 to 2 gm per kg intravenously infused over 30 to 60 minutes. Orbital massage is begun immediately, and any packing that has been inserted should be removed. Lateral canthotomy, Lynch incision, or both, with external ethmoidectomy, may be necessary.

A lateral canthotomy is performed by making a horizontal incision through all the lateral tissues at the lateral canthus, including the raphe. A lateral canthotomy should be performed before a medial decompression is attempted. The orbital pressure should be monitored with a Schiøtz tonometer. If the orbital pressure is not reduced, then a medial (Lynch) decompression should be attempted. The periorbita should be incised to help provide drainage and decompression.

The surgeon should decompress the optic nerve if there is evidence of optic foramen hemorrhage or tension injury.[18] Postoperatively, the patient should be monitored closely.

Miotic eyedrops can reduce intraocular pressure; however, they may interfere when one is trying to evaluate the pupillary response. The use of steroids has been controversial and is without support.

Diplopia is related to direct or indirect injury to the medial rectus muscle or its neurovascular supply. Some diplopia is related to edema and is temporary. However, persistent diplopia may require ophthalmologic surgical correction.

Other Major Complications

The following complications are extremely rare: cavernous sinus–internal carotid artery fistula, anterior fossa brain damage, anesthesia-related cardiac arrhythmias and death, intracranial hemorrhage, pneumocephalus, brain abscess, and malignant hyperthermia. Nevertheless, the surgeon should be aware that these complications have been reported to occur.

MINOR COMPLICATIONS

The following are minor complications of endoscopic sinus surgery: periorbital hematoma, subcutaneous orbital emphysema, epiphora, synechiae, and natural ostia closure.

Periorbital Hematoma

Periorbital hematoma may occur secondary to entering the lamina papyracea or periorbita. Close observation for signs of increased intraocular pressure is necessary. Ecchymosis usually resolves within 1 to 2 weeks.

Subcutaneous Orbital Emphysema

Subcutaneous emphysema occurs secondary to increased pressure forcing air through the lamina papyracea or periorbita or dehiscence. The pressure forcing air through this area is usually caused by nose blowing, sneezing, coughing, or straining. The air will usually resolve with light pressure and warm compresses within 1 week.

Epiphora

Epiphora is a rare complication of endoscopic sinus surgery, because even if the nasolacrimal duct is violated it will usually drain into the nose at the site of damage. However, if it occurs, it can be quite bothersome to the patient. The duct may be injured during antral irrigation or when performing a middle meatal antrostomy.

The nasolacrimal duct courses its way toward the inferior meatus in the lateral wall just lateral to the agger nasi cell superiorly and lateral to the anterior tip of the middle turbinate inferiorly. The duct itself is covered by the hard bone of the lateral wall. Therefore, in performing a middle meatal antrostomy, the surgeon should not open the antrostomy too far anteriad to the area of harder bone. This bone is harder than that of the natural ostia and maxillary sinus fontanelle. As well, osteitis of the lateral wall in the area of the nasolacrimal duct (i.e., the agger nasi cell) may cause a dacryocystitis. This may lead to epiphora or actual purulence seen coming from the opening of the puncta in the medial corner of the eye.

Ophthalmology consultation may be required. Initial treatment of late cases requires antibiotic-steroid eye cream, oral antibiotics, or both. A probe may need to be passed or a dacryocystotomy performed in cases of trauma or stenosis.

Synechiae

Noted as the most common complication with endoscopic sinus surgery, permanent synechiae usually can be avoided with meticulous postoperative cleaning. Thus the importance of postoperative care for the patient undergoing endoscopic sinus surgery cannot be overemphasized.

Adhesions commonly occur anteriorly, especially when the middle turbinate is preserved. They also occur in narrow nasal airways when the septum pushes the turbinate toward the lateral wall. If synechiae are present and the middle meatus is totally obstructed with return of disease, revision surgery may be required. Partial turbinectomy may be necessary, depending on the extent of the disease and the synechia formation.

In addition, synechiae and bony septa may form the scaffolding for re-epithelialization to cover over the frontal recess or to result in a very tight frontal recess with recurrence of or resultant frontal symptomatology. The importance of postoperative cleanings in this area cannot be overemphasized. If the recess becomes obstructed, a repeat CT scan and possible revision surgery may be required should postoperative cleaning fail to open

the area to provide adequate aeration and drainage.

Natural Ostia Closure

Middle meatal antrostomy closure rarely occurs but may lead to recurrent maxillary sinus symptomatology. Even large antrostomies can close. Good postoperative care usually assists in keeping the antrostomy open; however, closure may occur despite this.

Recirculation of mucus can occur if the middle meatal antrostomy is not connected with the natural ostium. This may occur either by synechiae formation separating the two or as a result of surgery not connecting the natural ostia with the middle meatal antrostomy. The recirculation can be responsible for continuation of symptoms regardless of how well-epithelialized the cavity appears. This can be corrected by connecting the two under direct visualization, using the backbiting forceps.

CASE STUDIES

Case 1

A 53 year old woman complained of recurrent right sinusitis. She had had functional endoscopic sinus surgery bilaterally at another institution one year previously. CT scan revealed persistent right ethmoiditis, with the remainder of her sinuses being relatively normal.

She underwent a revision right ethmoidectomy without incident. The next morning she called the office to say that her right eye was slightly proptotic. Upon questioning, she related that, despite being instructed not to blow her nose, she had been non-compliant.

Examination revealed a moderate proptosis with normal vision. CT scan revealed considerable orbital emphysema (Fig. 11–3). This resolved without treatment or sequelae.

Case 2

A 32 year old mother of four complained of frequent right-sided headaches. Evaluation by several physicians revealed no obvious cause.

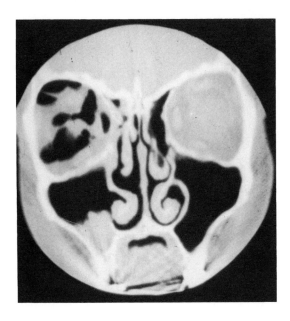

FIGURE 11–3. Orbital emphysema in coronal CT scan of Case 1.

Antibiotics did not alter the course. She was referred to an otolaryngologist–head and neck surgeon. His examination revealed a slightly deviated nasal septum, and a CT scan was normal. He recommended a septoplasty, right Caldwell-Luc, and transantral-transnasal ethmoidectomy.

In the recovery room, she was noted to have severe swelling of her right upper and lower eyelids. Her vision was reported to be normal, and she was discharged with instructions to return in 5 days.

When she returned 5 days later, she was noted to be blind with an exotropia. A CT scan revealed significant damage to the lamina papyracea (Fig. 11–4). There was no return of function.

Case 3

A 12 year old boy was referred to an otolaryngologist–head and neck surgeon for treatment of sinusitis. The patient underwent functional endoscopic sinus surgery and was noted postoperatively to have clear fluid running from his nose in significant volume, as well as a personality change. A CT scan showed pneumocephalus.

Conservative management was felt to be inadvisable because of the volume of the CSF leak. Subsequent frontal craniotomy revealed three openings in the fovea ethmoidalis with penetration into the brain substance to a depth of 5 cm.

Case 4

A 35 year old woman underwent bilateral functional endoscopic sinus surgery under general anesthesia. During the procedure, the scrub nurse noted that the respective eye moved while the operation was being performed. Postoperatively the patient was found to be blind bilaterally. No return of function occurred. A postoperative CT scan showed transection of both optic nerves (Fig. 11–5).

Case 5

A 35 year old man was evaluated for recurrent sinusitis. The otolaryngologist–head and neck surgeon who saw him recommended bilateral Caldwell-Lucs and transantral-transnasal ethmoidectomies. Postoperatively, the patient had diplopia for 9 months because of left medial rectus dysfunction, with gradual complete resolution.

Postoperative coronal CT scan (Fig. 11–6) revealed a large defect in the left lamina papyracea with some medial and inferior prolapse of the orbital contents.

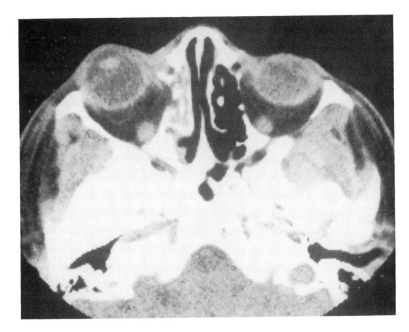

FIGURE 11–4. Right-sided damage to the lamina papyracea in axial CT scan of Case 2.

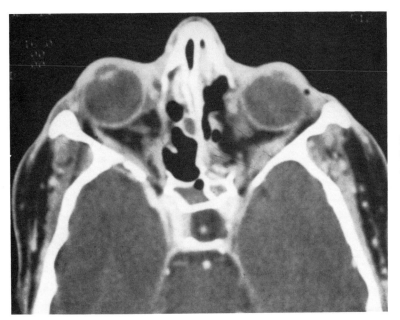

FIGURE 11–5. Transection of the optic nerves bilaterally in axial CT scan of Case 4.

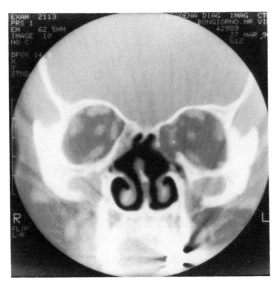

FIGURE 11–6. Prolapse of the orbital contents medially and inferiorly through a large defect in the lamina papyracea in coronal CT scan of Case 5.

Case 6

A 34 year old woman complained of recurrent left-sided frontal headaches that began after functional endoscopic sinus surgery was performed at another institution. An endoscopic examination revealed the frontal recess to be closed by bony septa, scar bands, and the re-epithelialization process.

This patient had not been having postoperative endoscopic cleanings following her original operation. In revision functional endoscopic sinus surgery, the frontal recess was reopened, and continued postoperative cleanings resulted in resolution of her headaches and an open, well-epithelialized frontal recess.

References

1. Kennedy DW: Functional endoscopic sinus surgery: Technique. Arch Otolaryngol 111:643–649, 1985.

2. Kennedy DW, Zinreich SJ, Rosenbaum A, et al: Functional endoscopic sinus surgery: Theory and diagnosis. Arch Otolaryngol 111:576–582, 1985.

3. Kennedy DW, Josephson JS: Functional Endoscopic Sinus Surgery: Atlas of Head and Neck Surgery. Vol 1. Philadelphia, BC Decker, 1989, pp 80–101.

4. Josephson JS, Linden BE: The importance of postoperative care in the adult and pediatric patient treated with functional endoscopic sinus surgery. Oper Tech Otolaryngol Head Neck Surg 2:112–116, 1990.

5. Messerklinger W: On the drainage of the normal frontal sinus of man. Acta Otolaryngol 63:176–181, 1967.

6. Messerklinger W: Endoscopy of the Nose. Baltimore, Urban and Schwarzenberg, 1978.

7. Mosher HP: The applied anatomy and intranasal surgery of the ethmoid labyrinth. Trans Am Laryngol Assoc 94:25–39, 1912.

8. Ritter RN: The middle turbinate and its relationship to the ethmoidal labyrinth and the orbit. Laryngoscope 92:479–483, 1982.

9. Kennedy DW: Complications in otolaryngology–head and neck surgery. In Johns ME (ed): Surgery of the Sinuses. Vol 2. Philadelphia, BC Decker, 1986, pp 71–82.

10. Stammberger H: Endoscopic endonasal surgery—concepts in treatment of recurring rhinosinusitis. Part II. Surgical technique. Otolaryngol Head Neck Surg 94:147–156, 1986.

11. Wigand ME: Transantral ethmoidectomy under endoscopical control. Rhinology 19:7–15, 1981.

12. Vleming M, de Vries N: Endoscopic paranasal sinus surgery; Results. Rhinology 4:13–17, 1990.

13. Stankiewicz JA: Complications of endoscopic intranasal ethmoidectomy. Laryngoscope 97:1270–1273, 1987.

14. Stankiewicz JA: Complications in endoscopic intranasal ethmoidectomy; An update. Laryngoscope 99:686–689, 1989.

15. Keros P: Über die praktische Bedeutung der Niveau—Unterschiede der Lamina Cribrosa des Ethmoids (1962). Cited in Naumann HH (ed): Head and Neck Surgery: Face and Facial Skull. Vol 1. Philadelphia, WB Saunders, 1980.

16. Anderson WM, Schwarz GA, Gammon GD: Chronic spontaneous CSF rhinorrhea. Arch Intern Med 107:723, 1961.

17. Mombelli G, et al: Gram-negative bacillary meningitis in neurosurgical patients. J Neurosurg 58:634–641, 1981.

18. Stankiewicz JA: Blindness and intranasal endoscopic ethmoidectomy: Prevention and management. Otolaryngol Head Neck Surg 101:320–329, 1989.

CHAPTER 12

Cleft Lip Surgery

MONTE S. KEEN, MD
HOWARD W. SMITH, DMD, MD

SECONDARY DEFECTS FOLLOWING PRIMARY CLOSURE OF UNILATERAL CLEFT LIPS

Defects in the upper lip following surgical cleft lip closure are variable. Some relate to the expertise of the operating surgeon, others to the condition of the existing defect, and still others to subsequent development following closure. The defects may relate to the vermilion, muscle, skin, or ala.

Early techniques designed to close the lip defect concentrated on the lip alone and provided for secondary repairs at the time of early social exposure, usually at age 6 to 8 years. On occasion the surgeon's expertise and the patient's subsequent growth produced a result that did not require preschool adjustment and left the nasal component for septal and rhinoplastic surgery at age 16 to 18 years.

The gradual development of extended techniques of single cleft lip closure and the development of new concepts provided for improvement in lip closure that created more symmetry in the nasal area. The technical surgical improvement was also enhanced by the use of pre- and postoperative orthodontic appliances and, on occasion, lip adhesion prior to definitive closure.

The concepts of rotation-advancement, muscle fiber realignment, alar cartilage suspension, alveolar bone grafts, and augmentation of the bony piriform base support of the ala are but a few of the great improvements over time that have reduced the need for surgical correction in the preschool period.

A random selection of examples of single lip defects existing following repair may be grouped into those related to surgical technique, those related to the severity of the original cleft, and those related to subsequent growth. This grouping would require knowledge of the preoperative cleft, the surgeon, the surgical technique used, the postoperative course, possible secondary operations, and the presence or absence of ancillary dental and orthodontic support.

In the absence of such knowledge, defects can be observed and the possible cause of

Text continued on page 151

143

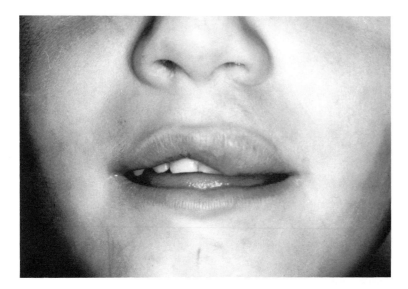

FIGURE 12–1. Inequality of lip length. The additional length of the lip on the cleft side appers to be primarily in the muscle tissue. The normal level of the vermilion border suggests a technical error rather than increased growth following closure. The alveolus pushing the lip out and down does not appear to be an underlying problem.

FIGURE 12–2. Lip excess at the junction of the wet and dry vermilion. This appears to result from a technical error in leaving an excess of tissue at the lower border at closure.

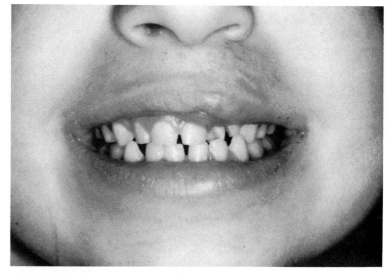

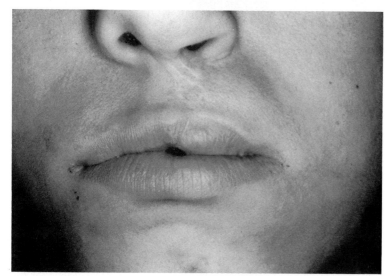

FIGURE 12–3. Fullness of the lip on the cleft side. This appears to be an increased growth of the cleft lip element secondary to closure. It is also possible that the fibers of the upper borders of the orbicular muscle of the mouth had not been dissected and reoriented in the upper portion of the lip closure.

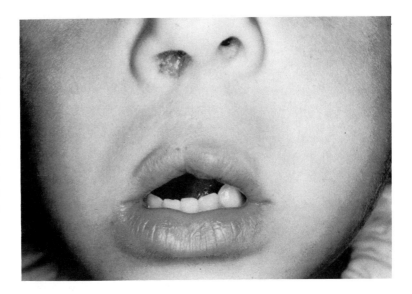

FIGURE 12–4. Flat lip on the cleft side. The position of the ala suggests that the cleft lip element was hypoplastic along with the right anterior portion of the body maxilla. It is also possible that there is some collapse of the alveolar arch. In addition, there is a notch at the vermilion border and the lip line.

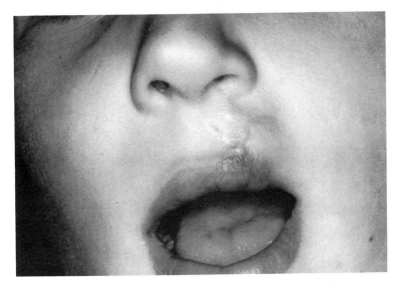

FIGURE 12–5. Disfiguring lip skin scar. The skin scar resulted from trauma to the lip shortly after adequate healing of the primary lip closure. The trauma extended into the vermilion portion of the lip, obscuring the border and causing a full thickness of scar tissue.

FIGURE 12–6. Suture rejection. The subcutaneous catgut sutures placed in the lip border and the columella base caused inflammation along the closure line, which resulted in a noticeable lip scar.

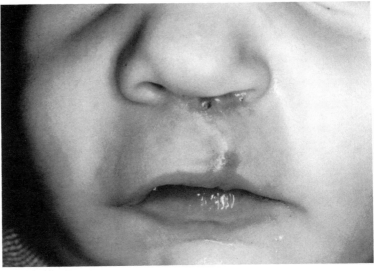

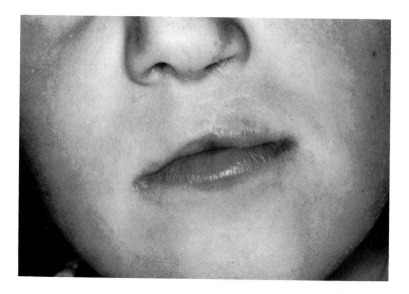

FIGURE 12–7. Notching at the lip border. In addition to the notch, there is a reversal of Cupid's bow. The closure line appears to be in the midline rather than at the peak of the bow on the cleft side. This appears to be a technical error in which the noncleft side was pared excessively and the cleft lip side pared insufficiently, leaving an excess of lip on the cleft side.

FIGURE 12–8. Lip notching. The defect extends from the lip border into the nostril floor. It appears that a good muscle closure was not achieved and that the floor of the nostril was not supported. Possibly the lateral lip element was not pared sufficiently to produce a lip element thick enough to match the noncleft side. It is also possible that the cleft lip element was not sufficiently mobilized, causing subsequent traction at the closure line, with separation of the muscle elements.

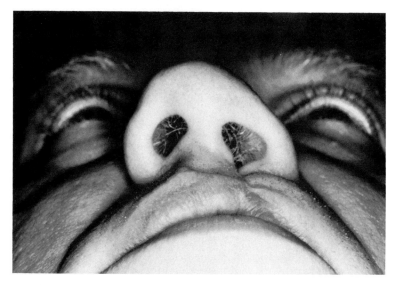

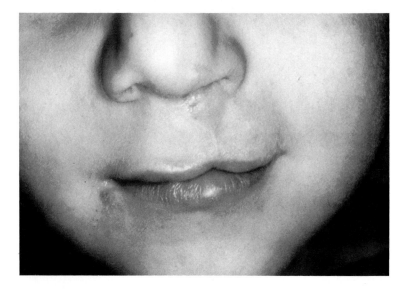

FIGURE 12–9. Notching. Apparently downward rotation of the noncleft element was insufficient to provide a closure line equal to that of the cleft lip side. Insufficient space for the advancement flap resulted, causing retraction of the lip scar and elevation of the lip border.

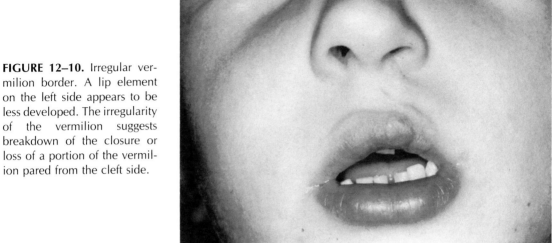

FIGURE 12–10. Irregular vermilion border. A lip element on the left side appears to be less developed. The irregularity of the vermilion suggests breakdown of the closure or loss of a portion of the vermilion pared from the cleft side.

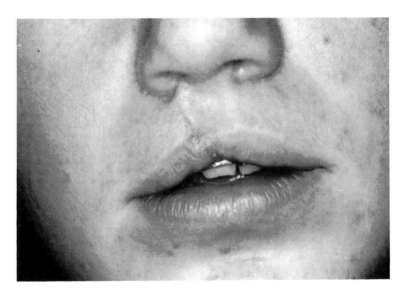

FIGURE 12–11. Retracted lip scar. The skin indicates that this was a straight line closure after paring the cleft edges. Rotation-advancement would have provided sufficient tissue in the upper lip to hold the lip border in position.

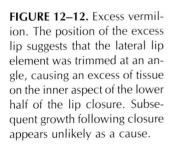

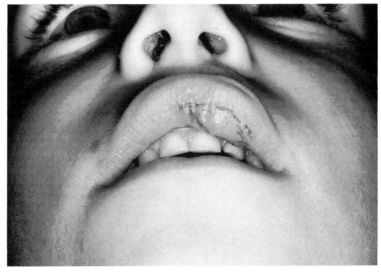

FIGURE 12–12. Excess vermilion. The position of the excess lip suggests that the lateral lip element was trimmed at an angle, causing an excess of tissue on the inner aspect of the lower half of the lip closure. Subsequent growth following closure appears unlikely as a cause.

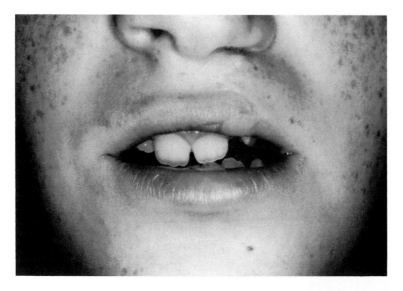

FIGURE 12–13. Depressed alar base. The position of the alar base indicates a failure to mobilize the ala and bring it forward. Development of the ala appears lacking, and a defect in the bony piriform base of the maxilla is seen. The skin scar suggests that a rotation-advancement closure was not employed; this would have supported the cleft side of the columella and provided medial support for the advanced alar base.

FIGURE 12–14. Horizontal nostril. The shape of the nostril is dependent superiorly on the location of the lower lateral cartilage and the position of the ala. No attempt was made to reorient and suspend the lower lateral cartilage. The upper fibers of the orbicular muscle of the mouth do not appear to have been mobilized, reoriented, and attached to the noncleft side. The bony piriform rim also appears to be deficient.

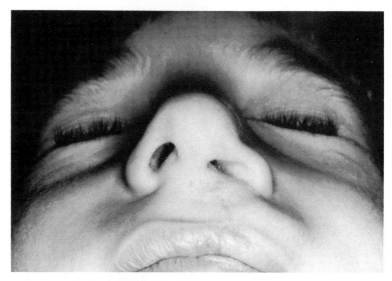

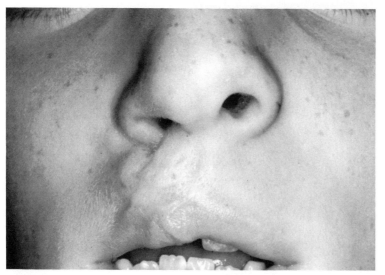

FIGURE 12–15. Unequal height of the ala. The cleft side ala appears to be unsupported. The cleft lip element appears to be hypoplastic and the underlying bone deficient. Possibly there is alveolar arch collapse, allowing the lip to fall in and distort the height of the cleft side alar base.

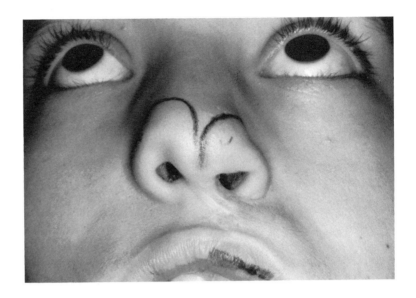

FIGURE 12–16. Depressed nostril floor. Muscle fibers in the upper lip suggest that the muscle was not carried medially in the closure, causing inadequate support of the floor. The nostril sizes appear nearly symmetric, which suggests that the alar advancement and skin closure of the nostril floor were adequate.

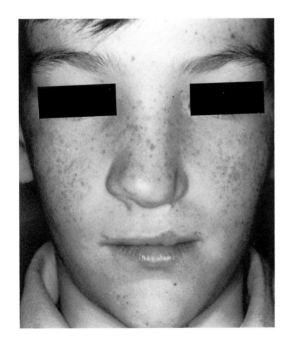

FIGURE 12–17. Elevated cleft side at peak of Cupid's bow. The elevation appears to result from scar contracture and inadequate downward rotation of the medial lip element.

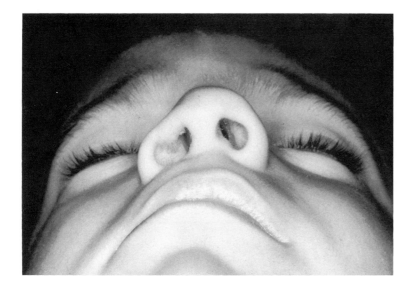

FIGURE 12–18. Buckled ala. The shape of the nostril suggests that this was a very wide cleft prior to primary closure. Apparently the floor of the nostril was left wide and the primary object was to obtain a good primary closure of the lip and leave the nasal distortion for subsequent operation.

FIGURE 12–19. Nasolabial fistula. Closure of the floor of the nose can be difficult. Often the tissue is torn in the process of elevating periosteal flaps. Two-layer closure is often not possible. Clefts that have been brought too close together with preoperative orthodontics can make the operation more difficult for lack of space and visibility.

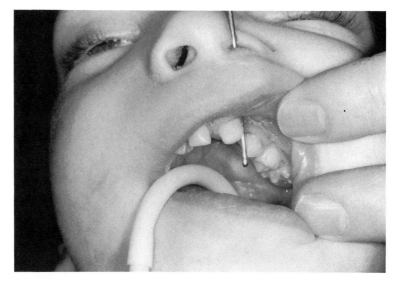

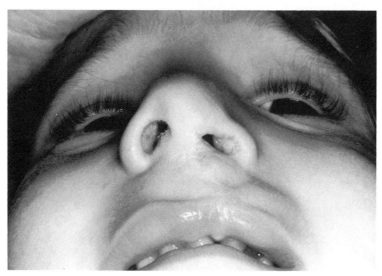

FIGURE 12–20. Muscle mass in the upper portion of the lateral lip element. Failure to dissect, reorient, and close the muscle fibers in the lateral lip element superiorly results in a bulge in the lip and a depression of the upper lip closure line. A 3-layer closure of the lip provided an opportunity to locate, reorient, and attach all elements to the medial side of the cleft.

the defect derived from observation. Many defects have been observed and photographs taken over the years, and from this group the following common defects are presented for observation and comment on possible causes.

The need for secondary repair of the single cleft lip closure at preschool age has decreased remarkably in the past 10 years. Techniques such as preoperative orthodontia, correction of the lower lateral cartilage position, greater use of the rotation advancement techniques, bone grafting, lip adhesion, muscle and orientation and improved soft tissue techniques have been employed with greater frequency. These techniques, along with postoperative orthodontia and continuing dental care, have allowed the single cleft lip patient to have a satisfactory, presentable appearance until the age of 16 years, when septorhinoplasty can be performed to achieve a near-normal facial appearance.

SUMMARY

Common defects following primary closure of the single cleft lips have been presented. Photographs of lips showing various problems were analyzed and the probable cause of each defect explained. Defects of these types have markedly decreased in the past 10 years owing to a number of factors relating to techniques, employment of ancillary disciplines, and a better understanding of the goals to be achieved at the time of primary closure.

CHAPTER
13

Salivary Gland Surgery

JAMES F. REIBEL, MD
PAUL A. LEVINE, MD

Surgical treatment of salivary gland disease represents a significant component of the otolaryngologist–head and neck surgeons' practice. Understanding of pathophysiology, accurate preoperative cytologic diagnosis, and advanced imaging techniques allow surgeons to better prepare the patient and themselves for the proposed treatment regimen. Because facial dysfunction is an obvious deformity, accurate surgical planning and patient counseling are imperative. This chapter will review complications of operations on the major salivary glands and suggest methods for handling these problems.

Infection

Although wound infection can complicate any operative procedure, wound infection following salivary gland surgery is uncommon. Langdon reports an infection rate of less than 2 per cent following parotidectomy.[1] Although infection complicated 9 per cent of submandibular gland resections, over 80 per cent of these procedures were per-

formed for recurrent infections.[2] Thus, routine antimicrobial prophylaxis for staphylococcal and anaerobic infection is not indicated, prophylaxis being reserved for those patients with a history of recurrent infection.[1, 3]

Hemorrhage and Hematoma

Hemostasis is an essential part of any operation. Significant bleeding is best avoided by careful dissection, isolation, and ligation of vessels. Many surgeons utilize thermal or laser instruments in dissection of glandular tissue to facilitate a dry surgical field. If a ligature slips or vessel injury occurs during salivary gland surgery, hasty clamping in the depths of the wound must be avoided to prevent inadvertent injury to the facial nerve. Digital pressure provides temporary control until the bleeding point is precisely identified and ligated. In this way injury to adjacent structures, especially the facial nerve, is avoided.

The reported incidence of hematoma varies

153

from 0.8 per cent to 16 per cent following salivary gland surgery.[1, 2, 4–6] Hematoma is accompanied by pain and fullness at the operative site. Neither suction drains nor passive drains with pressure dressings consistently prevent this complication. Once the diagnosis of hematoma is made, the patient should return to the operating room for an evacuation of the wound under sterile conditions and control of the offending vessels, which are not always found.

Aesthetic Concerns

Although parotid and submandibular gland operations involve an external scar, a fine, barely noticeable scar is possible with placement of the incision in skin folds, gentle handling of tissue, and cosmetic wound closure in which epithelial edges are accurately approximated before the placement of skin sutures. The Blair incision can be modified as in face-lift surgery, so that a portion of the vertical facial incision is hidden posterior to the tragal cartilage. Undesirable scarring and keloid formation in African Americans have been reported following 3 per cent to 4 per cent of parotid and submandibular procedures.[2, 4, 5] An accurate subcutaneous closure minimizes scarring, and a careful history and physical examination can identify the patient with a propensity for keloid formation. In keloid formers, the skin is injected with triamcinolone at the time of operation and again 4 to 6 weeks postoperatively.

Another source of aesthetic concern is the depression or hollow resulting from the parotid gland resection, particularly following total parotidectomy. Transfer of soft tissue to obliterate the defect[7] or modifications in the technique to remove the mass, e.g., enucleation with postoperative radiation,[8] have been advocated. These measures are inappropriate, however, since they can mask the recurrence of tumor and increase the risk of facial nerve injury.[9] With careful preoperative counseling, the deformity is readily accepted.

Resections for advanced malignant disease produce extensive defects requiring complex reconstruction. Fine-needle aspiration cytology permits a more accurate diagnosis of malignant disease preoperatively, and contemporary imaging techniques permit a better assessment of disease extent. They provide the surgeon with more accurate preoperative data to better predict the resulting deficits and plan appropriate reconstruction. Although these deficits are properly termed sequelae and not complications, their impact upon the patient is no less significant. A thorough discussion regarding anticipated deficits and the planned reconstruction is essential in these difficult cases.[10]

Sensory Changes

Cutaneous anesthesia and hypesthesia are very annoying sequelae of salivary gland surgery, particularly following parotid surgery. Anesthesia, hypesthesia, and paresthesia from greater auricular nerve transection occur routinely and should be discussed with the patient. Although recovery to normal or near-normal sensation does occur, it should be understood that it may take 6 to 9 months or more. Complaints about sensory changes following submandibular gland surgery are few, and almost always come from men who notice the deficit when shaving.

Occasionally a painful amputation neuroma develops. They occur in less than 1 per cent of submandibular gland procedures;[2] the reported incidence of neuromas following parotid procedures varies from 0 to 18 per cent.[4–6, 10] The surgeon must be wary of confusing these neuromas with recurrent tumor. Excision of the neuroma is curative.

Sialoceles and Salivary Fistulas

Sialoceles and salivary fistulas are uncommon complications of salivary gland surgery. The incidence ranges from 3 per cent to 6.5 per cent[1, 5] and 0.2 per cent to 3.3 per cent, respectively.[1, 2, 5, 11] Most are transient and respond to pressure dressings, with repeated aspirations proving necessary in the case of sialoceles. Glycopyrrolate assists in decreasing the volume of secretions, thus facilitating closure.

Woods emphasizes routine division of Stensen's duct without ligation, suggesting that the duct might provide additional drainage of the wound bed.[12] Langdon discusses two cases refractory to conservative treatment that required additional intervention, noting that both cases involved ligation of Stensen's duct.[1] Although this technical point will not eliminate complicating sialoceles and fistulas, it may reduce the number that require other than conservative management.

The persistent parotid fistula (which has failed treatment with pressure dressing and glycopyrrolate) represents an unusual complication to the patient and surgeon. Secondary closure is frequently unsuccessful, as evidenced by Langdon's patient whose fistula finally closed spontaneously after three failed attempts at surgical closure.[1] Although a second procedure to remove the deep lobe of the parotid can be curative, there is increased risk of facial nerve injury.[9] Radiation therapy has been successful,[1] but use of radiation therapy for benign disease presents its own risks. Tympanic neurectomy has been very successful in treatment of chronic fistulas provided a complete interruption of Jacobson nerve is performed.[13, 14] When wound care fails, this procedure is the treatment of choice.

Gustatory Sweating and Flushing

The reported incidence of localized gustatory sweating and flushing, Frey syndrome, following parotidectomy ranges from 2.6 per cent to 65 per cent[1, 5, 6, 11, 15–18] and may reflect the degree to which these symptoms are sought.[9, 16] Although only a minority of patients find these symptoms bothersome enough to seek treatment, it is not surprising that the minor starch iodine test is positive in all postparotidectomy patients[17, 18] (Fig. 13–1). A similar syndrome, chorda tympani syndrome, can follow submandibular gland excision and was observed in 1 per cent of the series reported by Milton and colleagues.[2] The aberrant regeneration of postganglionic parasympathetic fibers gives rise to these symptoms.[21]

Some have observed no "symptomatic" gustatory sweating and flushing following "limited surgery" or "local excision" for parotid tumors.[4, 16] Because of this, some surgeons have advocated the management of benign parotid neoplasms by "limited surgery."[4] Although the incidence of Frey syndrome is lower following these more limited procedures, it does occur.[6, 19] Because neoplasm recurrence and facial nerve injury are potentially greater using the abbreviated technique,[9] the argument for "limited surgery" to decrease symptomatic Frey syndrome is flawed. The one technical procedure that does not have an adverse impact upon facial nerve injury or recurrence and reduces the incidence of symptomatic Frey syndrome is the use of a thick skin flap when performing parotid surgery.[15]

Treatment for symptomatic gustatory sweating includes topical agents, radiation therapy, and various surgical procedures (Table 13–1).[17] Commercial antiperspirants are capable of controlling mild symptoms, but topical treatment of more severe symptoms requires anticholinergic preparations. Scopolamine,[17, 20] glycopyrrolate,[17, 20–22] and diphemanil methylsulfate[23] have been used. Fewer side effects have been noted with glycopyrrolate and diphemanil methylsulfate, both quaternary ammonium compounds that do not cross the blood-brain barrier. Unfortunately, neither of these two compounds has FDA approval for this usage. Topical glycopyrrolate is available in the United States for investigational use only (Table 13–2), though it appears to be the topical agent of choice for treatment of more severe symptoms. Because of the investigational nature of this usage, precautions regarding its use must be strictly adhered to (Table 13–3).

When topical therapy is ineffective or unacceptable to the patient, tympanic neurectomy is the next treatment choice. Satisfactory control was reported in 82 per cent of symptomatic patients reviewed by Hays.[17] As in its use for postparotidectomy fistulas, the key to success with this procedure is thorough middle ear exploration to assure interruption of all branches of the tympanic

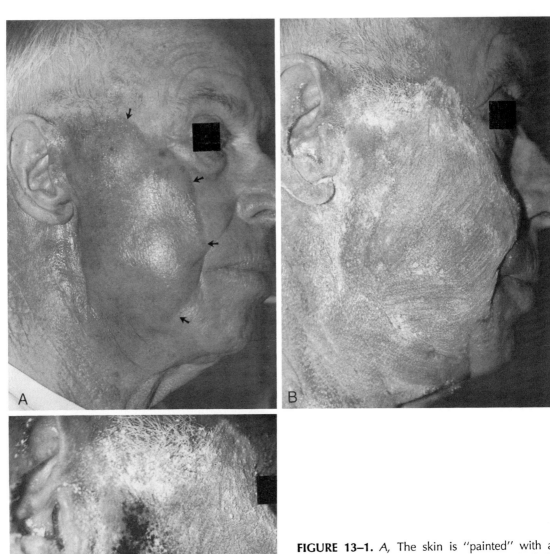

FIGURE 13–1. *A,* The skin is "painted" with a solution of iodine, castor oil, and absolute alcohol. *B,* Cornstarch is dusted onto the dried, painted area. *C,* A positive test was evoked after the patient chewed a lemon wedge for 5 minutes.

TABLE 13–1. Treatment Options for Frey Syndrome

I. Topical agents
  A. Commercial antiperspirants—generally effective only for milder symptoms
  B. Anticholinergic preparations—side effects similar to those that make systemic anticholinergics impractical for Frey syndrome are possible with topical agents; however, side effects from glycopyrrolate are less than with scopolamine
II. Radiation therapy
  Since a total treatment dose of approximately 50 Gy is needed to control gustatory sweating, use of this potentially carcinogenic treatment for this disorder is not justified except in very symptomatic patients for whom alternative treatments have failed or are contraindicated
III. Surgical procedures
  A. Skin excision—can be used only for localized and relatively small areas. Also risks facial nerve injury
  B. Auriculotemporal nerve section—risks facial nerve injury and may not provide permanent control
  C. Fascia lata interposition—also risks facial nerve injury
  D. Tympanic neurectomy—risks of facial nerve injury and significant morbidity virtually nil, and most patients can safely undergo outpatient surgery

(Modified from Hays LL: The Frey syndrome: A review and double blind evaluation of the topical use of a new anticholinergic agent. Laryngoscope 88:1796–1824, 1978.)

plexus.[13, 14, 17, 24, 25] Although chorda tympani section has been used to treat failures of tympanic neurectomy (nearly always in association with revision tympanic neurectomy), revision tympanic neurectomy alone is also effective.[17] Ross found no evidence to support chorda tympani section for treatment of symptomatic Frey syndrome.[25] Radiation therapy and surgical procedures with greater morbidity, including chorda tympani section, should be reserved for treatment failures after topical glycopyrrolate and tympanic neurectomy.

TABLE 13–2. Procedure to Obtain and Use Topical Glycopyrrolate

1. Obtain a Notice of Claimed INVESTIGATIONAL EXEMPTION for a NEW DRUG (IND Forms 1571 and 1572) from the Food and Drug Administration:

   United States Food and Drug Administration Center for Drug Evaluation and Research (HFD-008)
   5600 Fishers Lane
   Rockville, MD 20857

2. When an IND is granted, request glycopyrrolate from:

   Wyeth–Ayerst Laboratories
   Clinical Research and Development Division
   Box 8299
   Philadelphia, PA 19101

3. Prepare glycopyrrolate formulation in accordance with the method described by Hays et al[20]

(Modified from Hays LL, Novack AJ, Worsham JC: The Frey syndrome: A simple, effective treatment. Otolaryngol Head Neck Surg 90:419–425, 1982.)

Facial Nerve Dysfunction

Facial nerve paresis or paralysis is a dreaded complication of major salivary gland surgery. The recent literature shows only one large series reporting the incidence of this complication following submandibular gland excision (18 per cent transient marginal nerve deficit, 7 per cent permanent),[2] but many series report the incidence of postparotidectomy facial nerve dysfunction. These series require careful comparison regarding surgical indications and technique, as well as duration of facial nerve dysfunction. As mentioned, surgical sacrifice of a branch or of all the facial nerve may be necessary in treating parotid malignancy, and the resulting deficit is appropriately termed a sequela rather than a complication.

Since facial nerve sacrifice may be necessary for recurrent malignancies, high-grade primaries, and the unusually large and infil-

TABLE 13–3. Guidelines for Topical Glycopyrrolate Treatment

1. Minor starch iodine test confirms and localizes area to be treated (see Fig. 13–1)
2. Intact facial skin. Patients should not apply to cut or infected skin
3. Ophthalmologic consultation to exclude glaucoma
4. Review of medical history identifies patients with conditions contraindicating systemic anticholinergic medications: obstructive uropathy; gastric outlet obstruction; diabetes mellitus; or thyroid, cardiovascular, central nervous system, renal, or hepatic diseases
5. Dispense preparation with appropriate patient counseling and precautions
   a. Avoid application into mouth, nose, or eyes
   b. Emphasize careful application and thorough hand-washing after application
   c. Use child-resistant containers and caution patients to keep medication out of reach of children

(Modified from Hays LL: The Frey syndrome: A review and double blind evaluation of the topical use of a new anticholinergic agent. Laryngoscope 88:1796–1824, 1978; and Hays LL, Novack AJ, Worsham JC: The Frey syndrome: A simple, effective treatment. Otolaryngol Head Neck Surg 90:419–425, 1982.)

trating low-grade primaries,[10, 26] facial function will reflect the success of various methods of surgical rehabilitation. When series including parotid malignancies are evaluated, the accurate measure of facial dysfunction is the incidence of permanent deficits following attempts to preserve the nerve. In such series of both benign and malignant parotid lesions, the reported incidence of permanent facial nerve deficit varies from less than 1 per cent to 6.5 per cent.[1, 4, 27–29]

In parotidectomies performed for primary benign disease, the incidence of permanent facial dysfunction is 0 to 3 per cent, but transient deficits occur in 40 per cent to 58 per cent.[5, 6, 27, 29] Although the significance of a transient facial deficit to a patient with benign disease should not be discounted, the surgeon will do well to remember the words of Patey and Moffat:

The question of the prevention of functional facial paralysis after parotidectomy needs to be considered in proper perspective. Surgery of the parotid is performed to rid the patient of his disease. At times, even the complete sacrifice of the facial nerve and permanent facial paralysis may be a small price to pay for the attainment of this objective. Still less should fear of producing a temporary facial paralysis inhibit the surgeon in carrying out whatever operation is indicated on pathological grounds. Facial paralysis is, however, an unpleasant disability even if only temporary, and its avoidance is desirable if this can be achieved without prejudice to the success of the operation.[31]

Since transient facial palsy is common after

parotidectomy, the desire to reduce this temporary complication by more limited procedures is understandable.[4, 8] Although Owen and colleagues did not observe any transient or permanent facial palsy following their "limited surgery," 10 of the 16 patients so treated had incomplete excision of the tumor or gross tumor spill.[4] A review of parotid surgery in the northern United Kingdom showed the 3.7 per cent incidence of transient facial palsy following "local excisions" to be less than the 21.8 per cent following parotidectomy. There was no advantage for limited "local excision" with respect to permanent facial deficit, 0.9 per cent and 0.[32] Also reported was a 38.5 per cent incidence of incomplete excision or tumor spill with "local excision." Permanent facial deficits in 5.5 per cent to 7.8 per cent have been reported as a result of "limited" parotid procedures.[8, 29] These results show that any advantage with respect to decreased transient facial dysfunction is offset by the significantly increased likelihood of incomplete excision and tumor spill[4, 32] and by the greater possibility of permanent facial dysfunction.[8, 29] The only lesser procedure that may be reasonable is the partial superficial parotidectomy as described by Patey and Moffat.[31]

Surgical treatment of recurrent benign tumors places the facial nerve at risk. Ward noted a 71 per cent incidence of permanent facial nerve injury following parotidectomy for recurrent benign disease,[29] and Conley and Clairmont reported a 57 per cent regional facial weakness and 14 per cent incidence of radical parotidectomy with need for nerve grafting in their series of recurrent pleomorphic adenomata.[33] The incidence of facial dysfunction following surgical treatment of recurrent benign tumors reported by others ranges from 12.6 per cent to 39 per cent.[6, 11, 30, 34, 35] It is interesting that others, like Conley and Clairmont, report the need for radical parotidectomy with nerve grafting in approximately 14 per cent of their cases treated for recurrent pleomorphic adenomata.[6, 36]

Parotidectomy, either superficial or total, with facial nerve dissection and preservation is obviously the procedure of choice in treating benign conditions of the parotid gland. This procedure has been well described by many workers and need not be emphasized here. Just as in thyroid surgery, early identification and careful dissection of the nerve are the key points in all safe parotidectomy techniques. Unlike the recurrent nerve, the facial nerve can be approached and dissected centrifugally or centripetally, as dictated by the pathology. Depending on the disease location and extent, the surgeon must be prepared to use either approach, including identification of the vertical segment of the facial nerve in the mastoid. After identification of the nerve, care must be taken to avoid a stretch injury, particularly in cases involving deep lobe tumors with parapharyngeal extension. To avoid a stretch injury in these difficult cases, mandibulotomy,[37] facial nerve rerouting,[38] or facial nerve section and primary anastomosis[31, 38] may be required.

Tumor Recurrence

Dissatisfaction with the high incidence of tumor recurrence following enucleation led to the development of superficial and total parotidectomy sparing the facial nerve. The recurrence following primary surgery for pleomorphic adenoma has declined from a range of 20 per cent to 30 per cent[39, 40] to 0 to 7 per cent as superficial or lateral lobe parotidectomy has become the standard procedure.[5, 6, 11, 13, 27, 30, 41]

The Michigan and the Mayo Clinic series demonstrate the need for long-term follow-up, e.g., 25 to 30 years, in reporting recurrence rates for pleomorphic adenomata,[36, 40] and no doubt the recurrence rate of the more recent series will increase slightly with time. Donovan and Conley showed that parotidectomy became a de facto capsular dissection resulting from the dissection and preservation of the facial nerve in 61 of the 100 cases they studied.[42] Although in a single series report Gleave and associates demonstrated that a meticulous capsular dissection may yield recurrence rates comparable to those of parotidectomy with nerve dissection,[11] the risks of incomplete removal or capsular rupture are obvious. Reports by Maynard[5] and Lindsey and Hobsley[6] underscore the risk of recurrence when capsular rupture occurs during parotidectomy. Maynard mentions the use of liberal wound irrigation with sterile water and possible use of radiotherapy in these instances of operative capsular rupture.[5] In cases with tumor spill or when an adequate margin cannot be excised with the neoplasm, radiation therapy should be considered.

The treatment of recurrent benign mixed tumors may be a difficult task. Not only is the facial nerve at increased risk, but the potential for tumor control is reduced. Conley and Clairmont reported a 4.7 per cent failure in control in his series of recurrent pleomorphic adenomata.[33] Others cite secondary recurrence rates of 12 per cent to 35 per cent.[6, 11, 30, 34] Fee and associates showed that 70 per cent to 75 per cent of subsequent procedures fail to control the tumor.[34] Radiation therapy can be a helpful adjunct in controlling initial and subsequent recurrences.[43]

Parotid malignancies are more likely to fail locally than regionally or distantly. Spiro reported a 39 per cent incidence of locoregional recurrence, predominantly at the primary site.[41] The Mayo Clinic reported a decrease in local recurrence of from 50 per cent to 28 per cent after adopting a policy of more aggressive surgery, including facial nerve sacrifice.[16] Spiro's series confirms the importance of tumor staging and histology to patient survival.[41] Johns has outlined a protocol for management of parotid malignancies, which relies upon aggressive treatment of the primary tumor based on tumor extent, appropriate use of neck dissection determined by nodal sampling at the time of the parotidectomy, and adjuvant radiation therapy as indicated by tumor histology and extent.[10]

Conclusions

As surgical education has improved for the head and neck surgeon, the complication rate of operations has improved as well. Wound complications are uncommon and generally require only conservative treatment. The keys to successful surgery on the parotid and submandibular gland are identification and careful dissection of the facial nerve and its branches, avoidance of tumor spill or incomplete excision, and an understanding of tumor pathophysiology. With this technique, the incidence of permanent facial nerve dysfunction and tumor recurrence should be minimal when primary benign tumors and low-grade malignant tumors are treated. Recurrence after primary management increases the likelihood of facial dysfunction and decreases the likelihood of tumor control. Parotid malignancies of advanced stage and high grade require aggressive treatment, possibly requiring facial nerve sacrifice. Although the ultimate measure of success in these cases is patient survival, the expected deficits must be explained to the patient and rehabilitative measures undertaken. Full knowledge of the various techniques of facial reanimation assist in limiting the cosmetic and functional deficits associated with these resections.

References

1. Langdon JD: Complications of parotid gland surgery. J Maxillofac Surg 12:225–229, 1984.
2. Milton CM, Thomas BM, Bickerton RC: Morbidity study of submandibular gland excision. Ann R Coll Surg Engl 68:148–150, 1986.
3. Powell ME, Clairmont AE: Complications of parotidectomy. South Med J 76:1109–1112, 1983.
4. Owen ERTC, Banerjee AK, Kissin M, Kark AE: Complications of parotidectomy: The need for selectivity. Br J Surg 76:1034–1035, 1989.
5. Maynard JD: Management of pleomorphic adenoma of the parotid. Br J Surg 75:305–308, 1988.
6. Lindsey SK, Hobsley M: The treatment of pleomorphic adenomas by formal parotidectomy. Br J Surg 69:1–3, 1982.
7. Rankon RM, Polayes IM: Surgical treatment of salivary gland tumors. In Diseases of the Salivary Glands. Philadelphia, WB Saunders, 1976, p 239.
8. McEvedy BV, Ross WM: The treatment of mixed tumors by enucleation and radiotherapy. Br J Surg 63:341–342, 1976.
9. Johns ME, Shikhani AH: Surgery of the salivary gland. In Johns ME (ed): Complications in Otolaryngology–Head and Neck Surgery. Toronto, BC Decker Inc, 1986, pp 153–162.
10. Johns ME: Parotid cancer: A rational basis for treatment. Head Neck Surg 3:132–141, 1980.
11. Gleave EN, Whittaker JS, Nicholson A: Salivary tumours—Experience over thirty years. Clin Otolaryngol 4:247–257, 1979.
12. Woods JE: Parotidectomy: Points of technique for brief and safe operation. Am J Surg 145:678–683, 1983.
13. Mandour MA, El-Sheikh MM, El-Garem F: Tympanic neurectomy for parotid fistula. Arch Otolaryngol 102:327–329, 1976.
14. Chadwick SJ, Davis WE, Templer JW: Parotid fistula: Current management. South Med J 72:922–926, 1979.
15. Singleton GT, Cassisi NJ: Frey's syndrome: Incidence related to skin flap thickness in parotidectomy. Laryngoscope 90:1636–1639, 1980.
16. Woods JE, Chong GC, Beahrs OH: Experience with 1,360 primary parotid tumors. Am J Surg 130:460–462, 1975.
17. Hays LL: The Frey syndrome: A review and double blind evaluation of the topical use of a new anticholinergic agent. Laryngoscope 88:1796–1824, 1978.
18. Laage-Hellman JE: Gustatory sweating and flushing after conservative parotidectomy. Acta Otolaryngol 48:234–252, 1957.
19. Laage-Hellman JE: Gustatory sweating and flushing. Acta Otolaryngol 49:306–314, 1958.
20. Hays LL, Novack AJ, Worsham JC: The Frey syndrome: A simple, effective treatment. Otolaryngol Head Neck Surg 90:419–425, 1982.
21. Ford FR, Woodhall B: Phenomena due to misdirection of regenerating fibers of cranial, spinal and autonomic nerves. Arch Surg 36:480–496, 1938.
22. May JS, McGuirt WF: Frey's syndrome: Treatment with topical glycopyrrolate. Head Neck Surg 11:85–89, 1989.
23. Laccourreye O, Bonan B, Brasnu B, Laccourreye H: Treatment of Frey's syndrome with topical 2% diphemanil methylsulfate (Prantal[R]): A double blind evaluation of 15 patients. Laryngoscope 100:651–653, 1990.
24. Friedman WH, Swerdlow RS, Pomarico JM: Tympanic neurectomy: A review and an additional indication for this procedure. Laryngoscope 84:568–577, 1974.
25. Ross JAT: The function of the tympanic plexus as related to Frey's syndrome. Laryngoscope 80:1816–1833, 1970.
26. Eneroth CM: Classification and management of parotid gland tumors. In Fisch U (ed): Facial Nerve Surgery. Birmingham, AL, Aesculapius Publishing Co, 1977, pp 186–192.

27. Woods JE: Parotidectomy versus limited resection for benign parotid masses. Am J Surg 149:749–750, 1985.
28. Nichols RP, Stine PH, Bartschi LR: Facial nerve function in 100 consecutive parotidectomies. Laryngoscope 89:1930–1933, 1979.
29. Ward CM: Injury of the facial nerve during surgery of the parotid gland. Br J Surg 62:401–403, 1975.
30. O'Dwyer PJ, Farrar WB, Finkelmeiser WR, et al: Facial nerve sacrifice and tumor recurrence in primary and recurrent benign parotid tumors. Am J Surg 152:442–445, 1986.
31. Patey DH, Moffat W: A clinical and experimental study of functional paralysis of the facial nerve following conservative parotidectomy. Br J Surg 48:435–440, 1961.
32. Gunn A, Parrott NR: Parotid tumours: A review of parotid tumour surgery in the Northern Regional Health Authority of the United Kingdom 1978–1982. Br J Surg 75:1144–1146, 1988.
33. Conley J, Clairmont AA: Facial nerve in recurrent benign pleomorphic adenoma. Arch Otolaryngol 105:247–251, 1979.
34. Fee WE, Goffinet DR, Calcaterra TC: Recurrent mixed tumors of the parotid gland—Results of surgical therapy. Laryngoscope 88:265–273, 1978.
35. Maran AGD, Mackenzie IJ, Stanley RE: Recurrent pleomorphic adenomas of the parotid gland. Arch Otolaryngol 110:167–171, 1984.
36. Niparko JK, Beauchamp ML, Krause CJ, et al: Surgical treatment of recurrent pleomorphic adenoma of the parotid gland. Arch Otolaryngol 112:1180–1184, 1986.
37. Baker DC, Conley J: Surgical approach to retromandibular parotid tumors. Ann Plast Surg 3:304–314, 1979.
38. Fisch U, Mattox D: Microsurgery of the Skull Base. Stuttgart, George Thieme Verlag, 1988, pp 386, 389.
39. McFarland J: Three hundred mixed tumors of the salivary glands of which sixty-nine recurred. Surg Gynecol Obstet 63:457–462, 1936.
40. Kirklin JW, McDonald JR, Harrington SW, New GB: Parotid tumors: Histology, clinical behavior, and end results. Surg Gynecol Obstet 92:721–733, 1951.
41. Spiro RN: Salivary neoplasms: Overview of a 35-year experience with 2,807 patients. Head Neck Surg 8:177–184, 1986.
42. Donavan DT, Conley JJ: Capsular significance in parotid tumor surgery: Reality and myths of lateral lobectomy. Laryngoscope 94:324–329, 1984.
43. Dawson AK: Radiation therapy in recurrent pleomorphic adenoma of the parotid. Int J Radiat Oncol Biol Phys 16:819–821, 1989.

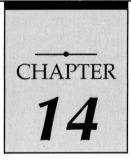

CHAPTER

14

Surgery of the Pharynx and Esophagus

MICHAEL F. PRATT, MD
GARY L. SCHECHTER, MD

Complications resulting from surgery of the pharynx and esophagus cover a wide range. Most of the surgical procedures performed in the pharynx and esophagus are designed to remove tumors. Due to the contaminated nature of the operative field, surgery for both benign and malignant disease is associated with significant risk of postoperative morbidity. This includes wound infection, poor tissue healing due to inadequate nutritional status or reduced vascularity, pharyngocutaneous fistula, bleeding, and nerve injury.

In recent years, major improvements have been made in pharyngoesophageal surgery. Advances in reconstructive techniques have allowed more extensive extirpative surgery and more rapid postoperative rehabilitation. The overall result has been shorter hospitalization periods, more rapid return of function, and reduced morbidity and mortality.

An organized and systematic approach is necessary for evaluation and management of complications to minimize the problems as-

sociated with this type of surgery. The surgeon can reduce the morbidity with expeditious management of the primary lesion and any complications that occur. Patients will then benefit from rapid rehabilitation and improved quality of life.

The most common errors in postoperative management are made when the surgeon fails to recognize the nature and extent of a complication. Failure to detect and treat a pharyngocutaneous fistula may lead to skin flap elevation, infection, and tissue necrosis. Failure to recognize and evacuate a hematoma or seroma may lead to abscess formation and soft tissue breakdown. Failure to detect necrosis of a buried myocutaneous flap may lead to massive infection that places the carotid artery at risk for rupture.

In this chapter we cover the common complications associated with pharyngeal and esophageal surgery. The discussion is separated into two broad categories: complications of primary closure and complications of pharyngeal and pharyngoesophageal reconstructive surgery. Early recognition and rapid correction of postoperative complications are stressed.

COMPLICATIONS OF PRIMARY CLOSURE

It is uncommon to find pharyngeal and esophageal lesions early enough to allow primary closure following resection. The most common problems associated with primary closure are caused by poor surgical judgment. A decision to close primarily when insufficient tissue remains after tumor ablation produces tension at the anastomosis. This usually results in poor healing, salivary fistula, tissue necrosis, and stenosis.

The often-stated rule that a pharyngoesophageal closure can be accomplished primarily if there is enough mucosa to close over a No. 18 nasogastric tube has resulted in more patients with stenoses and fistulas than with normally functioning systems.

Pharyngoesophageal (Zenker) Diverticulum (Table 14–1)

Zenker diverticulum requires special mention since it stands alone as one of the most

TABLE 14–1. Complications of Zenker Diverticulum Repair

Procedure	Complications
Endoscopic repair (Dohlman)	Mediastinitis Recurrent laryngeal nerve palsy Frequent recurrence
Diverticulectomy	Recurrence Recurrent laryngeal nerve palsy Fistula Sepsis Stricture Hematoma Pneumonia or atelectasis
Diverticulopexy	Dysphagia Fistula Stenosis

common benign problems of this area. This outpouching of the hypopharyngeal wall results from a weakened triangular area between the cricopharyngeus and the inferior thyropharyngeal portions of the inferior constrictor muscle. As Zenker originally described it, the diverticulum is caused by the absence of coordinated cricopharyngeus relaxation during swallowing.[1] Since there is a tendency for this lesion to occur in elderly and debilitated patients, surgical therapy can be hazardous.

Most surgeons espouse the single-stage diverticulectomy with or without cricopharyngeal myotomy as the treatment of choice. Conventional suturing techniques are usually employed, but excellent results also can be obtained with linear stapling devices.[2] Many patients have been treated with primary dilation or cricopharyngeal myotomy alone. Dohlman described endoscopic resection of the hypopharyngeal diverticular party wall, allowing the sac contents to flow into the esophagus.[3] Diverticulopexy with cricopharyngeal myotomy is also used in the treatment of these conditions. Although the literature contains many reports on the surgical treatment for Zenker diverticulum, few workers have discussed the therapy as it relates to the overall condition of the patient. The potential for postoperative complications with each procedure must be considered in this context.

Dohlman's procedure is associated with multiple complications, including mediastinitis, recurrent laryngeal nerve palsy, and frequent recurrence of the diverticulum. Although Overbeek and associates describe good overall results using this endoscopic procedure with either electrocautery or the CO_2 laser, most investigators find better results with alternative techniques.[4]

Excision of the diverticular sac is associated with a variety of complications. Maran and associates tabulated data from ten separate series reported between 1972 and 1986 on the complications of excision techniques.[5] The total complication rate was 18 per cent. Individual complications included recurrence (6 per cent), recurrent laryngeal nerve palsy (4 per cent), fistula (3 per cent), sepsis (3 per cent), stricture (1 per cent), cervical emphysema (1 per cent) and death (1 per cent). Causes of death include perforation, aspiration pneumonia, and carcinoma. Carcinoma is rarely found in the pharyngoesophageal pouch, but its occurrence certainly requires a more aggressive approach to the treatment of the patient. Donald and Huffman reported the 24th case of carcinoma in a Zenker diverticulum in 1979.[6] The patient was free of disease at 3 years following laryngopharyngectomy with cervical esophagectomy, mediastinal dissection, and full-course radiation therapy.

Konowitz and Biller recently delineated the advantages of using diverticulopexy and cricopharyngeal myotomy in the high-risk patient with a pharyngoesophageal diverticulum.[7] They reported 32 patients, of whom 12 had diverticulopexy and myotomy and 20 had a one-stage resection with myotomy. A nasogastric tube was not utilized with diverticulopexy. Patients were allowed oral intake on the first postoperative day, and they began ambulation immediately. The following complications were reported: one wound infection, one case of atelectasis, one salivary leak, and two hematomas in the diverticulectomy group; two cases of urinary retention and one case with dysphagia (resolved with alimentation) in the diverticulopexy group. Konowitz and Biller concluded that diverticulopexy with myotomy is the appropriate procedure for patients who possess risk factors making them unsuitable candidates for diverticulectomy. Given that the results were similar and that diverticulopexy is associated with less risk of fistula and stenosis, it is probably the procedure of choice and should be considered in the treatment of all patients with Zenker diverticulum.

Recurrent pharyngoesophageal diverticula occur in 3 per cent to 6 per cent of treated patients. They present the surgeon with major technical challenges. For the patient with progressively disabling and potentially life-threatening symptoms related to recurrent Zenker diverticulum, reoperation is essential. Because of extensive fibrosis, meticulous dissection under magnification is required to preserve major neural and vascular structures. The recurrent laryngeal nerve is frequently not identifiable. The diverticular sac is often friable and requires sharp dissection for mobilization. Suture techniques rather than stapling devices are recommended. Cricopharyngeal myotomy is difficult due to dense fibrous reaction between mucosa and muscularis.

A comparison of results achieved with primary and secondary operations is revealing. Of 325 primary and 31 secondary procedures reported from the Mayo Clinic over a 19-year period, morbidity was significantly higher in the secondary group.[8] The investigators reported the following differences: (1) vocal cord paralysis: 1.5 per cent primary, 19 per cent secondary; (2) wound infection: 1 per cent primary, 32 per cent secondary; (3) fistula: 1 per cent primary, 19 per cent secondary; (4) recurrent diverticulum: 3 per cent primary, 6 per cent secondary; and (5) mortality: 1 per cent primary, 3 per cent secondary. These figures notwithstanding, a good or excellent result was achieved in 96 per cent of secondary repairs, compared with 93 per cent of primary procedures.

Despite the inherent difficulties with Zenker diverticulum surgery, satisfactory results can be achieved and should be attempted in the significantly symptomatic patient whose medical condition warrants surgical intervention. In the properly selected patient, reoperation is often less hazardous than what appears to be the more conservative course of medical management, which is usually ineffective.

Excision of Pharyngeal and Esophageal Tumors

Possible complications of pharyngeal and esophageal surgery include wound infection and necrosis, bleeding, salivary fistula, carotid artery rupture, and death. Positive surgical margins and prolonged operative time have been related to an increased incidence of subsequent complications.[9] Shorter operating times decrease the duration of anesthesia, amount of blood loss, and tissue exposure to the damaging effects of desiccation and contamination. Routine use of perioperative antibiotics decreases the incidence of complications related to wound sepsis.

It is, of course, important to obtain clear resection margins from an oncologic point of view. If positive margins are present, one of the first signs may be that the suture line does not heal. Other negative factors include poor nutritional status, medical disease of vital organ systems (specifically cardiac, renal, pulmonary, and liver disease), and reduced response of stress hormones.[10, 11] Age does not appear to be a factor that correlates with postoperative complications.

It is important to consider the role of radiation therapy in the overall treatment plan for these lesions. Combined therapy is required for adequate treatment of advanced tumors. Preoperative or postoperative irradiation may be used. Although some workers have shown as much as a 15 per cent to 20 per cent increase in complications with preoperative radiation therapy, Driscoll and colleagues reported no significant difference between groups having combined therapy and groups having surgery alone.[12] Most of their radiation therapy was delivered preoperatively, and the numbers were small.

Simple skin wound infections usually do not create serious management problems. Preventable causes include poor closure, inadequate hemostasis, improper aseptic technique, and malfunctioning drains. Treatment consists of antibiotics and local wound care. Wound necrosis can be caused by poor flap design and closure under tension. Hematoma, seroma, infection, and radiation therapy may be contributing factors. Treatment involves adequate debridement, local wound care, and reconstruction if indicated. If the wound infection produces extensive necrosis of tissue, carotid coverage must be ensured.

Salivary fistula results from separation of the mucosal suture line and presents a potentially lethal problem. Contributing factors include failure to invert mucosal or flap edges, strangulating sutures, local tissue necrosis, infection, tension closure, systemic diseases, radiation therapy, and poor nutritional status. Small fistulas will heal spontaneously with exteriorization, aggressive local wound care, and maintenance of adequate nutrition and blood volume.[13] The wounds must be drained and debrided once they become infected. Transfusions must sometimes be given to maintain a hemoglobin level adequate for healing. Aggressive nutritional support by nasogastric tube, esophagostomy, gastrostomy, or parenteral hyperalimentation is necessary.

Some fistulas require reconstruction. A variety of methods are used for these repairs, including adjacent flaps, regional flaps, and distant flaps. Primary closure is usually unsuccessful unless bilateral inverting flaps to close the mucosa are possible prior to undermining and approximating the adjacent skin flap edges. A local inversion skin flap may be used for inner epithelial lining, whereas an advancement, rotation, or regional flap is used for skin resurfacing.

Large fistulas require compound tissues to effect good closure. This may be accomplished using a delayed cervical flap that is inverted to close the pharynx.[13] A regional flap, such as the deltopectoral or pectoralis major, is then used for external resurfacing. Regional tissue, such as the pectoralis major or latissimus dorsi myocutaneous flap, can be used for pharyngeal closure with a skin graft for closure of the exterior surface. In addition, free tissue transfers, such as the forearm or rectus abdominis flaps, may be used for internal lining in combination with some of the other techniques for skin coverage. A sternocleidomastoid myoperiosteal flap consisting of clavicular periosteum attached to muscle also has been described for closure of the mucosal defect in patients who have not had bilateral radical neck dissections.[14]

This is not meant to be an exhaustive discussion of pharyngocutaneous fistula reconstruction, but rather a summary of some available techniques. It is important to be familiar with multiple options and to take a systematic approach to managing this difficult complication. The simplest procedure that will work for each individual situation is often the best choice for the patient. It must be emphasized that prevention remains the best method of handling complication.

When fistulas and infection do occur, however, the patient should be managed both locally and systemically. Hasty employment of a reconstructive technique is ill advised. It is more appropriate to clean up the wound, create direct fistulas, correct systemic problems, and wait for local evidence of a good patient response, such as granulation, before traumatizing the wound with a reconstructive procedure.

COMPLICATIONS OF COMPLEX RECONSTRUCTIVE SURGERY

As mentioned, it is not common to find a situation in which hypopharyngeal tumor can be removed and the defect closed primarily. This is possible in some patients with small (T_1 or T_2) carcinomas of the superior aspect of the piriform fossa, but in most cases reconstruction is necessary. Many techniques have been proposed for reconstruction of pharyngoesophageal defects. This gives testimony to the fact that the ideal procedure has yet to be found. The best reconstruction would involve a one-stage operation that uses tissue outside radiation fields and requires only one anastomosis. In addition, it would not require an abdominal or thoracic procedure.

Most of the available techniques fall short of the ideal. Examples of procedures that have been used over the years with variable success rates include skin, mucosal and dermal grafts; local flaps such as cervical skin and tongue; axial pattern flaps (deltopectoral); myocutaneous flaps (pectoralis major and latissimus dorsi); gastric transposition; colon interposition; and free tissue transfer (fasciocutaneous flap or jejunum). It is important for the head and neck surgeon to consider several options for each case. The method selected should restore function quickly, provide acceptable appearance, and allow delivery of adjuvant radiotherapy within 4 to 6 weeks following surgery.

Partial Hypopharyngeal Reconstruction (Table 14–2)

There are two possible types of hypopharyngeal reconstruction: partial and total. Partial reconstruction requires leaving a strip of mucosa after the tumor is removed, whereas total reconstruction entails the complete circumferential restoration of the pharyngeal lining. Grafts and flaps are used more successfully in partial reconstructions.

For a posterior pharyngeal wall defect, a split-thickness skin graft or dermal graft may be used. Both provide pliability and minimal bulk.[11] Graft contracture is minimized by using an oversized graft supported by a bolus that is removed after 10 days. Lorře described a sliding posterior tongue flap for the anterolateral pharyngeal wall and a dermal graft for the posterior pharyngeal repair.[15] Defects of up to 8 cm could be repaired using this one-stage procedure. Supraglottic mucosa with a larynx autograft and epiglottis mucosa also have been described for the repair of partial pharyngeal defects.[16, 17] Larger lateral and posterolateral defects, however, require use of regional or free flaps.

Another management problem relative to graft and flap reconstruction of the pharynx has to do with the amount of pharyngeal wall that can be removed while preserving a normal larynx. Complications of dysphagia and aspiration are common when more than one third of the pharynx is replaced and the larynx is preserved.[11] Cricopharyngeal myotomy has not been helpful in these cases. When partial pharyngectomy with laryngeal preservation is performed, laryngeal dysfunction may occur if the flap used for reconstruction is sutured to the larynx.[18]

TABLE 14–2. Complications of Partial Hypopharyngeal Reconstruction

Procedure	Complications
Partial pharyngectomy with laryngeal preservation	Laryngeal dysfunction Dysphagia Aspiration Fistula
Laryngectomy with partial pharyngectomy	Fistula Stenosis

A recent report by Chang described the use of a partially tubed pectoralis major flap for reconstruction of posterior and lateral walls of circumferential hypopharyngeal defects. The flap was tacked to the prevertebral fascia and then sutured to the inner surface of the apron skin flap of the anterior neck.[19] This technique is used when the larynx is removed. Of eight patients who underwent this form of reconstruction, one developed a pharyngocutaneous fistula and subsequent stenosis at the pharyngoesophageal junction. The other seven patients had satisfactory swallowing and suffered no postoperative complications.

Complications directly related to reconstruction with grafts and local flaps usually involve fistulas and stenosis rather than necrosis. Pre-existing metabolic disorders relating to liver disease, diabetes, or malnutrition are significant factors that predispose to complications in these reconstructive efforts. Intravenous hyperalimentation should be considered for all patients with malabsorption or liver disease to minimize postoperative problems.[11] Multiple continuous suction catheters should be placed at critical locations along suture lines. Prolonged use of continuous suction often allows small leaks to close spontaneously.

Total Hypopharyngeal Reconstruction (Table 14–3)

In most cases of hypopharyngeal cancer, the larynx is removed and part of the cervical esophagus must be replaced as well. Complications are directly related to the procedure used for reconstruction of the resulting defect. One older technique for total pharyngeal reconstruction used split-thickness skin grafts over a supporting tubular stent. This method resulted in a high incidence of stenosis and should not be used to repair circumferential defects.[20] The tubed cervical skin flap method of reconstructing the hypopharynx and cervical esophagus was popularized by Wookey.[21] This was a staged procedure associated with limited tissue availability, fistula formation, stenosis, and

TABLE 14–3. Complications of Total Hypopharyngeal Reconstruction

Procedure	Complications
Tubed skin graft	Stenosis (high incidence)
Tubed skin flap (Wookey)	Fistula Stenosis (high incidence)
Modified Wookey	Fistula Stenosis (low incidence) Flap necrosis
Tubed myocutaneous flap	Fistula Stenosis (high incidence) Flap necrosis Dysphagia Decreased arm or shoulder motion
Visceral flaps	Organ necrosis Fistula Stenosis Death Wound infection Flap necrosis
Pharyngogastrostomy	Fistula Gastric reflux Dumping syndrome Injury to thoracic or abdominal viscera Organ necrosis Stenosis Pulmonary infection Diarrhea Bile regurgitation Gastric distention Hypoparathyroidism Hypothyroidism Death
Free jejunal graft	Graft necrosis Dysphagia Carotid rupture Fistula Stenosis Gastrointestinal bleeding Cervical bleeding Bowel obstruction Abdominal wound dehiscence Redundant bowel syndrome Death

prolonged hospitalization. The classic Wookey technique has no application today. A modified Wookey procedure may be used as a planned reconstructive effort or to salvage an unsuccessful reconstruction after the pharynx and esophagus are exteriorized. The modified Wookey technique involves a staged, tension-free closure of the pharynx and cervical esophagus using tubed cervical skin. A pedicled chest flap is used to close the cervical skin defect. Surkin and coworkers reported 31 such procedures, with many performed following radiotherapy.[22] Flap slough occurred in only one patient (3 per cent incidence). Many fistulas developed, but there was a low incidence of stenosis because the esophageal anastomosis was delayed.

Regional Flaps

Staged deltopectoral flap reconstruction of pharyngoesophageal defects was reported by Bakamjian.[23] Although this method was used extensively for many years, it has limited application today. The medially based deltopectoral chest flap is best reserved for skin coverage; other techniques are employed for visceral reconstruction.

A great impact on head and neck reconstructive surgery was made by the introduction of the pectoralis major myocutaneous flap by Ariyan.[24] A tubed pectoralis major flap was described by Withers and associates for the reconstruction of pharyngoesophageal defects.[25] Initial results were encouraging. Transient fistulas occurred in two of nine patients, and swallowing could be initiated after 12 days. No late strictures were reported.

In circumferential pharyngoesophageal repair, the tubed pectoralis major flap is associated with many postoperative reconstructive complications, such as fistulas, stenoses, and flap necroses. A complication rate of 67 per cent was reported by Surkin and colleagues in an initial report of 17 patients reconstructed by this method.[22] Adequate swallowing was achieved in only seven patients (41 per cent). The distal anastomosis is prone to stricture formation because it involves closure of the bulky flap to the thin, pliable mucosa of the esophagus, which has been mobilized out of the mediastinum. Strictures usually can be managed with periodic dilatation, but swallowing is often unsatisfactory. Baek and colleagues initially reported 14 cases of hypopharynx–cervical esophagus reconstructions using tubed pectoralis major flaps.[26] Of seven patients who underwent one-stage reconstruction, three had separation of the upper suture line requiring the creation of a secondary pharyngostoma. The other seven patients received a temporary lateral pharyngostoma which was closed at 7 to 14 days in a planned second stage. This latter group developed only minor complications.

Fabian recommended a two-stage modified Montgomery technique using a partially tubed pectoralis major flap for reconstruction of the pharyngoesophagus.[27] Partial resection of the ipsilateral clavicle was proposed to decrease pressure and torsion on the vascular pedicle. Of 35 patients evaluated, 11 (31 per cent) had complications directly related to reconstruction. All were fistulas, ten of which healed spontaneously and one required surgical closure. All patients could swallow initially; however, ten showed some degree of esophageal stricture that necessitated repeated esophagoscopies and dilatations.

The latissimus dorsi myocutaneous flap also can be used for pharyngeal and cervical esophageal reconstruction. Watson and colleagues reported its use in 16 patients.[28] A posterior mucosal strip was incorporated in three, six were total circumferential reconstructions under intact skin, and five were compound total reconstructions. A skin graft, a second latissimus dorsi, or a deltopectoral flap was used for skin closure in the compound reconstructions. A controlled pharyngostoma was used in two patients. There was one complete failure due to an inadequate tunnel that caused compression of the flap pedicle between the clavicle and the pectoralis major muscle. In this case, an adequate tunnel would have been ensured by detaching the clavicular origin of the pectoralis major muscle from the clavicle. A second latissimus dorsi flap and two deltopectoral flaps were required to salvage this repair. Three patients (19 per cent) developed salivary fistulas, two of which were large enough to require a second flap for reconstruction. One stricture at the lower anastomosis was successfully revised. This form of reconstruction provides a large, reliable skin paddle. The donor site may be closed primarily if the flap measures no more than 10 cm in width.

The latissimus dorsi flap is beneficial in

reconstruction after complications with other techniques that result in large areas of necrosis. It may be preferred to the pectoralis major flap in women with pendulous breasts or in hirsute men. Elevation of the latissimus dorsi flap may cause the patient difficulty in raising the arm if the spinal accessory nerve has been divided. The same postoperative complication may be noted with use of the pectoralis major flap if the spinal accessory nerve is removed in the neck dissection. The incidence of postoperative complications with the latissimus dorsi flap is comparable to that seen with other regional myocutaneous flaps.

Visceral Flaps

Abdominal viscera, such as colon, jejunum, and stomach, are used for reconstruction of the upper alimentary tract after resection of hypopharyngeal and cervical esophageal tumors. Complications associated with their use can be significant.

Goligher and Robin popularized the technique of reconstructing the pharynx with a pedicle flap consisting of transverse and left colon.[29] A survey of the literature between 1964 and 1980 (267 reported cases) reveals a mortality rate of 20 per cent.[22] The incidence of postoperative reconstructive complications was 25 per cent. These included organ necrosis, salivary fistula, and stenosis. A success rate of 68 per cent was achieved, with 45 per cent of patients experiencing at least one major complication related to abdominal, thoracic, or medical problems. The interval to oral alimentation was 10 to 30 days, and the duration of hospitalization was 4 to 9 weeks. With this method of reconstruction, there is a significant risk of wound infection as well as the disadvantage of three anastomoses. There is also a tendency for the colonic segment to become distended over time.

Technical problems are associated with colon interposition surgery. It is difficult to protect the vascular pedicle when the colon is mobilized for transfer to the cervical region.[30] If the segment is mobilized through the posterior mediastinum, there is the potential for vascular pedicle obstruction from bronchial compression. The retrosternal route sometimes requires sternoclavicular joint resection to prevent sternal compression of the pedicle. Since these technical problems are so common and the mortality and morbidity associated with colon interposition are so high, other methods of reconstruction are favored by most surgeons working in this field.

Gastric Transposition

Gastric transposition is a reliable one-stage method of reconstruction that promotes rapid healing. Mobilization of the stomach with preservation of right gastric and gastroepiploic vessels provides an excellent blood supply for optimal healing. This method carries some relative disadvantages. Gastric reflux and dumping syndrome are common. Abdominal and thoracic viscera, including the spleen, the great vessels, and the party wall of the trachea may be injured. Seriously debilitated patients may not tolerate the combined abdominal, thoracic, and cervical procedures without pulmonary or cardiovascular sequelae. Although gastric voice production is possible, it is sometimes unsatisfactory to the patient, requiring the use of an electrolarynx.

Many reports can be found describing gastric transposition for pharyngeal reconstruction following resection of large hypopharyngeal and esophageal carcinomas. The senior author (GLS) initially reported 15 patients treated by pharyngolaryngoesophagectomy with pharyngogastrostomy.[31] Three transient anastomotic leaks healed spontaneously with the assistance of continuous closed suction. There was one death on the seventh postoperative day from liver failure and *Pseudomonas* pneumonia. Two patients with cirrhosis had transient jaundice. One patient early in the series required secondary pyloroplasty to improve gastric emptying. Pyloroplasty is now performed in all cases. All patients were able to swallow well and produce intelligible gastric speech. The present Eastern Virginia Medical School series is composed of over 40 pharyngogastrostomies, with a continued low incidence of complications.

Other series of gastric transpositions published since 1972 report mortality rates of 6 to 11 per cent.[22, 31, 33] The average incidence of postoperative reconstructive complications is 7.5 per cent.[22] These include organ necrosis, salivary fistulas, and anastomotic stenosis. Much of the reported morbidity associated with this procedure is unavoidable. Chest tubes, which are necessary in some patients, may cause pulmonary effusion. Pulmonary infection is common in those with chronic bronchitis. Diarrhea, common with jejunostomy feeding, and bile regurgitation secondary to the new anatomic relationships, usually stop when oral alimentation is begun. Long-term problems with gastric distention are common.

A large series of 157 patients who received pharyngogastrostomies was reported by Lam and associates in 1981.[32] Their study covered 14 years and reported an overall mortality of 31 per cent. This decreased to 18 per cent in the last two years of the study. Mortality was higher in patients with poor cardiopulmonary status or with tumors extending into the vallecula requiring base of tongue resection. Postoperative swallowing was generally good, but speech rehabilitation was poor. The most common cause of long-term failure was the development of metastatic disease.

Laryngopharyngectomy often requires total exenteration of the neck, including the thyroid and parathyroid glands. Three recent studies reported a high incidence (up to 73 per cent) of postoperative hypoparathyroidism, requiring therapy.[34-36]

The patient's calcium levels should be evaluated pre- and postoperatively. The combined insult of total parathyroidectomy and altered enteral physiology can produce a profound medical management problem. Parathyroid autotransplantation should be performed whenever the glands can be retrieved without compromising the tumor resection. Thyroid replacement should not be given during the immediate postoperative period since it inhibits intestinal absorption of calcium. Treatment should be aimed at maintaining a normal ionized serum calcium. A total dose of 2 to 3 gm per day of elemental calcium in the form of water-soluble calcium gluconate is usually required via jejunostomy tube. Vitamin D therapy in the form of 1,25[OH]$_2$ cholecalciferol should be administered in a dosage of 0.5 to 2.0 mg per day (Calcitrol, Rocaltrol). Oral feedings are started when suture lines are secure and a swallowing study demonstrates no fistula. At this point, calcium requirements are usually reduced because passage of feedings through the duodenum and proximal jejunum improves the efficiency of calcium absorption. Continued monitoring of calcium levels is necessary, with medication adjustments made as required.

Although the morbidity and mortality associated with gastric transposition are significant, the rate compares favorably with other techniques used for reconstruction after laryngopharyngectomy. The procedure is versatile, and it provides excellent palliation for these patients who have a poor long-term prognosis. When an esophagectomy is required to obtain an adequate inferior margin, gastric transposition is the reconstructive procedure of choice. It is a single-stage technique with one anastomosis, rehabilitation is usually rapid, and the quality of survival is good.[37] It also may be used when other techniques, such as regional flaps, free skin transfers, and free jejunal grafts, have failed.

Free Tissue Reconstruction with Microvascular Anastomosis

The free jejunal interposition graft for pharyngoesophageal reconstruction was first described by Seidenberg and associates.[38] As microvascular techniques have become more widespread, this method of reconstruction has become more commonplace. It is an excellent reconstructive technique in appropriate circumstances but may be associated with significant complications.

The success of any microvascular free tissue transfer depends upon meticulous surgical technique and careful postoperative monitoring. The use of a monitor segment brought out through the neck wound has been quite helpful.[39] The pedicle to the monitor flap can be ligated and divided after the success of the free autograft is ensured (usually after 5 to 7 days). There are numerous potential complications related to the microvascular surgery. The vascular pedicle is very fragile and can be easily damaged while harvesting the segment from the thick, fatty mesentery. It is often difficult to find healthy recipient vessels in the neck, and size discrepancies between the mesenteric and external carotid vessels frequently exist. The microvascular anastomoses must be performed without producing tension or torsion. Vein grafts are occasionally required.

Three recent series of free jejunal graft reconstructions have demonstrated excellent reliability.[40–42] An overall success rate of 90 per cent was achieved in 141 patients. Fisher and coworkers reported a physiologic success rate of 86 per cent as determined by adequate swallowing function in 33 of 36 patients.[40] All the patients who died of recurrent disease in this report had excellent palliation.

Of all the potential complications associated with this technique, the most catastrophic is graft necrosis. If ischemia is diagnosed early, the microvascular anastomosis can be revised, or a new segment of jejunum can be harvested and placed. If the diagnosis of graft failure is delayed for many days, there is a great danger of carotid artery rupture.[43] Once the diagnosis of graft failure is made, immediate exploration is necessary. With delayed discovery of graft necrosis, it is imperative to determine the status of the great vessels. Some patients with graft necrosis may be managed without sacrifice of the carotid artery or jugular vein. In the presence of significant infection, however, prophylactic ligation is preferable.[42] Many graft failures have resulted in carotid artery or jugular vein rupture.

The overall mortality related to the free jejunal autograft is 8 per cent.[22] The incidence of postoperative reconstructive complications, including graft necrosis, salivary fistula and stenosis, is 35 per cent.[22] The average interval to oral alimentation is 10 to 12 days,

with a hospitalization period of 2 to 3 weeks in the uncomplicated patient. Other reported complications include gastrointestinal bleeding, cervical bleeding, bowel obstruction, and abdominal wound dehiscence.[44] All patients develop some edema of the jejunal segment, resulting in dysphagia that usually resolves within several months. "Redundant bowel syndrome" resulting in pooling of secretions and food can develop if the segment is too long.[42] Stenosis of the upper and lower segments has been reported. This usually responds well to dilatation. McCaffrey and Fisher reported a higher incidence of graft failure in patients who had received preoperative radiation therapy, presumably secondary to vessel thrombosis.[43]

Free fasciocutaneous flaps are also being used for pharyngoesophageal reconstruction. The radial forearm flap is the most familiar autograft in this category, but the lateral thigh flap also may be used. These methods provide thin, pliable skin that can be tubed with less risk of stenosis than the bulky myocutaneous flaps. Palliation is good and pharyngeal speech is often better than what can be achieved with jejunal reconstructions. Intra-abdominal complications are avoided. These procedures are associated with the same postoperative complications in the neck as those delineated for the free jejunal interposition graft. They each have the potential for unique donor site problems. As these techniques are relatively new, there are few published data on the long-term complications.

Functional complications related to pharyngoesophageal reconstruction in general involve swallowing and voice rehabilitation. Skin flaps, gastric pullup, and jejunal autografts all provide good palliation and acceptable function in the majority of patients. More detailed evaluation of functional results indicates that the gastric transposition provides the best overall tissue environment for swallowing and voice production. Gastric transposition and jejunal autograft are superior to the chest flap techniques.[45]

References

1. Bockus HL: Gastroenterology. Philadelphia, WB Saunders, 1974, pp 319–324.

2. Talmi YP, Finkelstein Y, Sadov R, et al: Use of a linear stapler in excision of Zenker's diverticulum. Head Neck 2:150–152, 1989.
3. Dohlman G: The endoscopic operation for hypopharyngeal diverticula. Arch Otolaryngol 71:744–752, 1960.
4. Overbeek JJM, Hoeksema PE, Edens E: Microendoscopic surgery of the hypopharyngeal diverticulum using electrocoagulation or carbon dioxide laser. Ann Otol Rhinol Laryngol 93:34–36, 1984.
5. Maran AGD, Wilson JA, Al Muhanna AH: Pharyngeal diverticula. Clin Otolaryngol 11:219–225, 1986.
6. Donald PJ, Huffman DI: Carcinoma in a Zenker's diverticulum. Head Neck Surg 2:71–75, 1979.
7. Konowitz PM, Biller HF: Diverticulopexy and cricopharyngeal myotomy: Treatment for the high-risk patient with a pharyngoesophageal (Zenker's) diverticulum. Otolaryngol Head Neck Surg 100:146–153, 1989.
8. Huang B, Payne WS, Cameron AJ: Surgical management for recurrent pharyngoesophageal (Zenker's) diverticulum. Ann Thorac Surg 37:189–191, 1984.
9. Gall AM, Sessions DG, Ogura JH: Complications following surgery for cancer of the larynx and hypopharynx. Cancer 39:624–631, 1977.
10. Nishi M, Hiramatsu Y, Hioki K, et al: Risk factors in relation to postoperative complications in patients undergoing esophagectomy or gastrectomy for cancer. Ann Surg 207:148–154, 1988.
11. Schechter GL: Complications of flaps and grafts in the oral cavity and pharynx. Laryngoscope 93:306–309, 1983.
12. Driscoll WG, Nagorsky MJ, Cantrell RW, Johns ME: Carcinoma of the pyriform sinus: Analysis of 102 cases. Laryngoscope 93:556–560, 1983.
13. Myers EN: The management of pharyngocutaneous fistula. Arch Otolaryngol 95:10–17, 1972.
14. Friedman M, Toriumi DM, Chilis T, et al: The sternocleidomastoid myoperiosteal flap for esophagopharyngeal reconstruction and fistula repair: Clinical and experimental study. Laryngoscope 98:1084–1091, 1988.
15. Loré JM: Total reconstruction of the hypopharynx with tongue flap and dermal graft. Ann Otol Rhinol Laryngol 83:476, 1974.
16. Asherson N: Pharyngectomy for post-cricoid carcinoma: One stage operation with reconstruction of the pharynx using the larynx as an autograft. J Laryngol Otol 68:550, 1954.
17. Sabri JA: Reconstruction of the pharyngoesophagus using mucosa of epiglottis. Otolaryngol Head Neck Surg 89:746, 1981.
18. Rees RS, Ivey GL, Shack RB, et al: Pectoralis major musculocutaneous flaps: Long-term follow-up of hypopharyngeal reconstruction. Plast Reconstr Surg 77:586–591, 1986.
19. Chang S: Reconstruction of circumferential defect of the hypopharynx: Experimental studies and clinical application of a new method. Laryngoscope 99:736–740, 1989.
20. Ballantyne AJ: Methods of repair after surgery for cancer of the pharyngeal wall, postcricoid area and cervical esophagus. Am J Surg 122:482–486, 1971.
21. Wookey H: The surgical treatment of carcinoma of the pharynx and upper esophagus. Surg Gynecol Obstet 75:499, 1942.
22. Surkin MI, Lawson W, Biller HF: Analysis of the methods of pharyngoesophageal reconstruction. Head Neck Surg 6:953–970, 1984.
23. Bakamjian VY: A two-stage method for pharyngoesophageal reconstruction with a primary pectoral skin flap. Plast Reconstr Surg 36:173, 1965.
24. Ariyan S: The pectoralis major myocutaneous flap—A versatile flap for reconstruction in the head and neck. Plast Reconstr Surg 63:73, 1979.
25. Withers EH, Franklin JD, Madden JJ, et al: Immediate reconstruction of the pharynx and cervical esophagus with the pectoralis major myocutaneous flap following laryngopharyngectomy. Plast Reconstr Surg 68:898, 1981.
26. Baek SM, Lawson W, Biller H: Reconstruction of hypopharynx and cervical esophagus with pectoralis major island myocutaneous flap. Ann Plast Surg 7:18–24, 1981.
27. Fabian RL: Reconstruction of the laryngopharynx and cervical esophagus. Laryngoscope 94:1334–1350, 1984.
28. Watson JS, Robertson GA, Lendrum J, et al: Pharyngeal reconstruction using the latissimus dorsi myocutaneous flap. Br J Plast Surg 35:401–407, 1982.
29. Goligher JC, Robin IG: Use of left colon for reconstruction of pharynx and esophagus after pharyngectomy. Br J Surg 42:283–290, 1954.
30. Silver CE: Surgical treatment of hypopharyngeal and cervical esophageal cancer. World J Surg 5:499, 1981.
31. Baker JW, Schechter GL, Jackson RT, et al: Reconstruction of combined pharyngolaryngoesophageal defects with stomach and jejunal autotransplantation. In Demester TR, Skinner DB (eds): Esophageal Disorders: Pathophysiology and Therapy. New York, Raven Press, 1985.
32. Lam KH, Wong J, Lim S, Ong GB: Pharyngogastric anastomosis following pharyngolaryngoesophagectomy—Analysis of 157 cases. World J Surg 5:509–516, 1981.
33. Harrison DRN, Thompson AE: Pharyngolaryngoesophagectomy with pharyngogastric anastomosis for cancer of the hypopharynx: Review of 101 operations. Head Neck Surg 8:418–428, 1986.
34. Krespi YP, Wurster CF, Wang TD, Stone DM: Hypoparathyroidism following total laryngopharyngectomy and gastric pull-up. Laryngoscope 95:1184–1187, 1985.
35. Price JC, Ridley MB: Hypocalcemia following pharyngoesophageal ablation and gastric pull-up reconstruction: Pathophysiology and management. Ann Otol Rhinol Laryngol 97:521–526, 1988.
36. Wei WI, Lam KH, Choi S, Wong J: Late problems after pharyngolaryngoesophagectomy and pharyngogastric anastomosis for cancer of the larynx and hypopharynx. Am J Surg 148:509–513, 1984.
37. Spiro R, Shah JP, Strong EW, et al: Gastric transposition in head and neck surgery. Am J Surg 146:483–487, 1983.
38. Seidenberg B, Rosznak SS, Hurwitt ES, et al: Immediate reconstruction of the cervical esophagus by a revascularized isolated jejunal segment. Ann Surg 149:162–171, 1959.
39. Tabah RJ, Flynn MB, Acland RD, Banis JC: Microvascular free tissue transfer in head and neck and esophageal surgery. Am J Surg 148:498–504, 1984.
40. Fisher SR, Cameron R, Hoyt DJ, et al: Free jejunal interposition graft for reconstruction of the esophagus. Head Neck 12:126–130, 1990.
41. McDonough JJ, Gluckman JL: Microvascular recon-

struction of the pharyngoesophagus with free jejunal graft. Microsurgery 9:116–127, 1988.

42. Gluckman JL, McCafferty GJ, Black RJ, et al: Complications associated with free jejunal graft reconstruction of the pharyngoesophagus—A multiinstitutional experience with 52 cases. Head Neck Surg 7:200–205, 1985.

43. McCaffrey TV, Fisher J: Effect of radiotherapy on the outcome of pharyngeal reconstruction using free jejunal transfer. Ann Otol Rhinol Laryngol 96:22–25, 1987.

44. Ferguson JL, DeSanto LW: Total pharyngolaryngectomy and cervical esophagectomy with jejunal autotransplant reconstruction: Complications and results. Laryngoscope 98:911–914, 1988.

45. Schechter GL, Baker JW, Gilbert DA: Functional evaluation of pharyngoesophageal reconstructive techniques. Arch Otolaryngol 113:40–44, 1987.

Tonsillectomy and Adenoidectomy

GADY HAR-EL, MD

MICHAEL NASH, MD

Serious complications of tonsillectomy and adenoidectomy (T&A) are uncommon. Nonetheless, because these operations are among the most commonly performed surgical procedures in the United States,[8, 45, 59, 68] the absolute number of complications is high enough to contribute significantly to the overall surgical morbidity rates in otolaryngology.

The purpose of this chapter is to help the surgeon prevent, recognize, diagnose, and manage potential complications associated with T&A. The focus is on statistics, life-threatening complications, common complications, uncommon complications, rare and anecdotal complications, long-term sequelae, and laser tonsillectomy.

STATISTICS

Reliable statistics regarding the incidence of T&A and the complication rate are difficult to obtain. A substantial number of T&As are still performed by physicians other than otolaryngologists;[60, 68] consequently, data collection is even more difficult. Overall indications are that the number of T&As performed annually in the United States has declined during the last three decades. The number of T&As performed in the early 1960s was 1,500,000 per year, which dropped to less than a million in 1972, to about 700,000 in 1977, and to 500,000 in 1983.[8, 28, 45, 59, 68] Different sources, however, report slightly different numbers. The most significant reason for the decline is probably an increasing awareness, in both the medical community and the general population, of the appropriate indications for the operation. Even so, T&As are still the most common surgical procedure in children[8, 45] and account for 38.5 per cent of all procedures performed by otolaryngologists.[60]

Reported morbidity rates are even less reliable, since parameters for reporting morbidities most likely vary among surgeons. Many surgeons might not report seemingly "minor" complications. A complication for one surgeon might be considered part of the accepted postoperative course by another. Time may be a factor as well. For instance, at what point after surgery are pain and dysphagia considered to be "significant" complications?

Rates quoted in the literature range from 1.5 per cent [28] of serious complications to 14 per cent of all complications.[64] Crysdale and Russel surveyed nearly 10,000 T&As and reported an 0.6 per cent incidence of delayed discharge, mostly due to postoperative complications.[16] However, this number does not include the immediate postoperative bleeding cases and 2400 other T&As that had other preoperative medical problems. Samuel Crowe and associates reported their experience during the years 1911 to 1917. In this study, the morbidity rate was 4.7 per cent and the mortality rate was zero![15]

LIFE-THREATENING COMPLICATIONS

Death

Mortality rates are difficult to estimate for the same reasons described for morbidity rates. Rates quoted in the literature range from 1:1000[72] to zero.[15] Several studies have narrowed the range down to 1:10,000 to 1:35,000 operations,[61, 71] and more than one investigator has reported the number to be 1:16,000.[1, 67, 71, 82] Rasmussen states that with high social and sanitary standards, current mortality rates should be in the range of 1:50,000 to 1:150,000 operations.[72]

The main causes of death were consistently described in the literature as hypovolemia due to bleeding (with a significantly high percentage of cases defined as "avoidable"), complications of anesthesia, and cardiac arrest.[22, 31, 66, 72]

Anesthesia

As a result of the establishment of strict guidelines regarding the indications for T&A

and the overall decline in the number of T&As performed in the United States, children operated on today are generally sicker and their anesthesia management is more difficult. Detailing all the possible complications during and after general anesthesia is beyond the scope of this chapter; only those specifically related to T&A will be discussed.

To avoid potential complications, it is imperative that all patients be screened by the anesthesiologist before the operation. Although children with any pre-existing disease are usually seen by a pediatrician, cardiologist, or another medical specialist before hospital admission, often the anesthesiologist can be the first to notice a previously unknown problem. Children may develop subclinical right heart failure and pulmonary hypertension because of their upper airway obstruction. These children are at high risk for intra- and postoperative complications, such as pulmonary edema.

The anesthesiologist should examine and record the condition of the teeth, temporomandibular joint, and upper airway. As will be discussed in detail later, significant nasal obstruction may complicate mask ventilation, and significant tonsillar hypertrophy can make intubation difficult. The severity of preoperative airway obstruction will determine what dosage (if any) of premedication should be prescribed. Excessive narcotic or hypnotic premedication may induce hypoventilation and hypoxia. As discussed later, proper premedication is generally recommended to reduce the psychologic trauma of any pediatric surgery. However, this prophylactic measure may present a problem in children with preexisting cardiopulmonary diseases; for such patients, it is recommended that, with the cooperation of the surgeon, anesthesiologist, and nursing staff, premedication be used with close monitoring. It might also be helpful, in these cases, to allow the parents to accompany the patient into the operating room suite.

Dysrhythmias. Atrial dysrhythmia in a patient undergoing T&A is not unusual and may be related to reflex vagal stimulation by the oro- and nasopharyngeal manipulations. Ventricular dysrhythmias are more serious and may indicate problems such as hypoxemia. Difficulty arises when premature atrial beats are blocked in the bundle branches and produce wide and unusual QRS complexes, which may appear to be ventricular dysrhythmia. By careful analysis of the QRS complex, the anesthesiologist should be able to determine quickly the cause of these QRS complexes and, at the same time, look for a possible cause of ventricular dysrhythmia. Dysrhythmias tend to be accentuated by halothane. Most atrial dysrhythmias respond to cessation of operative manipulation, releasing the mouth gag, and deepening the anesthesia.

Oxygenation. Many patients have significant nasal airway obstruction because of large adenoids. If the mouth is closed while the patient is being mask-ventilated during induction, hypoxemia will result. With the same fingers the anesthesiologist uses to hold the mask under the lower lip, he or she also should pull gently in a caudal direction to keep the mouth open.

Compression or kinking of the endotracheal tube during surgery is another potential cause of hypoxemia. The insertion and removal of the mouth gag should be done carefully, with the attention and assistance of the anesthesiologist. Accidental extubation with the removal of the mouth gag may also occur.

Use of a pulse oximeter, generally accepted as routine today in the United States, provides a simple, quick, reliable, noninvasive, and objective indicator of O_2 saturation. In adults, desaturation will be noted after several minutes of hypoxia. Children are more labile, and hypoxia will result in almost immediate desaturation. End-tidal CO_2 monitors are being increasingly used in operating rooms. These may be even more sensitive indicators of changes in respiration during T&A (and other) surgery.

Postoperative problems of oxygenation will be discussed under the specific cause (e.g., edema, dislodged clot, and so forth).

Laryngospasm. To avoid coughing, straining, and increased bleeding in the patient during awake extubation, many anesthesiologists prefer deep extubation. This approach, however, carries the possibility of aspiration of blood and laryngospasm. The decision of whether to use deep extubation should be based upon the nature of the drugs used for anesthesia and the likelihood of the patient's regaining consciousness quickly after extubation. Patients given opiates, thiopental, or halothane may take a considerable time to wake up and hence are at high risk for developing laryngospasm; they should be extubated when awake. Measures to prevent laryngospasm include gentle suctioning during emergence, extubation with the patient's head turned to the side to prevent blood from reaching the larynx, and, as recommended by some anesthesiologists, injection of intravenous lidocaine before extubation. Lidocaine may inhibit the cough reflex, which is an important protective mechanism at this time of possible bleeding. Patients with underlying respiratory or cardiac disease should not be extubated while in deep anesthesia.

Patients after T&A are transferred to the recovery room and kept there in a "tonsil position." The child should lie on the side with the head down below the shoulder level. The hips are raised by a pillow and the neck is extended. In this position, secretions and blood will drain out through the mouth and nose.

Teeth. Children, especially those 4 to 7 years old, may have loose primary teeth. Loosening or accidental extraction of a primary tooth during intubation is not a terrible complication as long as it is noticed immediately and the tooth is removed safely. Prevention is important. It includes preoperative evaluation (by the anesthesiologist) of the patient's dentition and identification of loose teeth; repeated examination just before and immediately after intubation, after removal of the mouth gag, and after extubation. Loose teeth may be tied around the crown with 2-0 silk and the loose ends taped to the cheek. This prevents dislodgement in case the tooth is pulled out. Extremely loose teeth should be extracted, and the necessary permission for this should be obtained from the parents preoperatively. Further details relating to teeth will be discussed later in this chapter.

Anesthesia for the Bleeding T&A. Taking a patient back to the operating room because of bleeding after T&A presents an extremely difficult problem to the anesthesiologist. If the patient is hypovolemic, establishing intravenous access may be very difficult. That is why we recommend keeping the IV cannula in place at least until the patient is back on the floor and, in cases of tonsillectomy, until the patient takes liquids orally.

All efforts should be made to correct hypovolemia before taking the patient back to the operating room. Blood loss is usually underestimated because the child swallows the blood, and quantifying the stomach contents is very difficult, especially in a semiawake child. The decision of whether to reoperate is not up to the surgeon alone. It is also the anesthesiologist's responsibility to monitor the child's color, oxygen saturation, heart rate, and peripheral circulation and to make the appropriate recommendation. There is no place for waiting and hoping for the bleeding to stop in a child because examination of the oropharynx, bedside manipulations, and blood loss estimation are difficult in children. Our policy is: when in doubt, reoperate.

No matter how insignificant the bleeding seems to be, blood should be cross-matched for possible transfusion.

In the operating room, the next difficult step is induction. Ventilation with a face mask may cause regurgitation of stomach contents and aspiration, which leads to immediate hypoxia-related and delayed infection-related respiratory complications. Regurgitation of a blood clot may cause an immediate airway problem. The patient should stay in the lateral "tonsil position" with the head down. If the patient is hypovolemic, the use of pentothal may precipitate severe hypotension. Ketamine is preferable in this situation.[3, 30] In immediate postoperative bleeding, the previous anesthesia and sedation make the induction shorter. After adequate preoxygenation, the patient should be intubated using the rapid sequence technique. Visualization of the pharynx and larynx may be difficult, and blood clots should be removed before intubation. Edema makes intubation even more difficult; thus a smaller size tube may be required. With cricoid pressure, the endotracheal tube should be rapidly inserted by an experienced anesthesiologist. Once the tube is secured and the lungs are adequately ventilated, a suction catheter should be passed through the tube to remove blood from the lungs. The stomach should be suctioned and irrigated with saline. This procedure is repeated at the end of the operation, before the patient awakes. It is impossible to empty the stomach completely; therefore, vomiting and aspiration may occur during emergence. Awake extubation is recommended in these cases. If a posterior pack has been placed for nasopharyngeal bleeding, the anesthesiologist and surgeon should evaluate the airway carefully before extubation, because too big or too loose a pack may compromise the oropharyngeal airway. Sedation and analgesia are contraindicated in a patient with posterior nasal packing during the immediate postoperative period to prevent hypoventilation or apnea. The patient is kept in "tonsil position" while being transferred to the recovery room. Pulse oximetry is highly recommended. Patients with posterior packs should be placed in an ICU setting. Repeated blood counts are necessary, as the result of one count done immediately postoperatively may be misleading.

In the Recovery Room. Many of the postoperative complications to be discussed later in this chapter, such as bleeding and airway obstruction, may occur in the recovery room where the patient is still under the anesthesiologist's care. The patient should stay in the "tonsil position" as long as he or she is still sleepy. Vital signs are monitored every 15 minutes. The nurses should look for and immediately report any oral or nasal bleeding and bloody vomitus.

It is important, though very difficult, to differentiate crying (usually due to pain, fear, and discomfort) from restlessness. The latter may indicate bleeding or hypoxemia or both. Treating restlessness with strong analgesics, without excluding a serious cause, may mask the warning signs and delay proper treatment.

Pulmonary Edema. Although not related

to the anesthesia itself, this complication may develop intraoperatively or in the recovery room, and the anesthesiologist is required to assist with its recognition, diagnosis, and management.

The underlying mechanism that brings about pulmonary edema is not fully understood. It is believed that, in children with long-standing adenotonsillar hypertrophy, expiration against the obstructed upper airway creates significant positive intrathoracic pressures (as does the Valsalva maneuver), which reduces venous return and pulmonary blood volume. Because the complete relief of this pressure is not possible, it remains during inspiration and balances the negative intrathoracic pressure generated by inspiration against the obstructed upper airway. The sudden surgical relief of the obstruction generates a sudden drop in intrathoracic pressure, which causes an increase in venous return, an increase in pulmonary blood volume, and increased hydrostatic pressure. The capillary hydrostatic pressure may rise beyond the threshold of transudation, and water from the intravascular space will shift to the interstitial and alveolar spaces.[20, 25]

Pulmonary edema may happen immediately after intubation or even several hours later. It should be recognized by the sudden oxygen desaturation, cyanosis, and increase in the amount of fluid suctioned from the endotracheal tube. Auscultation of the lungs, arterial blood-gas analysis, and the findings of a chest film will confirm the diagnosis.

Children with preoperative signs of right heart failure and pulmonary hypertension (cor pulmonale) should be monitored closely because acute heart failure may complicate their perioperative course. Since cor pulmonale can become more severe and pulmonary hypertension may reach a stage of irreversibility, this is one of the only situations in which delaying or canceling the surgery because of cardiopulmonary status is not advisable. In rare cases of cor pulmonale, emergency T&A may be necessary.

Treatment of postobstructive pulmonary edema depends upon severity. Intravenous diuretics may be enough for mild cases, though intensive care management with me-chanical ventilation is often required for severe heart failure.

Malignant Hyperthermia. This rare, but potentially fatal, complication has been reported to occur with T&A.[78, 79] Prevention depends on good history-taking and the detection of patients at risk. Continuous intraoperative core temperature monitoring will help in early diagnosis. The protocol for management, which includes immediate control of bleeding and termination of the surgical procedure, as well as nonspecific (immediate cessation of anesthetics; administration of oxygen; cooling) and specific (dantrolene) measures, should be known to all operating room personnel.

Bleeding

Bleeding from T&A is probably the most common serious complication of this type of surgery. The inherent nature of this surgery, in which adenoid tissue is "scraped" with a curette, or the tonsil removed by sharp dissection, and the complex vascular anatomy of the tonsils and adenoids make bleeding, to a degree, a recognized component of the surgery. Bleeding can range in severity from several drops of blood, necessitating only close observation, to life-threatening bleeding, which may even require carotid ligation for control. It can occur as a complication intraoperatively or can be seen at any time from the immediate recovery phase to several weeks postoperatively.

The rate for bleeding post-T&A (both immediate and delayed) is approximately 0.5 per cent to 1 per cent,[12] with a slightly higher incidence in the winter,[9] in adults (older than 20 years), and in girls aged 10 to 19 years.[9] Ranges vary from 0.1 per cent[2] to 8.1 per cent,[46] but the higher number may include cases that did not require operative intervention.[8] Incidences of bleeding resulting in mortality are approximately 0.002 per cent.[67] Fatal hemorrhages invariably occur within 24 hours of surgery.[9]

Anatomy. The rich vascular supply to the tonsils and adenoids undoubtedly contributes to the risk for T&A bleeding. The tonsillar area has a rich collateral system, including branches from both the internal (via the ophthalmic, middle meningeal, and infraorbital arteries) and external (branches of facial, lingual, ascending pharyngeal, and internal maxillary arteries) carotid systems, as well as collateral supply via the contralateral facial and lingual arteries. The adenoid area also has a very rich blood supply, with bilateral contributions from both internal and external carotid systems. The venous system is also rich, and includes channels to the pharyngeal venous plexus and tonsillar veins draining to the lingual vein.[62]

Intraoperative Bleeding. Excessive intraoperative bleeding must be recognized, assessed, and treated promptly. Blood suctioned during surgery should be collected and the volume quantified. Estimates should include and account for any irrigation used, in addition to an estimate for blood lost in sponges. The surgeon should always be aware of (1) the preoperative hemoglobin and hematocrit, (2) what degree of blood loss is dangerous, and (3) when consideration should be given to a transfusion. A useful formula for determining blood loss involves calculation of total blood volume based on weight: 80 to 85 ml/kg in infants; 70 to 75 ml/kg in children, and 60 to 65 ml/kg in adults. By these calculations, infants should be given a transfusion when 10 per cent of their total blood volume is lost. Children should get blood with a loss of 10 to 15 per cent of total blood volume (with consideration to the preoperative values and overall condition of the patient) and adults with a loss of 20 per cent or more. Carithers and colleagues reported the average blood loss in 2944 pediatric patients to be 49 ml (adenoidectomy = 2.6 per cent of total blood volume), 68 ml (tonsillectomy = 2.2 per cent), and 70 ml (T&A = 3.6 per cent).[8]

Control of Excessive Intraoperative Bleeding. Excessive bleeding during adenoidectomy is usually due to retained adenoid tissue. Digital palpation and visual examination of the nasopharynx usually will help localize the retained tissue, which then can be removed by punch forceps or curette. If all the adenoid tissue has been removed and bleed-

ing persists, it may be due to tears in the posterior pharyngeal wall musculature. This bleeding often can be controlled with prolonged pressure from a tonsil or dental roll or a nasopharyngeal pack. A good approach to T&A is to perform the adenoidectomy at the onset of the procedure, inspect and pack the nasopharynx, then perform the tonsillectomy. Assuming normal patient coagulation parameters, this approach usually will allow adequate time for pressure hemostasis in the nasopharynx. The pack is then removed from the nasopharynx and the head raised and flexed slightly to check for any further bleeding. Other methods of controlling excessive intraoperative adenoidectomy bleeding include (1) the use of pressure with sponges soaked in topical agents such as Neo-Synephrine or epinephrine; (2) other hemostatic agents such as Avitene, thrombin, Surgicel, or Gelfoam; (3) the suction cautery, if a specific bleeding point is evident; and (4) sutures of plain or chromic catgut (tapered needle) placed horizontally across the nasopharyngeal musculature.

Rarely, all measures fail to reduce or stop the bleeding. In these instances, a posterior nasopharyngeal pack must be placed, using dental or tonsil rolls or a Foley catheter. The pack is placed under tension, taking care to avoid alar or nasal septal necrosis. The patient may then be transferred to an ICU or monitored bed and placed on oxygen by mask. The posterior pack may be removed in 24 to 48 hours. Adults tend to tolerate this under local anesthesia, but general anesthesia in the operating room is often necessary for children.

Excessive intraoperative tonsillectomy bleeding may be controlled in a variety of ways. Initially, pressure with tonsil sponges, with or without hemostatic agents (adrenaline, Neo-Synephrine, bismuth, tannic acid, Avitene, thrombin, Surgicel, Gelfoam) should be attempted. Should this fail, the suction cautery is usually successful in controlling bleeding. Figure-of-eight sutures with plain or chromic catgut on a tapered needle often help control bleeding at the superior or inferior poles of the tonsil. Some have advocated clamping tissue at the superior pole of the tonsil and using catgut ties (slip knots) to help control bleeding. Rarely does excessive intraoperative tonsil bleeding result in a need for ligation of the external carotid or its branches. This is seen more often in delayed tonsil bleeding and will be discussed later. Some surgeons use the technique of suturing the anterior and posterior pillars at the inferior or superior pole (depending on the bleeding site) as a method for hemostasis. Others will suture at least the inferior pole routinely in every case.

Postoperative Bleeding. Postoperative T&A bleeding can be further subdivided into primary (early) hemorrhage and secondary (late) bleeding. Primary hemorrhage is that which occurs within the first 24 hours after operation, whereas secondary hemorrhage usually occurs within the first 7 to 10 days postoperatively. A smaller subset of patients with secondary hemorrhage bleed more than 10 days after surgery, possibly as a result of the slough of the eschar from the cautery used during surgery. There are indications[33] that immediate hemorrhage is on the decline, whereas the incidence of delayed hemorrhage remains stable. This is most likely due to surgeons' increased attention to hemostasis while the patient is still in the operating room, and possibly to an increase in the use of cautery for both the tonsillectomy and hemostasis.[33] Primary and secondary bleeding can range in severity from minor bleeding, which requires no more than evaluation by the surgeon and which can be observed even at home, to moderate or even severe bleeding, which requires hospital admission and intervention, possibly even in the operating room under anesthesia. Occasional blood-tinged sputum is quite common after T&A and may persist for up to several days after the procedure. If the surgeon is confident on examination that there is no active bleeding, and if the patient's vital signs are stable, the patient may be observed with periodic office visits, with instructions to return should further bleeding ensue.

Dark-colored blood, either in the sputum, from the nose, or vomited, usually represents old blood that was swallowed or clotted during or after the procedure. This condition also can be managed by observation.

Handler and associates note that persistent ear or lateral pharyngeal pain may herald a bleeding episode.[33] They recommend such patients returning to the office for a complete evaluation.

When a patient reports bleeding bright red blood, an attempt should be made to quantify the amount of blood loss. Estimations such as "a cupful" may give an indication of the volume lost. It must be emphasized, however, that children tend to swallow the blood, and there is a dangerous possibility that the parents and surgeon may underestimate the amount of blood lost. Further evaluation includes careful and frequent monitoring of vital signs. With increasing blood loss, the pulse rate may increase, and as the loss becomes more severe, the patient may become hypotensive. If blood loss is estimated to be significant, a large-bore intravenous line should be started and fluid replacement with crystalloid (lactated Ringer solution or normal saline 0.9 per cent) begun. All patients should be typed and cross-matched, and if more than 10 per cent (children) or 20 per cent (adults) of blood volume is lost, the patient should receive a transfusion with packed red blood cells or whole blood. The patient should be admitted to the hospital for careful observation, including a complete physical examination, with special attention to the head and neck.

If active bleeding is noted, any of the aforementioned methods may be used to attempt to stop the bleeding. In a cooperative patient, much may be accomplished in the treatment room. Pressure with use of topical hemostatic agents, chemical or electric cautery, or suctioning of a clot may stop the bleeding. Care must be taken to ensure that the patient's airway is secure at all times, and standby equipment, including an intubation set and tracheotomy tray, should be readily available.

When local methods fail, or if the patient is agitated or uncooperative, it is safer to attempt to stop the bleeding under controlled conditions, under anesthesia, in the operating room. Induction of anesthesia and reintubation of children with T&A bleeding is an extremely difficult and challenging procedure and is discussed at length in the section on anesthesia complications.

With the patient intubated, a careful examination is made to locate the site of bleeding. Adenoid bleeding is usually amenable to prolonged pressure. Any of the methods described earlier can be used to attempt to stop tonsillar fossa bleeding (e.g., pressure, cautery, suture ligation). If bleeding persists in spite of all attempts, consideration must be given to ligation of the external carotid artery or its branches or both. If time and circumstances permit, angiography may be helpful in localizing collateral flow and identifying which specific vessels should be tied off.[75]

External carotid ligation is performed through a standard lateral neck incision, reflecting the sternomastoid muscle to encounter the carotid sheath. The sheath is entered, and the carotid bifurcation identified. Care should be taken to identify and preserve cranial nerve XII, which crosses near the bifurcation. The external carotid is identified by locating at least two (even three) branches. The external carotid is then ligated with heavy silk sutures. Branches are ligated as needed.

Ogusthorpe and associates have reported a 1 per cent incidence of internal carotid artery tortuosity.[61] This anomaly places the vessel at risk during T&A surgery. They recommend careful palpation of the tonsillar fossa prior to tonsillectomy. If bleeding due to an anomalous internal carotid does occur, they recommend transoral vessel repair. If this approach fails, the artery may have to be ligated. The complications of internal carotid ligation are well known.

Physical and radiologic examination of the lungs should be done in all patients with excessive bleeding to determine whether aspiration has occurred. Sequelae of aspiration should be treated aggressively with pulmonary care, respiratory support, and antibiotics.

Prevention. The first and best treatment of T&A bleeding should be prevention. Meticulous hemostasis should be the goal in every procedure. No operation should be done during a period of acute inflammation, as vessels tend to be dilated during inflammation, and this dilation increases the risk of postoperative hemorrhage. Patients with previous episodes of peritonsillar abscess are also at increased risk for postoperative bleeding, because of tissue fibrosis (which makes surgical dissection difficult), as well as chronically dilated vasculature. Meticulously careful dissection should be done in these cases. The issue of whether to perform an "abscess tonsillectomy" has been discussed elsewhere in the literature.

Preoperative Screening. How much preoperative screening is too much (or too little)? Certainly this question is on the mind of every surgeon contemplating an operative procedure in which bleeding is a known risk. Insurance carriers and governmental agencies demand that surgeons take all measures necessary to reduce the risk of intra- and postoperative complications, though in the same breath they demand that costs be cut and the number of tests ordered be kept to a minimum. The first preoperative screen should be the history. It is inexpensive and noninvasive; moreover, assuming patient/parent reliability, it is highly accurate in detecting preoperative abnormalities. All pre-T&A parents/patients should be questioned about their complete medical history, including cardiovascular, metabolic, and other diseases. Careful questioning about bleeding tendencies is imperative. Any history of excessive or frequent bleeding, from any body orifice, in either the patient or the immediate family, should be a stimulus to the surgeon to initiate a complete hematologic work-up. Questions about the patient's medication history also must be carefully pursued. The patient should be asked specifically about salicylate products, since many patients do not regard aspirin and other anti-inflammatory drugs as "medicine." These and other preparations that increase bleeding (e.g., Coumadin) should be discontinued no later than 3 days prior to surgery, and sooner if possible. Adult patients should be instructed to stop all smoking and alcohol consumption 1 week prior to the operation date. All such medications (including cigarettes and alcohol) should not be used for at least 2 to 3 weeks after the surgery as well.

Any history of patient or family coagulopathy, such as sickle disease/trait, hemophilia, or anemia of unknown origin, should prompt a complete hematologic evaluation prior to the scheduled operations.

Laboratory Work-up. Routine preoperative screening includes the complete blood count (CBC) with platelet level and urinalysis. Other available tests include the prothrombin time (PT), which measures the extrinsic pathway of coagulation; the partial thromboplastin time (PTT), which measures the intrinsic clotting pathway; the bleeding and clotting times; and the clot retraction and thrombin times.[34] Sickle hemoglobin screens and specific factor assays are also available when indicated for evaluation. Tami and colleagues found no association of bleeding based on platelet counts in their series of 775 patients.[81] Of these patients, 763 also had preoperative PT and PTT screening, and 10 per cent of this group had abnormal results (though minimally so), all with a negative bleeding history. However, 24 per cent of those who bled after T&A did have abnormal clotting studies. Thomas and Arbon recommend that the PTT be part of the routine preoperative screening for tonsillectomy, despite no prolonged PTTs in 206 patients (23 of whom bled postoperatively).[84] Two studies have indicated that the PT and PTT do not add to the preoperative work-up in surgical patients;[24, 43] nonetheless, because of the special nature of T&A surgery related to bleeding, it may be prudent to include both the PT and PTT in the preoperative screen. In the event that T&A surgery is to be undertaken in a patient with a known clotting disorder, all necessary preparations should be taken prior to operation, including availability of platelets, whole blood, plasma, and cryoprecipitate. A colleague from the hematology service should follow the patient's course in hospital pre- and postoperatively.

General Versus Local Anesthesia. In past years many adult tonsillectomies were performed under local anesthesia. Currently, most otolaryngologists elect to use general anesthesia. Some of the halogenated gas anesthetics are known to correlate with an increased risk of bleeding. The question then arises of whether to inject local anesthetics (containing a dilute epinephine solution) even when using general anesthesia. Many anesthesiologists worry that the combination used in close proximity to significant vasculature may precipitate cardiac arrhythmias; consequently, they are reluctant to allow the surgeon to do so. Children may be able to withstand higher epinephrine doses than adults.[44] Broadman and associates evaluated the effects of peritonsillar infiltration with local epinephrine-containing anesthetic and epinephrine-containing saline and demonstrated significantly reduced intraoperative bleeding in both groups, most likely resulting from the vasoconstrictive effect of the epinephrine.[5] Volume injection with "plane dissection" and compression of vessels by volume may have played a role as well, given that plain saline infiltrated into the peritonsillar area also resulted in a decrease in intraoperative tonsillar bleeding.[5]

Light. It is imperative that adequate lighting be available for tonsillar and adenoid surgery. Overhead lights may cast shadows in the oral cavity (especially in small children) and a headlight worn by the surgeon, preferably with coaxial capability, is the light of choice. Adequate retraction is also imperative to allow the surgeon to visualize the upper and lower tonsillar poles, the depth of the tonsillar fossa, and the nasopharynx.

Dissection. Adenoidectomy is usually accomplished by curettage or by use of an adenotome. Because the adenoids are behind and superior to the soft palate, meticulous dissection under direct vision is difficult. The key to prevention of bleeding is to ensure that the instruments used are sharp and to try to remove the adenoids with as few passes as possible. This reduces the chances of bleeding from tears of the pharyngeal musculature. It must also be emphasized that complete removal of all adenoid tissue is imperative, as retained adenoid fragments are the most common cause of adenoid bleeding.

In tonsillectomy, one of the key maneuvers in reducing bleeding is to dissect very close to the tonsillar capsule, in the plane between the capsule and the pharyngeal musculature.

This approach reduces bleeding from torn muscles and makes it easier to identify vessels passing into the tonsil and to cauterize them. Older instruments, such as the Sluder tonsillotome and guillotine, do not allow for careful dissection and hence may increase the chance of bleeding. Current dissection techniques using a Hurd dissector, Fisher knife, or Metzenbaum scissors allow for more precision. Hemostasis then can be achieved by any one or more of the methods outlined earlier. The two most common methods used are the suction cautery and sutures. Many surgeons routinely suture either one or both of the upper and lower poles, and some also place a suture through the midportion of the tonsillar fossa. Plain 0 or 2-0 catgut on a taper needle is the usual suture of choice. Gardner warns that even this technique can be fraught with problems.[27] He has detailed five tonsillectomy "disasters" that occurred in spite of apparently careful suturing. This complication may derive, he thinks, from suture injury to the facial (external maxillary) artery. Based on his experience, Gardner advocates the prompt removal of any suture that appears to cause an increase in bleeding after it has been placed.

Suction (or nonsuction) electrocautery also can be used for hemostasis. The cautery can be used in a "spot" method or can be used to cauterize upper and lower poles and mid-fossa (corresponding to the suture areas noted above). Williams and Pope compared "spot" cautery and "site" cautery in two groups of patients.[93] The "spot" cautery group had a 2.8 per cent incidence of primary bleeding and a 3.6 per cent incidence of secondary bleeding. The site cautery figures were 0.2 per cent and 3.2 per cent, respectively. Papangelou also recommends the use of cautery for hemostasis, noting that it is faster and more efficient than ligation, cutting down on the operative time.[63] He has reported bleeding rates of 2.31 per cent for cautery and 1.44 per cent for ligation, which he considers a nonsignificant difference. One should note that pain may be increased when cautery is used extensively in the tonsil fossa.

The cautery (spatula or needle tip) also can be used to perform the entire tonsillectomy, as was advocated by Mann and colleagues, who demonstrated a significantly reduced blood loss, reduced operating time, and no increase in postoperative bleeding when the cautery was used.[55] However, they did find that cauterized tonsils were more painful, for a longer time.

Suturing the tonsillar fossa shut, or suturing a dental roll into the tonsillar fossa to achieve hemostasis also has been advocated in the past. It seems, however, that these methods might be prone to failure because motion of the pharyngeal musculature (due to swallowing, talking, coughing) would loosen the sutures. Any pack sutured in this manner then would be in danger of being aspirated or of obstructing the airway. These methods are not commonly in use today.

Laser. All types of laser are becoming increasingly common in otolaryngologic surgical usage and will likely be even more so in the future. CO_2 and KTP lasers have been advocated for use in tonsillectomy. The CO_2 laser is an excellent precision cutting tool and probably would result in decreased postoperative pain, but it is not a good instrument for hemostasis, especially in the tonsil area. The KTP is also a good cutting tool (less precise than the CO_2), as well as a hemostatic machine, and can be used in tonsillectomy. However, the time and effort needed to set up the laser properly, as well as the extensive safety precautions needed, probably make it less cost effective than any of the currently available methods, while it adds very little to the procedure. The CO_2 laser likely would be better for use in the excision of small tonsillar area tumors than in tonsillectomy. The KTP may be useful in tonsillectomy for those patients at risk for bleeding problems. Specific laser complications are discussed later in the chapter.

Postoperative Care. Postoperative care is also important in helping reduce the risk of post-T&A bleeding. Patients must be maintained in an adequate state of hydration, since excessive dryness of the healing fossa may contribute to bleeding. It is preferable that the patient drink by mouth, but this may not be possible due to pain or nausea. In these cases, appropriate analgesia and antiemetic preparations should be administered. If these methods fail, intravenous hydration should be administered for as long as needed. Severely dehydrated patients may even exhibit fever; these patients should be maintained on intravenous fluids overnight if necessary. The patient's state postoperatively should be checked by the surgeon, and documented in writing, especially if the patient is being discharged on an ambulatory basis. This practice will help avoid potential legal questions should a bleed occur later on.

Ambulatory T&A. Insurance carriers and governmental agencies are putting increasing pressure on surgeons to perform a greater number of procedures on an ambulatory basis, among which is T&A. Many surgeons tend to resist, however, citing the risk of postoperative bleeding as a reason for keeping patients in the hospital overnight. Needless to say, T&A must be performed on an inpatient basis in any person with a complex medical history, such as cardiovascular, pulmonary, or metabolic diseases; and, of course, in any person at risk for increased bleeding postoperatively. But what of otherwise "healthy" patients? A study by Carithers and colleagues on 2944 pediatric T&A patients attempted to determine how soon these patients could be released from the hospital postoperatively, while keeping the complication risk at or below 10 per cent.[8] (This assumes that a 10 per cent risk of further complication is acceptable.) Their results showed that 19 per cent of the patients could be released after 4 hours. Of those remaining, 85.9 per cent could be released at 8 hours, and 98.2 per cent at 10 hours. Assuming that a surgeon waits 10 hours to ensure that 98 per cent of the patients have a less than 10 per cent risk for further complications, patients would be sent home after 8 or 9 p.m.; any procedure that finished in the afternoon would have the patient discharged close to midnight. The cost of keeping patients 10 hours may not be significantly less than that of keeping them overnight until 7 or 8 A.M., especially if special post-T&A units are used.

The operating surgeon should base the decision on when to release patients on multiple factors, such as those used in the study just mentioned.[8] These include age, amount of blood loss, difficulty of operation, postoperative vomiting, and need to force fluids. Additionally, the surgeon should weigh social factors and general conditions in the decision. Reliable patients and parents, who live in proximity to a hospital, may be considered for ambulatory discharge; those less reliable or at great distance from the hospital are probably better being kept in. In severely inclement weather, no one should be sent home on the same day.[8] The decision concerning when to discharge T&A patients should be made carefully by the surgeon, considering all factors, on a case-by-case basis (rather than being arbitrarily mandated by insurance and bureaucratic agencies).

T&A in Infants. The indications for performing T&A are a discussion beyond the scope of this chapter. However, surgeons are often asked to perform either or both procedures on infants less than 2 or 3 years old. Because of the increased chance for complication in infants (higher proportion of blood volume to weight), when possible all medical measures available should be exhausted prior to scheduling operation. Nevertheless, there should be no problem with a trained, experienced surgeon performing T&A in infants, provided the proper indications exist and all measures are taken to reduce the risk of complications. The risks and benefits of the procedure(s) must be carefully explained to the parents, and if they understand and agree, the operation may be performed. Consideration should be given to observing infants overnight after T&A, in view of the increased chance for complications.

Airway Obstruction

Airway problems may arise before operation, during induction, during emergence, and after operation. There have been reports of patients requiring emergency tracheotomy because of extremely difficult intubation and worsening obstruction due to repeated attempts to intubate (e.g., during "hot" tonsillectomy in patients with infectious mononucleosis).[11, 76] As mentioned earlier, the status of the upper airway should be evaluated preoperatively by both the surgeon and the anesthesiologist. In difficult cases presenting a possible intubation problem and especially in cases of quinsy tonsillectomy or tonsillectomy for airway distress, the surgical team and operating room personnel should be prepared for all possible events. Smaller-size orotracheal tubes, as well as nasotracheal tubes, fiberoptic scopes, and, in extremely difficult cases, gowned and gloved surgeons with an open instrument tray are all highly recommended safety measures. Other anesthesia-related airway problems, especially laryngospasm, were discussed in the previous section.

Dislodged blood clots are a known cause of upper airway obstruction. This complication may happen early during emergence or right after extubation, or they can present as a delayed complication. The most important preventive measures during operation are complete hemostasis and the suctioning of the oro- and hypopharynx. When the procedure is completed, the surgeon should inspect the operative field for clots, release the mouth gag, raise the patient's head and watch for blood or blood clots coming down the posterior pharyngeal wall, and, as recommended by many surgeons, irrigate the nasopharynx via the nostrils. Before the mouth gag is finally removed, the hypopharynx is examined. During emergence, the oropharynx is suctioned, and, as recommended by many anesthesiologists, the hypopharynx and larynx are examined once more just before extubation.

Dislodged adenoid or tonsil tissue also may cause airway obstruction. Awareness, close observation, and maintaining the patient in the "tonsil position" are important to prevent airway obstruction caused by delayed dislodgement of nasopharyngeal or tonsillar clot/lymphoid tissue.

In the recovery room, before the supine patient is fully awake, the tongue may fall back and obstruct the airway. Proper positioning and use of oral or nasopharyngeal airways will help prevent this complication.

Postoperative edema can occur at different anatomic levels. Oropharyngeal edema is common but rarely is a cause of significant airway problem. The uvula may reach an unusually large size but rarely is the cause of airway obstruction. Tongue swelling is common and occasionally may require a nasopharyngeal airway tube. Donaldson and Stool describe a case of massive tongue swelling that required a tracheotomy.[22] Hypopharyngeal and, most important, glottic and subglottic edema are known complications of T&A.

Prevention of postoperative edema is based mainly on the avoidance of too much manipulation and trauma to the oropharyngeal tissues. For example, proper and careful handling and positioning of the suction tip reduce the chance of the uvula being caught in it. Meticulous surgical technique and careful dissection prevent trauma to the tonsillar pillars and the palate. Strenuous retraction of the palate also should be avoided. Prevention of glottic and subglottic edema requires the proper selection of endotracheal tube size, atraumatic intubation, and avoidance of excessive manipulations of the tube during operation.

Delayed airway obstruction is rare. The senior author (GHE) had the unfortunate experience of treating a child who developed a retropharyngeal cellulitis/abscess after an adenoidectomy (Fig. 15–1). Although dysphagia and pain were present throughout the postoperative period, mild respiratory distress appeared only on the fourth postoperative day. Retropharyngeal hematoma may present earlier in the postoperative course.

Prevention of delayed airway obstruction requires awareness and close observation, especially during the first 24 hours. Due to pain and discomfort, a muffled voice is very common and therefore is not a reliable early sign of airway compromise. It is the stridor or the increased inspiratory effort that should alert the surgical and nursing staff to a problem. Humidification, nebulized drug therapy, insertion of a soft nasopharyngeal tube, and systemic steroids are the most common and most effective treatment modalities currently used. Reintubation or tracheotomy are

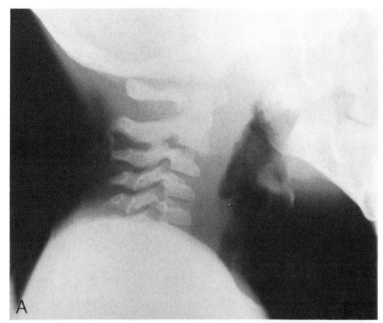

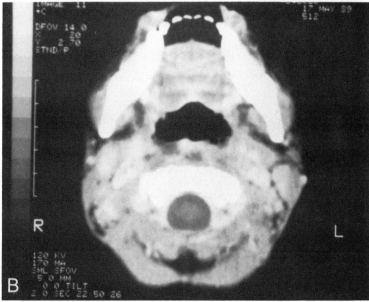

FIGURE 15–1. Retropharyngeal cellulitis/abscess after adenoidectomy in a 2.5-year-old boy (postoperative day 5.) A, Lateral neck radiograph B, Axial CT scan.

reserved for the severe cases. Retropharyngeal hematoma is treated conservatively unless it is progressive or causing respiratory distress. Retropharyngeal abscess requires operative drainage.

The list of foreign bodies that can cause airway obstruction during or after T&A is almost endless. Sponges, teeth, broken instruments, and needles are the most common ones. Needless to say, a careful count of sponges and instruments at the end of the operation is the most important preventive measure.

Cranial nerve injury complicating T&A is a very rare cause of airway obstruction. Anecdotal case reports will be mentioned later. Mediastinal emphysema and pneumothorax are other rare complications of T&A that cause airway (tracheal) obstruction.[65, 69]

Late nasopharyngeal airway obstruction is a rare, slowly progressive, yet not life-threatening complication of adenoidectomy. It may cause difficulties with nasal breathing and hyponasal speech. The cause is scarring, stenosis, and even complete obliteration of the nasopharynx.[13, 31, 57] Scarring and cicatrix formation are also possible at the oro- and hypopharygeal levels following tonsillectomy. Prevention is basically the avoidance of unnecessary trauma to the surrounding tissues during surgery. This is especially important in the nasopharynx, choanae, posterior pharyngeal wall, tonsillar pillars, soft palate, and base of the tongue. If airway obstruction or hyponasality is severe, treatment is indicated. This requires widening the naso-, oro-, or hypopharyngeal spaces by resecting scar tissue or using local flaps and Z-plasty with or without stenting.

COMMON COMPLICATIONS

Sore Throat

Sore throat is very common after T&A. In most cases, it is a self-limited problem, and most patients, especially children, respond well to acetaminophen. Aspirin and nonsteroidal anti-inflammatory medicines should *not* be used.

Many workers believe that the use of electrocautery for hemostasis increases the severity of postoperative pain.[52, 55] The use of electrocautery for the entire procedure, dissection, and hemostasis may cause significant postoperative pain. We have tried intraoperative injection of bupivacaine into the tonsillar bed after electrodissection tonsillectomy, but we have not seen a significant reduction in pain. Topical anesthetics should not be used as they increase the risk of aspiration. It has been stated, but not proved, that laser tonsillectomy causes less pain than conventional or electrodissection tonsillectomy.[56]

Significant pain beyond the first 24 to 48 hours should alert the physician to the possibility of other complications such as infection.

Sore throat should not be considered a minor problem because it is a major one to

the patient and the parents. Certain postoperative complications may be secondary to the pain. Among them are dysphagia, dehydration, psychologic sequelae, and worried, dissatisfied parents.

Otalgia

Otalgia is a common complaint and is usually due to referred pain from the tonsillar fossae. If persistent, it should alert the physician to the possibility of purulent otitis media.

Fever

Fever is common during the first 18 postoperative hours.[94] In a study of 9409 T&As, 245 patients (2.6 per cent) had temperatures higher than 38.5°C.[16] Only 17 patients (0.18 per cent) had their scheduled discharge delayed because of fever. Fever is most probably caused by the combination of the effects of anesthetics, stress, and transient bacteremia. Temperatures above 38.0°C that persist beyond 24 hours should alert the physician to the possibility of infection. Infection may be relatively simple to diagnose and treat, such as local pharyngitis (persistent fever with *increasing* pain) or acute otitis media, but the rare possibility of other infections, which are more difficult to diagnose, should be kept in mind. These will be discussed later and include pneumonia, meningitis, and lymphadenitis, among others.

Fever leads to increased loss of body water. This water loss should be accounted for when calculating the fluid maintenance. The combination of fever and dysphagia may lead to dehydration.

Some surgeons believe that the routine use of postoperative antibiotics reduces the incidence of pain and fever.[83]

Dysphagia

Dysphagia and odynophagia are expected sequelae of T&A. The tonsil-adenoid areas are richly supplied by the pharyngeal plexus nerves (branches of nerves IX and X). The very nature of the surgery disturbs the underlying muscle fibers, irritating the nerve plexus and causing pain and dysphagia. Spasm of the pharyngeal constrictors from the surgical procedure also contributes to postoperative dysphagia.[73]

Most cases of dysphagia after T&A are short-term and resolve within 7 to 10 days following the procedure. By the second or third postoperative day, patients are usually able to consume fluids and soft food by mouth. By the tenth postoperative day most patients are eating a normal diet.

Rarely, dysphagia may be a prolonged problem. This complication may occur when the operation excessively traumatizes the pharyngeal musculature. Scarring can potentially result and thus lead to long-term swallowing difficulties. Psychologic factors also may contribute to long-term dysphagia in certain patients.

Dehydration

Patients who experience pain after T&A may refuse to drink and take adequate hydration postoperatively. If this progresses for several days, the patient may become dehydrated. In children, fever caused by dehydration may ensue. Vomiting, possibly resulting from the emetic effect of blood swallowed during operation or from a reaction to the anesthesia, may compound the problem. Adequate hydration, either orally or intravenously or both will usually reverse this process. Acetaminophen (*not* aspirin or related nonsteroidal anti-inflammatory medicines) given around the clock (not just as needed) may help reduce the pain so that adequate oral fluid intake may be established. Codeine preparations are reserved for as needed use in cases of severe pain. Fluids taken should be lukewarm to cool but not hot. Citrus products will increase the pain and should be avoided. In severe cases of dysphagia and dehydration, the patient may need hospital admission for intravenous hydration until adequate oral intake resumes.

Salassa and colleagues have reported that oral sodium dantrolene (normally used for prophylaxis against malignant hyperthermia) is potentially useful in reducing postoperative pain.[73] However, Wackym and Abdul-Rasool note that dantrolene may have significant side effects.[90]

Infection

Bacteremia. T&A leads to a transient bacteremia that is usually of no clinical consequence. Special attention should be given to patients with congenital or acquired heart disease. Prophylactic treatment against bacterial endocarditis is recommended. The reader is referred to the recommendations made by the American Heart Association.

Local. T&A may cause a localized infection in the pharynx or in the tonsillar bed. The patient will complain of excessive pain, and bleeding may be noted. The patient may also exhibit systemic signs of toxicity, including lethargy, generalized myalgia, and high fever. Appropriate throat and blood cultures[38, 87] should be obtained, and broad-spectrum antibiotic therapy should be initiated and adjusted based on culture results.

Neck. Local infection may also result in lymphadenitis. This can occur in cervical lymph nodes or less frequently in the retropharyngeal lymph nodes. Adenoidectomy itself also has been shown to cause retropharyngeal adenitis. In either of these cases the infection can progress to form an abscess (deep neck or retropharyngeal),[66, 85] and the patient will usually exhibit signs of systemic toxicity. External neck swelling will be present. Edema and swelling within the airway may result in airway compromise, necessitating urgent intubation or tracheotomy. CT scan is usually diagnostic in cases of an abscess. Appropriate antibiotic therapy should be instituted before and after surgical intervention and continued until the resolution of the abscess.

Peritonsillar. Peritonsillar abscesses (quinsy) also have been reported after tonsillectomy.[70] These may be caused by retained tonsil remnants. Treatment includes antibiotics, incision and drainage, and later excision of tonsil remnants.

Ear. Otitis media (both suppurative and serous) also can occur after T&A. However, otalgia as a symptom is not absolutely diagnostic for otitis, since pain post-T&A may be referred from the tonsil fossa. Otitis may occur if swelling and edema obstruct the eustachian tube opening[22] or if reflux of microorganisms occurs up the now open eustachian tube. (The bulk of the adenoid tissue may "protect" an overly patulous eustachian tube.[22]) Holt and colleagues theorized that surgery disturbs peritubal lymphatic drainage, causing stasis and engorgement.[37] This, together with muscle incoordination, may lead to abnormal middle ear function, evidenced by abnormal tympanograms and acoustic reflexes.

The Uvula

Swelling of the uvula is very common. It contributes significantly to the dysphagia and "hot potato" voice that are common during the first 12 to 18 postoperative hours. Rarely does it become a problem that needs to be addressed specifically. Pratt recommends making an incision through the dorsal surface of the uvula to allow the escape of fluid and relieve the edema.[66] We had the experience of a patient who required a partial uvulectomy for an extremely long uvula that became very swollen, in order to make extubation possible. Three attempts to extubate the patient, before the uvulectomy, failed. However, this is an extreme case, if the swollen uvula interferes with extubation, a soft rubber nasopharyngeal airway usually will suffice.

Prevention requires the avoidance of trauma to the uvula during surgery. Trauma may be due to sharp instruments and also to the suction tip. It is important not to excise the anterior and posterior pillars too close to the uvula. Doing so will reduce the venous return from the uvula and lead to edema.

When using the tonsil snare, unplanned uvulectomy is a possible complication.[66] This usually results only in a cosmetic, not a functional, problem.

Hypernasality

Velopharyngeal insufficiency (VPI; rhinolalia aperta; hypernasality) occurs when the velopharyngeal inlet is incompetent. This may be caused by congenital lesions (clefts), to muscular dysfunction (palate and pharyngeal muscles), or to surgical trauma (T&A). Sudden "opening" of the nasopharynx and lateral ports by the removal of enlarged tonsils and adenoids, even in the absence of excessive surgical trauma, may result in hypernasality. The palate and uvula do not abut the posterior pharyngeal wall (ridge of Passavant), and air escapes from the nose, resulting in hypernasal speech and possibly in the regurgitation of food and fluid. The incidence of VPI following T&A is estimated to be between 1 in 1500 to 1 in 10,000 operations.[95] In a study of 137 patients, it was reported that 30 per cent had preoperative factors, such as submucous cleft; history of nasal regurgitation; family history of VPI, cleft, or hypernasality, that increased the risk for postoperative VPI. Of these 137 patients, 13 per cent improved with no treatment, 37 per cent improved with only speech therapy, whereas 50 per cent required surgical correction.[95]

Croft and coworkers studied 120 patients with post-T&A hypernasality.[14] A total of 74 per cent had normal or minimally hypernasal speech preoperatively, which worsened postoperatively. The remaining 26 per cent were hypernasal preoperatively and remained so after surgery. Causes included occult or evident submucous cleft in 46 per cent, "short palate" (also possibly representing occult submucous cleft) in 30 per cent, neurologic disorders in 14 per cent, functional problems in 7 per cent, and surgical trauma in 3 per cent.

Careful preoperative history (to elicit the aforementioned potential risk factors) and physical examination (inspection and palpation of the oral cavity and palate) are good preoperative screening methods. Multiview videofluoroscopy[14] or fiberoptic endoscopy to evaluate the velopharyngeal inlet should be added to the workup in patients in whom palatal pathology is suspected. In those patients at risk for VPI, lateral adenoidectomy may relieve nasopharyngeal obstruction while still allowing for adequate velopharyngeal closure.

Most cases of postoperative VPI are of limited duration. Recovery may take weeks to several months, by which time speech returns to normal. Observation or speech therapy, along with reassurance, is usually sufficient in these cases. In patients at risk (with the predisposing conditions noted earlier), and rarely in normal patients, the VPI may be prolonged, or even permanent. Speech therapy should be prescribed in these cases for up to 1 year postoperatively. Improvement may occur in a significant number of cases.[95] After 1 year, if speech therapy and all other methods of conservative treatment fail to improve the problem, pharyngoplasty (either by superiorly or inferiorly based flaps) is helpful in alleviating the hypernasality and regurgitation.[53]

Psychologic Sequelae

It is very difficult to evaluate the nature and estimate the occurrence of the effects of T&A on the child's short- and long-term behavioral development. In a retrospective study, Levy found that T&A, among other operations, commonly precipitates behavioral disorders.[51]

Psychologic trauma may manifest itself immediately after surgery. The child is frightened of separation from the parents; he or she may experience nightmares, fear of the dark, insomnia, bed-wetting, or even withdrawal and regression. Fortunately, these are usually self-limited problems.[19, 22, 31, 42]

To avoid psychologic sequelae, it is recommended that operation not be performed on children younger than the age of 3 years—or even 5 years, according to Joseph and Templer.[42] At these ages, the child should be given a full explanation, preferably with demonstration (for instance, trying the mask during the preoperative anesthesia examination) and illustrated books of the pre- and postoperative routines. Adequate sedation is recommended on the way to the operating room. Parents should be allowed to stay with the child in the holding area and immediately after operation. Adequate control of postoperative pain is important. The parents also should be given all the necessary information, especially regarding the anticipated immediate postoperative course. An overworried parent cannot give the child good support.

UNCOMMON COMPLICATIONS

Teeth

Because T&A involves intraoral retraction, instrumentation, and manipulation, dental trauma is a possible complication. Teeth may be cracked, broken, loosened, or accidentally extracted. If extracted, teeth may be swallowed, may be aspirated, or, at worst, may simply disappear without being noticed by the surgeon. The patient or the parents will find out the next day that a tooth is missing. A time- and money-consuming radiologic search for the missing tooth is then required. This may be followed by legal actions taken by the patient or family. All these problems can be avoided by awareness, prevention, recognition, and proper management.

All patients undergoing T&A should be evaluated by the anesthesiologist and the surgeon, and the number and condition of all teeth should be recorded. The fate of loose teeth should be discussed and decided upon by the surgeon and patient and parents before surgery. Elective extraction may be indicated in cases of loose upper deciduous incisors.

The most commonly injured teeth are the maxillary incisors. Children with overbite are especially vulnerable. The inclination of their upper incisors is such that even a slight pressure from the mouth gag may dislodge them.

The double-bite mouth gags and the McIvor gag rest on the canines and premolars. We prefer these gags over the single-bite one that rests on the central incisors. Careful placement and removal of the mouth gag are important. The condition of the teeth should be re-examined after removal of the mouth gag, but before extubation. Permanent teeth that become loose should be splinted. Teeth that were dislodged should be replaced immediately, preferably by an experienced dentist, who may elect to perform root canal treatment before reinsertion. Replacement and splinting may be done with acrylic or wire.

A tooth that has disappeared should be searched for before extubation. If not found, radiographs should be taken on the operating room table. If the tooth is found in the stomach, the parents should be notified. If the tooth is in the airway, immediate bronchoscopy is indicated.

Tonsil and Adenoid Recurrence

Adenoid tissue may recur or "regrow" from nearby lymphatic tissue. If the symptoms that led to the initial procedure recur, secondary adenoidectomy may be necessary. As adenoids tend to involute by puberty, those removed at an earlier age may have a higher tendency to recur.

Tonsil tags may be found in 15 per cent to 28 per cent of tonsillectomy patients.[72] Patients may notice a "lump" in the tonsil fossa, or be concerned that their tonsil(s) are regrowing. Only 6 per cent to 8 per cent experience recurrent throat infections. Peritonsillar abscesses may occur.[70] Four to seventeen per cent of these patients develop recurrent chronic pharyngitis or "pharyngitis tonsillopriva."[72] In asymptomatic patients, reassurance is sufficient. In certain patients with recurrent infections or abscess, secondary (tag) tonsillectomy may be needed.

The Eustachian Tube

It has been theorized that adenoidectomy can cause irreversible injury to the eustachian tube, with subsequent scarring and stenosis that may result in middle ear effusion and conductive hearing loss. This delayed complication is most probably one of the reasons

for "failed" adenoidectomy.[22, 36] It usually responds only to insertion of tympanostomy tubes. Injury to the eustachian tube can be prevented by avoidance of aggressive curettage at the torus tubarius region. Some surgeons do not use the adenotome or curette at all at this region. They prefer the punch forceps, which is used under direct vision with the palate retracted or with the help of a mirror.

An overly patulous eustachian tube that has been protected by the adenoid tissue may be uncovered by adenoidectomy. This outcome has been mentioned as a possible mechanism for postoperative recurrent acute otitis media.[22]

Injury to Adjacent Structures

Face and Mouth. Laceration of the lips is an avoidable, though not a rare, complication. The lips should be released from the mouth gag before the gag is widely opened. Injury to the eye is much less common but a far more serious complication. Application of ointment and taping the eyelids shut will help prevent injury to the eye.

Cautery burns of the lips, facial skin, and buccal mucosa are becoming increasingly common. Prevention includes proper draping of the patient and shielding of the cautery tips.

Neck. In addition to pain referred from the tonsillar fossa and nasopharynx, neck pain may be caused by hyperextension and manipulation during surgery. Placing the patient in the Rose position with a shoulder roll requires support of the head. This positioning can prevent postoperative neck pain.

The surgeon also should be aware of the uncommon immediate or delayed complication of atlantoaxial dislocation.[28] The patient presents with significant neck pain, limited motion, and torticollis (Grisel disease) within a few days to a week after surgery. The cause of delayed atlantoaxial dislocation is most probably decalcification of bone and laxity of anterior ligaments between C1 and C2, both caused by inflammation, hyperemia, and possible infection of the posterior nasopharyngeal wall following adenoidectomy. Patients with Down syndrome are predisposed to traumatic delayed atlantoaxial subluxation. Positioning these patients should be done carefully; hyperextension should be avoided; and posterior nasopharyngeal curettage should be gentle and not deep.

Diagnosis of atlantoaxial subluxation is done by lateral neck film. Treatment, which is usually successful, includes immobilization with a soft neck collar.

An unusual case of osteomyelitis of C2 and C3 has been described by Tami and associates; this complication may have been caused by the combination of nasopharyngeal inflammation/infection and surgical positioning and manipulation.[80] Sipila and colleagues described the possible relation between local anesthesia and atlantoaxial infection and subluxation.[77]

Eagle Syndrome. One of the explanations for the uncommon complaint of chronic, usually unilateral, throat and neck pain after T&A is irritation of an elongated styloid process caused by fibrosis at the oropharyngeal level.[96] Injury to the styloid tip is another possible mechanism. The pain may be referred to the ear, a fact that may make the diagnosis difficult. Diagnosis is made by palpation and radiograph (Panorex). Treatment options range from reassurance and symptomatic therapy to local injection of long-acting steroid. Definitive treatment involves the surgical removal of the styloid tip.

Temporomandibular joint. The combination of muscle relaxants and maximal opening of the jaw by the mouth gag may result in dislocation of the temporomandibular joint (TMJ). This dislocation should be recognized—immediately after removal of the mouth gag—by the inability to close the mouth. Reduction should be performed immediately. This procedure is done with the surgeon's two thumbs in the mouth pressing against the mandibular alveolar ridge as close to the angle as possible, and both index fingers pressing against the inferior aspect of the mandible outside the mouth at the mental region. Reduction is performed by first pulling the entire jaw downward and then rotating it by pushing the rami and condyles backward and pulling the body and mentum upward. With or without apparent dislocation during surgery, patients may complain of postoperative TMJ pain. This problem is usually self-limited, requiring no more than soft diet and mild analgesics. It should be considered as a possible cause of postoperative otalgia when the otoscopic examination is normal.

Hypoglycemia

Though not clinically apparent, postoperative hypoglycemia is much more common than appreciated.[7] Ware and Osborne suggest a "rebound hypoglycemia" phenomenon after the hyperglycemia induced by surgery.[91] This rebound happens about 4 hours after the operation. Secondary electrolyte imbalance may result from hypoglycemia, which is more serious than the hypoglycemia itself and may cause electrocardiographic changes. It is possible to overlook the symptoms and signs of hypoglycemia in a semi-conscious postoperative child.

Prevention is based on the shortening, as much as possible, of the pre- and postoperative starvation period. Children should be operated on during the early morning hours. Postoperative feeding should start as soon as possible. Fry and Ibrahim have shown that with the use of metoclopramide to aid gastric emptying, food can be given orally until 2 hours before surgery.[26]

Pulmonary Infection

Pneumonia and lung abscess used to be relatively common complications of T&A. The most likely cause was aspiration of bloody clots and infected fragments of adenotonsillar tissue. The role of bacteremia in the etiopathogenesis of infectious pulmonary complications is unclear. A thorough review of the literature reveals that it was *not* the introduction of antibiotics that reduced the incidence of pulmonary complications. It was the significant improvement in instrumentation, patient's positioning, and surgical technique, as well as the introduction of modern anesthesia, that resulted in the near disappearance of these complications during the 1920s and 1930s. By 1954, the incidence of lung abscess dropped to 0.04 per cent, and by 1969 the incidence of pneumonia was 0.5 per cent and that of lung abscess was zero.[10] In a (1986) study of 9409 T&As, six cases of pneumonia (0.06 per cent) were recorded.[16] Thus, the possibility of this complication still exists and should be included in the differential diagnosis of persistent postoperative fever with rising leukocyte count.

RARE AND ANECDOTAL COMPLICATIONS

As a consequence of the extremely large number of T&As performed in the last 70 years, many rare, anecdotal, and unpredictable complications have been seen and reported. The reader may not encounter any of these complications during his or her entire professional career. The following list will provide the reader with the relevant literature that may be referred to if such a rare complication is encountered.

Necrosis of the uvula may be caused by an overly aggressive palate excision that includes the arterial blood supply to the uvula.[35] Pneumothorax, pneumomediastinum, and subcutaneous emphysema have been described and may be attributed to rupture of a pulmonary alveolus or bleb.[65, 69] Atelectasis with basal or segmental pulmonary hypoaeration that is clinically significant is also a rare complication. Dong[23] and Derkay and associates[21] describe cases of persistent postoperative torticollis resulting from an Arnold-Chiari malformation type I. An injection site abscess that complicated intramuscular injection during tonsillectomy has been described by Jacobson and associates;[39] Tovi and group described a pseudoaneurysm of the internal carotid artery secondary to tonsillectomy.[86] Fracture of the mandibular condyle, attributed to overstretching of the lower jaw by the mouth gag in an attempt to obtain a larger operative field, has also been described.[32]

Surgical trauma to cranial nerves is another rare complication. There have been reports of nerve injuries that involved the glossopharyngeal, hypoglossal, lingual, facial, recurrent laryngeal, and phrenic nerves.[22, 85] Surgical trauma to the sympathetic chain has been described as the cause of Horner syndrome.[97] In one case report, the combined sympathetic, hypoglossal, and superior laryngeal nerve injury is attributed to a carotid sheath abscess that followed tonsillectomy.[97] In another case, bilateral vocal cord paralysis is attributed to posterior nasal packing following adenoidectomy.[22]

Bicknell and Wiggens described two patients who had taste disorders after tonsillectomy.[4] Both patients responded to zinc therapy. Tolczynski reviews the literature on complications of T&A, in a report in which he also details his own experience.[85] His list of rare and anecdotal complications includes tetany, meningitis, optic neuritis, acute myocarditis, salivary fistula from the sublingual gland to the tonsillar fossa, and amputation of the anterior third of the tongue. Holzer describes a case of post-tonsillectomy anaerobic septicemia,[38] and Vorhies describes transient parotid swelling following tonsillectomy.[89] Donaldson and Stool mention blindness as a possible complication of intraoperative injection of steroids into the tonsillar fossa.[22]

LONG-TERM SEQUELAE

The tonsils and adenoids have a role in the human immune system. Locally, these lymphoid tissues act as the first immunologic barrier against different antigens that are constantly introduced transorally and transnasally. Immunoglobulin A probably has an important role in the local defense system.[41] Other types of antibodies are produced in the tonsil tissue and are released, together with T cells, into the lymphatic and blood systems. These findings have led many investigators to suspect increased immunologic risks in patients after T&A. However, the few studies showing increased incidence of certain diseases have not been validated. These diseases include poliomyelitis,[92] Hodgkin disease,[50, 88] thyroid cancer,[6] leukemia,[17] multiple sclerosis,[18] and rheumatoid arthritis.[29, 54]

Kristiansen and Elverland found that a significantly higher number of post-T&A patients than controls became carriers of *Neisseria meningitidis*.[49] Rasmussen, however, doubts if this finding is of any clinical significance.[72] He points out that only a few case reports in the Russian literature had linked meningitis to T&A.

Lingual tonsil hyperplasia is an uncommon entity that is most probably related to T&A. Almost all patients with lingual tonsil pathology, especially hyperplasia, described in the literature had undergone T&A in the past. In the single largest series of lingual tonsil disease, presented by Krespi and colleagues, 84 per cent of the patients had undergone palatine tonsillectomy.[48] It has been speculated that lingual tonsil hyperplasia is a compensatory mechanism of Waldeyer ring following T&A.

Shenoy believes that the incidence of allergic rhinitis increases after T & A.[74] This complication is manifested by the aggravation of symptoms in patients who had allergic rhinitis before T&A and by the new onset of allergic rhinitis in post-T&A patients. He postulated that decreased T suppressor cell function after T&A causes a relative increase in nasal mucosal IgE levels, resulting in symptomatic rhinitis. This hypothesis has not been tested yet by immunologic or epidemiologic studies.

LASER TONSILLECTOMY

With the advancement of laser technology, it was only natural for otolaryngologists to try to perform tonsillectomies with the laser. Surgeons who perform laser tonsillectomy state that it has two major advantages: first, less intraoperative bleeding makes the surgery easier, safer, and faster, and second, there is less postoperative pain or discomfort.[56] Jake recommends laser T&A, especially

for patients with hematologic disorders.[40] Other surgeons argue that the laser does not significantly change the outcome and postoperative course of T&A patients, and, therefore, the extra time, personnel, and expensive equipment required for laser surgery cannot be justified.[47] Use of the laser, however, does contribute to the array of possible intra- and postoperative complications.

The most dramatic complication is laser-ignited explosion of the endotracheal tube. This is a life-threatening event. It is caused by the laser beam striking the tube, and is related to the power and duration of the beam, the type of tube and the material it is made of, the quality and effectiveness of the tube's protective wrapping, and the FiO_2 within the tube. It is best prevented by using a special laser tube or a properly wrapped Rusch (red rubber) tube, by inflating the cuff with saline and methylene blue, by protecting the tube with wet gauze, and by close cooperation between the anesthesiologist and the surgeon throughout the procedure.

In case of fire, the endotracheal tube must be removed immediately, the oxygen flow must be disconnected, and the fire extinguished by instillation of saline solution. Once the fire has been extinguished, the patient is ventilated with 100 per cent oxygen via a mask, and an oral airway is placed. Muscle relaxants are given to prevent laryngospasm. Reintubation is performed with a small tube, or a bronchoscope is introduced with the ventilating apparatus connected to its side port. The degree of pharyngeal and tracheal injury is assessed, and lavage is performed with saline to remove the debris. The surgeon then must decide whether tracheotomy or steroids and antibiotics are needed.

Laser-specific surgical complications are rare. It is possible to penetrate too deeply with the laser beam and cause bleeding. This problem is best avoided by starting with a low wattage setting, increasing it as needed under direct visualization. Laser burns to the pharynx, buccal mucosa, and tongue are prevented by careful handling of the handpiece, by activating the laser only after the aiming beam is directed at the target spot, and by releasing the foot control before the aiming beam is removed from the target spot. All efforts should be made to avoid accidental movement of the patient, table, or microscope. The use of nonreflecting instruments will prevent injury to healthy tissue. Burns to the lips, face, and eyes are prevented by proper covering with moist towels. Personnel injury is avoided by proper handling of the handpiece or microscope, by the use of eyeglasses or goggles, and by giving "laser privileges" only to specially trained physicians, nurses, and other operating room personnel.

The laser handpiece or microscope should not be brought into the surgical field before all drapes and wet towels and packs are in place. The laser is the first instrument to be turned off and *then* removed from the surgical field at the end of the procedure. Silence is important during laser surgery. All orders for laser settings are given by the surgeon alone, and they are repeated loudly and clearly by the nurse who operates the control box. Strict enforcement of these simple safety procedures in the operating room during a laser procedure will help prevent potentially serious complications.

CONCLUSION

The best way to manage complications is to prevent them, and the best prevention, of course, is to avoid operation. Most T&As are not performed to save a life but rather to improve the quality of life. Thus, strict adherence to the guidelines regarding indications for T&A is strongly recommended. In patients with an increased surgical risk because of an underlying problem, such as a bleeding disorder or cardiac or pulmonary disease, the risks of operation should be carefully weighed against the benefits. Even with clear indications for T&A, the surgeon and family may find it safer to avoid operation.

T&A should not be considered a minor procedure. Indeed, T&A is considered major surgery by many malpractice insurance carriers.[58] T&A should be performed only by surgeons who have been trained specifically in this surgical field and are capable of recognizing and managing all possible complications.

References

1. Alexander D, Graff T, Kelly E: Factors in tonsillectomy mortality. Arch Otolaryngol 82:490, 1965.
2. Allen TH, Steven IM, Sweeney DB: The bleeding tonsil—anesthesia for control of hemorrhage after tonsillectomy. Anaesth Intensive Care (6):517–520, 1973.
3. Battersby EF: Paediatric anaesthesia. In Kerr AG (ed): Scott Brown's Otolaryngology. 5th ed. Vol 6. London, Butterworths, 1987, pp 503–526.
4. Bicknell JM, Wiggens RV: Taste disorder from zinc deficiency after tonsillectomy. West J Med 149:457–460, 1988.
5. Broadman LM, Patel RI, Feldman BA, et al: The effects of peritonsillar infiltration on the reduction of intra-operative blood loss and post-tonsillectomy pain in children. Laryngoscope 99:578–581, 1989.
6. Bross IDJ, Shimaoka K, Tidings J: Some epidemiological clues in thyroid cancer. Tonsillectomy, acne, allergy, ethnicity. Arch Intern Med 128:755–760, 1971.
7. Capper JWR: Postoperative hypoglycemia in children undergoing adenotonsillectomy. J Laryngol Otol 95:519–521, 1981.
8. Carithers JS, Gebhart DE, Williams JA: Postoperative risks of pediatric tonsilloadenoidectomy. Laryngoscope 97:422–429, 1987.
9. Carmody D, Vamadevan T, Cooper SM: Post tonsillectomy hemorrhage. J Laryngol Otol 96:635–638, 1982.
10. Catlin FI: Pulmonary complications of tonsillectomy as originally described by Samuel J. Crowe, MD. Laryngoscope 91:52–62, 1981.
11. Catling SJ, Asbury AJ, Latis M: Airway obstruction in infectious mononucleosis. Anaesthesia 39:699–702, 1984.
12. Chowdhury K, Tewfik TL, Schloss MD: Post tonsillectomy and adenoidectomy hemorrhage. J Otolaryngol 17:46–49, 1988.
13. Cotton RT: Nasopharyngeal stenosis. Arch Otolaryngol 111:146–148, 1985.
14. Croft CB, Shprintzen RJ, Ruben RJ: Hypernasal speech following adenotonsillectomy. Otolaryngol Head Neck Surg 89(2):179–188, 1981.
15. Crowe SJ, Watkins SS, Rothholz AS: Relation of tonsillar and nasopharyngeal infections to general systemic disorders. Bull Johns Hopkins Hosp 28:1–25, 1917.
16. Crysdale WS, Russel D: Complications of tonsillectomy and adenoidectomy in 9,409 children observed overnight. Can Med Assoc J 135:1139–1142, 1986.
17. Cuneo JM: Tonsillectomy and leukemia. Lancet 1:846, 1972.
18. Currier RD, Martin EA, Woosley PC: Prior events in multiple sclerosis. Neurology 24:748–754, 1974.
19. Davenport HT, et al: The effect of general anesthesia surgery and hospitalization on the behavior of children. Am J Orthopsychiatry 40:806–824, 1970.
20. DeDio RM, Hendrix RA: Postobstructive pulmonary

edema. Otolaryngol Head Neck Surg 101:698–700, 1989.

21. Derkay CS, Kenna MA, Pang D: Refractory torticollis: An uncommon complication of adenotonsillectomy. Int J Pediatr Otorhinolaryngol 14:82–93, 1987.

22. Donaldson JD, Stool SE: Complications of tonsillectomy and adenoidectomy. In Conley JJ (ed): Complications of Head and Neck Surgery. Philadelphia, WB Saunders, 1979, pp 227–238.

23. Dong ML: Arnold Chiari malfunction type I appearing after tonsillectomy. Anesthesiology 67:120–122, 1987.

24. Eisenberg JM, Clark JR, Sussman SA: Prothrombin and partial thromboplastin times as preoperative screening tests. Arch Surg 117:48–51, 1982.

25. Feibert AN, Shabino CL: Acute pulmonary edema complicating tonsillectomy and adenoidectomy Pediatrics 75:112–114, 1985.

26. Frye ENS, Ibrahim AA: Hypoglycemia in pediatric anesthesia. Anaesthesia 31:552, 1976.

27. Gardner JF: Sutures and disasters in tonsillectomy. Arch Otolaryngol 88:551–555, 1968.

28. Gibb AG: Unusual complications of tonsil and adenoid removal. J Laryngol Otol 83:1159–1174, 1969.

29. Gottlieb NL, Page WF, Appelrouth DJ, et al: Antecedent tonsillectomy and appendectomy in rheumatoid arthritis. J Rheumatol 6:316–323, 1979.

30. Gregory GA: Pediatric anesthesia. In Miller RD (ed): Anesthesia. 2nd ed. Vol 3. New York, Churchill-Livingstone, 1986, p 1755.

31. Grundfast KM: Complications of tonsillectomy and adenoidectomy. In Johns ME (ed): Complications in Otolaryngology–Head and Neck Surgery. Vol II. Toronto, BC Decker, 1986, pp 111–119.

32. Gupta SC, Singh R, Misra T, Misra VP: Fracture of the mandibular condyle as a complication of tonsillectomy. Ear Nose Throat J 68:477–479, 1989.

33. Handler SD, Miller L, Richmond KH, Baranak CC: Post tonsillectomy hemorrhage: Incidence, prevention and management. Laryngoscope 96:1243–1247, 1986.

34. Harvey AM, Johns RJ, McKusick VA (eds): The Principles and Practice of Medicine. 20th ed. New York, Appleton-Century-Crofts, 1980, pp 523–525.

35. Hibbert J: Acute infection of the pharynx and tonsils. In Kerr AG (ed): Scott Brown's Otolaryngology. 5th ed. Vol 5. London, Butterworths, 1987, pp 76–98.

36. Hibbert J: Tonsils and adenoids. In Kerr AG (ed): Scott Brown's Otolaryngology. 5th ed. Vol 6. London, Butterworths, 1987, pp 368–383.

37. Holt GR, Watkins TM, Yoder MG, Garcia A: The effect of tonsillectomy on impedance audiometry. Otolaryngol Head Neck Surg 89(1):20–26, 1981.

38. Holzer NJ: Post tonsillectomy anaerobic septicemia. NY State J Med 79(4):763, 1979.

39. Jacobson JT, et al: Injection site abscess caused by group A beta hemolytic streptococcus. An unusual complication of tonsillectomy and intramuscular injection. Am J Infect Control 12:293–296, 1984.

40. Jake GJ: State of the art of otolaryngology. Lasers Surg Med 6:384, 1986.

41. Jeschke R, Stroeder J: Continual observation of clinical and immunological parameters, in particular of salivary IgA in tonsillectomized children. Arch Otorhinolaryngol 226:73–84, 1980.

42. Joseph DJ, Templer J: Tonsillectomy and adenoidectomy. In English GM (ed): Otolaryngology. Vol 3. Philadelphia, JB Lippincott, 1989, Chapter 28.

43. Kaplan EF, Scheiner LB, et al: The usefulness of preoperative laboratory screening. JAMA 253:3576–3581, 1985.

44. Karl HW, Swedlow DB, Lee KW, et al: Epinephrine-halothane interactions in children. Anesthesiology 58:142–145, 1983.

45. Kavanagh KT, Beckford NS: Adenotonsillectomy in children: Indications and contraindications. South Med J 81:507–511, 1988.

46. Kerr AIG, Brodie SW: Guillotine tonsillectomy: Anachronism or pragmatism? J Laryngol Otol 92:317–323, 1978.

47. Krespi YP, Har-El G: Laser palatine and lingual tonsillectomy. In Ossoff RH, Duncavage JA (eds): Lasers in Otolaryngology–Head and Neck Surgery. St. Louis, CV Mosby, in press.

48. Krespi YP, Har-El G, Levine TM, et al: Laser lingual tonsillectomy. Laryngoscope 99:131–135, 1989.

49. Kristiansen BE, Elverland H: Increased meningococcal carrier rate after tonsillectomy. Br Med J 288:974, 1984.

50. Langman AW, Kaplan MJ: Hodgkin's disease and tonsillectomy. Otolaryngol Clin North Am 20:399–404, 1987.

51. Levy DM: Psychic trauma of operations in children. Am J Dis Child 69:7–25, 1945.

52. Linden BE, Gross CW, Long TE, Lazar RH: Morbidity in pediatric tonsillectomy. Laryngoscope 100:120–124, 1990.

53. Lindsay WK: Pharyngoplasty. Ann Plast Surg 2:511–516, 1979.

54. Linos A, O'Fallow NW, Worthington JW, Kurland LT: The effect of tonsillectomy and appendectomy on the development of rheumatoid arthritis. J Rheumatol 13:707–709, 1986.

55. Mann DG, St. George C, Schelner E, et al: Tonsillectomy—some like it hot. Laryngoscope 94:677–679, 1984.

56. Martinez SA, Akim DP: Laser tonsillectomy and adenoidectomy. Otolaryngol Clin North Am 20(2):371–376, 1987.

57. McDonald TJ, Devine KD, Hayles AB: Nasopharyngeal stenosis following tonsillectomy and adenoidectomy. Arch Otolaryngol 98:38–41, 1973.

58. Medical Liability Mutual Insurance Company (New York): Malpractice Rate Tables, 1988.

59. Moore FD, Pratt LW: Tonsillectomy in Maine. Ann Surg 194:232–241, 1981.

60. Nickerson RJ, Hauck WW, Bloom BS, Peterson OL: Otolaryngologists and their surgical practice. Arch Otolaryngol 104:718–725, 1978.

61. Ogusthorpe JD, Adkins WY Jr, Putney FJ, Hungerford DG: Internal carotid artery as source of tonsillectomy and adenoidectomy hemorrhage. Otolaryngol Head Neck Surg 89:758–762, 1981.

62. Paff G: Anatomy of the Head and Neck. Philadelphia, WB Saunders, 1973, p 177.

63. Papangelou I: Hemostasis in tonsillectomy: A comparison of electrocoagulation and ligation. Arch Otolaryngol 96:358–360, 1972.

64. Paradise JL, et al: Efficacy of tonsillectomy for recurrent throat infections in severely affected children: Results of parallel randomized and non-randomized clinical trials. N Engl J Med 310:674, 1984.

65. Podoshin L, Persico M, Fradis M: Post-tonsillectomy emphysema. Ear Nose Throat J 58:73–82, 1979.

66. Pratt LW: Infections of the lymphoid tissue. In

English GM (ed): Otolaryngology. Vol 3. Philadelphia, JB Lippincott, 1989, Chapter 27.

67. Pratt LW: Tonsillectomy and adenoidectomy: Mortality and morbidity. Trans Am Acad Opthalmol Otolaryngol 74:1146–1154, 1970.

68. Pratt LW, Gallagher RA: Tonsillectomy and adenoidectomy: Incidence and mortality, 1968–1972. Otolaryngol Head Neck Surg 87:159–166, 1979.

69. Pratt LW, Hornberger HR, Moore V: Mediastinal emphysema complicating tonsillectomy and adenoidectomy. Ann Otol Rhinol Laryngol 71:158, 1963.

70. Randall CJ, Jefferis AF: Quinsy following tonsillectomy. Five case reports. J Laryngol Otol 98:367–369, 1984.

71. Ranger D: Tonsillectomy and adenoidectomy. Lancet 1:1205, 1968.

72. Rasmussen N: Complications of tonsillectomy and adenoidectomy. Otolaryngol Clin North Am 20:383–390, 1987.

73. Salassa JR, et al: Oral dantrolene sodium for post-tonsillectomy pain; A double blind study. Otolaryngol Head Neck Surg 98:16–33, 1988.

74. Shenoy P: Allergic rhinitis after tonsillectomy. Arch Otolaryngol Head Neck Surg 115:1134–1135, 1989.

75. Shoelevar J, Hunsicker RC, Stool SE: Arteriography in post-tonsillectomy hemorrhage. Arch Otolaryngol 95:581–583, 1972.

76. Simcock AD, Prout BJ: A patient with respiratory obstruction in glandular fever. Thorax 29:145–146, 1974.

77. Sipila P, Palva A, Sorri M, et al: Atlantoaxial subluxation. An unusual complication after local anesthesia for tonsillectomy. Arch Otolaryngol Head Neck Surg 107:181–182, 1981.

78. Snow JC, Healy GB, Vaughan CW, Kripke BJ: Malignant hyperthermia during anesthesia for adenoidectomy. Arch Otolaryngol 95:442–447, 1972.

79. Souliere CR Jr, Weintraub SJ, Kirchner C: Markedly delayed postoperative malignant hyperthermia. Arch Otolaryngol Head Neck Surg 112:564–566, 1986.

80. Tami TA, Burkus JK, Strom CG: Cervical osteomyelitis. An unusual complication of tonsillectomy. Arch Otolaryngol Head Neck Surg 113:992–994, 1987.

81. Tami TA, Parker GS, Taylor RE: Post-tonsillectomy bleeding: An evaluation of risk factors. Laryngoscope 97:1307–1311, 1987.

82. Tate N: Deaths from tonsillectomy. Lancet 7:1090–1091, 1963.

83. Telian SA, Handler SD, Fleisher GR, et al: The effect of antibiotic therapy on recovery after tonsillectomy in children. Arch Otolaryngol Head Neck Surg 112:610–615, 1986.

84. Thomas GK, Arbon RA: Pre-operative screening for potential tonsillectomy and adenoidectomy bleeding. Arch Otolaryngol 91:453–456, 1970.

85. Tolczynski B: Tonsillectomy; its hazards and their prevention. Eye Ear Nose Throat Monthly 48:71–80, 1969.

86. Tovi F, Leiberman A, Hertzanu Y: Pseudoaneurysm of the internal carotid artery secondary to tonsillectomy. Int J Pediatr Otorhinolaryngol 13:69–75, 1987.

87. Van Eyck C: Bacteremia after tonsillectomy and adenoidectomy. Acta Otolaryngol 81:242–243, 1976.

88. Vianna NJ, Davies JNP, Harris S, et al: Tonsillectomy and childhood Hodgkin's disease. Lancet 2:338–339, 1980.

89. Vorhies PE: Transient swelling of the parotid glands following tonsillectomy. AANA J 46:611–614, 1978.

90. Wackym PA, Abdul-Rasool IH: Oral dantrolene sodium for tonsillectomy pain (letter). Otolaryngol Head Neck Surg 99:607, 1988.

91. Ware S, Osborne JP: Postoperative hypoglycemia in small children. Br Med J 2:499, 1976.

92. Weinstein L, Vogel ML, Weinstein N: Study of relationship of abscess of tonsils to incidence of bulbar poliomyelitis. J Pediatr 44:14–19, 1954.

93. Williams JD, Pope TH Jr: Prevention of primary tonsillectomy bleeding: An argument for electrocautery. Arch Otolaryngol 98:306–309, 1973.

94. Withers BT, Nail BM Jr: Pyrogenic reaction following tonsillo-adenoidectomy. Texas J Med 60:897–899, 1964.

95. Witzel MA, Rich RH, Margar-Bencal F, Cox C: Velopharyngeal insufficiency after adenoidectomy. An 8 year review. Int J Pediatr Otorhinolaryngol 11:15–20, 1968.

96. Zalzal GH, Cotton RT: Adenotonsillar disease. In Cummings CS (ed): Otolaryngology–Head and Neck Surgery. Vol II. St. Louis, CV Mosby, 1986, pp 1189–1211.

97. Zollner B, Herrmann IF: Horner-, Hypoglossus- und Rekurrensparese als entzundlich Spatkomplikation nach Tonsillektomie. Monatsschr Uhrenheilkd Laryngorhinol 105:228–232, 1971.

CHAPTER 16

Thyroid and Parathyroid Surgery

GORDON W. SUMMERS, DMD, MD

Thyroid and parathyroid operations should be accomplished with minimal morbidity and mortality. These procedures result in little patient discomfort and usually allow discharge from the hospital within 2 days following surgery. The close proximity of the parathyroids and thyroid, recurrent laryngeal nerves, superior laryngeal nerves, laryngotracheal complex, esophagus, and carotid vessels creates considerable potential for complication; however, the actual incidence is quite low when surgical procedures are performed by experienced neck surgeons (Table 16–1).

Injury to any of the nerves innervating the larynx can be particularly devastating to the person who depends on extensive use of the voice or who is a professional singer. Severe airway problems from combinations of various nerve injuries also may occur. Postoperative hypoparathyroidism, if permanent, is a serious complication that requires constant medical management to alleviate troublesome and sometimes disabling symptoms. Hemorrhage, wound infection, keloid for-

mation, and unsightly neck scars are additional complications. Thyroid storm, once a frequent complication of thyroidectomy for hyperthyroidism, is now very rare because of better preoperative medical management.

A thorough understanding of surgical anatomy and the pathologic conditions to be expected, combined with skillful surgical technique, should help prevent complications. Prompt recognition and treatment of complications are essential to prevent worsening of the patient's condition and prevent death. This chapter discusses the prevention, recognition, and management of complications from thyroid and parathyroid surgery.

PREOPERATIVE EVALUATION AND COUNSELING

It is not within the scope of this presentation to discuss all the various diagnostic studies in common use, except to emphasize that fine needle aspiration biopsy has proved to

TABLE 16–1. Incidence of Complications in Thyroid-Parathyroid Surgery

	Per Cent
Permanent hypoparathyroidism	2.4–5.0
Permanent nerve paralysis	
Unilateral recurrent laryngeal	0.8–2.0
Bilateral recurrent laryngeal	0.25
Superior laryngeal	?
Postoperative hemorrhage	0.2
Wound infection	0.2
Surgical thyroid storm	<0.01
Scar, keloid	?
Operative mortality	0.03–0.1

be the most valuable single test in the evaluation of thyroid nodules. Advance insight into the precise histopathologic nature of a thyroid mass allows the surgeon to predict more accurately the extent of surgery necessary and the potential problems. With this knowledge the surgeon is better prepared to present an informed consent discussion to the patient and appropriate family members.

Vocal cord function must be assessed by indirect laryngoscopy both before and after thyroid-parathyroid operations. Reliance upon a "normal" speaking voice is not adequate, particularly in reoperations. Unless routine indirect laryngoscopy is performed, some cases of cord impairment will not be discovered. Occasionally an idiopathic vocal cord paralysis is encountered, and the patient may have a fairly good speaking voice through overcompensation of the normal cord. Vocal cord paralysis has even been reported as a result of endotracheal tube cuff pressure.[9] If the patient has had previous neck surgery in the remote past, the postoperative hoarseness and breathy voice symptoms may have long been forgotten. A fairly "normal" speaking voice may have returned over time as the uninvolved vocal cord developed compensatory overadduction. It is extremely important to document this impaired vocal cord function preoperatively, not only because of medicolegal implications but also because of the possibility

of injury to the only remaining functional recurrent nerve.

ANESTHESIA

General endotracheal anesthesia is the accepted standard of practice in thyroid and parathyroid surgery. Patients with hypothyroidism who require emergency operation are usually given lower doses of premedication because of slower metabolism. In patients with suspected hyperthyroidism who require emergency operation, the anesthesiologist should be aware of the possibility of thyroid crisis or storm.

Thyroid storm is a life-threatening exacerbation of thyrotoxicosis, characterized by fever, severe tachycardia, and the exaggeration of all its metabolic manifestations. Proper preoperative preparation of thyrotoxic patients with thionamide drugs and iodide has essentially eliminated "surgical storm." It is generally recommended that thyrotoxic patients not be operated on electively until the thyroxine (T_4) and triiodothyronine (T_3) levels have stabilized in the normal range for at least 4 to 6 weeks.[72] This additional time allows all the unmeasured metabolic derangements of the thyrotoxicosis to have a chance to be corrected. If surgical storm develops, the surgeon must stop manipulating the thyroid gland and initiate prompt therapeutic measures. Malignant hyperthermia must be ruled out, for which dantrolene is specific therapy. The first drug of choice is usually propranolol, given intravenously (4 to 10 mg/kg, not to exceed 1 mg/min) with appropriate electrocardiographic monitoring. Other adrenergic blocking drugs include reserpine (2.5 mg IM) and guanethidine (50 to 150 mg orally daily). Sodium iodide (1 to 2.5 gm IV every 8 hr), propylthiouracil (600 mg stat and 200 mg every 6 hr), and hydrocortisone (100 mg stat followed by 300 mg daily) are also administered. Other supportive measures include oxygen, intravenous glucose, fluids, and induced hypothermia.

In a hypertensive patient who is being operated on for a thyroid mass, the possible coexistence of medullary thyroid cancer and pheochromocytoma should be kept in mind. These conditions should be diagnosed before operation because of the possibility of precipitating a hypertensive crisis. Such a hypertensive crisis is treated with nitroprusside.

PATIENT POSITION AND EXPOSURE

The neck is hyperextended, which moves the laryngotracheal complex with its overlying thyroid gland in a cephalad and anterior direction. The head of the operating table is elevated slightly to reduce venous engorgement.

Symmetric placement of the incision is critical to avoid unsightly scars. The incision should follow the natural skin wrinkle lines and extend the same distance on each side of the midline. Incisions that are too curved are more noticeable, as are incisions that are too straight. This "collar" incision can be marked out with a marking pen or a ligature pressed against the neck. The incision should be about 2.5 cm or 2 fingerbreadths above the sternal end of the clavicles in the hyperextended position. In men, this incision will be covered by a shirt collar, and in women, it will follow the "necklace line." Incisions that are too low and fall down over the manubrium may widen and become unsightly. If a neck dissection is necessary, then a parallel Macfee incision can be made higher in the neck, which is cosmetically more acceptable than a vertical extension of the collar incision.

The upper and lower flaps are elevated in the avascular subplatysmal plane in a bloodless manner, utilizing traction and the electrocautery unit. The midline fascia between the strap muscles also can be divided with the electrocautery to facilitate their lateral retraction. It is seldom necessary to divide the strap muscles for exposure. The thyroid gland is thus exposed, and at this point the mobilization and surgical removal of the pathologic lobe or process can begin. The middle thyroid vein is ligated, and then the lobe can be retracted medially with either a deeply placed traction suture or a Babcock clamp. The posterior surface of the thyroid lobe is then dissected meticulously.

It is not necessary to type and cross-match blood in patients undergoing thyroid and parathyroid operations. In a series of over 450 such operations, I have never given a transfusion.

RECURRENT LARYNGEAL NERVE

Anatomy

The right recurrent laryngeal nerve, after branching from the vagal trunk, crosses the undersurface of the subclavian artery and ascends superomedially in the tracheoesophageal groove along the posterior capsular surface of the thyroid lobe. The left recurrent laryngeal nerve passes posteriorly around the arch of the aorta and ascends superomedially into the neck in the tracheoesophageal groove until it enters the larynx in the same fashion as the right nerve. On the right side, a rare anomaly may exist where the nerve branches directly off the vagal trunk at the level of the thyroid gland to enter the larynx without recurring around the subclavian artery. The reported incidence of a nonrecurrent laryngeal nerve is 0.3 per cent to 1.0 per cent.[4, 34] A nonrecurrent laryngeal nerve also can occur on the left side if there is transposition of the great vessels.

Each recurrent nerve, accompanied by a branch of the inferior thyroid artery, passes deep to or between the leaves of the posterior suspensory ligament (Berry ligament) and enters the larynx deep to the lower border of the inferior constrictor muscle just behind the cricothyroid joint. The lowermost fibers of the inferior constrictor muscle arise from the cricoid and blend in with the lower fibers of the cricothyroid muscle. The palpable tip of the inferior horn of the thyroid cartilage serves as a guide to the point of entrance of the recurrent laryngeal nerve into the larynx.

The cricothyroid muscle arises from the external surface of the arch of the cricoid cartilage and divides into an anterior and superior portion and into a posterior and inferior, oblique portion. The anterior inserts on the lower border of the thyroid cartilage, whereas the posterior inserts along the inferior horn and inner surface of the thyroid cartilage. This muscle tilts the thyroid cartilage forward and the cricoid cartilage backward through the cricothyroid joint, thus lengthening and tensing the vocal cords. The posterior cricothyroid muscle is innervated by the external branch of the superior laryngeal nerve.

Lore has stressed the critical importance of the posterior suspensory ligament in performing total thyroid lobectomy.[49] This bilateral ligament extends from the cricoid, the first tracheal ring, and sometimes the second tracheal ring, to the posteromedial aspect of each thyroid lobe (Fig. 16–1).

Proximal to the suspensory ligament, the recurrent nerve usually divides into two or more branches and is closely related to the inferior thyroid. This nerve-artery relationship is quite variable and is seldom similar on the two sides of the neck. The nerve or its branches may be posterior or anterior to, or in between, the branches of the artery.

The inferior thyroid artery arises from the thyrocervical trunk and ascends posterior to the common carotid artery, passes deep to this artery, and curves anteromedially to enter the thyroid gland along its posterolateral surface. The inferior thyroid artery and the superior thyroid artery (external carotid) provide the main blood supply to the thyroid. The inferior thyroid artery usually supplies both parathyroid glands, although occasionally the superior parathyroid gland derives some arterial supply from the superior thyroid artery. Usually a branch of the inferior thyroid artery traverses the posterior suspensory ligament, which can result in troublesome bleeding during total thyroid lobectomy.

Injury Prevention

Most surgeons advise that the recurrent nerve be identified, protected, and kept in view to prevent iatrogenic injury during thyroid lobectomy. Lore recommends initial identification of the main trunk just above the superior thoracic inlet in the triangle formed by the trachea, common carotid ar-

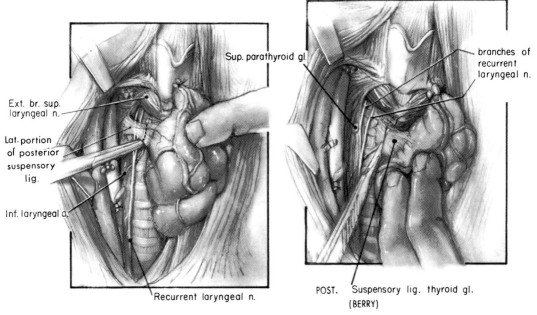

FIGURE 16–1. Relationship of the posterior suspensory ligament to the recurrent laryngeal nerve. (From Lore JM Jr (ed): Atlas of Head and Neck Surgery. 3rd ed. Philadelphia, WB Saunders, 1988, p 775.)

tery, and the lower pole of the thyroid.[49] The nerve can then be traced cephalad. Attie and Khafif[3] and Karlan and associates[44] prefer to identify the nerve just inferior to the thyroid artery and then proceed with the dissection. If these above approaches are not satisfactory, the nerve can be exposed and identified at the level of the inferior border of the thyroid cartilage.[73] Complete dissection of the recurrent laryngeal nerve, from below the inferior thyroid artery to its passage into the larynx below the inferior border of the inferior constrictor muscle, is necessary for the safety and preservation of this structure. Injury results from severing, crushing, ligating, stretching or applying electrocautery to the nerve trunk or its branches. Medial traction on the gland can "tent up" the nerve, making it more susceptible to injury. Indiscriminant clamping of bleeders close to the nerve and along the suspensory ligament can result in injury. The nerve is most vulnerable to injury over the last 2 cm of its course prior to entering the larynx. Once the recurrent nerve is completely exposed, the parathyroid glands can be dissected away from the thyroid capsule, preserving an intact blood supply.

UNILATERAL INJURY

Unilateral recurrent laryngeal nerve paralysis results in a vocal cord that assumes a median or paramedian position and does not abduct on inspiration. If the ipsilateral superior laryngeal nerve is intact, then cricothyroid muscle contraction will adduct the cord to some extent upon phonation. Early on, a patient with a unilateral recurrent laryngeal nerve paralysis usually exhibits a weak, breathy voice, ineffective cough, and some tendency to aspirate. With time, glottic closure improves by overcompensation of the contralateral vocal cord and the action of the ipsilateral cricothyroid muscle, which tenses the cord. Some patients with unilateral recurrent laryngeal nerve paralysis are asymptomatic and actually may go undetected unless subjected to a careful laryngoscopic examination. This again emphasizes the importance of indirect laryngoscopy before thy-

roid or parathyroid surgery to document vocal cord function.

The reported incidence of permanent recurrent laryngeal nerve paralysis following thyroidectomy varies from 0 to 10.5 per cent.[3, 13, 18, 55, 61, 68, 69] Most workers agree that the incidence should be 2 per cent or less.[13, 27, 31, 46, 50] A survey of recent literature reveals a composite incidence of 0.8 per cent (Table 16–2). Reoperations increase this incidence to as high as 17 per cent in the presence of thyroid cancer.[5] Temporary vocal cord paresis occurs occasionally, even in the hands of the most experienced surgeons, presumably because of operative nerve edema. Delayed nerve paralysis is also occasionally observed after thyroidectomy due to edema and postoperative inflammation. In this instance, complete resolution is often expected within 6 weeks.

At operation, if thyroid cancer is found invading a recurrent laryngeal nerve that is already paralyzed, then the nerve is intentionally sacrificed to facilitate en bloc resection of the tumor. However, if the nerve is still functional, as demonstrated by normal vocal cord motion preoperatively, then the nerve may be dissected free from the tumor and postoperative radioactive iodine relied upon to destroy residual tumor. If a recurrent laryngeal nerve is inadvertently divided during surgery, the surgeon should reanastomose it using microsurgical technique.[6, 28, 62, 67]

Adequate recovery of vocal cord function after direct nerve repair has been documented, particularly when performed immediately after injury.[3, 21, 22, 37, 39] In 1970, Doyle reported the results of ten recurrent laryngeal nerve repairs in humans.[23] Six of these repairs were performed within 5 days of injury. Five vocal cords showed recovery of normal function, and one showed no recovery. Four repairs performed between 3 months and 2 years following injury showed improved adduction with resulting excellent voice, but in no case was recovery of abduction complete. Ezaki and colleagues performed immediate end-to-end anastomosis of severed recurrent laryngeal nerves in seven thyroid cancer patients.[30] The length of nerve resected because of cancer infiltra-

TABLE 16–2. Incidence of Recurrent Laryngeal Nerve Paralysis After Thyroidectomy

	Ref. No.	No. of Patients	No. of Nerves at Risk	Permanent Paralysis of Recurrent Laryngeal Nerve
Shemen and Strong, 1989	68	64	128	1
Calabro et al, 1988	12	66	132	0
Lore, 1988	50	375	488	2
Lennquist, 1987	46	197	394	2
Reeve et al, 1987	65	115	230	1
Harness et al, 1986	37	404	808	10
Martensson and Terins, 1985	54	514	749*	27
			76†	7
VanderSluis and Wobbes, 1985	70	46	92	1
Karlan et al, 1984	44	1000	2000	0
Jacobs et al, 1983	42	213	426	0
Fenton, 1983	32	117	126	1
Clark, 1982	13	82	164	0
Attie and Khafif, 1975	3	249	498	0
TOTALS		3442	6311	52 (0.8%)

*Primary thyroidectomy.
†Secondary thyroidectomy.

tion was about 1 cm in length. All 7 patients had normal vocal cord function prior to the cancer resection. Follow-up revealed no return of motion in five patients; however, one patient exhibited almost normal cord motion and one developed slight motion. None of the seven patients demonstrated paradoxic motion of the cords despite the possibility of misdirected regeneration of the nerve fibers. When compared with a group of patients with unilaterally severed unrepaired recurrent nerves, all seven repaired patients had better voice quality and less severe hoarseness. The patients with repaired nerves also had prolonged phonation time and little or no visible atrophy of the involved vocal cord. Thus, immediate primary repair of a severed recurrent laryngeal nerve can be expected to produce a stronger voice and prevent vocal cord atrophy.

Satisfactory recovery of abductor function is infrequent and unpredictable. Inconsistent and unsatisfactory results reported both in dog nerve repair experiments and human case reports, attributed mostly to misdirected nerve regeneration, have led many surgeons to direct their efforts toward rehabilitation of the larynx rather than the injured recurrent laryngeal nerve.[31] Removal of ligatures or sutures entrapping the nerve has resulted in complete recovery of recurrent laryngeal nerve function.[22, 38] Again, as in nerve repair, the earlier this can be done, the better the recovery. Therefore, immediate paralysis noted after thyroidectomy deserves immediate wound re-exploration, not only to exclude nerve severance but also to relieve physical involvement of the nerve by sutures or ligatures.

The timing of re-exploration for possible recurrent laryngeal nerve injury is critical. If delayed beyond 10 to 14 days, the scarring and fibrosis will make nerve repair very difficult. If more than 3 weeks elapse before re-exploration and repair, then recovery of abduction will probably not be adequate for airway maintenance in a bilateral nerve injury case. Some recovery of adduction and muscle tone is obviously of value for voice production. Delayed exploration and repair after several months has elapsed is probably not indicated.[24, 25] Observation for signs of recovery is then required for 6 to 8 months before secondary procedures are performed to improve glottic closure.

Injection of Teflon paste generally results

in predictable results and is the treatment of choice for most patients with unilateral recurrent laryngeal nerve paralysis.[20] Alternative procedures to medialize the affected cord, utilizing cartilage implants and grafts, have been reported.[48] Successful reinnervation utilizing nerve-muscle pedicle grafting techniques also have been reported.[20, 48]

BILATERAL INJURY

Bilateral recurrent laryngeal nerve injury as a result of thyroid or parathyroid surgery is fortunately very rare.[17] It is a disastrous complication that will be evident in the immediate postoperative period when the patient is extubated. Both vocal cords are paralyzed in a paramedian position, causing laryngeal airway obstruction. The patient's voice may be normal or exhibit a peculiar monotone interrupted by stridorous inspiration. Inspiratory stridor, cyanosis, and impending asphyxia will lead to emergency reintubation to maintain a satisfactory airway. At this point, consideration should be given to re-exploration of the wound to confirm nerve integrity. Ruling out nerve severance will have important long-term implications regarding laryngeal rehabilitation. Any ligatures or sutures involving the nerves may be removed. Re-exploration of the nerves in a careful, atraumatic manner will not be deleterious and may be of great benefit if correctable nerve injury is found. Stimulation of the main nerve trunk below the level of the thyroid dissection can also help confirm nerve continuity.

Once it is established that the nerves are intact, parenteral steroid therapy may be given in the hope that the acute paralysis is due to surgical edema. Trial extubation, observation, and indirect laryngoscopy after several days will establish whether there is satisfactory vocal cord abduction to provide an adequate airway. If not, tracheotomy will ultimately be necessary. If there is no return of vocal cord function over the next 6 to 12 months, secondary surgical rehabilitation of the larynx will be required. Numerous procedures have been described and include external arytenoidectomy, arytenoidopexy, laryngoscopic arytenoidectomy, cordectomy, laser arytenoidectomy, and nerve-muscle pedicle graft reinnervation techniques.[26, 48] Successful decannulation is the goal of all these various approaches, with preservation of a serviceable voice.

It must be recognized that creation of an adequate glottic airway in this instance will always be detrimental to voice quality; however, the alternative is permanent tracheotomy. Endoscopic laser arytenoidectomy using the technique reported by Ossoff and colleagues is the most satisfactory arytenoid procedure in the management of the patient with bilateral vocal cord paralysis.[60]

SUPERIOR LARYNGEAL NERVE

Anatomy

The superior laryngeal nerve arises from the nodose ganglion of the vagus and descends medial to the carotid sheath on its way to the larynx. It divides into internal and external branches about 2 to 3 cm above the superior thyroid pole. The internal branch enters the larynx through the thyrohyoid membrane and carries sensory and secretory fibers to the supraglottic larynx. The external branch follows the superior thyroid vessels along the investing fascia of the inferior constrictor muscle to the superior thyroid pole, then passes medially into the cricothyroid muscle. It innervates both the inferior constrictor and the cricothyroid muscles. The cricothyroid muscle acts as a tensor of the vocal cord. The external branch of the superior laryngeal nerve has a variable course in relationship to the superior thyroid artery.[47, 56] In about 20 per cent of subjects, the nerve has an intramuscular course in the region of the inferior constrictor muscle, making surgical identification very difficult. About 18 per cent of the nerves pass lateral to the superior thyroid artery or are intertwined with arterial branches in their course to the cricothyroid muscle.

External Branch Injury

Injury to the superior laryngeal nerve during thyroidectomy is probably more common than is generally recognized.[41, 57, 58, 76] It is highly vulnerable during ligation of the superior pole vessels. Massive high-bulk ligation of the superior pole vessels is more likely to result in superior laryngeal nerve injury than separate individual ligation of the vessels close to the superior thyroid pole.[45] Damage to the external branch of the superior laryngeal nerve is less conspicuous and more difficult to diagnose than lesions of the recurrent laryngeal nerve.[43, 76]

The true incidence of superior laryngeal nerve injury in patients with thyroid disorders undergoing surgery is unknown and is probably higher than previously thought. The use of high-speed photography, electromyography, and stroboscopic examination of the larynx has contributed to an understanding of the functional disability associated with injury to this nerve. In unilateral injury, the affected cord remains shorter and at a lower level than the normal cord. When the patient phonates, the glottis will have an asymmetric or oblique appearance. The posterior part of the glottis points toward the paretic side, and the vocal process of the arytenoid will, during phonation, assume a somewhat lower position on the paretic side. Aspiration is usually not a significant problem unless the injury has occurred higher in the neck and also has affected the internal branch of the superior laryngeal nerve. The person's voice may "crack" when shouting, and the singing voice may be permanently impaired. (Other names for this nerve are the "high-note" nerve or the "Amelita Galla Curci" nerve after the famous opera singer whose external laryngeal nerve was injured during a thyroid operation.[14]) Although there is no medical or surgical treatment for the patient with isolated superior laryngeal nerve paralysis, speech therapy may improve voice production. This injury may result in a minor, relatively unnoticeable disability in some, but it may be very significant in the heavy voice user or professional singer.

In bilateral injury, the larynx is symmetric; however, both cords fail to lengthen or tense during phonation. The cords appear flaccid and bowed and allow excess leakage of air during phonation. Bilateral injuries result in a weak, breathy voice with lower pitch. To avoid injury to this nerve, it is best to stay lateral to the cricothyroid muscle and pass clamps around the superior pole vessels in a medial to lateral direction so that the nerve is not caught in the tip of the clamps. Individual vessel ligation close to the superior pole is advised to avoid injury to this nerve. Gentle lateral and downward traction on the superior pole also aids in the dissection.

LARYNGEAL NERVE PARALYSIS

Unilateral Superior and Recurrent Nerves

If both the internal and external branches of the superior laryngeal nerve are paralyzed along with the ipsilateral recurrent laryngeal nerve, the vocal cord will be flaccid, motionless and positioned laterally. Phonation will produce a weak, breathy voice due to air leakage. The airway will be better than that observed with a unilateral recurrent laryngeal nerve paralysis alone, since the affected vocal cord assumes a more lateral position than the typical paramedian position. The affected cord may appear bowed. Phonation produces glottic asymmetry with lengthening and tensing of the normal cord. The paralyzed cord will be at a lower level than the normal cord. The posterior larynx shifts toward the paralyzed side. Aspiration may be severe due to the sensory loss in the ipsilateral supraglottic larynx.

If the internal branch of the superior laryngeal nerve is intact, then the appearance of the larynx will be the same; however, aspiration is usually not a problem. Voice changes and the airway will be similar. Since the affected vocal cord is at a lower level than the normal cord, Teflon injection does not usually achieve a satisfactory glottic closure.

Bilateral Superior and Recurrent Nerves

In combined complete bilateral superior and recurrent laryngeal nerve paralysis, the larynx is motionless, with the cords bowed and in the lateral cadaveric position. The voice is extremely weak and breathy. The airway is adequate, but aspiration is usually so severe that tracheotomy is necessary to manage secretions, and gastrostomy is necessary for feeding.

Ward pointed out that since both recurrent and both superior laryngeal nerves are at risk in total thyroidectomy procedures, a total of 16 possible combinations (4 × 4) of pure paralysis exists.[77] Varying degrees of injury, recovery, and regeneration create a multitude of combinations of paresis and paralysis. It is easy to recognize complete unilateral recurrent laryngeal nerve paralysis by indirect mirror laryngoscopy; however, the more subtle changes of partial paralysis and combined paresis of various laryngeal nerves are difficult to evaluate and require specialized techniques. Using high-speed photography, stroboscopy, and electromyography, Ward has made a significant contribution to the definition and evaluation of laryngeal morbidity secondary to nerve paresis and paralysis.

POSTOPERATIVE HYPOPARATHYROIDISM

Incidence

The reported incidence of permanent hypoparathyroidism after total thyroidectomy varies from 0.4 per cent to 29 per cent.[3, 18, 44, 61, 68, 69] Higher incidence rates are generally found in the older literature. A survey of the recent literature reveals incidence rates of between 0.4 per cent and 4.3 per cent, with a composite rate of 2.4 per cent (Table 16–3). Most workers state that the incidence of this complication should be less than 5 per cent.[3, 4, 27, 31, 50]

Anatomy

Parathyroid glands may be located ectopically anywhere from the angle of the mandible down into the mediastinum; however, they are most commonly adjacent to or within the posterior capsular surface of each thyroid lobe. Autopsy studies reveal four glands in about 84 per cent of subjects, with 13 per cent having more than four glands and 3 per cent having fewer than four glands.[1] Normal glands weigh less than 65 mg, excluding surrounding fat, and average 5 × 3 × 2 mm in size.[74] They are usually oval, bean-shaped, or oblong, although sometimes they are elongated and leaflike. Color varies from light yellow to light chestnut brown or caramel. Parathyroid glands may be located beneath the capsule of the thyroid gland and infrequently are completely within the thyroid lobe. In a study of cadaver thyroid glands, at least one of the parathyroid glands was found to be intrathyroidal 1.3 per cent of the time. In one case of 356 specimens, all four parathyroid glands were found to be within the thyroid parenchyma.[19]

The blood supply to both the superior and inferior glands is from the inferior thyroid artery in 86 per cent of patients.[36] In the remainder, both glands are supplied by the superior thyroid artery or by an anastomotic arch from the superior and inferior thyroid vessels. The superior thyroid may be the sole blood supply to both glands on the right side 0.6 per cent of the time and on the left side 2.8 per cent of the time.[2]

After the middle thyroid vein is divided and the thyroid lobe retracted medially, meticulous dissection of the posterior capsule is necessary to identify the parathyroid glands. This search for parathyroids is carried out simultaneously as the recurrent laryngeal nerve is being carefully exposed. All arterial branches are ligated close to the thyroid capsule. The parathyroid glands are atraumatically swept off the surface of the thyroid gland, preserving as broad a vascular pedicle as possible. Parathyroid glands should not be grasped with a forceps. If a gland is devascularized, it will turn jet black. It should

TABLE 16–3. Incidence of Permanent Hypoparathyroidism After Total Thyroidectomy

	Ref. No.	No. of Patients	Permanent Hypoparathyroidism
Shemen and Strong, 1989	68	64	1
Lore, 1988	50	66	2
Lennquist, 1987	46	197	2
Reeve et al, 1987	65	115	2
Wingert et al, 1986	78	221	9
Harness et al, 1986	37	404	16
VanderSluis and Wobbes, 1985	70	46	2
Karlan et al, 1984	44	457	2
Jacobs et al, 1983	42	213	6
Clark, 1982	13	82	1
Attie and Khafif, 1975	3	249	8
TOTALS		2114	51 (2.4%)

then be removed, diced into small pieces, and transplanted into a suitable muscle. Glands that are separated from their vascular pedicle and glands found by inspecting the resected thyroid specimen are likewise auto-transplanted.[51] Successful preservation of the parathyroid glands is aided by the use of magnifying loupes or the operating microscope. Frozen section confirmation on a small biopsy sample also can be of benefit in questionable situations.

Clinical Course

If the vascular supply to the parathyroid glands is irreversibly compromised or the glands are inadvertently removed, the patient will develop hypocalcemia. Early symptoms develop within 12 hours and may be due in part to the rate of calcium decline rather than the absolute serum level. The earliest symptoms are usually numbness and tingling of the extremities and perioral area, malaise, and anxiety. A reduction in the ionized calcium concentration leads to heightened neuromuscular activity. Tetany or cramping of extremity muscles and carpopedal spasms develop as hypocalcemia worsens. Severe hypocalcemia may lead to laryngeal stridor and generalized convulsions. Anxiety-induced hyperventilation can also produce paresthesias and tetany, so determination of the serum calcium level is important to confirm the presence of hypocalcemia. Facial nerve irritability elicited by tapping over the main nerve trunk anterior to the ear lobe (Chvostek sign) and carpal spasm elicited by occlusion of the arm's arterial blood supply (Trousseau sign) are both reliable clinical tests to detect tetany.

Temporary hypocalcemia is common after both subtotal and total thyroidectomy procedures.[78] Many patients are only mildly symptomatic and hypocalcemia resolves within several weeks to several months. Patients with permanent hypoparathyroidism are those who require continuous calcium and vitamin D to control symptoms lasting beyond 6 months. Patients with hyperthyroidism, medically controlled Graves disease, and thyroid cancer will have a higher incidence of postoperative hypoparathyroidism. Repeat operations and more extensive cancer operations, including neck dissections, increase the incidence of postoperative hypoparathyroidism.

Treatment

Acute severe symptoms should be treated with intravenous calcium. A bolus of 10 ml of a 10 per cent calcium gluconate solution (1 ampule) can be administered slowly over 4 to 5 minutes, or the 10-ml ampule of 10 per cent calcium gluconate can be diluted in 250 to 500 ml of saline and given as a continuous

TABLE 16–4. Oral Calcium Preparations

Proprietary Name	Generic Name	Unit Dosage (mg)	Elemental Calcium (mg)
Tums	Calcium carbonate	500	200
Tums Ex	Calcium carbonate	750	300
Os Cal	Calcium carbonate	500	200
Os Cal 500	Calcium carbonate	1250	500
Os Cal 250 + D	Calcium carbonate + D	625	250 & 125 U vit D
Os Cal 500 + D	Calcium carbonate + D	1250	500 & 125 U vit D
Titralac	Calcium carbonate	400	160
Neo-Calglucon	Calcium glubionate	1 tsp = 1.8 gm	115

drip. Oral calcium therapy in the form of calcium carbonate, calcium lactate, or calcium glubionate is initiated (Table 16–4). Less severe symptoms are easily managed by oral calcium preparations (calcium carbonate, 2 to 12 gm in divided doses, or NEO-Calglucon, 1 to 3 tablespoons three times a day). Serum calcium should be monitored twice daily while the patient is hospitalized. Vitamin D is added to promote intestinal calcium absorption (Table 16–5). In patients with resistant hypocalcemia, aluminum hydroxide gel is given four times daily to bind dietary and intestinal phosphates. Hyperphosphatemia depresses the serum calcium level further. Dairy products and other high-phosphorus foods should be excluded from the diet.

Hypocalcemia will stimulate whatever residual parathyroid tissue is left. It may be advantageous to keep the serum calcium at or slightly below normal during the recovery phase. One should adjust the therapy to relieve the patient's symptoms and prevent hypercalcemia from vitamin D intoxication.

The patient should be stable and free of symptoms on oral therapy at the time of discharge from the hospital. Depending on the severity of the postoperative hypocalcemia, serum calcium may be monitored weekly, bimonthly, and then monthly until the patient is weaned from all medication. This generally takes 8 to 12 weeks in most patients with temporary hypoparathyroidism. If medication is required past 6 months postoperatively, then the condition most likely is permanent.

POSTOPERATIVE HEMORRHAGE

Hemorrhage after thyroidectomy can result in tracheal compression and acute airway obstruction. An arterial bleeder can certainly produce an expanding hematoma within the closed space of the thyroidectomy wound. The trachea in older patients is more commonly calcified and more rigid than in younger patients, in whom it is quite soft and compressible. The presence of a wound drain may signal that excessive bleeding is occurring, but it will not always prevent the development of an expanding hematoma caused by an arterial bleeder. If an expanding hematoma is detected, the wound should be opened immediately to relieve pressure on the trachea and prevent an acute airway obstruction. It may be necessary to open the

TABLE 16–5. Vitamin D Preparations

Proprietary Name	Generic Name	Unit Dosage	Onset of Maximal Action
Ergocalciferol	Vitamin D	1200 mg = 50,000 Units	30 days
Dihydrotachysterol	Dihydrotachysterol	400 mg	15 days
Calciferol	25-Hydroxyvitamin D_3	50 mg	15 days
Rocaltrol	1,25-Dihydroxyvitamin D_3	1 mg	3 days

wound in the recovery room or on the ward and then return the patient to the operating room for an orderly wound exploration to control the bleeding vessel.

The incidence of postoperative hemorrhage that requires wound exploration should be 1 per cent or less.[4, 68, 71]

WOUND INFECTION

This is a rare complication following routine thyroid and parathyroid operations. Incidence rates from 0 to 2 per cent have been reported in the literature; however, most workers feel that an acceptable rate is about 0.2 per cent.[3, 4, 42, 68] Treatment with specific antibiotics, drainage when indicated, and local wound care are essentially the same as in all wound infections.

EXCESS SCAR AND KELOID FORMATION

This is a rare complication of thyroid and parathyroid surgery. Proper incision placement and attention to proper detail in wound closure and management will prevent unsightly scars most of the time. Appropriate treatment may include scar revision and intralesional steroid therapy for keloids.

SPECIAL CONSIDERATIONS IN PARATHYROID SURGERY

Primary Hyperparathyroidism

The overall success rate for the surgical treatment of primary hyperparathyroidism is between 95 and 97 per cent.[11, 64] In patients who undergo removal of a single adenoma, the incidence of persistent or recurrent hyperparathyroidism is 1 per cent, and the incidence of permanent hypoparathyroidism

is less than 0.5 per cent.[66] Among patients undergoing subtotal parathyroidectomy for multiple gland involvement, persistent or recurrent disease occurs in about 8 per cent of patients without multiple endocrine neoplasia syndromes and in as many as 30 to 50 per cent of patients with multiple endocrine neoplasia syndrome type 1.[8, 63] The incidence of permanent hypoparathyroidism after this operation is about 3.4 per cent.[66]

As in repeat thyroidectomy procedures, reexploration for recurrent or persistent hyperparathyroidism is likewise associated with increased technical risks and therefore higher complication rates. The most common complication of reoperative parathyroid surgery is permanent hypoparathyroidism.[29, 75] Reported to occur in 10 per cent or more of cases, it usually occurs because the normal parathyroid glands have been devascularized or removed in the first operation in the mistaken belief that they are hyperplastic, and then subsequent removal of the elusive and often ectopic adenoma removes the last functioning parathyroid tissue.[10, 35] Parathyroid autotransplantation of tumor grafts into the forearm musculature eventually can result in a eucalcemic state. If tissue cryopreservation facilities are available, some of the tumor can be saved for eventual transplantation if necessary. Recurrent hypercalcemia due to hyperplasia of the parathyroid implant can be controlled by subtotal resection under local anesthesia.

Secondary Hyperparathyroidism

Secondary hyperparathyroidism with varying degrees of parathyroid hyperplasia is present in most, if not all, patients with chronic renal failure. Chronic hypocalcemia is the major stimulus for parathyroid hyperplasia. Phosphate and magnesium retention, altered vitamin D metabolism, decreased calcium absorption in the intestine, skeletal resistance to the hypercalcemic action of parathyroid hormone, and impaired degradation of parathyroid hormone are associated factors that lead to the development of secondary hyperparathyroidism. Skeletal complications (renal osteodystrophy) include immobilizing bone pain, skeletal deformities, progressive bone demineralization, and fractures. Medical management is effective in controlling most cases of secondary hyperparathyroidism; however, approximately 5 per cent to 10 per cent require surgical treatment because of symptoms or metabolic complications.[15] Indications for parathyroidectomy include severe pruritus, extensive soft tissue calcifications, calciphylaxis, bone pain, spontaneous bone fractures, psychoneurologic disorders, a serum calcium level × phosphate level product consistently greater than 70, and a serum calcium level greater than 11 mg/dl.[16, 59]

Subtotal parathyroidectomy, removing 3.5 glands, and total parathyroidectomy with autotransplantation are equally successful procedures.[7, 52] All four, or more, parathyroid glands are exposed and examined before any are removed. Removal of the thymus gland is recommended because as many as 15 per cent of patients with hyperplastic glands will have a fifth parathyroid gland, and about 10 per cent of patients with hyperparathyroidism will have parathyroid glands within the thymus.[53] After examining all the glands, the most normal-sized parathyroid gland is subtotally resected, preserving about 50 mg (the size of a normal parathyroid gland) of tissue. This remnant is marked with a hemostatic clip, and it is observed for viability before all the other glands are resected. If total parathyroidectomy with autotransplantation is planned, then multiple diced 1-mm fragments of parathyroid tissue are placed into separate muscle pockets on the nondominant forearm at a site not required for future hemodialysis.

Patients who have increased serum alkaline phosphatase levels and severe renal osteodystrophy are more likely to develop tetany following parathyroidectomy because of "bone hunger" for calcium.[40] Considerable calcium supplementation is usually required both intravenously and orally as calcium and phosphate are being deposited back into the mineral-depleted bones. Frequent monitoring of serum calcium, potassium, phosphate, and magnesium levels is necessary during the postoperative stabilization period.

OPERATIVE MORTALITY

Foster surveyed 24,108 thyroid operations performed during 1970 and reported 72 deaths, for an overall operative mortality of 0.3 per cent.[33] This was estimated to be one third of all the thyroid operations performed in the United States for that year. Mortality increased with age, being less than 0.1 per cent for those younger than 50 years of age and 2 per cent for those 70 years of age and older. Only one death occurred in the 3442 thyroidectomy patients surveyed in the recent literature (see Table 16–2), for an operative death rate of 0.03 per cent. The mortality rate probably cannot be expected to reach zero since an occasional death will inevitably occur from causes unrelated to the operation or anesthetic. Rarely a death may occur in the immediate postoperative period owing to acute airway compromise secondary to hemorrhage. A number of workers state that the operative death rate from thyroid-parathyroid surgery should be 0.1 per cent or less.[4, 13, 27, 31, 37, 42, 44, 50, 70, 71]

References

1. Akerstrom G, Malmaeus J, Bergstrom R: Surgical anatomy of human parathyroid glands. Surgery 95:14, 1984.
2. Alveryd A: Parathyroid glands in thyroid surgery. I. Anatomy of parathyroid glands. II. Postoperative hypoparathyroidism—identification and autotransplantation of parathyroid glands. Acta Chir Scand Suppl 389:1–120, 1968.
3. Attie JN, Khafif RA: Preservation of parathyroid glands during total thyroidectomy. Am J Surg 130:399–404, 1975.
4. Beahrs OH: Complications in thyroid and parathyroid surgery. In Conley JJ (ed): Complications of Head and Neck Surgery. Philadelphia, WB Saunders, 1979, pp 239–245.
5. Beahrs OH, Vandertoll DJ: Complications of secondary thyroidectomy. Surg Gynecol Obstet 117:535–539, 1963.
6. Bernedes J, Miehlke A: Repair of the recurrent laryngeal nerve and phonation: Basic considerations and techniques. Int Surg 49:319–329, 1968.
7. Blake DP, O'Brien TJ, Smith CL, et al: Surgical treatment of renal hyperparathyroidism. Surg Gynecol Obstet 157:325–331, 1983.
8. Block MA, Frame B, Kleerekoper M, et al: Surgical management of persistence or recurrence after subtotal parathyroidectomy for primary hyperparathyroidism. Am J Surg 138:561–566, 1979.
9. Brandwein M, Abramson AL, Shikowitz MJ: Bilat-

eral vocal cord paralysis following endotracheal intubation. Arch Otolaryngol Head Neck Surg 112:877–882, 1986.

10. Brennan MF, Norton JA: Reoperation for persistent and recurrent hyperparathyroidism. Ann Surg 201:40–44, 1985.

11. Bruining HA, VanHouten H, Juttman JR, et al: Results of operative treatment of 615 patients with primary hyperparathyroidism. World J Surg 5:85–89, 1981.

12. Calabro S, Auguste L, Attie JN: Morbidity of completion of thyroidectomy for initially misdiagnosed thyroid carcinoma. Head Neck Surg 10:235–238, 1988.

13. Clark OH: Total thyroidectomy: The treatment of choice for patients with differentiated thyroid cancer. Ann Surg 196:361–370, 1982.

14. Clark OH: Endocrine Surgery of the Thyroid and Parathyroid Glands. St. Louis, CV Mosby, 1985, p 268.

15. Clark OH: Endocrine Surgery of the Thyroid and Parathyroid Glands. St. Louis, CV Mosby, 1985, p 241.

16. Clark OH: Secondary and tertiary hyperparathyroidism. In Najarian JS, Delaney JP (eds): Endocrine Surgery. New York, Symposia Specialists Inc Publications, 1980, p 239.

17. Colcock BP, King ML: The mortality and morbidity of thyroid surgery. Surg Gynecol Obstet 114:131, 1962.

18. Crile G, Antunez AR, Esselstyn CB, et al: The advantages of subtotal thyroidectomy and suppression of TSH in the primary treatment of papillary carcinoma of the thyroid. Cancer 55:2691–2697, 1985.

19. Croyle PH, Oldroyd JJ: Incidental parathyroidectomy during thyroid surgery. Am J Surg 44:559–563, 1978.

20. Crumley RL: Update of laryngeal reinnervation; concepts and options. In Bailey BJ, Biller HF (eds): Surgery of the Larynx. Philadelphia, WB Saunders, 1985.

21. Doyle PJ: Surgical treatment of bilateral abductor laryngeal paralysis. Proc Can Otol Soc 18:68–75, 1964.

22. Doyle PJ, Everts EC, Brummett RE: Treatment of recurrent laryngeal nerve injury. Arch Surg 96:517–520, 1968.

23. Doyle PJ: Recurrent laryngeal nerve repair. Proceedings of the IX International Congress of Oto-Rhino-Laryngology, Mexico City. Excerpta Medica, 1970, p 297.

24. Doyle PJ: Vocal Cord Paralysis. American Academy of Otolaryngology, Continuing Education Manual, 1979.

25. Doyle PJ: Personal communication, 1990.

26. Doyle PJ, Morrison MD, Schramm VL: Management of the patient with vocal cord paralysis. American Academy of Otolaryngology, Continuing Education Manual, In press.

27. Edis AJ, Beahrs OH: Surgery of the thyroid gland. In Lore JM Jr (ed): Head and Neck Surgery. Philadelphia, Harper and Row, 1982.

28. Edis AJ: Prevention and management of complications associated with thyroid and parathyroid surgery. Surg Clin North Am 59:83–92, 1979.

29. Edis AJ, Sheedy PF II, Beahrs OH, et al: Results of reoperation for hyperparathyroidism, with evalua-

tion of preoperative localization studies. Surgery 84:384–393, 1978.

30. Ezaki H, Ushio H, Harada Y, Takeichi N: Recurrent laryngeal nerve anastomosis following thyroid surgery. World J Surg 6:342–346, 1982.

31. Farrar WB: Complications of thyroidectomy. Surg Clin North Am 63:1353–1361, 1983.

32. Fenton RS: The surgical complications of thyroidectomy. J Otolaryngol 12:104–106, 1983.

33. Foster RS Jr: Morbidity and mortality after thyroidectomy. Surg Gynecol Obstet 146:423–429, 1978.

34. Friedman M, Toriumi DM, Grybauskas V, Katz A: Nonrecurrent laryngeal nerves and their clinical significance. Laryngoscope 96:87–90, 1986.

35. Grant CS, VanHeerden JA, Charboneau JW, et al: Clinical management of persistent and/or recurrent primary hyperparathyroidism. World J Surg 10:555–565, 1986.

36. Halstead WS, Evans HM: The parathyroid glandules. Their blood supply and their preservation in operation upon the thyroid gland. Ann Surg 46:489–506, 1907.

37. Harness JK, Fung L, Thompson NW, et al: Total thyroidectomy: Complications and technique. World J Surg 10:781–786, 1986.

38. Holl-Allen RTJ: A new approach to the surgical management of paralysis of the laryngeal nerve after thyroidectomy. Surg Gynecol Obstet 163:543–546, 1986.

39. Horseley JS: Suture of the recurrent laryngeal nerve with report of a case. Trans South Surg Gynecol Assoc 22:161, 1909.

40. Hruska KA, et al: The predictability of the histologic features of uremic bone disease by noninvasive techniques. Metab Bone Dis Relat Res 1:39, 1978.

41. Hunt CJ: The superior and inferior laryngeal nerve as related to thyroid surgery. Am Surg 27:548–552, 1961.

42. Jacobs JK, Aland JW, Ballinger JF: Total thyroidectomy—A review of 213 patients. Ann Surg 197:542–549, 1983.

43. Jansson S, Tisell LE, Hague I, et al: Partial superior laryngeal nerve lesions before and after thyroid surgery. World J Surg 12:522–527, 1988.

44. Karlan MS, Catz B, Dunkelman D, et al: A safe technique for thyroidectomy with complete nerve dissection and parathyroid preservation. Head Neck Surg 6:1014–1019, 1984.

45. Lekalos NL, Miligos ND, Tzardis PJ, et al: The superior laryngeal nerve in thyroidectomy. Am Surg 53:610–612, 1987.

46. Lennquist S: The thyroid nodule: Diagnosis and surgical treatment. Surg Clin North Am 67:213–232, 1987.

47. Lennquist S, Cahlin C, Smeds S: The superior laryngeal nerve in thyroid surgery. Surgery 102:999–1008, 1987.

48. Levine HL, Tucker HM: Surgical management of the paralyzed larynx. In Bailey BJ, Biller HF (eds): Surgery of the Larynx. Philadelphia, WB Saunders, 1985.

49. Lore JM Jr: Practical anatomical considerations in thyroid tumor surgery. Arch Otolaryngol 109:568–574, 1983.

50. Lore JM Jr: Atlas of Head and Neck Surgery. 3rd ed. Philadelphia, WB Saunders, 1988, p 738.

51. Lore JM Jr, Pruet CW: Retrieval of the parathyroid

glands during thyroidectomy. Head Neck Surg 5:268–269, 1983.

52. Malmaeus J, Akerstrom G, Johansson H, et al: Parathyroid surgery in chronic renal insufficiency: Subtotal parathyroidectomy versus total parathyroidectomy with autotransplantation to the forearm. Acta Chir Scand 148:229–238, 1982.

53. Malmaeus J: Secondary hyperparathyroidism in chronic renal failure. Scand J Urol Nephrol (Suppl) 70:1, 1983.

54. Martensson H, Terins J: Recurrent laryngeal nerve palsy in thyroid gland surgery related to operations and nerves at risk. Arch Surg 120:475–477, 1985.

55. Mazzaferri EL, Young RL, Oertel JE, et al: Papillary thyroid carcinoma: The impact of therapy in 576 patients. Medicine 56:171–196, 1977.

56. Mooseman DA, DeWeese MS: The external laryngeal nerve as related to thyroidectomy. Surg Gynecol Obstet 126:1011–1016, 1968.

57. Moran RE, Castro AF: The superior laryngeal nerve in thyroid surgery. Ann Surg 134:1018–1021, 1951.

58. Newman AN, Becker SP: Superior laryngeal nerve paralysis and benign thyroid disease. Arch Otolaryngol Head Neck Surg 107:117–119, 1981.

59. Ogg CS: Parathyroidectomy in the treatment of secondary renal hyperparathyroidism. Kidney Int 4:168, 1973.

60. Ossoff RH, Sisson GA, Moselle HI, et al: Endoscopic laser arytenoidectomy for the treatment of bilateral vocal cord paralysis. Laryngoscope 94:1293–1297, 1984.

61. Perzik SL: The place of total thyroidectomy in the management of 909 patients with thyroid disease. Am J Surg 132:480–483, 1976.

62. Peters LL, Gardner RJ: Repair of recurrent laryngeal nerve injuries. Surgery 71:865–867, 1972.

63. Prinz RA, Gamvros OI, Sellu D, et al: Subtotal parathyroidectomy for primary chief cell hyperplasia of the multiple endocrine neoplasia type I syndromes. Ann Surg 193:26–29, 1981.

64. Purnell DC, Scholz DA, Beahrs OH: Hyperparathyroidism due to single gland enlargement: Prospective postoperative study. Arch Surg 112:369–372, 1977.

65. Reeve TS, Delbridge L, Cohen A, Crummer P: Total thyroidectomy. Ann Surg 206:782–786, 1987.

66. Rossi RL, ReMine SG, Clerkin EP: Hyperparathyroidism. Surg Clin North Am 65:187–209, 1985.

67. Sato F, Ogura JH: Neurorrhaphy of the recurrent laryngeal nerve. Laryngoscope 88:1034–1041, 1978.

68. Shemen LJ, Strong EW: Complications after total thyroidectomy. Otolaryngol Head Neck Surg 101:472–475, 1989.

69. Thompson NW, Olsen WR, Hoffman GL: The continuing development of the technique of thyroidectomy. Surgery 73:913–927, 1973.

70. VanderSluis RF, Wobbes T: Total thyroidectomy: The treatment of choice in differential thyroid carcinoma? Eur J Surg Oncol 11:343–346, 1985.

71. VanHeerden JA, Groh MA, Grant CS: Early postoperative morbidity after surgical treatment of thyroid carcinoma. Surgery 101:224–227, 1987.

72. Waldstein SS: Medical complications of thyroid surgery. Otolaryngol Clin North Am 13:99–107, 1980.

73. Wang C: The use of the inferior cornu of the thyroid cartilage in identifying the recurrent laryngeal nerve. Surg Gynecol Obstet 140:91–94, 1975.

74. Wang CA: The anatomic basis of parathyroid surgery. Ann Surg 183:271–275, 1976.

75. Wang CA: Parathyroid re-exploration: A clinical and pathological study of 112 cases. Ann Surg 186:140–145, 1977.

76. Ward PH, Berci G, Calcaterra TL: Superior laryngeal nerve paralysis: An often overlooked entity. Trans Acad Ophthalmol Otolaryngol 84:78–89, 1977.

77. Ward PH: Complications of thyroid surgery: Their prevention, recognition and management. In Chretien PB, Johns ME, Shedd DP, et al (eds): Head and Neck Cancer. St. Louis, CV Mosby, 1985, pp 247–251.

78. Wingert DJ, Friesen SR, Iliopoulous JI, et al: Postthyroidectomy hypocalcemia: Incidence and risk factors. Ann J Surg 152:606–610, 1986.

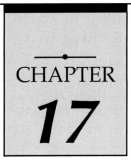

Laryngeal Surgery

YOSEF P. KRESPI, MD
UMANG KHETARPAL, MD

As with any other cancer, the surgical management of laryngeal cancer necessitates complete extirpation of the tumor. A significant change in the surgical management of laryngeal cancer over the last century has been the shift from total laryngectomy to conservation partial laryngectomy. The increasing enthusiasm for this is because this treatment is "radical" and at the same time preserves laryngeal function, resulting in an intact upper respiratory tract. The amount of larynx that can be preserved depends on the extent of the tumor and its location. It is estimated that up to 70 per cent of all laryngeal cancers are amenable to conservation procedures.[1, 2] The spectrum of conservation laryngeal and laryngopharyngeal surgery is large, ranging from minimal excisions like vocal cord stripping, partial cordectomy, and epiglottectomy to subtotal or near total laryngectomy and partial laryngopharyngectomy.

A greater tumor burden is associated with a greater extent of surgery and a larger number of complications.[3–5] Although Schechter[2] estimates the overall complication rate after supraglottic laryngectomy at 10 per cent, other workers report rates of up to 50 per cent after supraglottic laryngectomy (SGL) and its modifications.[4, 6–8] For vertical partial laryngectomy, the complication rate appears to be somewhat lower, varying from 1.5 per cent to 26 per cent.[2, 9–11] Most reports of both horizontal and vertical partial resections do not include minor complications like wound infection, asymptomatic aspiration, or poor voice in their reporting. It is not surprising that surgical craftsmanship and experience also affect the overall results. Generally, although not always, the incidence of complications is higher when radiation therapy is used as an adjunct to operation. The perioperative mortality rate varies from 0 to 6 per cent and is attributed to myocardial dysfunction; severe bleeding from the wound, carotid, or stomach; acute pulmonary edema; wound infection; and septicemia.[6–8, 11–13]

Prevention of complications starts at the preoperative stage. Patient selection is of primary importance. Patient evaluation must include accurate assessment of the lesion and its extent, lymphadenopathy, cord mobility, and associated aspiration, regurgitation, or swallowing disorders. Voice analysis and a visit to the speech therapist are helpful in providing baseline information, in building a rapport between the therapist and the patient, and in postoperative speech and swallowing rehabilitation. Radiologic studies include laryngeal contrast radiography, computed tomography scan or magnetic resonance imaging for tumor mapping, chest radiograph, and barium swallow to rule out any associated swallowing disorders or other primary lesions. Endoscopic evaluation of the upper aerodigestive tract is mandatory. Alcohol consumption and smoking should be curbed preoperatively. Cardiovascular, nutritional, and metabolic problems, such as diabetes, hypertension, and liver dysfunction, should be evaluated and treated prior to surgery. In conservation surgery, the patient's psychologic and physiologic fitness is of greater merit than the chronologic age.[1] Assessment of pulmonary function (PFT) is done using flow loop studies and spirometry. Some workers propose that patients with 50 per cent to 60 per cent of their predicted pulmonary function should not undergo this type of surgery.[14, 15] Controversy exists about the predictive value of these percentages and PFTs on the whole. Chow and associates reported that FEV_1, vital capacity, and COPD (chronic obstructive pulmonary disease) did not reliably predict the postoperative pulmonary complications after partial laryngectomy.[16]

Ogura suggested that the "stairs" test is a more reliable clinical indicator of lung function.[17] Flores and associates stated that PFTs are needed only when there is a serious ventilatory impairment detected from history or physical examination.[18] Therefore, clinical assessment of patients' pulmonary status should remain the major method in evaluating potential candidates for a partial laryngeal procedure. Although pulmonary function tests may provide additional information, their predictive value needs to be confirmed by well-designed prospective clinical trials.

The complications associated with conservation laryngeal surgery can be classified broadly into general and specific. General complications may occur after any major head and neck procedure and include wound infections, fistulas, hemorrhage, keloids, and systemic complications. Specific complications include those specific to conservation laryngeal surgery, such as glottic insufficiency, aspiration, postoperative voice poorer than predicted, web formation, and deglutition problems.

PHONATORY PROBLEMS

Voice quality depends on the subject's ability to generate adequate subglottic pressure and on properly vibrating vocal cords, the primary phonatory structures. Sphincteric function of the supraglottic structures provides adjunctive phonatory function by augmenting the phonatory pressure and enabling the cord to vibrate better.[19] Aggressive stripping of the cord results in scarring of Reinke space, atrophy, and poor mobility of the vocal cord mucosa. Following cordectomy, the larynx compensates for the nonvibrating cord by hyperkinesia of the supraglottic folds. The compensatory hyperkinesia may result in supraglottic hypertrophy or constriction.[19, 20] However, in attempting to preserve the vibratory mechanism in the glottic area, the supraglottic sphincter may act as a generator of noise, thereby disturbing the phonatory effect. After supraglottic laryngectomy (SGL), the loss of adjunctive phonatory function of the supraglottic structures results in a subnormal voice, even in the presence of a normal glottis. Supraglottic webbing or constriction at the base tongue suture line may worsen the voice further. Avoidance of tight wound closure could obviate this possible complication. Frequently, the postoperative voice quality is complicated by the development of granulation tissue, scar formation, glottic incompetence, and paralysis of laryngeal nerves.

Our review of voice results in the literature is hampered by the lack of detailed stroboscopic and spectral analysis. Many workers, using entirely arbitrary subjective criteria, report their results as excellent, good, fair, functional, or intelligible in a large majority of their cases. Neel and associates documented a 3.3 per cent poor voice rate after vertical partial laryngectomy (VPL) or cordectomy.[11] In extended VPL, the arytenoid may be resected in addition to one or both cords. This tissue loss results in an adynamic healed hemilarynx and a voice poorer than normal. Guerrier and Jazouli stated that the voice quality in their patients usually ranged from medium to excellent.[10] The criteria used in these studies were not mentioned. Vega subjectively assessed postoperative voice quality and reported that 86.5 per cent of his patients had a "good" voice, 8.5 per cent a "fair" voice, and 5 per cent a "bad" voice.[21] However, Kittel estimated that almost 80 per cent of Vega's patients would have moderate or severe dysphonia according to an objective dysphonia scale.[19] Tucker and associates reported that 60 per cent of their patients had a hoarse but functional voice after near-total laryngectomy with epiglottic reconstruction. A more objective assessment came from Moore, who stated that in almost all cases of vertical partial laryngectomy and in many cases of supraglottic laryngectomy the voice is poorer than normal.[23] The need to standardize criteria for comparing voice results is therefore great.

It is generally believed that reconstruction of the glottic region can improve glottic and supraglottic function even though the reconstructed substitute is unable to vibrate. In all cases of vertical partial laryngectomy and extended supraglottic laryngectomy, fixation of the sacrificed cord, arytenoid, or neocord in the midline is an important step that may minimize glottic insufficiency and poor voice. A compendium of techniques are available for neocord reconstruction. Laryngoplasty methods for arytenoid/cord replacement include, among others, sternohyoid muscle flaps; free and pedicled muscle insertion using omohyoid, digastric, or palmaris brevis tendons; omohyoid musculo-osseous insertion; thyroid cartilage–inferior constrictor muscle transfer; thyroid cartilage perichondrium; and pedicled skin flaps.[19, 24–31] Commonly used techniques for resurfacing the

neocord include skin grafts and pedicled flaps, mucosal flaps from the piriform sinus and postcricoid area, as well as cervical fascia grafts and flaps. The sternohyoid fascia has been claimed as an excellent surfacing material because of its ability to resist postoperative complications and decrease the incidence of granulation tissue formation.[32] The objective of resurfacing the neocord is to simulate the vocal cord mucosa for vibration. In most cases, however, the resurfacing material tethers to the underlying tissue because of scarring, making it a poor substitute. Krajina showed that the new fold formed after laser cordectomy vibrated synchronously and in phase with the contralateral normal vocal fold.[33] Although its amplitude was shorter and varying degrees of hoarseness were observed, the glottal periodicity was preserved in all six operated cases. That laser usage may be associated with lesser scarring and better neocord function remains to be confirmed by other objective studies.

The sacrifice of anterior commissure in frontal and frontolateral partial laryngectomy results in shortening of the glottis and loss of anterior support. The larger and deeper male larynx can tolerate this more easily than the small and broad female larynx.[34] In either sex, attempts must be made to reconstruct the anterior angle and anteroposterior diameter.[2] Anterior commissure reconstitution has been attempted using pedicled skin flaps, mucosal grafts, and cartilage and bone grafts, with marginal success. The epiglottic reconstruction technique reportedly has been more successful than others because it is a one-stage operation, providing excellent support as well as a mucosa-lined lumen.[35–38] The amount of epiglottis used depends on the extent of cordal and commissure resection.

Other intraoperative surgical maneuvers that may improve phonatory results are reattachment of the base of the epiglottis after extralaryngeal cordectomy[39] and reconstitution of the violated cricothyroid or thyrohyoid membrane with connective tissue.[39, 40] Due to cartilage resorption and muscle atrophy, secondary glottic reconstruction with cartilage or muscle implants is frequently unsuccessful.[2] Therefore, if glottoplasty is to be effective, it should be performed along with the primary surgery. Recently, thyroplasty procedures designed for phonatory improvement appear promising. Teflon injection of the vocal cords has met with marginal success. Preservation of the laryngeal and glossopharyngeal nerves enhances postsurgical phoniatric treatment. Postoperatively, all patients should be followed up with a phoniatrist for serial voice analysis and phonatory rehabilitation. The latter perhaps is the most crucial step in postoperative vocal recovery.

ASPIRATION AND GLOTTIC INSUFFICIENCY

The removal of a cord, hemilarynx, or more laryngeal tissue after vertical partial resections results in an abnormally large glottic chink, which allows air escape, aspiration, and breathiness of voice. The loss of supraglottic sphincteric function after supraglottic laryngectomy increases the potential for aspiration. In patients with good pulmonary reserve and adequate cough reflex, it is a matter of time before the glottis compensates for the loss of this adjunctive protective and phonatory tissue. In elderly patients and those with borderline pulmonary function, this process may be somewhat prolonged. The greater the sacrifice of laryngeal sphincters, the greater the predisposition to aspiration. Unless the anatomic potential for glottic closure is surgically restored by reconstruction and until the patient compensates for the inadequacy or learns to use the newly fashioned structures, aspiration remains a threat.[34] All patients undergoing conservation surgery aspirate to some extent.[34] In most patients the aspiration is mild and short-lived, allowing decannulation 1 to 3 weeks after surgery. Prolonged aspiration in others results in longer hospitalization and may necessitate extended nasogastric feeding or gastrostomy. Persistent severe aspiration with recurrent bouts of pneumonia may require, in a few cases, additional procedures to prevent aspiration or a completion laryngectomy.[34, 41]

The incidence of aspiration varies with the extent of arytenoid resection, tongue base excision, the success of reconstruction, and a prior history of radiation.[4, 34, 42–44] Other factors believed to contribute to aspiration are paralysis of laryngeal, hypoglossal, and pharyngeal branches of the vagus nerve, improper healing leading to granulation or scarring, and glottic edema from inflammation or radiation.[34] Ward and associates investigated the etiologic role of these factors in aspiration following conservation laryngeal surgery.[45] They concluded that paralysis of the superior or recurrent laryngeal nerves is one of the major causes. The external branch of the superior laryngeal nerve (SLN) innervates the cricothyroid muscle, which is responsible for tilting the thyroid cartilage upon the cricoid cartilage and for tensing and indirectly adducting the vocal cord, thus minimizing aspiration. The surgeon must make every effort to identify and preserve all branches of the superior and recurrent laryngeal nerves not involved by tumor. Preserving the external branch of the SLN is of primary importance during supraglottic laryngectomy.

Since many investigators include only severe aspiration with lung infection in their complications, it is difficult to determine the true incidence of aspiration. Additionally, the incidence of aspiration varies with the criteria used: clinical, endoscopic, or radiologic. The reported aspiration rate varies from 0 after cordectomy to 20 per cent after vertical partial laryngectomy.[2, 9, 11] Som[46] and Bocca[47] reported a 2.1 per cent and 1.2 per cent aspiration rate, respectively, after standard supraglottic laryngectomy. Other workers report a 4 to 41 per cent incidence of aspiration after SGL and its modifications.[2, 6, 8, 13, 48] A radiologic study using cineradiography and manometry documented a 34 per cent aspiration rate in horizontal partial laryngectomees.[49] In Pearson's series of near-total laryngectomy, the true incidence of aspiration was 29 per cent, whereas that of symptomatic aspiration was 12 per cent.[50] Tucker and associates reported a 22 per cent incidence of chronic aspiration and a 4 per cent rate of aspiration pneumonia in their near-total laryngectomy series.[22]

Although laryngeal reconstruction is frequently advocated to minimize glottic insufficiency-aspiration and its sequelae, no single surgical procedure has been uniformly agreed upon. As mentioned in the section on phonation, numerous techniques are available for replacement of the sacrificed cord and/or arytenoid. Those used more commonly include free and pedicled muscle transfers, cartilage grafts (helical, rib, thyroid), composite cartilage-muscle flaps, mucosal advancement, and rotation flaps and bone grafts. Resurfacing the reconstructed hemilarynx or arytenoid may be done using skin, hypopharyngeal mucosa, dermis, or cervical fascia. Denecke states that the use of skin and mucosal grafts has not proven effective in the long term and advocates the use of pedicled flaps in an area constantly subject to movement due to breathing, coughing, and swallowing.[31] He also suggests that in larger defects, where pedicled cervical skin and subcutaneous tissue flaps are used, a strip of thyroid cartilage may have to be resected to prevent postoperative compression of pedicle between the cartilage edges.

Teflon injections for glottic insufficiency have not proved useful because of extensive scarification and lack of potential space for augmentation. Cartilage implantation has been more successful. After supraglottic laryngectomy, one of the major causes of aspiration is the failure of the larynx to elevate toward the tongue base. Attempts to suspend the larynx during operation have had partial success.[51, 52] Good wound closure and modified SGL with preservation of hyoid or suprahyoid musculature may enhance laryngeal elevation during deglutition. In problem cases an infrahyoid/sternothyroid myotomy may help by canceling the unopposed downward laryngeal pull of these muscles.

To minimize aspiration, particular attention must be paid to oral rehabilitation following any conservation surgery. The time of removal of the nasogastric feeding tube varies between studies from 3 to 10 days and also with the extent of the operation. The process of re-educating the patient for swallowing is soon begun (10 to 14 days).[7] Radio-logic studies have shown that aspiration occurs more readily with liquids than with foods of thick consistency.[53] It is therefore necessary that patients be told to swallow liquids forcefully and rapidly. The patient also should be discouraged from using a straw or nibbling food. Vega recommends that during the process of swallowing re-education, the patient should receive only oral foods that dissolve after entering the bronchial tree, e.g., boiled potatoes.[7] Kothary and Dev recommend eating smaller amounts of food and initiating a cough at the end of each swallow.[40] Since the laryngeal sensations may be partially sacrificed during any conservation surgery, it may help to recruit the assistance of oropharyngeal and hypopharyngeal sensations by eating foods that have extremes of temperature, taste, and texture.[2] Decannulation prior to oral rehabilitation is important as it allows the generation of adequate subglottic pressure for coughing and also adequate elevation of the larynx during deglutition.

LATE GLOTTIC INSUFFICIENCY

Delayed postoperative glottic incompetence may be due to a number of factors. The reconstructive techniques used may be unsuccessful due to inadequate reconstruction. Over a period of time the muscular flaps may undergo atrophy. Where the resected hemilarynx or cord was not reconstructed primarily, healing by secondary intention may be inadequate, allowing laryngeal spillover and air escape if the contralateral normal cord does not compensate. Where cartilaginous grafts have been utilized, the cartilage may become infected or resorbed or may have been placed too far laterally. After partial arytenoid resection, the arytenoid remnant resurfaced with a mucosal flap may fibrose to the thyroid lamina and produce a V-shaped posterior glottic defect.[54] Postoperative radiation may lead to perichondritis and chondritis with resorption or necrosis. Cricoarytenoid joint fixation may occur in postsurgical irradiated patients. Occasionally late intralaryngeal granuloma formation[55] may lead to airway obstruction, glottic insufficiency, and delayed vocal recovery. However, this pathology is usually short-lived and in the majority of patients resolves spontaneously.

Czigner reported a 3 per cent incidence of permanent or late laryngeal incompetence after supraglottic laryngectomy.[8] Krajina indicated that late glottic insufficiency occurring after 6 months was seen in 1.2 per cent of patients after vertical partial resections (with or without radiation) and in 6.4 per cent of patients after combined partial resection (three quarter laryngectomy) with or without radiation.[56] Accurate incidence estimation necessitates prolonged follow-up and a meticulous search for late glottic complications.

As mentioned, Teflon injection of the neocord has been largely unsuccessful due to tethering of mucosa to underlying tissue and the possibility of infection after extrusion of the injected material.[23, 54] Various surgically corrective approaches have been described by different workers and are briefly reviewed here. For overall glottic incompetence (anterior and posterior), placement of cartilaginous graft in the inner subperichondrial pocket of the thyroid cartilage at the level of the true cord has been effective in medializing the neocord. Access to the thyroid cartilage internal perichondrium may be achieved through the cricothyroid space[57] or via an anterior thyrotomy.[58] The cartilage graft may be obtained from the thyroid cartilage[57, 58] or the costal cartilage.[59] The exact placement of the implant is confirmed by direct laryngoscopy. One technique for posterior glottic incompetence correction is mobilization and medial repositioning of the laterally placed arytenoid.[60] The medialized arytenoid is then fixed to the cricoid cartilage with permanent sutures at or just beyond the midline. Creating a bed for the medialized arytenoid by removing a small piece of cricoid cartilage at the same level as the contralateral normal arytenoid may be beneficial. Biller and associates advocated placing a thyroid cartilage graft, contoured like an arytenoid, in the subperichondrial pocket of the cricoid carti-

lage to correct posterior glottic incompetence.[61] The steps of the operation are (1) cutting the inferior constrictor, (2) disarticulating the cricothyroid joint, and (3) elevating the piriform sinus mucosa to expose the posterior body of cricoid cartilage. (4) A subperichondrial pocket is then dissected and (5) the cartilage implant is fixed in the midline by 28-gauge stainless steel wire. Biller and associates reported successful use of this technique in four of six patients with posterior glottic insufficiency. When aspiration persists despite primary and secondary reconstruction with cartilage grafts, Biller and Urken have successfully employed the cricoid collapse technique.[62] In principle, this technique corrects the glottic incompetence by segmentation of the hemicricoid on the affected side, resulting in its collapse and a narrowed glottis. This operation was successful in all four of their patients.

In a very small number of cases, all secondary reconstructive techniques may fail in controlling persistent aspiration and recurrent pulmonary complications. Complete diversion of the airway from the food passage may be necessary. Finally, completion laryngectomy may be indicated to prevent deadly pulmonary complications.

PULMONARY COMPLICATIONS

There is little doubt that patients who have had a successful partial laryngectomy are in a better functional and psychologic state than those who have had a total laryngectomy. The case for functional partial laryngectomy is therefore very strong. However, most proponents of partial laryngectomy stress the difficulty encountered in preventing its specific postoperative complications, such as laryngeal spillover and deglutition problems. Aspiration of saliva and food particles into the tracheobronchial tree may lead to acute and chronic pneumonitis, atelectasis, progressive chronic fibrosis, worsening of preexisting chronic bronchitis, and development of lung abscess. If left untreated, pulmonary insufficiency, debilitation, and death may ensue. Although the study of Chow and associates[16] showed poor correlation between pulmonary function tests and postoperative pulmonary complications, it is generally believed that smokers and patients with poor pulmonary reserve are at higher risk of pulmonary complications.

Although it is commonly believed that "extended" partial laryngectomies, which include the arytenoid and/or hypopharyngeal structures, are associated with a higher risk of pulmonary complications,[53, 58, 63] few comparative data exist on these parameters. One such study by Stell and associates reported a higher incidence of pulmonary complications, deglutition problems, and prolonged hospitalization in those patients who had excision of the arytenoid or the true cord along with supraglottic laryngectomy than in those who underwent a standard SGL.[4] It is not surprising that the greater the aspiration, the higher the incidence of lung complications.[64] The degree of aspiration also depends on the success of reconstruction and any associated esophageal dysfunction.

The incidence of pulmonary complications varies from 0 to 13 per cent after vertical partial resections[1, 11, 16] and usually from 1 per cent to 25 per cent after SGL and its modifications.[2, 6, 7, 16, 46–48] However, in Murray's radiologic study, half (50 per cent) of the nonirradiated SGL patients were found to have repeated chest infections and associated pulmonary disease.[65] Almost a fifth (19.4 per cent) of the patients in this series died of pneumonia. Stell and associates' review of several papers mentioning pulmonary complications revealed that 16 per cent of the patients died of pulmonary disease or developed pneumonia after SGL.[4] In near-total laryngectomy with epiglottic reconstruction[22] and myomucosal shunt,[50] aspiration-related pulmonary complications were reported in 4 per cent and 7 per cent, respectively. Czigner[12] and Shaw[55] found that 50 per cent and 39 per cent, respectively, of their patients had lung infections after salvage conservation horizontal and vertical laryngectomy for tumor recurrence following failed radiation. Much lower pulmonary infection rates have been reported by other workers for salvage VPL following failed irradiation.[66–68]

Since pulmonary complications are almost entirely aspiration related, prevention of aspiration is the surgeon's foremost responsibility. Appropriate patient selection and reconstruction of the glottis are important steps in preventing aspiration. The various reconstructive techniques employed have been outlined in the section on aspiration. The role of intraoperative or postoperative cricopharyngeal myotomy in preventing aspiration is controversial. Some advocate its usefulness,[4, 53, 58, 63, 69] whereas others report its value as doubtful.[47, 55] Flores and associates reported equivocal results with it.[18] However, it is a simple step that may assist swallowing and adds little to the operative time. All efforts must be made to preserve the laryngeal, glossopharyngeal, and hypoglossal nerves as well as pharyngeal branches of the vagus nerve. Tamponading the larynx[31] or usage of a cuffed tracheostomy tube in the early postoperative period is helpful in preventing soilage of the tracheobronchial tree. Dietary measures outlined earlier also may be beneficial. Sufficient air humidity should be provided, and chest physiotherapy should be started in the first few days after the operation. Repeated endoscopic follow-up is necessary to detect early tumor recurrence and mild asymptomatic aspiration.

Dysphagia due to edema, cricopharyngeal dysfunction, or obliteration of the piriform sinus may worsen the aspiration. A feeding gastrostomy or cervical esophagostomy may be of some benefit in this situation. Lung infection should be treated with antibiotics, vigorous tracheobronchial toilet, and chest physiotherapy. In patients with chronic aspiration and recurrent pneumonia or progressive interstitial fibrosis, surgically diverting the spillovers into the esophagus may be necessary. Alternatively, closure of the glottis or subglottis or laryngotracheal separation with stump closure can be tried.[70] The cited advantage of some of these procedures is their reversibility. Prior to any of these operations, surgical measures to correct glottic insufficiency should be undertaken. In most cases this would mean refixing the affected neocord in the midline or medializing the cord by cartilage implantations as described in the previous section, or both. In uncontrolled cases, completion laryngectomy may have to be performed.[2, 4, 34, 41, 55, 68]

DEGLUTITION PROBLEMS

The major requirements of deglutition are apposition of the larynx to tongue base, closure of the laryngeal sphincters, and a patent esophagus to avoid delay in passage of bolus through the cricopharynx.[71] Other factors that influence deglutition are the extent of inferior and posterior mobility of the tongue, coordination between propulsive power of the tongue and pharynx and relaxation of the pharyngoesophageal sphincter, and efficient peristalsis of the pharyngoesophageal musculature.[49] Depending on the extent of partial laryngeal or laryngopharyngeal surgery, one or more of these mechanisms may be compromised. The degree of swallowing dysfunction will accordingly manifest as mild, moderate, or severe.

The possibility of impaired deglutition increases with sacrifice of arytenoid, tongue base, and hypopharynx. A shorter and shallower piriform fossa after operation further increases the likelihood of dysphagia.[40] Both Flores[18] and Hirano[72] and their associates studied the effects of various parameters on postoperative deglutition. In the former study, arytenoid resection contributed significantly to the deglutition problems, and piriform sinus resection was suspected to be responsible. The latter study found that the extent of arytenoid removal and asymmetric removal of false cords showed statistically significant relationships with the duration of nasogastric intubation. Both studies concluded that resection of tongue base or hyoid bone did not worsen the swallowing function. The rate of failure of re-establishment of adequate deglutition following supraglottic laryngectomy and its modifications is reportedly between 2 per cent and 20 per cent.[18, 63, 72–74]

Mozolewski and associates studied the pharyngeal phase of deglutition following "standard" and "extended" supraglottic lar-

yngectomy by cineradiography and manometry in 53 patients.[49] They found the time course of pharyngeal deglutition prolonged in about 80 per cent of the cases, and in some this was up to 10 seconds long. Their study indicates that although the postsurgical disturbance in swallowing physiology is high, the incidence of symptomatic swallowing disorders is much lower. Thawley reported a higher incidence of pharyngoesophageal stricture/prolonged nasogastric intubation after partial laryngeal and laryngopharyngeal procedures with or without planned radiation in comparison with total laryngectomy with planned radiation.[9] In Tucker and associates' near-total laryngectomy patients, 20 per cent had delayed deglutition beyond 2 months, and 4 per cent had permanent dysphagia to solid foods.[22]

In all patients with extensive partial laryngeal resection, a nasogastric tube should be inserted. Within 10 to 14 days after operation, re-education of swallowing should be started. In most patients the postoperative edema subsides by the second or third week, at which time patients are successfully decannulated and relieved of their nasogastric tube. As tight wound closure may contribute to postoperative dysphagia, the surgeon should try to avoid this by mobilizing available tissue or transposing a healthy distal tissue into the defect. As mentioned in an earlier section, the role of cricopharyngeal myotomy in assisting deglutition postoperatively is uncertain. Prospective case-matched studies are required to clarify the exact role of this procedure in improving deglutition or preventing aspiration. Such studies should include serial radiography and pharyngoesophageal manometric analysis. Not placing any sutures in the pharynx or arytenoid region after supraglottic laryngectomy has been claimed to result in rapid resolution of postoperative deglutition problems.[73]

If swallowing is not established by 6 weeks, a feeding gastrostomy is indicated. If a stricture is the cause of dysphagia, repeated bougienage and dilatations are done. Rarely the dilatation is unsuccessful and the stenotic segment may have to be replaced with a myocutaneous flap, stomach, or a piece of jejunum. In all patients with significant dysphagia, the surgeon must guard against dehydration. Serafini performed total laryngectomy in 3 per cent of his patients with absolute dysphagia after supraglottic laryngectomy.[6]

LARYNGEAL EDEMA, STENOSIS, AND DELAYED DECANNULATION

Postsurgical laryngeal edema is seen in almost all patients, which may take a few weeks to subside. In irradiated tissue this edema tends to persist for a much longer period. In a small number of cases, excess scar formation after operation results in overclosure or stenosis. Some of the factors causing excessive scarification are impaired healing, foreign body in the tissue, inadequate reconstruction, wound infection, excessive tissue removal, perichondritis, chondritis, and chondronecrosis. Although glottic stenosis is the commonest, both supraglottic and subglottic stenosis may be seen after partial laryngeal surgery. After hemilaryngectomy and no reconstruction, glottic stenosis may result from excessive scar formation and collapse of surrounding soft tissues. Where reconstruction has been performed, laryngeal obstruction may be due to excess bulk of transposed tissue, mucosal flap edema, or collection under the resurfacing flaps. Patients with persistent laryngeal edema or early stenosis usually have problems with decannulation of the trachea. Patients with delayed laryngeal stenosis or recurrent edema during postoperative radiotherapy may present with respiratory distress and stridor and may need recannulation. These patients generally have a good voice but may or may not swallow without difficulty.[9] If neglected, the airway obstruction may be fatal.

Marks and associates recorded a 1.4 per cent incidence of supraglottic stenosis in their patients treated predominantly with low-dose radiation and supraglottic laryngectomy.[44] Staffieri reported a 5 per cent incidence of vestibular stenosis after standard SGL without radiation.[13] He also noted a 5 per cent incidence of early glottic edema and a 5 per cent incidence of late tracheostomy in his study. Two per cent of his patients could not be decannulated. In other studies, the incidence of persistent laryngeal edema and stenosis with delayed decannulation or late recannulation has varied from 2 per cent to 15 per cent after horizontal partial resections.[8, 9, 46, 48, 56, 73] and from 1 per cent to 20 per cent after vertical partial resections with or without radiation.[11, 55, 56, 68] Krajina documented an 11 per cent late stenosis rate after combined vertical and partial (three quarters) laryngectomy,[56] and Pearson noted a 7.3 per cent composite shunt stenosis rate after near-total laryngectomy.[50] Myers encountered stenosis only in cases that underwent three-quarter laryngectomy or subtotal vertical laryngectomy in which only the contralateral arytenoid and part of the membranous cord were left behind.[69] He emphasized that the cricoid cartilage should be preserved in routine vertical partial laryngectomy as its removal predisposes to stenosis. Variations of standard SGL which leave behind a part or all of the false cords increase the possibility of persistent edema in the remaining larynx and preferably should be avoided.[69]

Although little detailed information is available on the comparative incidence of late postoperative complication (such as stenosis) with or without laryngoplasty, the consensus of opinion is that careful, planned reconstruction is the most important factor in preventing laryngeal incompetence and stenosis. Immediate treatment of wound infections, perichondritis, and chondritis may prevent later stenosis. If radiation is to be used as an adjunct to conservation surgery, it should always be planned in such a manner that not more than 4 to 6 weeks elapse between the completion of radiation therapy and operation. Planned radiotherapy is associated with a much lower incidence of complications.[9] Once stenosis has set in, its progress may be retarded by repeated steroid injections into the immature scar tissue. In a mature, mild-to-moderate stenosis, endolaryngeal microsurgical excision and coagulation of the scar may restore the air passage in a majority of patients.[8] The CO_2 laser is a valuable tool for scar excision and should be utilized wherever available.[75] A more severe stenosis may require scar excision through an open thyrotomy, followed by transposition of a healthy mucosal flap for resurfacing. Postoperative stenting may be required for up to 4 months. The role of vascular/avascular cartilage and bone implants in repair of these stenoses is unclear. If all attempts to restore the air passage are unsuccessful, the patient will have to become reconciled to living with a permanent valved tracheostomy.

WEBS AND SYNECHIAE

Webbing and synechiae formation are frequently seen after conservation laryngeal surgery. The factors responsible for these are similar to those mentioned for stenosis. Aggressive bilateral cord stripping and laser surgery may result in anterior web formation. When operation is done on both vocal cords, it is preferable to keep them apart till reepithelialization takes place. The anterior web also may be prevented if stripping and laser work are restricted to the membranous cord, and the anterior commissure is protected. Anterior commissure webbing is a particular problem after frontal and frontolateral laryngectomy, and some workers have advocated leaving the anterior laryngeal wound open for 2 to 3 weeks to prevent this.[31] Anterior commissure restitution is done secondarily. Resurfacing the area with pedicled cervical skin flaps, with mucosal grafts, or with the epiglottis may help prevent this annoying complication. It has also been proposed that the anterior fibrosis following frontolateral laryngectomy is preventable by using internal tubular molds or interpositioning devices, like a T-shaped Silastic lamina or McNaught's keel.[39] Although the glottis is the commonest site for web formation, occasionally supraglottic webs may be observed after partial laryngectomies.[75] The formation of supraglottic webs may be minimized by precise removal of supraglottic structures just above the true cords. Both

webbing and synechiae impair laryngeal function, compromising voice quality and leading to aspiration.

Guerrier and Jazouli reported an anterior synechiae incidence of 6 per cent after unilateral cordectomies for T_{1a} tumors, 30 per cent after bilateral cordectomy for T_{1b} tumors, 19 per cent following frontolateral resections for T_2 glottic tumors, and 14 per cent following hemiglottectomies for T_2 tumors.[10] They reported that this webbing may be seen up to 5 years after surgery. Neel and associates found laryngeal webs in 0.5 per cent of their nonradiated vertical partial laryngectomees.[11] Krajina noted late synechiae formation (6 months to 10 years postoperative) in 3.3 per cent of the patients after vertical partial and frontolateral partial resection and in 2 per cent after horizontal partial laryngectomy.[56]

Web and synechiae formation are minimized by meticulous surgery and the methods just outlined. Once developed, they may be excised microsurgically or with a CO_2 laser through an endoscope.[10, 75] If unsuccessful, an extralaryngeal approach is indicated to excise the web, resurface the defect, and place a laryngeal keel. Secondary closure is done after 8 to 12 weeks.

LARYNGEAL GRANULOMAS

Yet another complication that may compromise voice and deglutition results is the formation of excessive granulation tissue or an intralaryngeal granuloma. Diabetes, radiation, foreign bodies such as silk sutures, tissue infection, and inadequate reconstruction with incomplete coverage of defect all may result in impaired healing and glottic or subglottic granuloma formation. The commonest sites are the anterior commissure and anterior third of the neocord.[10]

Glottic granulomas with scar formation were seen by Guerrier and Jazouli in 4.9 per cent of their patients after unilateral cordectomy, in 3 per cent after bilateral cordectomy, and in 5 per cent after frontolateral resection.[10] They noted these granulomas up to 2 years after surgery. In about 70 per cent of their cases, the granulomas resolved spontaneously, and the remainder underwent surgical excision. Neel's incidence of laryngeal granuloma after vertical partial laryngectomy without radiation therapy was 11 per cent.[11] He stated that laryngoscopy and granuloma excision were done in all 20 patients, usually 3 to 4 months after operation, without any evidence of tumor recurrence. A 13 per cent incidence of prolonged edema with or without granulation tissue was seen by Czigner in 226 horizontal partial resections.[8] In another report, he noted that 7 of 16 patients (44 per cent) undergoing salvage VPL for tumor recurrence after failed high-dose radiation developed persistent edema or granulation tissue or both.[12] Granulomas usually develop a few months after operation, and a majority of them resolve spontaneously. Besides causing glottic insufficiency, persistent hoarseness, and obstruction, they are important in that they may represent an early tumor recurrence. Meticulous follow-up is therefore necessary. Initially they may be observed for a short period, and if they do not resolve, microlaryngeal biopsy and laser excision should be done.

Steiner claims that prevention of adhesions and scar formation after anterior commissure surgery is possible by the application of a special solution containing alphachymotrypsin, cortisone, and gentamicin twice weekly to the resected area until healing is complete.[76] His theory is that vigorous painting of the wound with this solution disturbs and delays healing (incipient granulation tissue formation), allowing the wound to epithelialize from the surrounding healthy mucosa.

WOUND INFECTIONS AND FISTULAS

A small percentage of all surgical wounds is associated with wound infections, minor and major. The incidence is probably higher after oral cavity, pharyngeal, or laryngeal operation, due to soilage of the wound by saliva or tracheal, pulmonary, or regurgitated gastric secretions. Gall and associates reported that patients with hypopharyngeal lesions had higher complication rates than patients with glottic and supraglottic lesions.[77] Predisposing factors for wound infection are systemic disease such as diabetes or immune compromised states, inadequate antibiotic coverage, tight wound closure, and presence of foreign body in the wound. Collections of blood, serum, wound secretions, and saliva invite bacterial infection. Radiation induces fibrosis and obliterative end-arteritis, resulting in a decrease in local vascularity. Infection may lead to wound breakdown and fistula formation. Extensive necrosis and sloughing are infrequent and usually appear around the 7th postoperative day. The general condition worsens, temperature rises, and the wound is malodorous. In radiated and diabetic patients, this may occur a little later (10 to 14 days). Faulty healing following large-scale wound breakdown or extensive necrosis may result in granulomas, webbing, excessive scarification, and stenosis. Flap necrosis and hemorrhage from wound margins are more common in infected tissues. Septicemia and carotid artery bleeding are ominous sequelae.

Fistula formation following laryngeal or laryngopharyngeal surgery is one of the most dreaded complications. The factors that predispose to infection also predispose to fistula formation.[69, 78]

Perhaps the single most important factor contributing to fistula formation is tight wound closure, especially in patients undergoing partial laryngopharyngectomy and supraglottic laryngectomy.[9] Myers states that pharyngocutaneous fistulas are much more common after total laryngectomy than after supraglottic laryngectomy, extended SGL, or vertical partial laryngectomy. Because of ease of closure, fistula is rarely seen in hemilaryngectomy patients.[9] Bocca and associates[79] and Som[80] state that development of a cutaneous fistula is very rare after an ordinary supraglottic laryngectomy.

Gall and associates reported a 1 per cent incidence of infection after various laryngeal and laryngopharyngeal procedures.[77] Other series found a 2.7 per cent to 18 per cent infection rate.[7–9, 44, 47, 55] The rate of infection and fistula formation seems to be around 1 per cent to 2 per cent after hemilaryngectomy and vertical partial resections.[9, 11] Thawley reported a 6.7 per cent rate of infection and an 8 per cent fistula rate after partial laryngopharyngectomy and radiation therapy with or without neck dissection, and a 4.7 per cent infection rate and a 2.2 per cent fistula rate after total laryngectomy and radiation therapy with or without neck dissection.[9] There seems to be a trend for higher fistula rates in irradiated tissues. Laryngocutaneous and pharyngocutaneous fistula rates of up to 50 per cent have been reported in patients undergoing salvage partial laryngectomy for tumor recurrence after failed full-dose radiation.[12, 66, 67]

Various factors may help prevent infections and fistulas: proper antibiotic coverage, meticulous handling of tissue, good aseptic technique, appropriate placement of skin incisions, control of diabetes and other systemic diseases prior to surgery, and good planning and execution of flaps. Inclusion of platysma in the skin flap helps prevent flap necrosis. Adjunctive radiation, if necessary, should be planned. Tight wound closure must be avoided. This may be prevented by usage of a pharyngostome or by transposing a healthy flap into the defect. Banfai suggested dissecting the tongue base transversely to create a superficial and deep tongue layer that can be used separately in the wound closure after SGL, thus strengthening the closure.[81]

Once developed, wound infection and fistula should be treated with meticulous wound care and antibiotics. Oral feeding should be stopped and oral suctioning of saliva done to prevent further soilage of the wound. Small fistulas usually close spontaneously in a few weeks. Large scale wound breakdown and larger fistulas will require vascularized cutaneous or myocutaneous flap for reconstruction.

PERICHONDRITIS AND CHONDRITIS

Another feared complication of conservation laryngeal surgery is perichondritis and its attendant sequelae. In partial laryngectomy, usually the transected cartilage is covered with a mucosal or skin flap or by the closure itself. If the surgical closure or the coverage is inadequate or compromised, the bare cartilage is exposed to pharyngeal and pulmonary secretions with resultant infection. The organisms frequently responsible for cartilaginous contamination are *Staphylococcus aureus, Pseudomonas, Proteus*, and other coliforms.[34] Radiation may induce perichondrial fibrosis, diminish its vascularity, and impair its ability to resist infection.[82] Smoldering perichondritis may manifest as local pain, erythema, and dysphagia or odynophagia. The local temperature may be raised. If untreated, perichondritis may progress to chondritis and chondronecrosis, producing laryngeal incompetence or stenosis, preventing decannulation, or necessitating recannulation. The chondritic cartilage frequently sequesters and extrudes into the pharyngeal lumen or externally, resulting in a fistula.[9, 12]

The incidence of perichondritis and chondritis after partial laryngectomy varies from 0 per cent to 7 per cent.[8, 9, 11, 55, 67] Its reported incidence of 32 per cent in patients treated with salvage vertical partial laryngectomy for cancer recurrence after full-dose radiation[12] should caution the surgeon in the selection of patients for partial surgery after failed radiation.

The postoperative occurrence of perichondritis may be minimized by meticulous surgical care. Avoiding perichondrial tearing, cleanly transecting the cartilage, and efficient coverage of bare cartilage during surgery may be preventive. Tight wound closure should be avoided after supraglottic laryngectomy. Additionally, the bur holes placed in the thyroid cartilage should preferably be at different levels.

Correct antibiotic therapy, local toilet, and reducing soilage of bare cartilage constitute the early management of perichondritis. Infection that has not responded to antibiotics must be managed with subperichondrial resection of laryngeal cartilages. Operation is performed via a midline incision, elevating perichondrial flaps and removing the thyroid and cricoid cartilages piecemeal. Perichondrium and intralaryngeal mucosa are preserved. Removal of the avascular cartilages allows healing and may prevent the need for total laryngectomy. Hyperbaric oxygen therapy, if available, is a valuable adjunct.[83] Once cartilage necrosis has occurred, sequestrectomy and excision of the dead cartilage should be carried out and the defect reconstructed with a vascularized cutaneous (deltopectoral), muscular (sternomastoid), or myocutaneous (pectoralis major myocutaneous) flap.[84, 85] If the cartilage and soft tissue destruction are extensive, total laryngectomy is the only choice.

POSTOPERATIVE HEMORRHAGE

Postoperative bleeding may be from the wound margins, tongue base, or neck or tracheostomy related. A postoperative local hemorrhage rate of up to 12.5 per cent has been reported.[6, 7, 11, 12] If bleeding is not controlled or the blood loss not replaced, exsanguination and death may occur. The overall rate of carotid artery rupture after head and neck surgery varies from 0 to 7 per cent.[8, 77, 86, 87] In patients with positive microscopic surgical margins, carotid artery rupture occurs more frequently.[77] After conservation surgery, a rupture rate of up to 2 per cent has been reported.[6, 8] Meticulous surgery and wound closure, coverage of the carotid artery with dermal or muscular flaps, and prevention of infection may minimize the incidence of postoperative bleeding. Preoperative coagulation studies might detect patients with blood dyscrasias. Postoperative hemorrhage may necessitate blood replacement and return to the operating room for vessel ligation. A mortality rate related to postoperative bleeding of up to 2 per cent has been reported, most of which is usually preventable.[6, 8]

RADIATION AND CONSERVATION LARYNGEAL SURGERY

It is common knowledge that radiation or conservation laryngeal surgery alone can control 75 per cent to 95 per cent of mobile vocal cord cancer. However, when the role of radiation in combination with conservation laryngeal surgery is concerned, two important questions need to be considered:

(1) Is limited laryngeal surgery still oncologically feasible after curative radiotherapy?
(2) How well does the patient tolerate postoperative radiation after partial laryngeal resection or partial laryngectomy after radiation?

In answer to the first question, studies have shown that 70 per cent to 85 per cent of glottic cancer failures can be salvaged by vertical partial laryngectomies if specific criteria are followed.[66–68, 88–92] This rate is similar to or better than the 64 per cent to 78 per cent local tumor control rate reported for salvage total laryngectomy after irradiation failure.[93, 94] Although the opinion that early supraglottic carcinoma should be treated primarily with supraglottic laryngectomy seems to be well established, the benefit of planned preoperative radiotherapy at this stage remains controversial. There is reasonable evidence that in larger superior hypopharyngeal and supraglottic carcinomas, planned postoperative radiotherapy decreases the incidence of cervical metastasis and neck recurrence.[95, 96] Some practitioners of primary curative radiotherapy for supraglottic carcinoma have reported 50 per cent to 60 per cent local control with salvage supraglottic laryngectomy for recurrence following irradiation.[66, 92] Most surgeons believe that the poor success along with the high complication rate precludes performing SGL for radiation failures.

The ability of a patient to tolerate radiation depends on the quality of radiation (megavoltage versus orthovoltage) total dose, duration of treatment, fraction dose size, and individual response.[97] Orthovoltage radiation carries a higher risk of bone and cartilage necrosis. The risk of serious complications caused by radiotherapy increases with the total dose. Harwood and Tierie reported that the dose cure curve for early glottic cancer was flat over a dose range of 5500 to 7500 rads, but once the 7500-rad dose was exceeded, the risk of major complications like laryngeal edema, stenosis, and necrosis rose quite rapidly.[98] High-fraction dose and larger field size of radiation also increase the risk of complications. So do diabetes and other metabolic diseases, especially at higher doses.[97]

Some studies have reported a higher incidence of wound infection, fistula, and iatrogenic neural damage in irradiated tissues after operation than after operation alone.[99, 100] The fistula and overall complication rates also increase when one goes from low-dose to high-dose radiation therapy.[95, 101] However, the complication rate is lower if radiation and surgery (partial or total) are used in a planned combined program; in some studies it equals the complication rate of surgery alone.[9, 56, 77, 97, 101, 103] Most studies conclude that complication rates are disportionately higher in salvage laryngeal or laryngopharyngeal surgery for residual or recurrent carcinoma after failed curative radiation. The higher overall complications in this group are due mainly to increased incidence in wound infections, delayed wound healing, perichondritis and chondronecrosis, and laryngeal stenosis. Persistent postsurgical laryngeal and pharyngeal edema, so common in this group, results in delayed decannulation, deglutition problems, and prolonged rehabilitation. The unacceptably high complication rate after salvage surgery, particularly supraglottic laryngectomy, prompted Stell to conclude that a patient who once had radiotherapy for supraglottic cancer cannot then have a supraglottic laryngectomy.[104]

Denecke suggests that one solution to the prolonged edema after surgical intervention in the irradiated larynx is use of pedicled flaps.[105] The flaps presumably function as draining tissues in the early postoperative period. After an interval of 3 to 4 months, the lymphatic drainage recovers, the edema decreases, and the previous fixed arytenoid may resume its function.[105] In contrast, Shaw concluded that sophisticated reconstructive procedures such as cartilage transposition, muscle transplants, or fat and fascial grafts have no place after full-dose radiation.[55]

It is apparent from this discussion that if complications are to be minimized, radiotherapy is best used in a planned fashion with conservation laryngeal surgery. Once complications have developed, they should be managed as outlined in the previous sections of this chapter.

SUMMARY

There is increasing evidence that a majority of laryngeal cancers will be controlled by conservation laryngeal surgery in the future. Careful lesion mapping and patient evaluation preoperatively are mandatory in selecting potential candidates for this surgery. If indicated, radiotherapy should be used in a planned treatment program. Specific reconstructive measures after excisional surgery are necessary to correct resultant structural deficits. The specific acoustic and temporal parameters of voice to be used for comparing phonation results between different surgical studies and between radiation alone and conservation laryngeal surgery alone should be standardized. There is good evidence that vocal cord cancers of the anterior one third differ from those of the middle third, which differ from the posterior third cancers. The most appropriate therapeutic modality for these specific sites still needs to be defined. The role of cricopharyngeal myotomy in assisting postoperative deglutition and minimizing aspiration also needs to be clarified by prospective case-matched studies. Since the overall functional and oncologic results of partial laryngeal surgery or radiation (in glottic cancer) are good, the treatment modality should be tailored according to the facilities available, the experience of the surgeon and radiotherapist, and, more importantly, the patient's need. Many of the minor and most major complications of conservation laryngeal surgery are preventable by paying particular attention to surgical techniques, reconstructive procedure, and postoperative follow-up.

References

1. Tucker HM: Conservation laryngeal surgery in the elderly patient. Laryngoscope 93:237, 1983.

2. Schechter GL: Conservation surgery of the larynx. In Cummings CW, Frederickson JM, Harker LA, (eds): Otolaryngology–Head and Neck Surgery. Vol III. St. Louis, CV Mosby, 1986, pp 2095–2115.

3. Yonkers AJ: Complications of conservation surgery of the laryngopharynx. Laryngoscope 93:314, 1983.

4. Stell PM, Morton RP, Singh SD: Functional complications after supraglottic laryngectomy. In Wigand ME, Steiner W, Stell PM (eds): Functional Partial Laryngectomy. Berlin, Springer Verlag, 1984, pp 301–305.

5. Sellars SL, Mills EED, Seid AB: Combined preoperative telecobalt therapy and supraglottic laryngectomy. J Laryngol Otol 95:305–310, 1981.

6. Serafini I: Results of supraglottic horizontal laryngectomy. In Wigand ME, Steiner W, Stell PM (eds): Functional Partial Laryngectomy. Berlin, Springer Verlag, 1984, pp 223–225.

7. Vega MF: Early and late complications after partial resections of the larynx. In Wigand ME, Steiner W, Stell PM (eds): Functional Partial Laryngectomy. Berlin, Springer Verlag, 1984, pp 295–298.

8. Czigner J: Early and late complications after supraglottic partial resection of the larynx. In Wigand ME, Steiner W, Stell PM (eds): Functional Partial Laryngectomy. Berlin, Springer Verlag, 1984, pp 298–301.

9. Thawley SE: Complications of combined radiation therapy and surgery for carcinoma of the larynx and inferior hypopharynx. Laryngoscope 91:677–700, 1981.

10. Guerrier Y, Jazouli N: Vertical partial laryngectomy—results. In Wigand ME, Steiner W, Stell PM (eds): Functional Partial Laryngectomy. Berlin, Springer Verlag, 1984, pp 145–149.

11. Neel HB, Devine KD, DeSanto LW: Laryngofissure and cordectomy for early cordal carcinoma: Outcome in 182 patients. Otolaryngol Head Neck Surg 88:79–84, 1980.

12. Czigner J: Vertical and horizontal partial resections of the larynx after radiotherapy. In Wigand ME, Steiner W, Stell PM (eds): Functional Partial Laryngectomy. Berlin, Springer Verlag, 1984, pp 280–284.

13. Staffieri A: Horizontal supraglottic laryngectomy: Results. In Wigand ME, Steiner W, Stell PM (eds): Functional Partial Laryngectomy. Berlin, Springer Verlag, 1984, pp 219–222.

14. Mohr RM, Quenelle DJ, Shumrick DA: Verticofrontolateral laryngectomy (hemilaryngectomy). Arch Otolaryngol 109:384–395, 1983.

15. Alajmo E, Fini-Storchi O, Agostini V, Polti G: Conservation surgery for cancer of the larynx in the elderly. Laryngoscope 95:203–205, 1985.

16. Chow JM, Block RM, Friedman M: Preoperative evaluation for partial laryngectomy. Head Neck Surg 10:319–323, 1988.

17. Ogura JH: Discussion. Laryngoscope 87:1999, 1977.

18. Flores TC, Wood BG, Levine HL, et al: Factors in succesful deglutition following supraglottic laryngeal surgery. Ann Otol Rhinol Laryngol 91:579–583, 1982.

19. Kittel G: Voice and respiration before and after partial laryngeal resections. In Wigand ME, Steiner W, Stell PM (eds): Functional Partial Laryngectomy. Berlin, Springer Verlag, 1984, pp 174–176.

20. Vecerina S, Krajina Z: Phonatory function of the larynx following partial laryngectomy. In Wigand ME, Steiner W, Stell PM (eds): Functional Partial Laryngectomy. Berlin, Springer Verlag, 1984, pp 230–231.

21. Vega MF: Oncological and functional results of horizontal partial laryngectomy. In Wigand ME, Steiner W, Stell PM (eds): Functional Partial Laryngectomy. Berlin, Springer Verlag, 1984, pp 226–228.

22. Tucker HM, Benninger MS, Roberts JK, et al: Near-total laryngectomy with epiglottic reconstruction. Arch Otolaryngol Head Neck Surg 115:1341–1344, 1989.

23. Moore GP: Voice problems following limited surgical excision. Laryngoscope 85:619, 1975.

24. Biller HF, Lucente FE: Reconstruction of the larynx following vertical partial laryngectomy. Otolaryngol Clin North Am 12:761, 1979.

25. Dedo HH: A technique for vertical hemilaryngectomy to prevent stenosis and aspiration. Laryngoscope 85:978, 1975.

26. Bailey BJ: Glottic reconstruction after hemilaryngectomy. Bipedicle muscle flap for larynygoplasty. Laryngoscope 85:960, 1975.

27. Blaugrund S, Kurland S: Replacement of the arytenoid following vertical hemilaryngectomy. Laryngoscope 85:935–941, 1975.

28. Quinn H: Free muscle transplant method of glottic reconstruction after hemilaryngectomy. Laryngoscope 85:985–986, 1975.

29. Park NH, Major JW, Sauers PL: Hemilaryngectomy and vocal cord reconstruction with digastric tendon graft. Surg Gynecol Obstet 155:153, 1982.

30. Ogura JH, Dedo HH: Glottis reconstruction following subtotal glottis–supraglottic laryngectomy. Laryngoscope 75:865, 1975.

31. Denecke HJ: The role of laryngoplasty in vertical partial laryngectomies. In Wigand ME, Steiner W, Stell PM (eds): Functional Partial Laryngectomy. Berlin, Springer Verlag, 1984, pp 89–94.

32. Krajina Z, Kosokovic F: Experiences with vertical partial laryngectomy with special reference to laryngeal reconstruction by sternohyoid fascia. In Wigand ME, Steiner W, Stell PM (eds): Functional Partial Laryngectomy. Berlin, Springer Verlag, 1984, pp 108–112.

33. Krajina Z: Phonatory function following unilateral laser cordectomy. In Wigand ME, Steiner W, Stell PM (eds): Functional Partial Laryngectomy. Berlin, Springer Verlag, 1984, pp 152–153.

34. Ward PH: The Second Joseph H. Ogura Memorial Lecture. Complications of Laryngeal Surgery: Etiology and Prevention. Laryngoscope 98:54–57, 1988.

35. Kambic V: Epiglottoplasty: A new technique for laryngeal reconstruction. Radiol Yugoslav (Suppl II):33–43, 1977.

36. Tucker HM, Wood BG, Levine HL, et al: Glottic reconstruction after near-total laryngectomy. Laryngoscope 89:975–984, 1979.

37. Thawley SE: Epiglottic reconstruction of the vocal cord following hemilaryngectomy. Laryngoscope 93:237, 1983.

38. Schechter GL: Epiglottic reconstruction and subtotal laryngectomy. Laryngoscope 93:729, 1983.

39. Traissac L: Vertical partial resection. Oncological and functional results. In Wigand ME, Steiner W, Stell PM (eds): Functional Partial Laryngectomy. Berlin, Springer Verlag, 1984, pp 156–162.

40. Kothary P, Dev R: Horizontal supraglottic laryngectomy with total glossectomy—Oncological and functional results. In Wigand ME, Steiner W, Stell PM (eds): Functional Partial Laryngectomy. Berlin, Springer Verlag, 1984, pp 235–242.

41. Myers EN, Ogura JH: Completion laryngectomy. Ann Otol Rhinol Laryngol 88:172, 1979.

42. DiSantis DJ, Balfe DM, Koehler RE, et al: Barium examination of the pharynx after vertical hemilaryngectomy. Am J Radiol 141:335–339, 1983.

43. Padovan IF, Oreskovic M: Functional evaluation after partial resection in patients with carcinoma of the larynx. Laryngoscope 85:626, 1975.

44. Marks JE, Freeman RB, Lee F, Ogura JH: Carcinoma of the supraglottic larynx. Am J Radiol 132:255–260, 1979.

45. Ward PH, Berci G, Calcaterra TC: New insights into the causes of postoperative aspiration following conservation surgery of the larynx. Ann Otol Rhinol Laryngol 86:724–737, 1977.

46. Som ML: Conservation surgery for carcinoma of the supraglottis. Ann Otol Rhinol Laryngol 84:655–678, 1976.

47. Bocca E: Supraglottic cancer. Laryngoscope 85:1318–1326, 1975.

48. Robbins KT, Davidson W, Peters LJ, Goepfert H: Conservation surgery for T_2 and T_3 carcinomas of the supraglottic larynx. Arch Otolaryngol Head Neck Surg 114:421–426, 1988.

49. Mozolewski E, Jack K, et al: Cineradiographic and manometric measurements of deglutition following horizontal partial laryngectomy. In Wigand ME, Steiner W, Stell PM (eds): Functional Partial Laryngectomy. Berlin, Springer Verlag, 1984, pp 242–243.

50. Pearson B: Near-total laryngectomy. In Cummings CW, Frederickson JM, Harker LA, et al (eds): Otolaryngology—Head and Neck Surgery. St. Louis, CV Mosby, 1986.

51. Goode RL: Laryngeal suspension in head and neck surgery. Laryngoscope 86:349, 1976.

52. Calcaterra TC: Laryngeal suspension after supraglottic laryngectomy. Arch Otolaryngol 102:716, 1976.

53. Staple TW, Ogura JH: Cineradiography of the swallowing mechanism following supraglottic subtotal laryngectomy. Radiology 87:226–230, 1966.

54. Sacks S, Lawson W, Biller HF: Correction of late glottic insufficiency. Otolaryngol Clin North Am 21(4):761–769, 1988.

55. Shaw HJ: A view of partial laryngectomy in the treatment of laryngeal cancer. J Laryngol Otol 101:143–154, 1987.

56. Krajina Z: Late complications and recurrences after partial resections of the larynx. In Wigand ME, Steiner W, Stell PM (eds): Functional Partial Laryngectomy. Berlin, Springer Verlag, 1984, pp 305–308.

57. Kamer FM, Som ML: Correction of the traumatically abducted vocal cord. Arch Otolaryngol 95:6–9, 1972.

58. Sessions D, Ogura JH, Ciralsky RH: Late glottic insufficiency. Laryngoscope 85:950–959, 1975.

59. Waltner JG: Surgical rehabilitation of the voice following laryngofissure. Arch Otolaryngol 67:99–101, 1958.

60. Morrison LF: The "reverse King" operation. Am Otol 57:944–956, 1948.

61. Biller HF, Lawson W, Sacks S: Correction of posterior glottic incompetence following partial laryngectomy. Ann Otol Rhinol Laryngol 91:448–449, 1982.

62. Biller HF, Urken M: Cricoid collapse, a new technique for management of glottic incompetence. Arch Otolaryngol 111:740–741, 1985.

63. Litton WB, Leonard TR: Aspiration after partial laryngectomy: Cineradiographic studies. Laryngoscope 79:887–908, 1969.

64. Staple TW, Ragsdale EF, Ogura JH: The chest roentgenogram following supraglottic subtotal laryngectomy. Am J Roentgenol 100:583–587, 1967.

65. Murray GM: Pulmonary complications following supraglottic laryngectomy. Clin Otolaryngol 1:241–247, 1976.

66. Nichols RD, Stine PH, Greenwald KH: Partial laryngectomy after irradiation failure. Arch Otolaryngol 90:571–575, 1980.

67. Rothfield RE, Johnson JT, Myers EN, Wagner RL: Hemilaryngectomy for salvage of radiation therapy failures. Otolaryngol Head Neck Surg 103:792–794, 1990.

68. Croll GA, Brock PVD, Tiwari RM, et al: Vertical partial laryngectomy for recurrent glottic carcinoma after irradiation. Head Neck Surg 7:340–393, 1985.

69. Myers EN: Complications in cancer of the larynx and their treatment. In Ferlito A (ed): Cancer of the Larynx. Vol III. Boca Raton, FL, CRC Press, 1985, pp 167–182.

70. Nash M: Swallowing problems in tracheotomized patient. Otolaryngol Clin North Am 21(4):701–709, 1988.

71. Ogura HJ, Thawley SE: Complications of laryngeal surgery. In Conley JJ (ed): Complications of Head and Neck Surgery. Philadelphia, WB Saunders, 1979, pp 246–273.

72. Hirano M, Kurita S, Tateishi M, Matsuoka H: Deglutition following supraglottic horizontal laryngectomy. Ann Otol Rhinol Laryngol 96:7–11, 1987.

73. Steiner W: Oncological results of supraglottic horizontal partial laryngectomy (Alonso operation). In Wigand ME, Steiner W, Stell PM (eds): Functional Partial Laryngectomy. Berlin, Springer Verlag, 1984, pp 232–234.

74. Kurokawa H: Swallowing function after partial laryngectomy. Clinical and roentgenological investigations. Otol Fukuoka 18:94–111, 1972.

75. Lawson W, Biller HF: Cancer of the larynx. In Suen JY, Myers EN (eds): Cancer of the Head and Neck. New York, Churchill Livingstone, 1981, p 434.

76. Steiner W: Transoral microsurgical CO_2 laser resection of laryngeal carcinoma. In Wigand ME, Steiner W, Stell PM (eds): Functional Partial Laryngectomy. Berlin, Springer Verlag, 1984, pp 121–125.

77. Gall AM, Sessions DG, Ogura JH: Complications following surgery for cancer of the larynx and hypopharynx. Cancer 39:624–631, 1977.

78. Dedo DD, Alonso WA, Ogura JH: Incidence, predisposing factors and outcome of pharyngocutaneous fistula complicating head and neck surgery. Ann Otol Rhinol Laryngol 84:833, 1975.

79. Bocca E, Pignataro O, Masciaro O: Supraglottic surgery of the larynx. Ann Otolaryngol 77:1005–1026, 1968.

80. Som ML: Discussion of roles and limitations of conservation surgical therapy for laryngeal carci-

noma. Can J Otolaryngol CCLC Workshop 6:419, 1975.
81. Banfai I: Anatomische Rekonstruktion des Kehlkopfs nach horizontaler Resektion. Z Laryngol Rhinol 42:32–38, 1963.
82. McGovern FH, Fitz-Hugh JS, Constable W: Postradiation perichondritis and cartilage necrosis of the larynx. Laryngoscope 83:808–815, 1973.
83. Hart GB, Mainous E: The treatment of radiation necrosis with hyperbaric oxygen. Cancer 37:2580–2585, 1976.
84. Oppenheimer RW, Krespi YP, Einhorn RK: Management of laryngeal radionecrosis: Animal and clinical experience. Head Neck Surg 11:252–256, 1989.
85. Litton WB: Preservation of a radionecrotic larynx by excision of thyroid cartilage with flap coverage. Laryngoscope 88:1947–1949, 1978.
86. Ketcham AS, Hoye RC: Spontaneous carotid artery hemorrhage after head and neck surgery. Surg Gynecol Obstet 110:649–655, 1965.
87. Stell PM: Hemorrhage after major neck surgery. Br J Surg 56:525–527, 1989.
88. Biller HF, Barnhill FR, Ogura JH, Perez AC: Hemilaryngectomy following radiation failure for carcinoma of the vocal cords. Laryngoscope 80:249–253, 1970.
89. Burns H, Bryce DP, Van Nostrand AW: Conservation surgery in laryngeal carcinoma and its role following radiotherapy: A histological and clinical study of 32 cases. Arch Otolaryngol 105:234, 1979.
90. Harwood AR: Cancer of the larynx—the Toronto experience. J Otolaryngol 11(Suppl 11):1–21, 1982.
91. Norris CM, Peale AR: Partial laryngectomy for irradiation failure. Arch Otolaryngol 84:558–562, 1966.
92. Sorensen H, Hansen HS, Thomsen KA: Partial laryngectomy following irradiation. Laryngoscope 90:1344–1349, 1980.
93. Ballantyne AJ, Fletcher GH: Surgical management of irradiation failures of nonfixed cancers of the glottic region. Am J Roentgenol 120:164–168, 1974.
94. Hawkins NV: The treatment of glottic carcinoma. An analysis of 800 cases. Laryngoscope 85:1485–1493, 1975.
95. Vandenbrouck C, Sancho H, Fur RL, et al: Results of a randomized clinical trial of preoperative irradiation versus postoperative in treatment of tumors of the hypopharynx. Cancer 39:1445–1449, 1977.
96. Eisbach K, Krause CJ: Carcinoma of the pyriform sinus: Comparison of treatment modalities. Laryngoscope 87:1904, 1977.
97. Sauer R: Combined radiation therapy and surgery for limited carcinoma of the larynx. In Wigand ME, Steiner W, Stell PM (eds): Functional Partial Laryngectomy. Berlin, Springer Verlag, 1984, pp 276–280.
98. Harwood AR, Tierie A: Radiotherapy of early glottic cancer—II. Int J Radiol Oncol Biol Phys 5:477–482, 1979.
99. Marchetta FC, Sako K, Maxwell W: Complications after radical head and neck surgery performed through previously irradiated tissues. Am J Surg 114:835–838, 1967.
100. Habel DW: Surgical complications in irradiated patients. Arch Otolaryngol 82:382–386, 1965.
101. Skolnik EM, Martin LO, Wheatley MA, et al: Combined therapy in the management of laryngeal carcinoma. Can J Otolaryngol 4:236–245, 1975.
102. Joseph DL, Shumrick DA: Risks of head and neck surgery in previously irradiated patients. Arch Otolaryngol 97:381–384, 1973.
103. Cummings CW, et al: Complications of laryngectomy and neck dissection following planned preoperative radiotherapy. Ann Otol 88:745–750, 1977.
104. Stell PM: Discussion of roles and limitations of conservation surgical therapy for laryngeal carcinoma. Can J Otolaryngol CCLC Workshop 6:406, 1975.
105. Denecke HJ: Radiotherapy and partial laryngectomy. In Wigand ME, Steiner W, Stell PM (eds): Functional Partial Laryngectomy. Berlin, Springer Verlag, 1984, pp 284–285.

CHAPTER

18

Laryngotracheal Devices

ISAAC ELIACHAR, MD
FRANCIS A. PAPAY, MD

Laryngotracheal devices are employed in a variety of local and systemic conditions ranging from routine endotracheal intubation for general anesthesia, maintenance of the tracheostomy tract, and internal support of the reconstituted or reconstructed laryngotracheal complex. The most common devices, the standard endotracheal and tracheostomy tubes, are well tested and optimally designed for short-term applications. In the majority of cases they perform well with minimal transient clinical sequelae.

Advances in surgical technology and growing efficiency of emergency services and intensive care units have led to sustenance and increased survival of patients who otherwise would have perished. Since the mid 1960s, long-term intubation has become the preferred method of treatment for prolonged maintenance of the airway, control of secretions, and assisted ventilation. Tracheostomy is currently reserved for patients difficult to intubate or manage and whenever more protracted management is indicated. Patients undergoing tracheostomy inevitably suffer higher risks for emergence of eventual com-

plications. Understanding the pathologic processes that lead to complications may prevent oversight, persistence, or repetition of injury. Combinations of separate or overlapping lesions may be encountered, requiring precise assessment prior to surgical management.

Problem patients should be identified. Some may have been treated conservatively or endoscopically because their conditions were initially considered insignificant. Others may have undergone major reconstructive surgery that failed, resulting in persistence or even aggravation of their condition. Medical conditions that prohibit major surgical intervention or lack of ample healthy tissue for reconstruction must be preoperatively identified. Such patients may have to be sustained by means of long-term devices, such as fenestrated tracheostomy tubes or Silastic Montgomery T-tubes. In some cases, the tracheostomy has to be modified to accommodate the devices for prolonged periods or even permanently.

Many devices or prostheses have been designed to correct or to maintain the airway

233

in these very complex pathologic conditions. The literature and commercial catalogs contain an abundance of ingenious tubes, splints, and devices produced from multiple materials in a variety of designs. Each of these products has a specific applicability in certain circumstances. None offer universal solutions. None are free of complications.

This chapter presents common complications resulting from endotracheal and tracheostomy tubes, keels, or splints and intraluminal supporting devices. Concepts and methods to prevent, restrict, or correct these complications are discussed.

ENDOTRACHEAL TUBES

The endotracheal tube for delivery of anesthesia was introduced by McEwen in 1868. Intubation of the laryngotracheal lumen has provided physicians with complete control of airway and ventilation. Atraumatic short-term cannulation of the laryngotracheal lumen with various types of endotracheal tubes leads to minimal postextubatory sequelae. In emergency situations, there may be little time to "select" the correct endotracheal tube. Under rushed circumstances, iatrogenic trauma to the airway mucosa can initiate a cascade of wound healing events that evolve into permanent changes of the airway lining and architecture, with subsequent ventilatory compromise.

The two available airway conduits for administration of prolonged ventilation are endotracheal tube intubation and tracheostomy. Prolonged endotracheal tube intubation has become the standard method over tracheostomy, since by comparison it has lower morbidity.[1] Endotracheal intubation is not a benign modality. Injury to the laryngotracheal lumen takes place by different biomechanical processes.[2] During introduction, the technician may avulse the delicate lumen mucosa, disrupt the cricoarytenoid joint, and tear the true vocal cords. Once the tube is in position, it rests against certain pressure points within the lumen. Current endotracheal tube designs do not take into

account the shallow S curve of the subglottic trachea or the natural cross-sections and narrowing of the glottic chink and the subglottic segment.[3–5]

Ideally, tubes used for prolonged intubation should (1) minimize tracheal and laryngeal irritation, (2) reduce cuff pressure, (3) provide a no-leak ventilation system, and (4) resist kinking.

Unfortunately, few current endotracheal tubes meet these ideals; many characteristics are mutually exclusive. One study compared eight different endotracheal tubes with variations of characteristics. The results indicated that polyvinyl chloride (PVC) and silicone rubber tubes are most flexible and cause the least pressure injury after long-term exposure.[4, 6] Therefore, these materials would be most preferable for prolonged intubation. The red rubber tube, in contrast, is relatively nonflexible, causing a higher incidence of pressure point necrosis. On the other hand, its stiffness may facilitate emergency intubation. Therefore, an endotracheal tube should be chosen not only for its design, ease of insertion (i.e., stiffness), lumen diameter, and length but also for patient tolerance during prolonged ventilatory assistance. The constructing materials and their tensile characteristics should be taken into consideration.

Physical characteristics that have direct impact on mucosal injury by endotracheal tubes include inertness, compliance and rigidity of the material, outer diameter, and cross-section and design curvature of the tube.[7] Component materials may have toxic effects on the mucosa. Leaching of toxic chemical additives used in manufacturing and sterilization cause mucosal cell death. Allergic inflammatory response to PVC tubes has been documented after 12 hours of intubation, compared with little response to silicone tubes.[8, 9] Factors responsible for airway morbidity from endotracheal tubes are listed in Table 18–1.

Probably two or more factors are responsible for any one case of laryngotracheal stenosis caused by endotracheal tube morbidity. The most common and important factor involved in laryngotracheal stenosis, secondary to intubation, is duration of the tube

TABLE 18–1. Predisposing Factors for Laryngeal Stenosis from Endotracheal Tubes

Duration of intubation
Tube size and design
Type of tube (physical and chemical)
Cuff pressure and design
Shearing motion
Sterilization techniques
Infection
Patient's hemodynamics
Reintubation
Nasogastric tube
Gastroesophageal reflux
Insertion by inexperienced personnel
Systemic factors:
  Diabetes mellitus
  Nutrition

placement[10–12] (Table 18–2). A poll in 1984 revealed the average acceptable duration of prolonged endotracheal tube placement to be approximately 14 days. The trend is to tolerate increasingly prolonged intubation for up to 3 to 4 weeks before considering alternative methods of airway access.[13–16] Unfortunately, these long episodes of endotracheal intubations are not benign.

Injuries secondary to the tube occur predominantly at two levels. At the glottic level, the endotracheal tube normally leans upon the posterior commissure, causing pressure necrosis of the mucosal membrane overlying the cricoid lamina and splaying the arytenoids. Ventilatory motions, swallowing, and coughing cause further shearing of the membranes, with eventual exposure and involvement of the cartilage.[17, 18] Symmetric ulceration of the true vocal cords over the vocal processes of the arytenoids with granuloma formation is frequently found. These "intubation granulomata" often appear immediately after extubation. The granuloma may develop at a later stage secondary to chronic inflammation and infection. However, it usually regresses spontaneously with time.

More inferiorly, tracheal injury is due to excessive prolonged pressure generated by the inflated cuff. Pressure sores, necrosis, and exposure of the perichondrium and cartilage with ensuing inflammation and infection lead to excessive scarring and eventual stricture.[19–22]

Despite the use of modern flexible tubes with high-volume–low-pressure cuffs and meticulous respiratory care, clinical studies have shown that the frequency of laryngotracheal injuries is still high.[3, 15, 20, 23] The advent of high-volume–low-pressure cuffs unfortunately has not decreased the clinical incidence of postintubatory subglottic and tracheal stenosis.[21, 22, 24–28] Cuff pressure management is discussed further in the tracheostomy tube section.

In one study, approximately one third of the patients showed signs of early postextubation subglottic and tracheal stenosis. Chronic established postintubatory tracheal stenosis is usually found in about 10 per cent. Studies suggest that routine tracheal assessment be performed 4 to 6 weeks after extubation for every patient exposed to factors predisposing to laryngotracheal injury. Since severe stenosis may occur soon after extubation, it is advised that any patient with even mild symptoms of airway obstruction have immediate endoscopic examination.[2, 28]

Tracheoesophageal fistula is a rare complication, often associated with high cuff pressures.[29, 30] Tracheal granulomas at the level of the tube tip result from mucosal damage owing to piston-like movements during ventilation. These were once regarded as rare, though one study reported 30 per cent of patients as having minor granulations. The tip of the tube may probe and erode the tracheal wall, eventually piercing into the mediastinum or a major vessel, or causing further stenosis.[2]

Damage to the posterior commissure remains common. Autopsy studies have

TABLE 18–2. Pathophysiology of Endotracheal Tube Injury

Mucosal edema, lacerations, ulcerations
Pressure necrosis
Mucociliary dysfunction and stasis
Secondary infection
Perichondritis
Cartilage exposure and breakdown
Inflammation, granulation tissue
Healing by second intention
Scarring, fibrosis, and stricture

(From Cotton, Hawkins.)

shown ulcers on the posterior aspect of the true vocal cords and along the interarytenoid space in more than 50 per cent of patients who died after endotracheal intubation.[1, 4] The incidence of posterior commissure stenosis reported in the literature is 2.4 per cent to 6.2 per cent.[31, 32]

Pharyngeal and laryngeal anatomy makes it difficult to avoid this trauma. Less damage would be expected following nasotracheal intubation compared with orotracheal intubation because of the more favorable anatomic relationship and better fixation of the tube.

The triangular shape of the glottis in transverse section tends to force the endotracheal tube toward the posterior commissure. Furthermore, the posterior half of the larynx is not oval and therefore does not readily accommodate the tube. The tensile properties of the vocal cords and the repetitive movements associated with swallowing also contribute to this problem. In the supine position, the tongue slumps backward and further potentiates the trauma to the posterior commissure.

We recently designed an endotracheal tube that reduces the pressure concentrated at the posterior commissure.[3] This is achieved by displacement of the tube anteriorly at the level of the glottis, away from the sensitive area of the tube-tissue interface at the posterior commissure. This is achieved by means of an additional, low-pressure, eccentrically inflatable cuff located on its posterior aspect at the level of the hypopharynx, above the laryngeal introitus (Fig. 18–1). When inflated, this cuff reduces pressure and potential damage to the posterior commissure. It transfers the pressure from the larynx to the pharynx, which is less critical and sensitive. An air-tight seal will still be obtained with the standard tracheal cuff. No damage was incurred by the hypopharyngeal cuff in canine experiments.[3]

Prolonged nasotracheal intubation may induce complications away from the larynx and trachea. Paranasal sinusitis and eustachian tube dysfunction may result. A high index of suspicion must be held whenever sepsis of unknown etiology is encountered.[33–38]

NASOGASTRIC TUBES

Nasogastric tubes, although they are not laryngotracheal devices, may cause aspiration, reflux of gastric juices, depressed cough reflex, and injuries to the arytenoids and

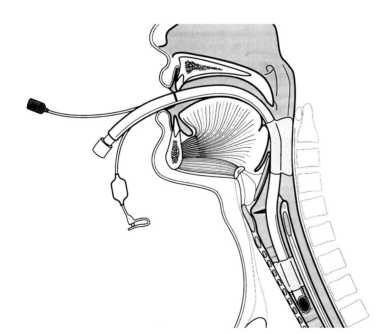

FIGURE 18–1. An endotracheal tube for prevention of posterior commissure stenosis. Expanding the asymmetrically inflatable cuff lifts the tube away from the posterior commissure.

posterior laryngeal commissure. Laryngeal changes were found in up to 30 per cent of patients after only a few days of nasogastric intubation.[39–41]

TRACHEOSTOMY TUBES

The first recorded tracheostomy was performed in 124 B.C. Tracheostomy tubes are designed to secure the patency of the surgical tract by connecting the cervical trachea with the ambient air through the soft tissues at the suprasternal notch. Tracheostomy provides the shortest and most effective route to bypass obstruction at the bottleneck of the airway (i.e., the larynx and hypopharynx). It reduces air flow resistance and ventilatory dead space. Tracheostomy tubes facilitate direct introduction of irrigation and catheters to evacuate secretions. They provide ready connection to assisted ventilatory devices.[42] Cuffed tracheostomy tubes are employed to seal the airway during artificial positive pressure ventilation and to limit influx of aspirated contaminants into the lower airway, where they may obstruct the lumen with adverse effects on the pulmonary parenchyma. Choice of material and design of the tube are determined by its goals and benefits. Unfortunately, all tracheostomies become infected within 24 to 72 hours postoperatively. Infection is unavoidable but can be restricted by use of nonirritating designs and materials that limit tissue injury. Indications for prophylactic antibiotics are controversial.[43–46]

The complications of prolonged tracheostomy are often regarded as unavoidable side effects of intensive care modalities, without which patients would not survive. Although this attitude is acceptable in relation to intensive care units, it should not be tolerated in short-term tracheostomies or in ambulatory patients. Damage occurring at the tracheostomy site can be minimized by modifications of surgical techniques and postoperative methods of sustaining the tracheostomy tract.

Tracheostomy tubes historically have been curved to be shaped as segments of a circle. This accommodates insertion and removal of the tube itself, its obturator/introducer, and an inner safety cannula. Furthermore, the curved design facilitates passage of suction tubes for clearance of secretions. The original constructing material had been metal, particularly silver. This allowed the design of thin walls, including an inner cannula. Currently, rubber or plastic materials, such as Teflon, silicone, and PVC, provide alternatives to metals. The preference for plastic tubes has been initiated by the search for lighter, safer, more flexible designs in an attempt to incorporate safely the inflatable cuff. PVC tubes are commonly used because of their flexibility, secure bonding with the thin expansile cuff, low price, dispensability, and ease of production. In general, the new flexibility and relatively safe materials are less traumatic and reduce sequelae.[47, 48]

Further progress is achieved through introduction of designs applicable to anatomic and managerial needs. Even though the standard curved design serves well in short-term tracheostomies (2 to 4 weeks), it often causes significant morbidity when employed for longer periods.

The curved tracheostomy tube enters through the anterior tracheal wall at an acute angle, requiring enlargement of the port of entry. The convex superior surface of the tube is in constant apposition with the anterior tracheal wall superior to the stoma (Fig. 18–2). In the supine patient, the weight of the tube compounds with the transmitted rhythmic deforming forces of assisted ventilation. The to-and-fro movement of the tube synchronous with the ventilatory cycle is superimposed on movements of the neck and those of the larynx during respiration, coughing, and swallowing, resulting in gradual erosion, posterior buckling, and collapse of the suprastomal anterior tracheal wall. Secondary infection causes further tissue breakdown, granulation tissue, fibrosis, and contracture above the tracheostomy site. This simultaneously compromises the lumen of the trachea in the anteroposterior dimensions. Squamous epithelium and granulation tissue may grow inward along the upper margin of the tube, resulting in the formation

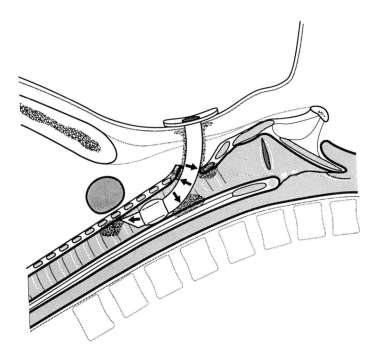

FIGURE 18–2. The variety of potential injuries inflicted on the trachea by the curved tracheostomy tube is marked by arrows.

of a valvelike flap causing intermittent obstruction.[49, 50]

Posterior buckling of the anterior suprastomal tracheal wall is, in our experience, the most common cause of failure to wean tracheotomized patients. This process also obstructs fenestrated tracheostomy tubes, resulting in failure to produce voice and speech. Tracheal granulations have been blamed incorrectly on fenestrated tubes. The granuloma often precedes the introduction of the fenestrated tube, although it may be further provoked by the irregularity of the fenestra[46, 51] (Fig. 18–3).

The anterior upper trachea may erode in patients with predisposing anatomy, such as short neck, low position of the larynx, and barrel chest. These may increase the acute angle at which the tube enters the trachea. In time, curved tubes may migrate superiorly toward the larynx, damaging the cricoid arch, cricothyroid membrane, and even the thyroid cartilage. Inflammatory involvement of the conus elasticus results in subglottic stenosis.[51] Fiberoptic endoscopy or lateral radiographs (preferably xeroradiographs) provide timely diagnosis. These destructive sequelae may ensue despite proper surgical technique and correct management.

Some degree of stenosis is present in all patients following tracheostomy; however, only 20 per cent have symptoms, with 10 per cent being disabled. The majority of these patients have difficulty in clearing secretions. These symptoms precede dyspnea and stridor. Since tracheostomy is often performed for lung disease, symptoms may be attributed to the underlying pulmonary condition rather than the post-tracheostomy stenosis or malacia.

Tracheal narrowing at the level of the stoma is typically concentric, with a tendency to be triangular in cross-section. The apex of the triangle is in the front where segments of the cartilage rings have been excised. After long-standing tracheostomy, the narrow lumen at the level of the tracheostoma is also flattened anteroposteriorly due to erosion and collapse of the anterior tracheal wall. Fibrosis and thickening of the membranous posterior tracheal wall further augment this narrowing. In general, tracheal stenosis is more common after tracheostomy than after intubation. It more often presents above the stoma than below it. As expected, the incidence of complications and their severity is compounded whenever tracheostomy follows prolonged intubation.[46, 51]

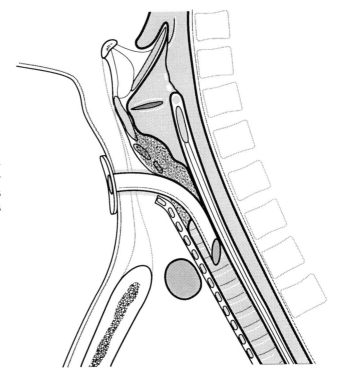

FIGURE 18–3. Typical presentation of tracheal injury after long-term tracheostomy with assisted ventilation. The shaded areas within the trachea represent pressure necrosis and granulation tissue.

Angled tubes have been introduced in an attempt to prevent the injurious effects of the standard curved tracheostomy tube[47] (Fig. 18–4). They enter the trachea at right angles to reduce the size of the fenestra, exerting less pressure against the anterior tracheal wall. Conversely, they have several inherent deficits. The segment of the angled tube intended to bridge across the soft tissues to the tracheal lumen may be either exces-

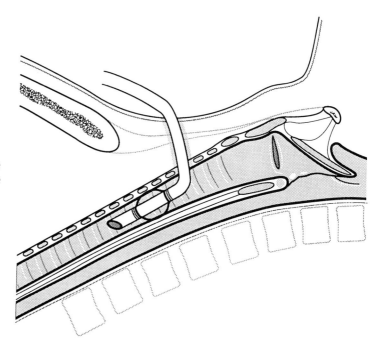

FIGURE 18–4. Angled tubes are designed to prevent trauma to the anterior tracheal wall.

sively long or too short. When short, it erodes the anterior tracheal wall below the tracheal stoma, also causing pressure necrosis of the skin under the neck plate. When too long, posterior membranous tracheal wall injury will occur, leading to cicatricial stenosis or to tracheal esophageal fistula. It is difficult to pass suction tubing through the acute angle at the knee of these tubes. Angled tubes are difficult to fit with an inner cannula. A wider internal diameter is therefore employed, defeating benefits of this design. Malleable inner cannulas have been incorporated but resisted insertion or removal.

One of the most versatile designs is manufactured by the Rusch Company (Ultra Tracheal Flex Tube). Constructed of spiral stainless steel, with a silicone rubber coat, this flexible armored tube with an adjustable neck plate is highly flexible yet retains an angled point of entry into the trachea. The neck plate is adjustable and may be secured at variable lengths. Different versions of this tube may allow various lengths of penetration into the trachea to pass beyond segments of stenosis or tracheomalacia.[47] Interposition of gauze padding beneath the neck plate may further modify its angle of entry. This change in angle may be a double-edged sword, trading one pressure point for another. In general, we suggest avoidance of gauze padding over the tracheostomy site as it accumulates secretions that become contaminated. The gauze irritates the underlying tissue and covers up granulations and pressure sores.

The hazards of the inflatable cuff have been dealt with in the discussion of endotracheal tubes. The following points pertain to cuffed tracheostomy tubes. The once popular "slip-on" cuff should not be used as it tends to slip off, occluding either the trachea or the distal opening of the tube. Use of high-volume–low-pressure cuff versus the sponge-filled variation (i.e., Bivona cuff tube) is determined by the patient's anatomy and the indications for tracheostoma. Cuff integrity must be predetermined. The sponge-filled cuffs may be abused by forced inflation, resulting in tracheomalacia and eventual stenosis. Cuffs that inflate irregularly are discarded. Thin-walled cuffs are better tolerated as they achieve seal at lower pressures. Cuff pressures should be monitored regularly. Cuff pressure should not exceed 20 to 30 cm of water. Periodic 10-minute depressurization is impractical in most cases. Automatic constant monitoring and regulation of cuff pressures appears to be the safest way to minimize tissue damage. However, this method is complicated and is not widely employed. The "just seal" or "minimal leak" methods are alternatives when performed by experienced personnel. Frequent periodic checking of cuff pressures is mandatory in intensive care units.

Double-cuffed tracheostomy tubes have been promoted. The concept was that the traumatic effect would be restricted by periodic alternation of the pressure points. This approach appeared promising but was not effective in reducing the complication rate. In essence, most tracheostomy tubes are too short to accommodate two high-volume–low-pressure cuffs.

Tracheal damage unfortunately occurs despite effective preventive measures. It is often caused by variations in blood pressure, infections, malnutrition, and systemic disease.

Postoperatively, it is wise to introduce cuffed tubes with built-in 15-mm hub connectors to ventilatory machines. These ought to be maintained in position for 24 to 48 hours until the patient and the tracheostoma are stable, allowing assisted ventilation for effective resuscitation and preventing aspiration. The cuffed tube should be withdrawn and replaced by a noncuffed design as soon as the patient's status is stable.

On principle, the smallest effective outer tube diameter should be applied. Frequent fiberoptic monitoring may detect heralding signs of impending stenosis.

Humidification and frequent irrigation of the tube will prevent crusting and obstruction of the lumen. The need for tracheostomy tubes with inner safety cannulas is determined by the patient's postoperative care. In the intensive care unit, where moisture exchange is controlled, an inner tube may not be mandated. Similarly, filter humidifiers, heat and moisture exchangers, may obviate the need for an inner cannula. These filter humidifiers act by capturing the patient's exhaled vapor and returning it upon the next inspiration.[53-55] Under normal conditions these devices may replace heated nebulizers or humidifiers. They are lightweight and adapted for use in children and adults. The thickness and nature of the patient's secretions are also determining factors in achieving better results, as are the patient's dexterity and the commitment or experience of the nursing staff. An uncuffed tube with the smallest effective diameter and inner cannula is the best choice in ambulatory patients. Disposable inner cannulas are now available for ease of management and sterility.

The surgeon may determine whether to use a curved or an angled tube, depending on the match between the patient's anatomy and the tube as demonstrated radiologically. The design of the neck plate is also considered to accommodate cervical anatomy, whether flat, horizontal, or winged. The connection of the neck plate to the tube should be swivel-type rather than rigid.

Guidelines for Tracheostomy Management

Determine:
1. Tube design and building material to best achieve goals and benefits.
2. Size—internal and external diameters, length of tube.
3. Choice of tube with inner cannula.
4. Availability of ventilator connectors.
5. Indications for a cuff.
6. Cuff type and design.
7. Cuff pressure and duration, with ability to monitor cuff pressures.
8. Indication and availability of valved or fenestrated tracheostomy tube.
9. Swivel-type adjustable neck plate.
10. Humidification—heat and oxygen, ability to employ a filter humidifier.
11. Local treatment and suction.

In general, the choice of the appropriate tube for any particular patient is difficult, requiring compromise and determination of priorities. A wide variety of tubes must be in stock in operating rooms, intensive care units, wards, and outpatient clinics. The choice should be guided by the indications, benefits, and goals set by the team of managing physicians. The tube causing the least trauma is preferred. Angled or cuffed tubes should not be applied if they are not specifically indicated, and the smallest effective diameter is preferred.

Communication in the Tracheotomized Patient

Loss of speech is devastating to the ventilatory-dependent patient. A number of options are available to re-establish effective, nontiring, intelligible communications.[56] Cuffed fenestrated tracheostomy tubes may be applied with assisted ventilation or in aspirating patients. The inner cannula is usually nonfenestrated to provide an airtight seal during assisted ventilation. When the inner cannula is temporarily removed, the patient may produce voice and generate speech even when the cuff is inflated. Cough also may be produced to clear the airway above the tube. Patients who are not ventilatory-dependent and who do not aspirate may use cuffless fenestrated tubes with single or double cannulas to produce voice while the airway is secured by the tracheostomy.[57] Fenestrated tubes may require custom designs to adapt and fit patients with unusual anatomic features.

A unique tracheostomy tube design is available for patients requiring uninterrupted assisted ventilation and therefore constant inflation of the cuff (Comunitrach, Implant Technologies, Inc.). This single-cuff, double-lumen tube, manufactured of PVC, was conceived to provide speech capability while the patient is on the ventilator. A special air channel directs controlled airflow from an outside source, other than the ventilator, toward the vocal cords. The patient or an attendant may control the flow of air through the glottis, providing patients with a normal vibratory mechanism with the ability to phonate. This same device is claimed to be

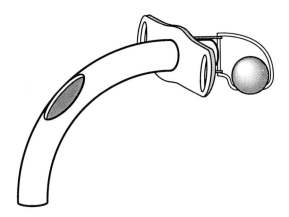

FIGURE 18–5. This drawing depicts the principle of a ball speaking valve mounted on a fenestrated curved tracheostomy tube.

effective in clearing secretions accumulated above the inflated cuff. This well-designed tube is effective and beneficial when properly applied and serviced. Unfortunately, its maintenance is time consuming and sometimes cumbersome, with frequent obstruction of the special air channel and its parts. Most patients receiving ventilation therapy are too sick to benefit from these devices.[58–60]

SPEAKING VALVES

Speaking valves operate by initiating unidirectional inspiratory air flow. Designed as one-way valves attached to tracheostomy tubes, they serve patients who can produce voice when the expired air is directed through their glottis. Such patients are dependent on the tracheostomy for inhalation (Fig. 18–5). These patients must otherwise speak by occluding the tube with a finger. This is one of the major discomforts of tracheostomy. The valves are attached to a standard tracheostomy tube. The built-in valve opens during inhalation and closes during exhalation to direct and force the air through the vocal cords. Valves such as the Trach-Talk, Olympic, Passy-Muir, Silicone Membrane Tracheal Cannula Valve by Boston Medical, Inc., and the Ball-Valve designed by Hood are all effective and very useful in voice and cough production. The valve must open with a minimal effort of approximately

−2 cm of water upon inspiration. These valves may become occluded by secretions and must therefore be readily detachable for cleaning. A secure means of attaching the valve must be included, otherwise it may be readily coughed out and lost. Trap-door designs have been successfully used in metal tracheostomy tubes; however, they are expensive and produce a loud audible click when in use.[52, 61, 62]

THE T-TUBE

Historically, laryngologists have sought effective means to maintain the airway through the tracheostomy site, simultaneously providing support and protection to the anterior superior tracheal wall (Fig. 18–6). The early 1960s saw the development of a soft, malleable, T-shaped tube, predominantly designed for introduction through the tracheostomy.[63–65] The T-tube is retained in position by virtue of its design, obviating the need for ties or sutures to prevent its expulsion or aspiration. The Montgomery silicone T-tube is one of the most commonly applied laryngotracheal stents. It is designed to maintain adequate tracheal airway and speech while providing internal support for reconstituted or reconstructed segments of the laryngotra-

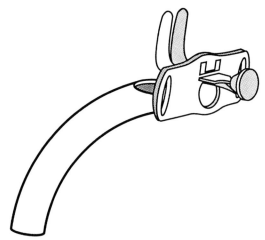

FIGURE 18–6. An example of a modified curved tracheostomy tube designed to support the anterior tracheal wall from within, thus preventing buckling.

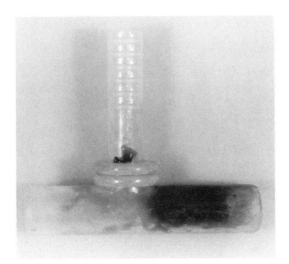

FIGURE 18–7. Occlusion of a Montgomery Safe-T-Tube by inspissated secretions.

cheal complex. Introduced endoscopically or through the tracheostomy, it often obviates the need for open surgery. Support of the tracheal and lower subglottic larynx facilitates passage of transglottic air for production of voice.

Because T-tubes lack an internal cannula, they are difficult to manage; they become occluded by encrusted and inspissated secretions. Thus they require frequent and continuous postoperative and ambulatory care. Lu-

minal obstruction can create potentially life-threatening situations. The outcome of the reconstructive surgical procedure may be jeopardized by premature removal (Fig. 18–7). While the free upper and lower margins of T-tubes must extend beyond the stenotic lesions, they should not be in close proximity to the glottis or to the carina. In both cases this may cause edema, inflammation, granulation tissue, and eventual extension of the stenosis. Whenever the glottis itself must be stented, it is preferable to extend the T-tube's superior limits above the vocal cords. The superior margin may abut the epiglottis, resulting in reactive granuloma (Fig. 18–8). Many patients aspirate when the upper orifice of the tube is not protected by functioning true vocal cords. However, some tolerate this relationship, particularly when the upper margin rises significantly above the glottis—about 1 to 2 cm. This also prevents erosion of the laryngeal surface of the epiglottis.

T-tubes may be trimmed for adaptation to the patient's particular anatomy and requirements. The newly formed margins must be carefully smoothed to prevent the emergence of additional points of irritation that can result in further pathology. Continuity and smoothness of the free margins must be retained, otherwise tears and breakdown en-

FIGURE 18–8. A silicone T-tube stenting stenotic lesions above and below the level of the tracheostomy site (*block shades*). Note the tip eroding the laryngeal surface of the epiglottis. A resulting granuloma may occlude the upper orifice.

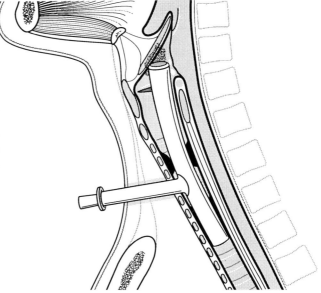

sue. A special cutting device for smoothing the free margins of the T-tube is available (Boston Medical Products, Inc.).[62] The medical and paramedical personnel in charge of a patient with a T-tube must be well acquainted with its design and management, knowing how to clean it, suction it, or even pull it out should it fail.

Safe Insertion

Insertion of the silicone T-tube is facilitated by its flexibility and design. The technique was clearly described by Montgomery.[65] This routine technique for insertion and exchange of T-tubes proved adequate and safe. However, there are exceptions. Inexperience and lack of confidence on the part of the surgeon may prolong the procedure, resulting in extended periods of apnea. The tube may fail to pass through the stenosed segments despite adequate preliminary dilatation. In particular, the upper limb may fail to snap into position in the presence of stenosis at or above the tracheal fenestra. Under such circumstances even instrumental traction through the endoscope may prove insufficient to complete the maneuver with minimal delay. Prolonged periods of apnea cause anxiety and distress to both surgeon and anesthesiologist. The following pre-emptive measures may safely expedite the process of insertion (Fig. 18–9).

A 0.5-cm umbilical tape is woven into the external limb of the T-tube, extending out through the upper orifice. This is in turn threaded into the trachea via the tracheostomy site and grabbed by alligator forceps to be pulled out through a rigid bronchoscope. A well-lubricated infant-sized cuffed endotracheal tube is passed through the lateral limb of the T-tube, extending down, through, and beyond the lower orifice of the inferior limb. This tube provides adequate oxygenation and constant ventilation throughout the procedure. In addition, the relatively narrow endotracheal tube extending beyond the lower margins of the T-tube acts as a guide and trocar. The lower limb is introduced first through the tracheostomy, sliding over the pediatric endotracheal tube, through which ventilation is maintained. The upper limb is guided into the larynx, being coaxed into position by tugging on the umbilical tape (Fig. 18–10). These modifications have been extremely helpful in compromised patients.[66]

Accidental Aspiration

Aspiration of T-tubes into the trachea, even though it seems improbable, has occurred

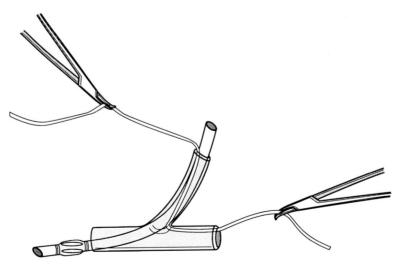

FIGURE 18–9. Safe insertion of the T-tube using a 0.5-cm umbilical tape together with a narrow, cuffed endotracheal tube.

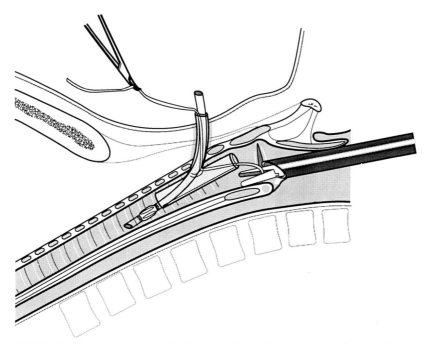

FIGURE 18–10. Safe insertion of a T-tube, with endoscopic control and assistance.

even in experienced hands. The first description of this complication was published by Marlowe and Eliachar in 1976.[68] Since then, additional instances have been encountered.[69] This extremely hazardous complication may ensue whenever the T-tube becomes partially obstructed by secretions. The patient or the attendant may push the tube down into the trachea while attempting to perform suction or to clear the obstructions. This may be compounded with a simultaneous strained inspiration by the anxious and irritated patient.

Awareness of this complication has led to development of T-tubes with a reinforced junction between the vertical and horizontal limbs, together with the addition of rings and washers on the horizontal segment that extends through the tracheostomy site (Safe-T-Tube, Boston Medical Products, Inc.). These modifications are generally effective; however, two of the seven instances of T-tube aspiration occurred with Safe-T-Tubes.[69] Furthermore, the lateral horizontal limb of the T-tube may not extend far enough beyond the surface at the tracheostomy site, as encountered in obese, kyphotic, and emphy-sematous patients. Such conditions may prompt aspiration of the tube contents or obstruction of its external orifice.[70]

THE MONTGOMERY SILICONE TRACHEAL CANNULA

This is one of several "tracheal buttons" designed to maintain stoma patency for suctioning and ventilation. This silicone tracheal tube closely resembles the Montgomery Safe-T-Tube.[62, 71] Instead of the vertical inner tube, it includes only two short inner flanges fashioned at a 27-degree angle to the long axis of the cannula to accommodate the angle of the anterior tracheal wall at the tracheostomy site. Its main advantage is that no foreign body projects into the inner lumen of the trachea. It is intended for use in patients with sleep apnea, bilateral vocal cord paralysis, chronic lung disease, and neurologic disorders, and following removal of T-tubes.

A unique method of insertion is provided by means of a metal tracheal fenestrator, consisting of an outer trephine knife fitted over the inner metal cannula (Boston Medical Products, Inc.). The fenestrator is used to establish the exact-sized opening in the anterior tracheal wall. Suction applied through the inner metal tube during the fenestrating process aspirates the cored-out segment of the trachea in a simple and exact manner. This results in a perfectly round fenestration that snugly accepts the tracheostomy cannula. Circumferential barb ridges and rings on the shaft of the silicone cannula are designed to prevent its displacement while serving to secure a silicone face plate in the appropriate position at the level of the cervical skin.

A one-way valve may be applied to the external margin of the cannula to serve patients with insufficient inspiratory air flow and adequate expiratory air flow, such as patients with bilateral vocal cord paralysis.[62]

The tracheal cannula appears to be an ideal method for the performance and maintenance of long-term tracheostomy. However, the concept of its application lacks formation of a circumferential skin-lined tract down to the level of the tracheal fenestra. Prolonged application of the tracheal cannula resulted in growth of granulation tissue along the shaft, and within the trachea at the point of

penetration (Fig. 18–11). A modified cannula in which the barbs were removed and the rings restricted to a minimum reduces, but does not prevent, the irritation of the tracheostomy tract.[71, 72]

THE ELIACHAR STOMA STENT

We have introduced a relatively new stoma stent in an attempt to improve upon imperfections in design and maintenance of the Montgomery tracheal cannula.[52] Made of biocompatible medical-grade silicone, stoma stents are flexible and not irritating to the skin and tracheal mucosa. Several designs and sizes are available. This single-unit prosthesis is provided with either an attached plug or a one-way valve (Figs. 18–12 and 18–13). A flexible external shield assists in proper placement of the stent, simultaneously preventing aspiration of the tube into the lower trachea. Two highly malleable and flexible inner flanges, extending vertically at the inner surface of the anterior tracheal wall, maintain the stent in position and prevent its expulsion during cough and speech. The stoma stent may be readily applied approxi-

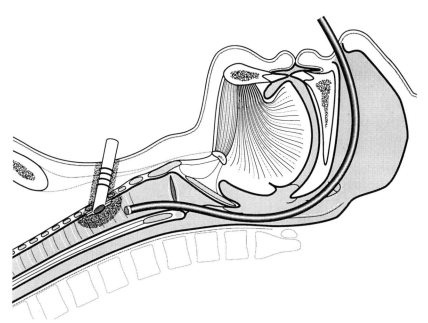

FIGURE 18–11. The Montgomery silicone tracheal cannula in position. The shaded area surrounding the cannula depicts areas where granulation may proliferate. This is best observed by means of fiberoptic endoscopy, as illustrated.

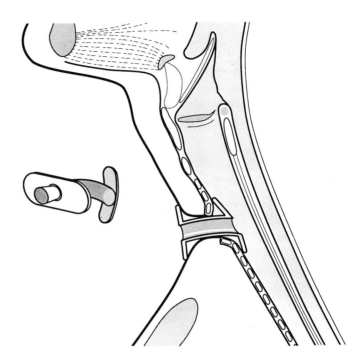

FIGURE 18–12. Sagittal projection of the airway showing the stoma stent in position. A plugged stent is also shown. Note absence of lumen compromise.

mately 3 weeks after the performance of a long-term flap tracheostomy (Fig. 18–14). It is well tolerated by the majority of patients. Easy insertion and extraction of the stent obviate the need for an inner cannula, promotes local hygiene, and prevents formation of granulation tissue and local irritation of the tracheostomy site and tract.

Its initial application was limited to patients with long-term or permanent tracheostomy. Currently, it is also applied in established short-term tracheostomy or in the weaning process after removal of tracheostomy tubes, stents, or silicone T-tubes. This stent is by no means applicable to every patient with a tracheostomy. Customized designs are occasionally required. No significant complications or side effects were encountered. Additional improvements and developments of the basic designs are anticipated, together with a wider variety of sizes. Other designs include the Olympic and the Kistner "buttons," each of which has its advantages and flaws.

DEVICES FOR EMERGENCY TRACHEOSTOMY

Several devices have been proposed for emergency transcervical access to the airway.

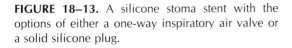

FIGURE 18–13. A silicone stoma stent with the options of either a one-way inspiratory air valve or a solid silicone plug.

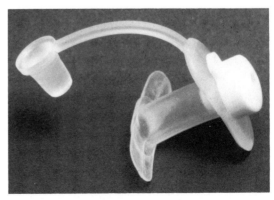

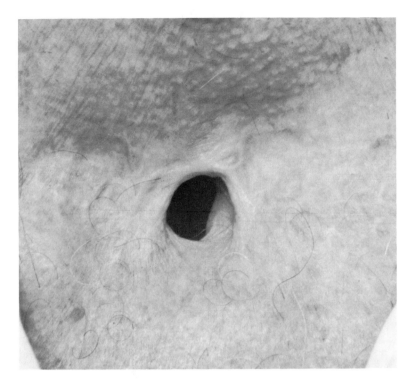

FIGURE 18–14. A well-healed long-term flap tracheostomy. Note the circumferential mucocutaneous junction, lack of granulation, and short skin-to-trachea tract. This condition must be achieved to ensure patient compliance and tolerance of stoma stents and buttons.

This may be achieved through sharp incision of the cricothyroid membrane (coniotomy) or by blind penetration of the anterior tracheal wall.[73, 74] All the available devices combine sharp metal blades with either sharp trocars or guide wires incorporated with a sliding internal or external overriding tube (e.g., NU-Tracke and Rapitrac Trach) (Fig. 18–15).

These instruments may be judiciously and effectively applied by trained and experienced surgeons. However, attempts to use these sharp devices by the inexperienced are potentially hazardous, bearing dangers of esophageal, neurologic, vascular, and pleural injuries. These devices should not be considered as alternatives to formal tracheostomy

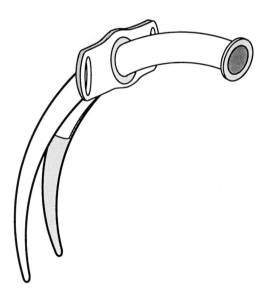

FIGURE 18–15. The author's preferred device for emergency tracheostomy. Note the double blades, introduced into the airway in the abutting position. Once the device is inside the trachea, an inner cannula splays the blades apart, extending beyond the sharp tips to prevent injury.

and definitely should not be recommended for use by any but experienced hands.

Recent publications prescribed cricothyrotomy over formal tracheostomy. It must be kept in mind that cricothyrotomy is in effect a laryngotomy.[75-77] Therefore, it is our contention that whenever cricothyrotomy is performed, it *must* be supplemented by a properly performed open tracheostomy within 12 to 24 hours. Otherwise, significant, sometimes irreversible, damage may affect the cricoid arch, thyroid cartilage, conus elasticus, and vocal cords.

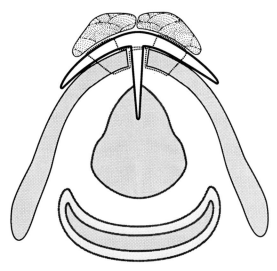

FIGURE 18–16. The Montgomery silicone "umbrella" keel.

INTRALARYNGEAL KEELS

Treatment of intralaryngeal webs is usually by surgical division of the fibrous tissue at the area of the anterior commissure. If such scar tissue is divided with no subsequent treatment, the webs tend to reform rapidly. Various techniques have been described to maintain separation of the vocal cord surfaces while re-epithelialization occurs. Open laryngeal procedures have used a laryngeal fissure approach to divide the web and enable insertion of devices such as the McNaught tantalum keel.[78] Tantalum is a soft, malleable metal, with minimal foreign body reaction. It is usually custom fashioned ad hoc at the operating room table. It is retained in position by virtue of its design without dislodgement or tensile strength breakdown.

The tantalum keel has been successfully used for extensive webs, but the technique itself requires invasive surgery that produces its own scar and a second procedure to extract the keel. A markedly improved silicone laryngeal keel was introduced by Montgomery[62-68] (Fig. 18–16). This umbrella-shaped prosthesis is soft and flexible to conform to soft tissue and minimize injury. It is indicated in the prevention and treatment of laryngeal stenosis limited to the anterior commissure of the vocal cords. A midline thyrotomy approach is also used to resect the stenosis and insert the keel. Two figure-of-eight 4-0 monofilament plastic sutures are applied to approximate the thyroid lamina and secure

the keel. These sutures bear the remote potential of trauma to the thyroid cartilage. Keels should be surgically removed under local anesthesia, not longer than 14 to 21 days after insertion; otherwise, granulation tissue is formed.[62]

Other such procedures are performed endoscopically. Following division of the anterior commissure web, solid or rolled Silastic stents can be inserted through the endoscope to provide separation of the vocal cords. Foreign body reaction to their presence may disrupt healthy endolaryngeal tissues surrounding the treated area.

Modified flat Teflon keels are found to be less traumatic than winged keels. These flat keels are inserted endoscopically, to be maintained in position by wire or nylon sutures that are in turn secured externally to the skin surface through onlay cutaneous buttons.[79]

Another version, an endoscopically introduced keel, has a tubular anterior segment attached longitudinally to a flat posterior wing. It may be trimmed to the size of the particular patient. Fixation is by means of nylon suture threaded through an intravenous cannula into the larynx at the cricothyroid and thyrohyoid membranes.[80] The suture secures the keel by its passage through the anterior tubular lumen. We caution that edema, pressure, trauma, and granulation tissue may develop. Prophylactic steroids and antibiotics may be considered.

Complications of intralaryngeal keels consist of aspiration, local granulation tissue, restenosis, extensive scarring, and infection caused by transcutaneous sutures.

ENDOLARYNGEAL CUFF FOR DILATING TRACHEAL AND TRACHEOSTOMY STENOSES

The cuff usually blamed for the development of tracheal stenosis may be applied for safe, atraumatic tracheal and stomal retrograde bougienage for dilation and relief of airway obstruction. Patients with tracheostomal or tracheal stenosis often present in emergency rooms, hospital wards, or a doctor's office, where instrumentation and anesthesia are absent. The airway obstruction must be relieved immediately. Under such emergency conditions, effective safe dilation is essential in order to break through the stenotic segment and allow insertion of a tube or cannula. Widening or re-establishing

a stenosed tracheostomy tract may be achieved with a series of trocars provided with tracheostomy tubes. These come in several sizes and may be applied progressively to expand the narrowed tract. Dilation by means of standard filiform rigid bougies is safe only when performed in the operating room by an experienced endoscopist working with the full cooperation of an anesthesiologist. Episodes of apnea during this type of bougienage are unavoidable and may further endanger an already critically ill patient.

We have safely used on numerous occasions a technique of tracheal dilation that eliminates the dangers of apnea and subsequent anoxia[81] (Fig. 18–17).

A narrow-cuffed red rubber or PVC endotracheal tube (internal diameter of 4 to 5 mm) is well lubricated and passed into the trachea, either through the mouth or through the tracheostomy site beyond the stenotic segment. After adequate ventilation of the patient, this tube is exchanged for one that is cuffed and of a similar diameter. Once the cuff has passed beyond the narrow segment, it is fully inflated and pulled back through the stenosis, dilating it in the process. This procedure of retrograde tracheal or tracheos-

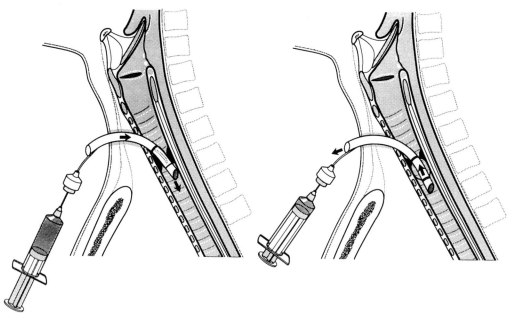

FIGURE 18–17. Safe retrograde bougienage, employing the inflated endotracheal tube cuff to overcome tracheal or tracheostomal stenosis.

tomal bougienage is repeated several times with successively growing increments in cuff pressure. Subsequently, an endotracheal tube of a larger diameter may replace the first, and the entire procedure is repeated until the tracheal lumen is wide enough to allow the safe introduction of an efficient hollow stent, T-tube, wide endotracheal tube, or tracheostomy cannula. Lubrication with an anesthetic gel is of great value. Note that throughout this procedure, the patency of the airway is maintained, and adequate ventilation coupled with bronchial toilet is made possible.

This technique may be used not only in the operating theater but also under topical anesthesia in emergency rooms, clinic offices, and wards, particularly in the presence of a tracheostomy. Once the acute emergency has been overcome, elective surgery may be undertaken with adequate time for proper work-up and preparation.

Dilation by bougienage is only of temporary value. However, safe, prompt dilation may be life-saving in acute emergency cases. This technique will not solve all the problems in the treatment of the severe, acutely stenosed tracheostoma or trachea, but it may buy time if properly utilized. It also may be applied repeatedly to dilate chronic cases in preparation for end-to-end tracheal anastomosis or laryngotracheal reconstruction.

LARYNGOTRACHEAL STENTS

The term *stent* is used to designate a splint that provides support for the purpose of keeping grafts in position or for maintaining the lumen of tubular structures. Stent was a 19th century English dental surgeon who described the application of a hard-setting resinous material to support and maintain the position of grafts. This term is now widely used as a noun, adjective, and verb ("to stent a stenotic lesion").

Stents have been applied widely as "lumen keepers" of the laryngotracheal complex in the management of acute trauma, following endoscopic dilatation, after open surgical re-

construction of laryngotracheal stenosis, or after conservation tumor surgery. Ideally, they should secure the airway and insure unrestricted ventilation while providing internal splinting and support. These devices must be well tolerated over extended periods. Their design should be as close as possible to the internal contours and dimensions of the laryngotracheal complex, to provide prolonged dilatation of stenosed or reconstructed segments of the airway, eventually resulting in a self-sustaining, stable lumen.

Stents are commonly introduced through an open surgical procedure, in conjunction with tracheostomy. Owing to development of well-tolerated biocompatible malleable materials, some stents may be introduced endoscopically, transorally, or through the tracheostomy tract. The length of the stent should be slightly longer than the stenosed segment under treatment. Its free margins should extend beyond the lesion, not irritating healthy tissue or structures above and below. Fixation in position to avoid migration, aspiration, or expulsion must be atraumatically secured for prolonged periods. Many methods have been used, including passage of retaining sutures through the laryngeal or tracheal skeleton or passage of ties around the tracheostomy cannula (Fig. 18–18).

Aspiration has to be contended with whenever internal support of the glottic or supraglottic levels is indicated. It has been thought that the portion of the stent reaching through and above the vocal cords must be sealed unless the stent is of a solid design.[82] As an alternative, an open-end stent must rise high above the glottis to avoid spillage into the airway.

Following surgical reconstruction of extensive comminuted transglottic and tracheal pathology, the surgeon is presented with unique stenting requirements. These cases often include revision and transposition of a previous existing tracheostomy, requiring internal support from the supraglottic level down to the upper mediastinum. In such cases, support of the larynx, upper trachea, and newly formed tracheostomy requires special stenting techniques. Special laryngo-

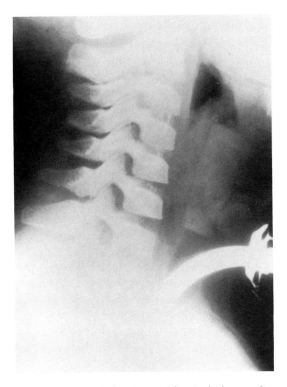

FIGURE 18–18. Soft tissue, midsagittal plane radiograph of the neck, demonstrating a solid laryngeal stent held in position by sutures tied to silicone retaining buttons.

tracheal stents must be integrated with the tracheostomy tube to provide the intended continuous support throughout the full extent of the larynx and the trachea.[83] Long T-tubes may serve well in these conditions if tolerated by the patient; however they may obstruct.[65] The angled designs and lack of inner safety cannulas prohibit effective cleansing of obstructing secretions, necessitating premature removal of the stent.

Ambulatory patients are more safely managed by a laryngeal stent combined with a standard curved tracheostomy tube that incorporates an inner safety cannula. These laryngeal stents are usually designed as solid inlays of the normal internal contours of the larynx and upper trachea.[65] As such, they are effective in preventing aspiration; however, at the same time they also prohibit production of voice. They are anchored in position by sutures fixed to the overlying skin or to the strap muscles. These sutures may damage the laryngeal cartilages and mucosa.[84]

Most stents described in the literature were designed and produced ad hoc of materials available to otolaryngologists in the operating room. Segments of endotracheal tubes,[82] silicone or metal tubes, and acrylic and tantalum mesh are commonly used. These are usually stabilized in position by sutures passed through the larynx or trachea to the skin by "collar buttons."[65] For instance, a PVC endotracheal tube may be trimmed to size, with one end melted shut over a flame to prevent aspiration. Crimping of the tube at the intended level of the glottis may be achieved by a hemostat. Heating the tube in the autoclave with a clamped hemostat on it, followed by rapid cooling, retains the desired design.

A modification of the PVC stent provides a cut strip of the anterior wall of the tube extending through the upper margin of the tracheostoma for external anchoring of the stent.[82] Other workers have described combinations of stents with standard tracheostomy cannulas to maintain their position, together with a safe airway.[85, 86] Intralaryngeal stents placed superiorly to the standard curved tracheostomy tube may elicit several inherent complications. This assembly lacks continuous intraluminal support, neglecting segments of the laryngotracheal lumen. This may result in circumferential stenosis in these intervening spaces because of irritation at the free margins of the stent and cannula.

After several modifications, a new tubular, hollow laryngotracheal stent was developed[87] (Fig. 18–19). Designed to conform to the inner contours of the larynx and upper trachea down to the level of the tracheostomy tube, it is anchored in position by a strap of soft, malleable silicone extending from its anterior wall through the upper margin of the tracheostomy site. This strap is attached to a silicone shield as a belt to buckle and tied around the neck by means of cloth tape. A one-way valve is built into the dome of the stent, to allow venting of intraluminal air from within the trachea and larynx up into the hypopharynx. Passage of the air through the one-way valve may be utilized to clear secretions or to create vibrations for the production of voice. Consequently, patients can

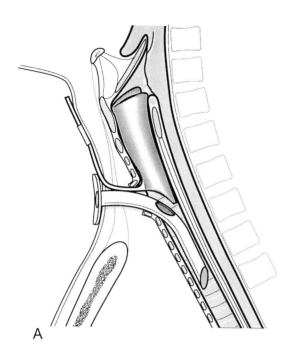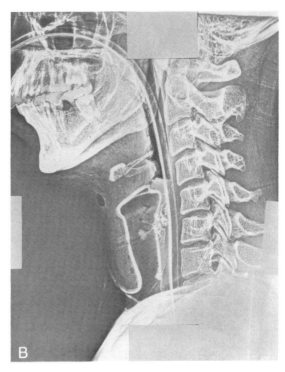

FIGURE 18–19. *A*, Drawing, and *B*, xeroradiograph of the hollow, vented laryngeal stent in position over a fenestrated tracheostomy tube.

communicate throughout the stenting period.

This newly designed laryngeal and upper tracheal stent is intended to be used in combination with a standard curved fenestrated tracheostomy tube, preferably with an inner safety cannula. These features eliminate risks of potential occlusion during prolonged periods of time, particularly in ambulatory settings. The design of the lower part of this stent protects the anterior superior tracheal wall and also prevents unstented gaps of tracheal and laryngeal mucosa encountered with the Teflon or PVC tubes and solid, Montgomery-type laryngeal stents. Furthermore, the lower part of the stent may be trimmed to accommodate various anatomic dimensions and relationships. We have used this stent in over 35 patients for postoperative internal support and for the control of incessant aspiration (Fig. 18–20).[88]

Endoscopically Placed Tracheobronchial Stents

Advances in endoscopy from a diagnostic to interventional modality have led to the development of tubular stents that may maintain the lumen not requiring tracheostomy. This technique has been applied initially in the management of laryngeal tumors and tracheal stenosis. Problems encountered are lumen obstruction by inspissated secretions, displacement of the tube, edema, and growth of either granulation tissues or the tumor beyond the margins. The availability of well-tolerated materials such as silicone rubber and the effectiveness of laser surgery in conjunction with fiberoptic rigid and flexible telescopy will in time lead to perfection of this technique. The main problems to solve are how to have continuous visual control of the insertion process and adequate, well-monitored ventilation by the anesthesiologist.[89]

SUMMARY

Devices for management of the laryngotracheal complex abound. The plethora of prosthetic devices reflects upon limited success

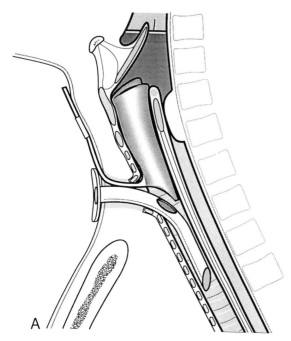
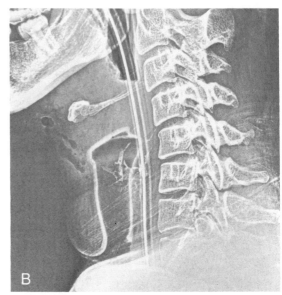

FIGURE 18–20. *A*, Drawing, and *B*, xeroradiograph depicting the laryngeal stent as a means of controlling aspiration. Note the pool of fluid in the hypopharynx, above the larynx.

and multiple complications. Management of the airway to avoid suffocation, provide effective ventilation and bronchial toilet, and prevent aspiration must employ devices and prostheses that ultimately may injure the larynx and the trachea. Adequate knowledge of these devices, familiarity with their variations, and experience in correct application may prevent many of the associated side effects and complications. We hope this chapter will contribute to a reduction in frequency and severity of side effects and complications, although so far there are no universal solutions to many of these complex problems.

References

1. Weymuller EA: Laryngotracheal injury from prolonged endotracheal intubation. Laryngoscope 98:1–15, 1988.
2. Kastanos N, Estopa-Miro R, Marin-Perez A, et al: Laryngotracheal injury due to endotracheal intubation: Incidence, evolution, and predisposing factors. A prospective long-term study. Crit Care Med 11(5):362–367, 1983.
3. Eliachar I, Roberts J, Olsen E, et al: Modified endotracheal tube for prevention of posterior commissure stenosis in long-term endotracheal intubation: A preliminary canine study. Otolaryngol Head Neck Surg 97(6):594–599, 1987.
4. Steen JA, Lindholm CE, Brdlik GC, Foster CA: Tracheal tube forces on the posterior larynx: Index of laryngeal loading. Crit Care Med 10(3):186–189, 1982.
5. Whited RE: A study of endotracheal tube injury to the subglottis. Laryngoscope 95(10):1216–1219, 1985.
6. Volpi D, Lin PT, Kuriloff DB, Kimmelman CP: Risk factors for intubation injury of the larynx. Ann Otol Rhinol Laryngol 96(6):684–686, 1987.
7. Alexopoulos C, Lindholm CE: Airway complaints and laryngeal pathology after intubation with an anatomically shaped endotracheal tube. Acta Anaesthesiol Scand 27(4):339–344, 1983.
8. Guess WL: Plastics for tracheal tubes. Int Anesthesiol Clin 8:805–814, 1970.
9. Stetson JB, Guess WL: Causes of damage to tissues by polymers and elastomers used in the fabrication of tracheal devices. Anesthesiology 33:635–652, 1970.
10. Hadden M, Ersoz CJ, Donnelly WH, Safar P: Laryngotracheal damage after prolonged use of protracheal tubes in adults. JAMA 207(4):703–708, 1969.
11. Via-Reque E, Rattenborg CC: Prolonged pro- or nasotracheal intubation. Crit Care Med 9(9):637–639, 1981.
12. Sellery GR, Worth A, Greenway RE: Late complications of prolonged tracheal intubation. Can Anaesth Soc J 25(2):140–143, 1978.
13. Watson CB: A survey of intubation practices in critical care medicine. Ear Nose Throat J 62:76–93, 1983.
14. Deane RS, Mills EL: Prolonged nasotracheal intubation in adults: A successor and adjunct to tracheostomy. Anesth Analg 49(1):89–97, 1970.

15. Lindholm CE: Prolonged endotracheal intubation. Acta Anaesth Suppl 33:1, 1969.
16. Harrison GA, Tonkin JP: Prolonged endotracheal intubation. Br J Anaesth 40:241–249, 1968.
17. Feder RJ: Early recognition and treatment of post-intubation dysphonia. Laryngoscope 93(8):1070–1072, 1983.
18. Whited RE: A study of post-intubation laryngeal dysfunction. Laryngoscope 95(6):727–729, 1985.
19. Cavo JW Jr: True vocal cord paralysis following intubation. Laryngoscope 95(11):1352–1359, 1985.
20. Weymuller EA, Bishop MJ, Fink BR, et al: Quantification of intralaryngeal pressure exerted by endotracheal tubes. Ann Otol Rhinol Laryngol 92:444–447, 1983.
21. Alexopoulos C, Jansson B, Lindholm CE: Mucus transport and surface damage after endotracheal intubation and tracheostomy. An experimental study in pigs. Acta Anaesthesiol Scand 28(1):68–76, 1984.
22. Schmidt WA, Schaap RN, Mortensen JD: Immediate mucosal effects of short-term soft-cuff, endotracheal intubation. A light and scanning electron microscopic study. Arch Pathol Lab Med 30(10):516–521, 1979.
23. Davies JE, Lesser TH, Cobley MA: Intubation trauma: A comparison of two different endotracheal tubes. J Laryngol Otol 102(9):822–823, 1988.
24. Cross DE: Recent developments in tracheal cuffs. Resuscitation 2:22–81, 1973.
25. Stanley TH: Nitrous oxide and pressures and volumes of high and low pressure endotracheal-tube cuffs in intubation patients. Anesthesiology 42:637–640, 1975.
26. Kamen JM, Wilkinson CJ: A new low-pressure cuff for endotracheal tube. Anesthesiology 34:482–485, 1971.
27. Greene SJ, Cane RD, Shapiro BA: A foam cuff endotracheal tube T-piere system for use with nitrous oxide anesthesia. Anesth Analg 65:1359–1360, 1986.
28. Stauffer JL, Olson DE, Petty TL: Complications and consequences of endotracheal intubation and tracheotomy. Am J Med 70:65–76, 1981.
29. Geha AS, Seegers JV, Kooner IJ, Lefrak S: Tracheoesophageal fistula caused by cuffed tracheal tube. Successful treatment by tracheal resection and primary repair with four-year follow-up. Arch Surg 113(3):338–340, 1978.
30. Bugge-Asperheim B, Birkeland S, Stren G: Tracheoesophageal fistula caused by cuffed tracheal tubes. Scand J Thorac Cardiovasc Surg 15(3):315–319, 1981.
31. Whited RE: Posterior commissure stenosis post long-term intubation. Laryngoscope 93:1314–1318, 1983.
32. Hedden M, Ersoz CJ, Donnelly HA, et al: Laryngotracheal damage after prolonged use of orotracheal tubes in adults. JAMA 207:703–708, 1969.
33. Deutschman CS, Wilton P, Simon J, et al: Paranasal sinusitis associated with nasotracheal intubation: A frequently unrecognized and treatable source of sepsis. Crit Care Med 14(2):111–114, 1986.
34. Dubick MN, Wright BD: Comparison of laryngeal pathology following long-term oral and nasal endotracheal intubation. Anesth Analg 57(6):663–668, 1978.
35. Inodel AR, Beckman JF: Unexplained fevers in patients with nasotracheal intubation. JAMA 248:868, 1982.
36. O'Reilly MJ, Reddick EJ, Black W, et al: Sepsis from sinusitis in nasotracheally intubated patients: A diagnostic dilemma. Am J Surg 147:601, 1984.
37. Pope TL, Stelling LB, Leitnen YB: Maxillary sinusitis after nasotracheal intubation. South J Med 74:610–612, 1981.
38. Berry FA, Blankenbaker WL, Ball CG: A comparison between bacteremia occurring with nasotracheal and orotracheal intubation. Anesth Analg 52:873–876, 1973.
39. Alessi DM, Berci G: Aspiration and nasogastric intubation. Otolaryngol Head Neck Surg 94(4):486–489, 1986.
40. Sofferman RA, Hubbell RN: Laryngeal complications of nasogastric tubes. Ann Otol Rhinol Laryngol 90:465–468, 1981.
41. Friedman M, Baim H, Shelton V, et al: Laryngeal injuries secondary to nasogastric tubes. Ann Otol Rhinol Laryngol 90:469–474, 1981.
42. Katz L, Crosby JW: Accidental misconnections to endotracheal and tracheostomy tubes. Can Med Assoc J 135:1149–1151, 1986.
43. Johnson JT: Antibiotics in tracheostomy. In Myers EN, Stool SE, Johnson JT (eds): Tracheostomy. New York, Churchill-Livingston, 1985, pp 171–176.
44. Niederman MS, Ferranti RD, Zeigler A, et al: Respiratory infection complicating long-term tracheostomy: The implication of persistent gram-negative tracheobronchial colonization. Chest 85:39–44, 1984.
45. Lepper MH, Kofman S, Blatt N, et al: Effect of eight antibiotics used singly and in combination on the tracheal flora following tracheotomy in poliomyelitis. Antibiot Chemother 4:829, 1954.
46. Sasaki CT, Horiuchi M, Koss NL: Tracheostomy-related subglottic stenosis: Bacteriologic pathogenesis. Laryngoscope 89:857, 1979.
47. Lindholm CE: Choice of tracheostomy tube. In Myers EN, Stool SE, Johnson JT (eds): Tracheostomy. New York, Churchill-Livingstone, 1985, pp 125–146.
48. Spooner TR: An evaluation of Silastic tracheostomy tubes. Laryngoscope 81:1132–1137, 1971.
49. Hughes M, Kirchner JA, Branson RJ: A skin-lined tube as a complication of tracheostomy. Arch Otolaryngol 94:568–570, 1971.
50. Myers EN, Stool SE: Complications in tracheostomy. In Myers EN, Stool SE, Johnson JT (eds): Tracheostomy. New York, Churchill-Livingstone, 1985, pp 147–169.
51. Eliachar I, Goldsher M, Joachims HZ, et al: Superiorly based tracheostomal flap to counteract tracheal stenosis: Experimental study. Laryngoscope 91:976–981, 1981.
52. Eliachar I, Oringher SF: Performance and management of long-term tracheostomy. Oper Tech Otolaryngol Head Neck Surg 1:56–63, 1990.
53. Myer CM: The heat and moisture exchanger in post-tracheostomy care. Otolaryngol Head Neck Surg 96:209–210, 1987.
54. Revenas B, Lindholm CE: The foam nose—a new disposable head and moisture exchanger. A comparison with other similar devices. Acta Anaesthesiol Scand 23:34–36, 1979.
55. Revenas B, Lindholm CE: Temperature variations in disposable head and moisture exchangers. Acta Anaesthesiol Scand 24:237, 1980.
56. Safar P, Grenvik A: A speaking cuffed tracheostomy tube. Crit Care Med 3(1):23–26, 1975.

57. Howsinger MJ, Yorkstone KM, Dowden PA: Communication options for intubated patients. Resp Man 17(3):45–51, 1987.
58. Beukelman DR, Yorkston KM, Dowden PA: Communication Augmentation: A Casebook of Clinical Management. San Diego, College Hill Press, 1985, pp 89–100.
59. Walsh JJ, Rho DS: A speaking endotracheal tube. Anesthesiology 63:703–705, 1985.
60. Blom ED, Singer MI, Markleroad BA: Self-activated pneumatic voicing system for ventilator-dependent patients. Presentation to the American Association for Respiratory Therapy, Annual Convention, New Orleans, 1982.
61. Passy V: Passy-Muir tracheostomy speaking valve. Otolaryngol Head Neck Surg 95(2):247–248, 1986.
62. Montgomery WW, Montgomery SK: Manual for use of Montgomery laryngeal, tracheal and esophageal prosthetics. Ann Otol Rhinol Laryngol 195(4):1–16, 1989.
63. Montgomery WW: T-tube tracheal stent. Arch Otolaryngol 82:320–321, 1965.
64. Meyer R: Reconstructive Surgery of the Trachea. New York, Thieme-Stratton, 1982.
65. Montgomery WW: Surgery of the Upper Respiratory System. Philadelphia, Lea & Febiger, 1973, p 2.
66. Eliachar I, Joachims HZ, Simon K: Safe insertion of tracheal T-tubes. Ann Rhinol Laryngol 8:228–229, 1978.
67. Landa L: The tracheal T-tube. In Grill HC, Eschapasse H (eds): Major Challenges (A Volume in the International Trends in General Thoracic Surgery Series). Philadelphia, WB Saunders, 1987, pp 124–132.
68. Marlowe FI, Eliachar I: Treatment of tracheal stenosis: An unusual complication. Laryngoscope 86(8):1268–1271, 1976.
69. Calhoun KH, Deskin RW, Bailey BJ: Near-fatal complication of tracheal T-tube use. Ann Rhinol Laryngol 97:542–544, 1988.
70. Solomons NB: Hazard of the tracheal T-tube: A method of removal. Int J Pediatr Otorhinolaryngol 14:171–173, 1987.
71. Montgomery WW: Silicone tracheal cannula. Ann Otol Rhinol Laryngol 89:521–528, 1980.
72. Strauss M: Use of modified silicone tracheal cannula for obstructive sleep apnea. Laryngoscope 100(2):152–154, 1990.
73. Holst M, Hedenstierna G, Kumlien JA, Schiratzki H: Five years' experience of coniotomy. Intensive Care Med 11:202–206, 1985.
74. Jakobsson J, Andersson G, Wiklund PE: Experience with elective coniotomy. Acta Chir Scand 520:101–103, 1984.
75. Sise MJ, Shackford SR, Cruickshank JC, et al: Cricothyroidotomy for long-term tracheal access. Ann Surg 200(1):13–17, 1984.
76. Boyd AD, Romita MC, Conlan AA, et al: A clinical evaluation of cricothyroidotomy. Surg Gynecol Obstet 149:365–368, 1979.
77. Holst M, Halbig I, Persson A, Schiratzki H: The cricothyroid muscle after cricothyroidotomy. Acta Otolaryngol (Stockh) 107:136–140, 1989.
78. McNaught RC: Surgical correction of the anterior web of the larynx. Laryngoscope 60:264–272, 1950.
79. Dedo HH: Endoscopic Teflon keel for anterior glottic web. Ann Otol Rhinol Laryngol 88:467–473, 1979.
80. Das Gupta AR, Parker DA: A preformed Silastic keel for the treatment of anterior laryngeal webs. ENT Technol 1:50–52, 1987.
81. Eliachar I, Simon K, Birkhan JH, Joachim HZ: Emergency management of tracheal stenosis. "Retrograde Tracheal Bougienage." Otol Rhinol Laryngol 42:46–48, 1980.
82. Passy V, Kulber H, Ermshar CB: The K.E.P. laryngeal tracheal stent. Laryngoscope 82:271–275, 1972.
83. Eliachar I, Joachims HZ: Reconstruction of the larynx and trachea with hyoid transposition. Surg Head Neck 2:259–265, 1981.
84. Weisberger EC, Huebsch SA: Endoscopic treatment of aspiration using a laryngeal stent. Otolaryngol Head Neck Surg 90:215–222, 1982.
85. Conley JJ: Tracheal prosthesis for stenosis. Arch Otolaryngol 82:433–436, 1985.
86. Aboulker P: Traitement des stenoses trachaels. Problemes actuel d'oto-rhino-laryngologie. Paris, Librairie Maloine, 1968, pp 275–295.
87. Eliachar I, Roberts JK, Hayes JD, Tucker HM: A vented laryngeal stent with phonatory and pressure relief capability. Laryngoscope 97(11):1264–1269, 1987.
88. Eliachar I, Nguyen D: Laryngotracheal stent for internal support and control of aspiration without loss of phonation. Otolaryngol Head Neck Surg 103:837–840, 1990.
89. Dumon JF: A dedicated tracheobronchial stent. Chest 97(2):328–332, 1990.

CHAPTER 19

Tracheotomy Complications

HUGH REILLY, MD
CLARENCE T. SASAKI, MD

Tracheotomy represents the surgical introduction of an artificial airway into the trachea to direct the pathway of airflow from the upper airway structures. Its long history begins before 100 B.C., when it was first described by Asclepiades, the Greek physician.[1] Its inherent dangers were recognized early and until the 19th century it was seldom performed because it was considered too hazardous. The term *trachea* is derived from the Greek "trachea arteria" or "rough artery," suggesting at least part of the hazards then encountered with the associated operative procedure. In 1909 Jackson described the technique largely as it is practiced today.[2]

Complications of tracheotomy frequently result from improper execution of the procedure or inadequate postoperative care of the tracheotomized patient. Most retrospective studies have addressed the incidence of overall complications, ranging from 5 per cent to 40 per cent.[3–13, 17] Representative studies suggest an overall complication rate approaching 15 per cent, with the most common of them being hemorrhage (3.7 per cent), tube obstruction (2.7 per cent), or tube displacement (1.5 per cent). Pneumothorax, atelectasis, aspiration, tracheal stenosis, and tracheoesophageal fistula occur with less than 1 per cent frequency each. Death occurs in 0.5 per cent to 1.6 per cent of cases and is most often caused by hemorrhage or inadvertent tube displacement. Moreover, emergency tracheotomy carries a two- to fivefold increase in the incidence of complications over an elective procedure.[9, 12, 13]

There is much controversy over the safety of prolonged orotracheal intubation and the timing of tracheotomy thereafter. The incidence of laryngotracheal complications is low with pretracheotomy intubation periods of up to 5 to 10 days but increases substantially thereafter.[11, 12] Pediatric populations uniformly have higher complication rates than adults, patient age being inversely related to complication rate.[14–16] The seriousness and frequency of tracheotomy-associated morbidity and mortality compare with those of major abdominal procedures, and in this respect tracheotomy must be considered a major operation.[5]

SURGICAL TECHNIQUE[18–20]

Adequate preparation and meticulous attention to the details of the procedure are imperative for safe and successful tracheotomy. The procedure can be performed at the bedside, preferably in the ICU or in the operating room. When emergent loss of the airway necessitates tracheotomy in the Emergency Department, cricothyroidotomy may be preferred. Under such circumstances the patient preferably should have adequate intravenous access; resuscitative medications and equipment should be present. The surgeon must have adequate lighting (headlight if at bedside) and suction equipment. In addition to securing the airway and insuring ventilation preoperatively, endotracheal intubation provides a recognizable target for the surgeon and helps protect the posterior tracheal wall and esophagus from inadvertent injury during entry of the trachea. Naso- and orogastric tubes should be removed, especially in infants, since they stiffen and distend the esophagus, causing it to resemble the trachea. The patient should be placed in the supine position, on a shoulder roll, with the neck extended and the occiput supported. This position brings the cricoid cartilage anterosuperiorly, aiding in its identification while drawing the trachea out of the mediastinum. Neck extension may have to be compromised in the trauma patient in whom cervical spine injury has not been excluded. Occasionally a patient with impending obstruction may not be able to tolerate the fully supine position. In this case a semireclining position may be necessary.

A midline vertical skin incision is made, beginning at the inferior border of the cricoid, and extended approximately 2 to 3 cm inferiorly. A vertical incision is favored since it avoids the transection of many vertically oriented subcutaneous vessels. More importantly, it allows the tracheotomy tube to glide unimpeded in the vertical plane as it ascends and descends during swallowing, without risk of being displaced from the trachea or pinned against the posterior tracheal wall. Straying off the midline can lead to transection of vessels, the esophagus, or recurrent laryngeal nerves. A tracheotomy placed too high can lead to injury of the cricoid or other laryngeal structures, causing late stenosis. Too low a tracheotomy may cause right main stem bronchial intubation, laceration, or later erosion of the innominate artery or entry into the apical pleura.[18] Excessive use of electrocoagulation to achieve hemostasis invites tissue destruction and should be avoided in favor of vessel ligation.

Layer-by-layer dissection of fascia is accomplished by having the assistant gently pick up the fascial tissues opposite the operator as each layer is divided. The thyroid isthmus is encountered at the level of the second and third tracheal rings. It is mobilized bluntly by inserting a hemostat from above and lifting it off the anterior tracheal wall. It is clamped on each side, divided, and its edges suture-ligated. Failure to divide the thyroid isthmus invites its erosion, bleeding, or tube displacement when the patient is taken out of neck extension. The pretracheal fascia is then lifted with a clamp and divided, exposing the anterior tracheal wall. Any dissection required below the isthmus should be done bluntly or with the scalpel blade pointing superiorly to minimize injury to the vascular structures of the mediastinum.

With a cricoid hook, upward traction is maintained by the assistant until the tube has been securely introduced into the tracheal lumen. In adults, a small window of cartilage is removed through the second and third tracheal cartilage, using a scalpel or heavy scissors while the segment to be removed is firmly grasped with a clamp. Entering the trachea by electrocautery is to be avoided to prevent ignition of the endotracheal tube. At this time the endotracheal tube or bronchoscope is pulled back just cephalad to the tracheal window, where it can be reinserted in the event initial tracheal cannulation fails. The posterior wall is quickly surveyed for damage and the tube carefully introduced under direct vision with the obturator in place to avoid "snowplowing" damage to the inner tracheal wall. While the assistant stabilizes the tube by holding the fixation plate, the obturator is removed, the inner cannula introduced, and the patient ventilated. Lungs should be auscultated for full bilateral breath sounds and the chest wall observed for symmetric excursions. The cricoid hook and the endotracheal tube can now be safely removed.

Excess secretions are suctioned, iodoform ointment is applied to the stoma, or an iodoform-moistened gauze is placed around the tube loosely and the fixation plate secured to the patient. The tracheotomy incision should be left open lest expired air become trapped and forced into the exposed fascial planes, causing expanding subcutaneous or mediastinal emphysema. A chest radiograph should be promptly obtained to verify the position of the tube and rule out undetected subcutaneous emphysema, pneumomediastinum, or pneumothorax.

Several modifications in technique are required in children. The subcutaneous tissue should be "defatted" to facilitate exposure and to allow easier tube reinsertion should premature accidental decannulation occur. Injury to the inferior thyroid vessels could lead to air embolism. In the infant the "trachea" should be palpated for pulsation prior to its entry, since the common carotid artery is of comparable size and can be mistaken for it. In children, a cartilage window should not be removed since this leads to an unacceptably high rate of tracheal stenosis. Instead, the trachea is entered through a vertical midline incision through the 2nd and 3rd cartilages. It is suggested that stay sutures placed on each side of the trachea will aid in obtaining access to the lumen in the event of accidental decannulation. Nonabsorbable sutures should be taped without tension to the anterior neck on each side and may be removed when a mature tract from skin to trachea has formed.

POSTOPERATIVE CARE

In the immediate postoperative period, the patient's respiratory status must be carefully monitored. Patients unable to speak need an alternative means of alerting others to distress. Agitation must not be prematurely regarded as psychologic distress, without assuring adequate ventilation to guard against overlooking early signs of hypoxia.

Tube patency is most often compromised by secretions or crusting. Inspired air should be sufficiently humidified, sterile saline irrigation should precede suctioning, and the patient should be kept adequately hydrated. These measures help prevent the thickening and drying of secretions. The inner cannula should be cleaned or replaced every 4 hours in the immediate postoperative period and three times a day thereafter. Suctioning removes secretions and small crusts, and the tube should be cleaned hourly for the first few postoperative days and at least several times a day thereafter. It must be done effectively but atraumatically. A soft tube with an open Y connector should be inserted and vacuum applied only during withdrawal to avoid mucosal injury to the trachea.

The monitored maintenance of tube position is important for two reasons. First, the tube must remain in a central position within the trachea so as to prevent occlusion of the lumen against the tracheal wall; a loose tube can be coughed out or dislocated. Improper positioning or movement of the tube will further aggravate damage to adjacent structures, leading to ulceration, infection, excessive scarring, or stenosis. The tracheotomy plate should remain flush against the anterior neck. Tracheotomy ties should be sufficiently tight to allow the interposition of two fingers between the tie and the neck. Tightness of fit should be closely monitored since changes in local swelling or body fluid content can dramatically alter this fit. The tracheotomy tube must be free of any possible traction that may result from poorly positioned ventilation tubing or by a thrashing, agitated patient. For these reasons, T-pieces should be avoided in favor of trach masks. Agitated patients may require sedation or restraint to prevent intermittent pulling against the tracheotomy tube. A spare tracheotomy tube (inner and outer) should always be available at the patient's bedside. Except for emergency situations, the ties and outer tube should not be removed during the first several days following tracheotomy placement. This interval will produce a stable tract allowing safe later removal of the entire apparatus.

Crusts, dried blood, or debris should be cleaned from the stoma with hydrogen peroxide or saline. Vigorous local wound care has been shown to prevent many infectious complications. Betadine ointment is applied to the stoma and a betadine-painted dressing placed over the stoma three times a day for the first 10 postoperative days (except in children in whom the dressing is omitted to insure tighter fit of the tube against the patient).

Some tracheotomy tubes are equipped with cuffs that are used to provide a seal between the tube and the tracheal wall. Such tubes also offer partial or temporary protection against massive aspiration. Although tracheal wall injury and stenosis was a frequent occurrence when small volume–high pressure cuff tubes were used, the advent of high volume–low pressure cuff tubes has lessened but not eliminated this problem. As will be detailed later, even the latter tubes can cause tracheal wall damage when mucosal capillary perfusion is compromised. In this regard, the cuff should be inflated only when necessary; cuff pressures should be monitored frequently and maintained below 15 mm Hg, if possible, but definitely below 25 mm Hg. At minimal occlusion pressures, the addition of even 2 cc of air can create pressures exceeding 30 mm Hg.

Finally, the patient and family must be informed of the principles of tracheotomy care. We utilize a clear plastic model of the airway to demonstrate such care. Only after demonstrated proficiency on the plastic model is the patient allowed to practice personal tracheotomy care in front of a mirror. In the event of airway obstruction unrelieved by suctioning, the patient is instructed to remove the inner cannula and to attempt vigorous coughing. If this is ineffective in expelling the mucous plug, the outer tube should then be removed to facilitate expulsion of plugs too large to pass through the constricted cannula.

EARLY COMPLICATIONS

HEMORRHAGE

Minor bleeding or oozing occurs in about 5 per cent of cases. The source is usually venous, involves the anterior jugular system or thyroid isthmus, and occurs near the stoma. Reducing venous pressure by raising the patient to a semirecumbent position and applying hemostatic gauze are usually sufficient treatments. Major hemorrhage is less common and usually involves the communicating branch of the superior thyroid artery. In this case immediate local exploration and ligation of the injured vessel are warranted.

Massive arterial hemorrhage is rare and usually indicates bleeding from the innominate artery. This is caused by erosion of the vessel by the distal end of the cannula in the presence of mediastinal infection or by intraoperative disruption when the artery is high lying or if the normal anatomy is distorted or obscured by tumor, previous operation, or radiation. The excessive use of electrocautery tends to obscure tissue planes and may contribute to accidental large vessel injury. In this instance the airway should first be secured by insertion of a longer tube—i.e., an endotracheal tube. Digital pressure is applied against the artery, and the patient is immediately returned to the operating room for arterial repair by a median sternotomy approach.

TUBE DISPLACEMENT

Whenever a new tracheotomy cannula is inserted, breath sounds should be assured by auscultation. Postoperative displacement of the cannula can cause a patient's demise rapidly and is reported to occur in about 2 per cent to 5 per cent of patients. It can occur at any time but is most common in the immediate postoperative period. It is particularly dangerous during the first 3 to 5 postoperative days before a stable tract has matured between the skin and tracheal lumen. Most frequently tube displacement is caused by failure to secure the tube adequately to the patient or by excessive traction applied to the tube from dependent ventilatory apparatus. Any force exerted on the tube by poorly designed horizontal skin flaps or an undivided thyroid isthmus can contribute to displacement of the tube out of the trachea or obstruct its lumen against the tracheal wall. These events are usually signaled by high airway resistance, decreasing oxygen saturation, inability to pass a suction catheter, air trapping, or, in the awake patient, signs of respiratory distress. These signs should prompt an immediate search for a misdirected tube.

The tube should be replaced under direct vision. Blind reinsertion invites the creation of a false passage in the pretracheal tissues that can further distort the anatomy and may also lead to subcutaneous emphysema, enormously amplifying the difficulty in re-establishing the airway. Since the diameter of the tracheotomy tube often approximates the size of the opening in the trachea, it may be difficult to insert the tube under direct vision. A smaller-caliber tube, such as a "red rubber" urinary catheter or even a No. 5 endotracheal tube, may be more easily inserted and used as a guide. The tracheotomy tube may then be passed over the guide into the tracheal lumen.

PNEUMOTHORAX

Pneumothorax occurs in 0 to 5 per cent of tracheotomies. It may be caused by aggressive dissection off the midline, especially in children and patients with chronic lung diseases when pleural apices can extend into the neck. An often overlooked cause of pneumothorax is overenthusiastic ventilation of the patient, which often occurs in situations of respiratory decompensation. Forceful and rapid ventilation prevents the passive exhalation of air, leading to breath stacking and the eventual rupture of alveoli, producing the entrance of air into the pleural space. A misplaced tracheotomy tube also can cause air to enter the soft tissues of the mediastinum and pleural space. Pneumothorax

causes decreased breath sounds and a hyperresonant chest wall and can be confirmed by chest radiograph. Treatment is based on the size of the pneumothorax and accompanying functional deficits. A small pneumothorax may require only observation by serial chest films. A large pneumothorax usually requires a thoracostomy tube. Should a tension pneumothorax occur, immediate pleural decompression is necessary to avoid potentially fatal depression of cardiac output.

SUBCUTANEOUS EMPHYSEMA

Subcutaneous emphysema results when air that normally escapes around the cannula is forced into loose fascial planes. It most often results from closing the wound too tightly. It may also be caused by tube obstruction or displacement. Soft tissue swelling and crepitus in the neck, face, and anterior chest wall usually herald impending respiratory decompensation. If minor, it may be alarming to the patient but is not dangerous and usually resolves spontaneously. If major, it can progress to pneumomediastinum. Treatment involves opening the tracheotomy wound to allow escape of air entrapped under pressure. Air entering mediastinal tissues can carry bacteria with it, allowing further contamination and subsequent mediastinitis.

MEDIASTINITIS

Mediastinitis can occur by either stomal contamination or an intraoperative esophageal perforation. The pretracheal fascia which is opened during the tracheotomy procedure extends into the mediastinum. Local wound care is necessary to prevent this complication. If contamination occurs, the loose areolar tissues in the mediastinum do not present a substantial barrier to infection. Fever, chills, dyspnea, tachycardia, back pain, and dull or pleuritic chest pain may signify this complication. Chest radiographs show widening of the mediastinal shadow. Septic shock and a fatal outcome may ensue rapidly. Treatment involves massive doses of broad-spectrum antibiotics and surgical drainage.

AEROPHAGIA

Aerophagia is more common in children but can occur in adults as well. Mechanical irritation from the cuff stimulates the sensation of a food bolus in the esophagus, resulting in reflex swallowing. Large amounts of air can be ingested, leading to gastric distention, increasing abdominal discomfort, and even respiratory embarrassment. The condition is effectively remedied by passage of a nasogastric tube to decompress the stomach.

CARDIOPULMONARY DYSFUNCTION

Cardiopulmonary arrest can occur during or soon after tracheotomy. Even a transitory period of oxygen desaturation in a hemodynamically unstable patient has the potential to trigger the collapse of vital functions. This can occur with any delay in obtaining an adequate airway by an improperly placed or dislodged tube, resulting in hypoxia and acidosis that can cause increased myocardial irritability, followed by an arrhythmic event or arrest. Pneumothorax or pneumomediastinum can impede cardiac output to a critical threshold with the same result. In certain situations, relieving airway obstruction itself can cause fatal respiratory depression. In the patient suffering from chronic upper respiratory obstruction, tracheotomy can cause a sudden loss of the hypoxic stimulation to which chemoreceptors have acclimated, leading to a loss of ventilatory drive. Ventilatory assistance may be required temporarily until chemoreceptors are reset to a lower level of Pco_2. Also, the sudden relief of upper airway obstruction may cause the sudden onset of pulmonary edema. The mechanism is incompletely understood but is thought to involve a rapid change in capillary-alveolar transmural pressure gradients and a catechol-mediated shift in pulmonary blood volume leading to a rapid egress of fluid out of the pulmonary capillary bed. Such patients should be maintained on continuous positive airway pressure ventilation in an intensive care unit and gradually weaned over 24 to 36 hours, depending on the arterial blood gas measurements. If CPAP is ineffective, fluids should be restricted and diuresis chemically induced.[22]

LATE COMPLICATIONS

Late complications are largely due to improper postoperative care and therefore are usually preventable.

TUBE OBSTRUCTION

Tube obstruction is a common cause of respiratory distress and is frequently due to mucus plugging. A combination of inadequate humidification, impaired mucociliary clearance, and diminished cough contributes to drying of mucous secretions in and around the tube. Crusts then accumulate and may become too large to expel. Total obstruction is preceded by audible air flow and increasing difficulty in passing a suction catheter. Increased humidification and more frequent irrigation should be instituted with a 5 per cent sodium bicarbonate solution or other mucolytic solutions such as acetylcysteine (Mucomyst). Oral guaifenesin also may help decrease mucus viscosity. In the situation of acute total obstruction unrelieved by suctioning or removal of the inner cannula, the entire tracheotomy appliance should be removed to allow the mucous plug to be coughed out. This technique may prove to be life-saving and should be taught to all patients and their families before discharge from the hospital. If the entire cannula requires changing in the first 5 postoperative days, it should be done by the surgeon as described previously under Tube Displacement.

INFECTION

The tracheotomy stoma is a moist, open wound and provides a ready portal for bacterial entry. Furthermore, the tube acts as a foreign body harboring mucus and crusts that serve as a nidus for infection.[23] Colonization of the trachea is virtually unpreventable.[24–26] Local cellulitis and purulent stomal exudate require aggressive local therapy. Sometimes systemic antibiotics may be required. Uncontrolled local infection can lead to several serious infectious complications, including mediastinitis, innominate artery rupture, sepsis, osteomyelitis, and necrotizing infections leading to extensive tissue loss.[27, 28] Stomal erosion caused by pressure from a malpositioned tube also can lead to necrosis, tissue loss, and erosion of adjacent structures. Granulation tissue frequently results from infected or eroded tissue and usually forms above the stoma where it can cause obstruction when the cannula is removed. Squamous epithelium often covers this granulation tissue, forming a tissue cast about the cannula that obstructs the airway upon inadvertent decannulation.

INNOMINATE ARTERY EROSION

Massive hemorrhage from innominate artery erosion is the most common delayed fatal complication of tracheotomy. Its incidence is 1 per cent to 2 per cent,[10] carrying a 10 per cent to 25 per cent survival rate.[29] It may be heralded by the so called "sentinel bleed," which should prompt a thorough investigation by fiberoptic tracheoscopy. Once massive bleeding occurs, immediate measures must be undertaken to prevent suffocation and exsanguination. Introduction of a longer endotracheal tube through the stoma can be lifesaving. Digital pressure should be applied between the anterior trachea and the manubrium to compress the artery. Simultaneously massive fluid resuscitation should be started and the patient immediately taken to the operating room for median sternotomy and vessel ligation.

TRACHEOESOPHAGEAL FISTULA

This complication is caused by pressure necrosis from malposition of the cannula, an overinflated cuff, or a malpositioned nasogastric tube. It occurs in less than 1 per cent of tracheotomies and should be suspected when there is a sudden increase in tracheal secretions, an air leak around the cuff, aspiration, and abdominal distention. The diagnosis is made by barium swallow or tracheoscopy. Many fistulas will heal with conservative treatment. A small-bore nasogastric tube should be placed for enteral feeding. If the fistula fails to heal, surgical repair may be necessary. Utilizing a lateral cervical incision, the tract is debrided and closed by the interposition of viable soft tissue.[30]

ASPIRATION

Aspiration following tracheotomy is reported to occur in about 2 per cent to 4 per cent of patients but probably goes unrecognized in many instances. Its occurrence raises the possibility of an unlikely tracheoesophageal fistula. The cause of aspiration is multifactorial. The tracheotomy appliance attached firmly to the neck can limit the upward excursion of the larynx, as occurs during normal swallowing. A horizontal incision can curtail this movement further by fixing the tube against the upper skin flap. Normally the larynx protects the lower airway by elevation of the glottis under the epiglottis, approximation of the false cords, and true vocal cord adduction. Tracheotomy has been shown to disrupt these glottic closure reflexes in dogs[21] (Figs. 19–1 through 19–6). Aspiration is a major cause of lower respiratory tract infections, including pneumonia and lung abscess. Soft solid foods are often tolerated better than liquids. Maintaining the patient in an upright position and inflating the tube cuff afford temporary protection, although hyperinflation encourages aspiration by obstructing the esophageal lumen. Patients having undergone major surgical procedures of the local structures may benefit from formal swallowing training with a speech therapist. Aspiration is a major cause of lower respiratory tract infections, including pneumonia and lung abscess.

PNEUMONIA

The tracheotomized patient's risk for the development of nosocomial pneumonia is greater than four times that of a nonintubated patient.[31] Tracheotomy bypasses defensive

A   **B**

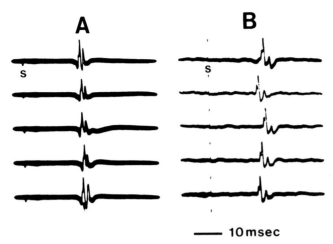

— 10 msec

FIGURE 19–1. Right thyroarytenoid muscle action potentials elicited by single shock stimulus applied to the right superior laryngeal nerve in *A*, control dogs, and *B*, chronically tracheotomized preparations (6–8 months). Note the latency shift in *B*. S represents stimulus artifact. (From Sasaki CT, Suzuki M, Horiuchi M, Kirchner JA: The effect of tracheostomy on the laryngeal closure reflex. Laryngoscope 87:1428–1433, 1977.)

FIGURE 19–2. *A*, Right thyroarytenoid muscle action potentials elicited by repetitive stimulation of the right superior laryngeal nerve (SLN) in control dogs. 8 Hz. *B*, Eight sweeps per second were recorded on moving film. Note the level of excitatory after-discharge activity produced by repetitive SLN excitation. 16 Hz. S represents stimulus artifact. (From Sasaki CT, Suzuki M, Horiuchi M, Kirchner JA: The effect of tracheostomy on the laryngeal closure reflex. Laryngoscope 87:1428–1433, 1977.)

A   **B**

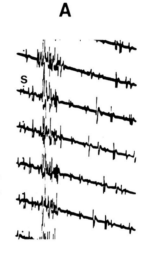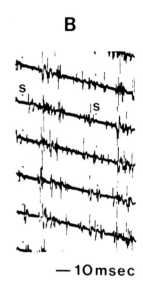

— 10 msec

A   **B**

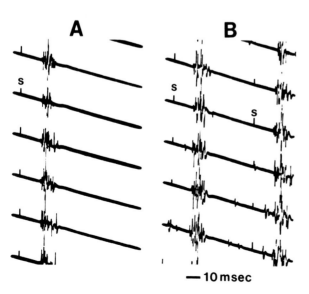

— 10 msec

FIGURE 19–3. *A*, Right thyroarytenoid muscle action potentials elicited by repetitive right superior laryngeal nerve stimulation. 8 Hz. *B*, Dogs tracheotomized for 2 months. Little after-discharge activity is observed. 16 Hz. S represents stimulus artifact. (From Sasaki CT, Suzuki M, Horiuchi M, Kirchner JA: The effect of tracheostomy on the laryngeal closure reflex. Laryngoscope 87:1428–1433, 1977.)

A

B

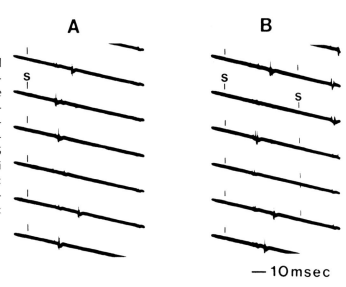

— 10 msec

FIGURE 19–4. *A,* Right thyroarytenoid muscle action potentials elicited by repetitive right superior laryngeal nerve stimulation. 8 Hz. *B,* Dogs tracheotomized for 6 to 8 months. 16 Hz. No afterdischarge activity is observed. Note attenuation of the primary evoked response. S represents stimulus artifact. (From Sasaki CT, Suzuki M, Horiuchi M, Kirchner JA: The effect of tracheostomy on the laryngeal closure reflex. Laryngoscope 87: 1428–1433, 1977.)

1

2

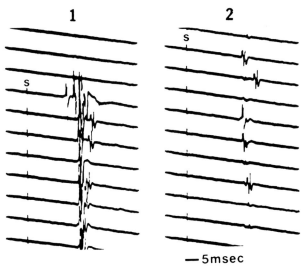

— 5 msec

FIGURE 19–5. Right thyroarytenoid muscle action potential elicited by repetitive right superior laryngeal nerve stimulation at 16 Hz in dogs tracheotomized for 6 to 8 months. Note that the primary evoked response attenuates within seconds of stimulus onset. *1,* Onset of stimulus train. *2,* One to two seconds after onset of stimulus train. S represents stimulus artifact. (From Sasaki CT, Suzuki M, Horiuchi M, Kirchner JA: The effect of tracheostomy on the laryngeal closure reflex. Laryngoscope 87:1428– 1433, 1977.)

A

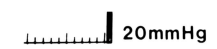

FIGURE 19–6. Glottic pressures caused by vocal cord adduction measured from a tambour placed within the laryngeal aperture. Cord adduction is produced by 16 Hz stimulation of the superior laryngeal nerve (SLN) in *A,* control dogs, and *B,* chronically tracheotomized dogs (6–8 months). Bar denotes duration of SLN stimulation. (From Sasaki CT, Suzuki M, Horiuchi M, Kirchner JA: The effect of tracheostomy on the laryngeal closure reflex. Laryngoscope 87:1428–1433, 1977.)

20mmHg

B

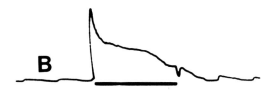

barriers in the upper airway, alters mucociliary clearance, depresses the cough reflex, and allows colonization by virulent organisms such as *Pseudomonas* and enteric gram-negative bacteria. In addition, these patients may be critically ill and malnourished, which are additional risk factors. Adequate local care of the stoma and sterile technique in tracheotomy care decrease the incidence of pneumonia. An increase in the quantity of sputum and a drop in lung compliance and arterial Po_2 herald the radiographic appearance of a lung infiltrate. Aggressive parenteral antibiotic therapy is warranted.

COMPLICATIONS ASSOCIATED WITH DECANNULATION

OBSTRUCTION BY GRANULOMA

Granulation tissue above the tracheotomy may go unrecognized until it causes airway obstruction upon decannulation. The obstruction often can be identified by lateral neck radiograph or xeroradiography. Early lesions are amenable to endoscopic removal by cupped forceps. Mature, fibrotic lesions may require endoscopic laser excision. Others may be endoscopically displaced within the existing tracheostoma for excision at the base by the surgeon's assistant.

PHYSIOLOGIC OBSTRUCTION

Normal inspiration requires the coordinated abduction of the vocal cords just before the descent of the diaphragm. Phasic abductor activity has been shown to decrease and eventually cease in tracheotomized animals (Figs. 19–7 through 19–10). It appears to be caused by a decrease in ventilatory resistance and can be re-established by a gradual increase in that resistance.[32] A freshly decannulated patient may exhibit nearly complete airway obstruction from the uncoordinated midline position of the vocal cords. Relief of obstruction and the gradual return of abductor activity are achieved by the gradual restoration of a ventilatory load. Sequential downsizing of the tracheotomy cannula will easily accomplish this. Eventually, when the patient will tolerate an adequate trial period with the cannula completely corked, he or she can be safely decannulated.

LARYNGEAL STENOSIS

Endotracheal tubes cause pressure-related damage at the true vocal cords, posterior commissure of the glottis, and the subglottis. When extubated, the normal movement of the vocal cords prevents their fusion. If, instead, the airway is converted to tracheotomy, the vocal cords can lie in apposition from the physiologic loss of vocal cord abduction. Scarring of the denuded surfaces can lead to fusion of the cords, requiring laryngeal dilatation and lysis of cord adhesions.[33]

SUBGLOTTIC STENOSIS

Subglottic stenosis is a more frequent consequence than vocal cord fusion but is thought to have a similar etiology involving

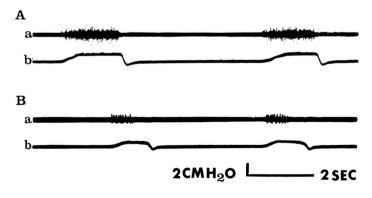

FIGURE 19–7. Acute study. *A*, Nose breathing. *B*, Mouth breathing. *a*, PCA activity. *b*, Intratracheal pressure. Note that upward deflection represents a negative pressure change. (From Sasaki CT, Fukuda H, Kirchner JA: Laryngeal abductor activity in response to varying ventilatory resistance. Trans Am Acad Ophthalmol Otolaryngol 77:403–409, 1973.)

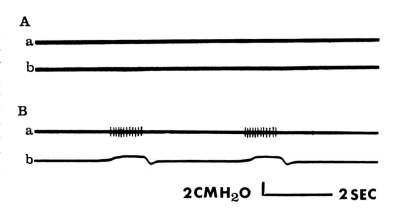

FIGURE 19–8. Acute study. *A,* Tracheostoma open. *B,* Tracheostoma partially closed. *a,* Posterior cricoarytenoid muscle activity. *b,* Intratracheal pressure. (From Sasaki CT, Fukuda H, Kirchner JA: Laryngeal abductor activity in response to varying ventilatory resistance. Trans Am Acad Ophthalmol Otolaryngol 77:403–409, 1973.)

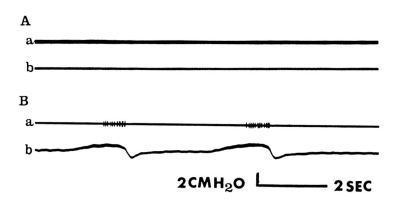

FIGURE 19–9. One week posttracheotomy. *A,* Tracheostoma open. *B,* Tracheostoma partially closed. *a,* Posterior cricoarytenoid muscle activity. *b,* Intratracheal pressure. (From Sasaki CT, Fukuda H, Kirchner JA: Laryngeal abductor activity in response to varying ventilatory resistance. Trans Am Acad Ophthalmol Otolaryngol 77:403–409, 1973.)

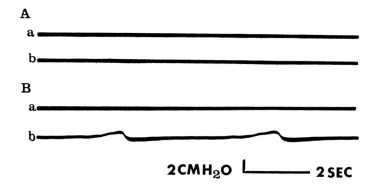

FIGURE 19–10. Four weeks posttracheotomy. *A,* Tracheostoma open. *B,* Tracheostoma partially closed. *a,* Posterior cricoarytenoid muscle activity. *b,* Intratracheal pressure. (From Sasaki CT, Fukuda H, Kirchner JA: Laryngeal abductor activity in response to varying ventilatory resistance. Trans Am Acad Ophthalmol Otolaryngol 77:403–409, 1973.)

the healing of damaged surfaces that have become secondarily infected. A tracheotomy placed too far superiorly, causing injury to the cricoid, predisposes to this type of injury. Children are particularly susceptible since this is the narrowest part of their airway. Infants less than 1 month on mechanical ventilators are at especially high risk.

An animal model has been used to study the role of tracheotomy in the development of subglottic stenosis in a previously injured larynx (Figs. 19–11 through 19–23). The authors' hypothesis was based on the understanding that the greater the imflammatory response, the greater the scar tissue produced.[34] In this study, all animals received a prescribed subglottic mucosal injury. At the injured site animals without tracheotomies were found to have low levels of bacteria present and exhibited normal mucosal healing. Animals that were tracheotomized had high levels of bacterial contamination, showed extension of the injury by infection

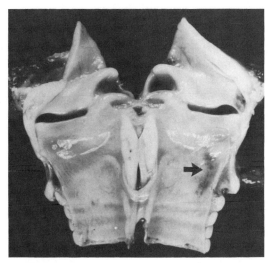

FIGURE 19–12. In untracheotomized dogs, the injured subglottic larynx (arrow) has healed by the second week postinjury. (Larynx opened anteriorly.) (From Sasaki CT, Horiuchi M, Koss N: Tracheostomy-related subglottic stenosis; Bacteriologic pathogenesis. Laryngoscope 89:857–865, 1979.)

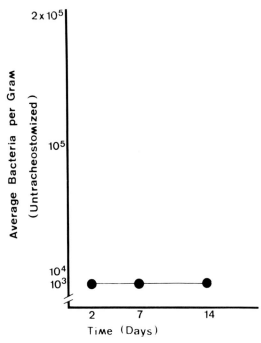

FIGURE 19–11. In Group I, untracheotomized dogs showed no increase in bacterial levels with respect to the postinjury interval. (From Sasaki CT, Horiuchi M, Koss N: Tracheostomy-related subglottic stenosis; Bacteriologic pathogenesis. Laryngoscope 89:857–865, 1979.)

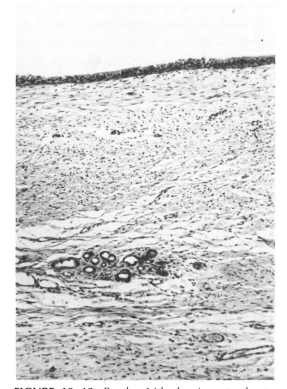

FIGURE 19–13. By the 14th day in untracheotomized dogs, the site of injury has become resurfaced by low columnar epithelium. × 100. (From Sasaki CT, Horiuchi M, Koss N: Tracheostomy-related subglottic stenosis; Bacteriologic pathogenesis. Laryngoscope 89:857–865, 1979.)

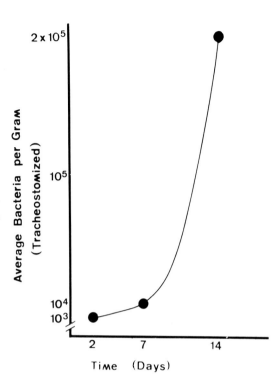

FIGURE 19–14. In Group II, tracheotomized dogs showed an exponential increase in bacterial levels with respect to the postinjury interval. (From Sasaki CT, Horiuchi M, Koss N: Tracheostomy-related subglottic stenosis; Bacteriologic pathogenesis. Laryngoscope 89:857–865, 1979.)

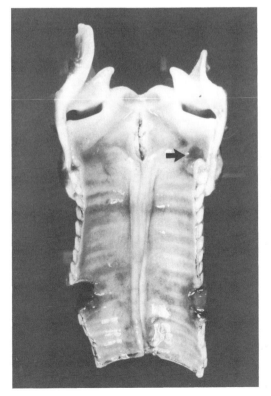

FIGURE 19–15. By the 7th day in tracheotomized dogs, the injured subglottic larynx is ulcerated and actively granulating (arrow). (From Sasaki CT, Horiuchi M, Koss N: Tracheostomy-related subglottic stenosis; Bacteriologic pathogenesis. Laryngoscope 89:857–865, 1979.)

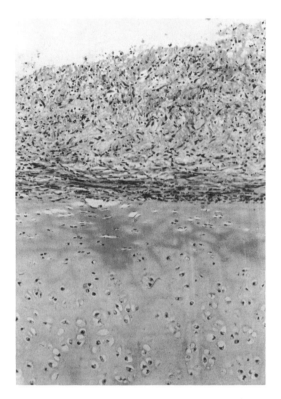

FIGURE 19–16. By the 7th day in tracheotomized dogs, the site of injury is actively granulating. Perichondrium is intact beneath the ulcer. × 100. (From Sasaki CT, Horiuchi M, Koss N: Tracheostomy-related subglottic stenosis; Bacteriologic pathogenesis. Laryngoscope 89:857–865, 1979.)

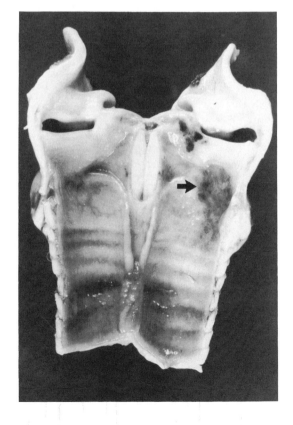

FIGURE 19–17. By the 14th day in tracheotomized dogs, the area of ulceration has extended beyond the site of initial injury (arrow). (From Sasaki CT, Horiuchi M, Koss N: Tracheostomy-related subglottic stenosis; Bacteriologic pathogenesis. Laryngoscope 89:857–865, 1979.)

FIGURE 19–18. By the 14th day in tracheotomized dogs, necrotic cartilage (arrow) is being replaced by new cartilage formation (NC). The perichondrium is disrupted beneath a granulating wound. × 40. (From Sasaki CT, Horiuchi M, Koss N: Tracheostomy-related subglottic stenosis; Bacteriologic pathogenesis. Laryngoscope 89:857–865, 1979.)

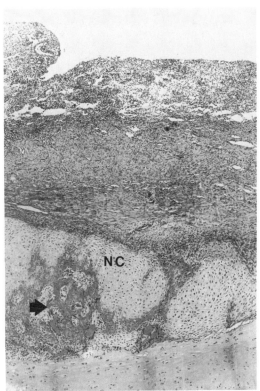

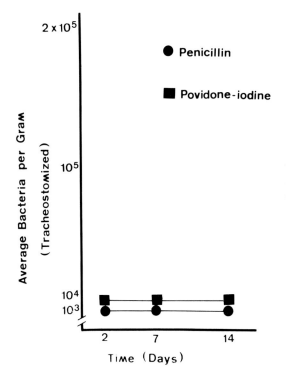

FIGURE 19–19. In Group III, tracheotomized dogs treated with systemic antibiotics or by meticulous stomal care exhibited bacterial levels below 5×10^3 per gram of injured tissue. (From Sasaki CT, Horiuchi M, Koss N: Tracheostomy-related subglottic stenosis; Bacteriologic pathogenesis. Laryngoscope 89:857–865, 1979.)

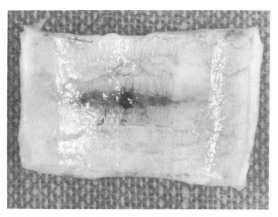

FIGURE 19–20. Submucosal injection of India ink demonstrated movement of carbon particles toward the paratracheal lymphatics. India ink did not cross the cartilaginous rings submucosally. (From Sasaki CT, Horiuchi M, Koss N: Tracheostomy-related subglottic stenosis; Bacteriologic pathogenesis. Laryngoscope 89:857–865, 1979.)

with disruption of perichondrium and active formation of new cartilage. The authors stated, "Significant laryngeal infection does not result from the trauma alone, but may be related to trauma and subsequent contamination by tracheotomy."[34] The mechanism of this contamination was demonstrated to be mucociliary flow from the stoma to the larynx. An additional group of tracheotomized subjects received antibiotic dressings to the stoma or parenteral antibiotics that prevented the subglottic contamination. The authors concluded, "Tracheotomy results in a contaminated wound, secondarily infecting a larynx which may have been injured . . . its effect on the larynx may be greatly influenced by our ability to control the level of stomal contamination."[34]

TRACHEAL STENOSIS

Tracheotomy-related tracheal stenosis is likely to occur at three distinct levels: the stoma, the cuff, or the tip of the tube. At the stoma, excessive trauma to the anterior cartilaginous support, neglected infection, chondritis caused by excessively large tubes, rigid connecting systems, and excessive tube traction are the usual etiologic factors. An im-

properly positioned incision or failure to divide the thyroid isthmus may cause indentation of the anterior tracheal wall, causing the cannula to compress the ring immediately above it. Stenosis is usually not appreciated until decannulation is attempted.

At the cuff site, excessive cuff pressure exceeds mucosal capillary perfusion pressure, leading to ischemic damage and mucosal ulceration over the rigid cartilaginous rings. Eventually the basement membrane is exposed, converting a superficial tracheitis to a deep one with exposure of cartilage. Persistent inflammation fosters chondritis and deterioration of cartilaginous support. An unstable wound with pus and granulation causes excessive scar formation and stenosis. Proper cuff management and timely discontinuance of its use help prevent this problem.

Stenosis at the tip of the tube is caused by

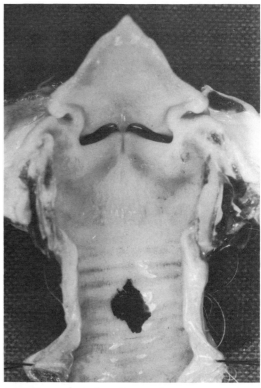

FIGURE 19–21. India ink was placed on the anterior tracheal wall. (From Sasaki CT, Horiuchi M, Koss N: Tracheostomy-related subglottic stenosis; Bacteriologic pathogenesis. Laryngoscope 89:857–865, 1979.)

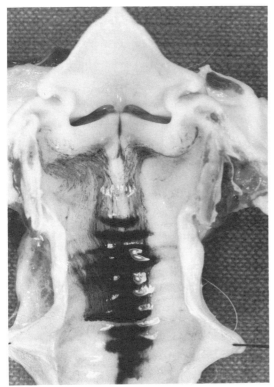

FIGURE 19–22. Within 3 to 5 minutes, carbon particles were swept upward across the subglottic larynx toward the posterior commissure. (From Sasaki CT, Horiuchi M, Koss N: Tracheostomy-related subglottic stenosis; Bacteriologic pathogenesis. Laryngoscope 89:857–865, 1979.)

friction of the tip against the tracheal wall, produced by faulty surgical technique or excessive tube movement. Injury at any level can cause loss of cartilaginous support and tracheomalacia. The effects of tracheal stenosis may become apparent only months following decannulation as fibrosis continues, producing a progressive decrease in exercise tolerance, dyspnea, and stridor. These symptoms should prompt evaluation of the airway by lateral neck radiographs, CT scans, and tracheoscopy. Fluoroscopy may be useful in the diagnosis of tracheomalacia.

Treatment of circumferential strictures depends on the length of the lesion. Patients with lesions less than 1 cm in length will respond favorably to serial dilatation. Endoscopic laser resection has also met with success. In large, fixed stenoses, segmental tra-

cheal resection with end-to-end anastomosis may be necessary. In young patients, a gap of 3 cm can be approximated without resorting to surgical release techniques.

Several methods have been described for securing additional tracheal length to obtain an end-to-end anastomosis free of excess tension. Intrathoracic release of the trachea can be accomplished by resection of the left main bronchus and reattachment to the right main bronchus. This allows the trachea to be moved superiorly up to 6 cm.[35] By suprahyoid release, the midportion of the hyoid bone is separated from the greater cornu on each side. This allows the body of the hyoid bone, the thyroid cartilage, the cricoid cartilage, and proximal trachea to drop inferiorly, adding up to 5 cm of additional length.[36]

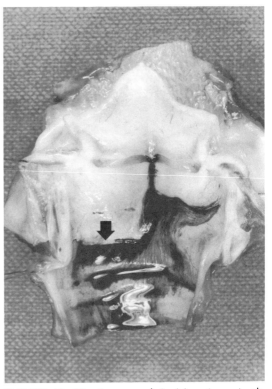

FIGURE 19–23. A mucosal incision (arrow) obstructed mucociliary transport, resulting in an accumulation of carbon particles at the site of injury. (From Sasaki CT, Horiuchi M, Koss N: Tracheostomy-related subglottic stenosis; Bacteriologic pathogenesis. Laryngoscope 89:857–865, 1979.)

TRACHEOCUTANEOUS FISTULA

Persistent tracheocutaneous fistula results from the downgrowth of squamous epithelium along the inside of the tracheotomy tract. It is caused by neglected infection and granuloma formation. An epithelium-lined fistula prevents healing of the stoma when the patient is decannulated. To allow wound closure, the epithelial lining must be excised from the skin to the trachea. If the skin is closed primarily, it must be approximated over a drain to prevent the subcutaneous dissection of trapped air.

References

1. Garrison FH: History of Medicine. Philadelphia, WB Saunders, 1917.
2. Jackson C: Tracheotomy. Laryngoscope 19:285–290, 1909.
3. Meade JW: Tracheotomy; Its complications and their management: A study of 212 cases. N Engl J Med 265:519, 1961.
4. Yarington CT, Frazer JP: Complications of tracheotomy. Arch Surg 91:652, 1965.
5. Skaggs JA, Cogbill CL: Tracheotomy: Management, mortality, complications. Am Surg 35:393, 1969.
6. Chew JV, Cantrell RW: Tracheotomy: Complications and their management. Arch Otolaryngol 96:538, 1972.
7. Dugan DJ: Tracheotomy: Present-day indications and techniques. Am J Surg 106:290, 1963.
8. Glas W: Complications of tracheotomy. Arch Surg 85:72, 1962.
9. Rogers L: Complications of tracheotomy. South Med J 62:1496, 1969.
10. Stauffer JL, Olson DE, Petty TL: Complications and consequence of endotracheal intubation and tracheotomy: A study of 150 critically ill adult patients. Am J Med 70:65, 1981.
11. Dayal VS, Masri WE: Tracheotomy in an intensive care setting. Laryngoscope 96:58, 1986.
12. Stock MC, Woodward CG, Shapiro BA, et al: Perioperative complications of elective tracheotomy in critically ill patients. Crit Care Med 14:861, 1986.
13. Eiseman B, Spencer FC: Tracheotomy: An underrated surgical procedure. JAMA 184:683, 1963.
14. Orlowski JP, Ellis NG, Amin NP, Crumrine RS: Complications of airway intrusion in 100 consecutive cases in a pediatric ICU. Crit Care Med 8:324, 1980.
15. Wetmore RF, Handler SD, Postic WP: Pediatric tracheotomy: Experience during the past decade. Ann Otol Rhinol Laryngol 91:628, 1982.
16. Kenna MA, Reilly JS, Stocl SE: Tracheotomy in the preterm infant. Ann Otol Rhinol Laryngol 96:68, 1987.
17. Goldstein SI, Breda SD, Schneider KL: Surgical complications of bedside tracheotomy in an otolaryngology residency program. Laryngoscope 97:1407, 1987.
18. Kirchner JA: Avoiding problems in tracheotomy. Laryngoscope 96:55, 1986.
19. Kirchner JA: Tracheotomy and its problems. Surg Clin North Am 60:1093, 1980.
20. Astrachan DI, Sasaki CT: Tracheotomy. In Bave A, Geha A, Hammand G, Loks H (eds): Thoracic and Cardiovascular Surgery. East Norwalk, CT, Appleton and Lange, 1988.
21. Sasaki CT, Suzuki M, Horiuchi M, Kirchner JM: The effect of tracheotomy on the laryngeal closure reflex. Laryngoscope 87:1428–1432, 1977.
22. Meyers EN, Stool SE, Johnson JT: Tracheotomy. New York, Churchill Livingstone, 1985.
23. Johnson JT: Antibiotics in Tracheotomy. In Johnson JT: Antibiotic Therapy in Head and Neck Surgery. New York, Marcel Dekker, 1987.
24. Bryant LR, Trinkle JK, Mobin-Uddin K: Bacterial colonization profile with tracheal intubation and mechanical ventilation. Arch Surg 104:647–651, 1972.
25. Brook L: Bacterial colonization, tracheobronchitis and pneumonia following tracheotomy and long-term intubation in pediatric patients. Chest 76:420–424, 1979.
26. Niederman MS, Ferranti RD, Ziegler A: Respiratory infection complicating long-term tracheotomy: The implication of persistent gram-negative tracheobronchial colonization. Chest 85:39, 1984.
27. Snow N, Richardson JD, Flint LM: Management of necrotizing tracheotomy infections. J Thorac Cardiovasc Surg 82:341, 1981.
28. Wang RC, Perlman PW, Parnes SM: Near-fatal complications of tracheotomy infections and their prevention. Head Neck 11(6):528–533, 1989.
29. Jones JW, Reynolds M, Hewitt RL, Drapanas T: Tracheoinnominate artery erosion: Successful surgical management of a devastating complication. Ann Surg 184:194, 1977.
30. Grillo HC, Moncure AC, McEnany MT: Repair of inflammatory tracheosophageal fistula. Ann Thorac Surg 22:112, 1976.
31. Cross AS, Roup B: Role of respiratory assistance devices in endemic nosocomial pneumonia. Am J Med 70:681, 1981.
32. Sasaki CT, Fukuda H, Kirchner JA: Laryngeal abductor activity in response to varying ventilatory resistance. Trans Am Acad Ophthalmol Otolaryngol 77:403–410, 1973.
33. Kirchner JA, Sasaki CT: Fusion of the vocal cords following intubation and tracheotomy. Trans Am Acad Ophthalmol Otolaryngol 77:403, 1973.
34. Sasaki CT, Horiuchi M, Koss N: Tracheotomy-related subglottic stenosis: Bacteriologic pathogenesis. Laryngoscope 89:857, 1979.
35. Grillo HC. The management of tracheal stenosis following assisted respiration. J Thorac Cardiovasc Surg 57:52, 1969.
36. Montgomery WW: Surgery of the Upper Respiratory System. 2nd ed. Vol 2. Philadelphia, Lea & Febiger, 1989, p 488.

CHAPTER 20

Rigid Endoscopic Procedures

JACK A. COLEMAN, Jr., MD

Doctor A has recently finished his residency and is starting out in practice in a small community. He is anxious to please his referring physicians and become a valued member of the medical community. He is presently in the operating room performing a direct laryngotracheobronchoscopy on an infant who has been referred to him by the local pediatrician for a stridor work-up. As Doctor A passes the endoscope down the trachea, he notes a mass compressing the anterior tracheal wall and compromising the airway. Pleased that he has found the problem, Doctor A reaches in with his cup forceps to get a piece of the mass for pathology. He grasps the mass and pulls—the airway fills with blood . . .

Doctor Z has been doing endoscopies for years. He is confident, competent, and comfortable with his endoscopic technique. Doctor Z is doing an esophagoscopy on one of his cancer patients for dysphagia. The barium swallow has shown a stricture of the midthoracic esophagus. As the stricture is encountered, Doctor Z notes that the lumen is almost, but not quite, big enough to pass the scope through. He has encountered this in the past and has been able to put light pressure on the scope and get through on those occasions. So Doctor Z pushes the scope gently against the stricture, which does not dilate. A little more gentle pressure and he is sure he will get through and . . . he tears the esophagus.

Both these physicians are fictitious, but the complications of their endoscopic procedures are not. These are things that have really happened to people, and the purpose of this chapter is to try to make the reader aware of what can happen, why it happens, how to avoid it, and what to do if it does happen.

The complications of Doctor A and Doctor Z are respectively caused by two things: inexperience and overconfidence. These two things are at the root of the majority of all surgical complications and, in fact, are probably at the root of most of the problems one will encounter in life. One cannot gain experience reading a book nor should one become too confident because one has read a book. These things come with experience. What one can get from a book and what this chapter will provide is some guidance to help the endoscopist along the way.

For the sake of this discussion, endoscopy will be defined as the examination of epithelium-lined body cavities in or directly contiguous to the head and neck by means of a rigid device that allows for direct line of sight examination of structures for the purpose of diagnostic or therapeutic intervention. Indirect techniques and flexible instrumentation will not be considered here. Complications associated with the delivery of electromagnetic radiation (lasers) are discussed elsewhere in this book. In addition to the usual laryngoscopy, bronchoscopy, and esophagoscopy discussion, otoscopy, sinusoscopy, and nasopharyngoscopy also will be covered. In an effort to maintain organization of such a large topic, the complications of the various techniques discussed will be divided into the general categories of immediate or intraoperative complications, immediate postprocedure or postoperative complications, and delayed complications or those that show up 24 or more hours after a procedure is performed.

COMPLICATIONS OF ENDOSCOPY

It is important that the surgeon be able to assess his or her own skills honestly in order to stay out of trouble. One should not be too proud to know when to back off and turn a case over to those more competent or when to seek consultation or further training from others. Also, in some instances what one does not do can be as important as what one does do. In other words, sins of omission can be as serious as sins of commission.

Most of our discussion will center on the sins of commission. The sins of omission generally can be categorized under the heading of "inadequate examination." The lesson is to remember to be thorough when doing a procedure. This does not necessarily mean that one will always have to do or be able to do a complete evaluation. Under some circumstances a complete examination cannot be done. An example is the intraluminal mass that the endoscope is too big to pass by. In this situation it is better to stop and consider

another diagnostic modality if knowing what is distal to the mass is important. It is therefore acceptable to do an incomplete examination when it is justified, as long as what is seen is adequately examined. It is never acceptable to do an inadequate examination. "Inadequate" and "incomplete" are words that the surgeon should take care in using—they mean two very different things.

Prevention is still the most effective way to deal with complications. The best prevention is firmly rooted in adequate training—of the surgeon and the other personnel in the operating room; in realization of level of experience; in realization of limitations—not only of the surgeon but of the institution's support services; in proper preparation of the patient, the surgeon, and ancillary personnel, as well as the equipment to be used; and in recognition of danger areas.

NASAL ENDOSCOPY AND NASOPHARYNGOSCOPY

Endoscopy of the upper respiratory tract has made a dramatic change in the way diseases of the nose and paranasal sinuses are diagnosed and treated in the United States since its introduction in the 1970s. No longer is physical diagnosis of the sinonasal tract limited to inspection of the anterior nasal airway with a speculum and the nasopharynx with a mirror. By use of nasal endoscopes or telescopes in combination with topical decongestion and anesthesia, the entire nasal airway, nasopharynx, and sinus ostia can be observed in the majority of cases. The more aggressive diagnostician may also inspect the maxillary sinus in the office using the telescopes through openings made by small trocars.

Surgery of the paranasal sinuses utilizing the endoscopes has provided practitioners with a better way to treat both limited and extensive sinus disease in the operating room. The introduction of these techniques has also created the potential for serious and even life-threatening complications to occur in relation to performing extensive nasal surgery.

HEMORRHAGE

Bleeding, both intraoperative and postoperative, is one of the most common problems associated with intranasal surgery. The physician performing this surgery must insure that, intraoperatively, hemostasis will be adequately maintained. Adequate preoperative precautions against hemorrhage must be taken. An essential step is to solicit an adequate history about bleeding problems, either in the patient or in the family, as well as a history of prescription and nonprescription medications taken. This should be done in the office and not the day of surgery in the holding area, so that any medications that could cause platelet dysfunction or other defects in the clotting mechanism can be stopped in plenty of time for normal coagulation function to return. Preoperative bleeding times, prothrombin time; and partial thromboplastin time should be obtained on patients, as well as a baseline complete blood count. Many hematologists feel that an adequate history is sufficient preoperative evaluation of the patient's ability to form clots and that further blood tests are redundant. Although this may be a cogent argument, in today's medical-legal climate it may still behoove the practitioner to document the patient's blood-clotting ability.

Packing the nose with vasoconstrictors, along with injection of the turbinates and mucosal membranes with vasoconstrictor substances, is also important. Some practitioners are also advocating intraoral injection of the sphenopalatine fossa; this is indeed useful to promote hemostasis but should be done with caution, as instances have been reported of transient and permanent blindness as a result of these injections. It is suggested that the needle not be advanced more than 1 centimeter into the fossa and that the injection site be aspirated first to insure that there is no injection into the lumen of a vessel. Injection into the area of the medial canthus to cause constriction of the anterior ethmoid artery is also popular among some surgeons. Again, caution should be taken not to go beyond 1 centimeter below the skin and to aspirate first. Injecting too deeply in this area has resulted in direct damage to the artery with subsequent hematoma formation. After injection, adequate time must be allowed for the vasoconstrictor to act. Many physicians are in the habit of administering the vasoconstrictors prior to draping the patient, to obtain the 5 to 10 minutes needed for the vasoconstriction to occur.

When one is contemplating a very long or extensive operation, it may be necessary to stagger the injections. This is done by injecting first the side or area upon which the operation is to begin. As that portion of the procedure nears completion, inject the area of the next step, and so on. This will accomplish three things. First, it will prevent the surgeon from injecting a very large dose all at once and perhaps causing a toxic reaction to the anesthetic agent if one is being used. Second, it will prevent some of the side effects often seen with the vasoconstrictors used, especially those effects on the heart rate and blood pressure that can be seen in the older patient. And third, it will allow continued vasoconstriction in the area being operated upon.

Electrocautery may be necessary during the procedure for control of bleeding of larger intranasal vessels. Lasers, especially the Nd:YAG and KTP, also have been found useful during these procedures to assist in achieving hemostasis.

Bleeding from the ethmoid arteries, usually the anterior ethmoid artery, also has been reported as a complication. Awareness of the anatomy and the fact that at times the arteries are not fully enclosed in bone will prevent this complication in most cases. Should this arise, cauterization is usually sufficient to bring the bleeding under control.

Another area with a bleeding problem is the posterior nasal artery, with its septal branches, which arises from the internal maxillary artery. This is often injured when the base of the sphenoid is approached. Also, in the posterior aspect of the inferior meatus are large vessels that may bleed. However, it is unusual that any dissection will be carried out in this area.

Often blood will ooze from several sites throughout the procedure. Patients who have had previous intranasal procedures, especially polypectomies, usually will have more fibrosis and vascularity in the operative field than those patients who have not. As would be expected, these patients will tend to bleed more, so hemostasis must be one of the primary concerns of the surgeon. It is not uncommon to have to pack the nose and work on one side until bleeding becomes a problem, pack that side and work on the other side, and alternate throughout the procedure to maintain adequate hemostasis. In those with severe polyposis, the bleeding is better controlled if the patient takes a course of steroids orally in the week prior to the procedure.

For limited procedures, packing of the nose often is not required, but for more extensive procedures it is almost always needed. Many methods and materials are available, and the selection depends on how much tamponade is necessary, airway management, patient tolerance, ease of removal, and length of time the packing will be in place. A petrolatum-based packing material bears the possibility of myospherulosis.[2] Toxic shock syndrome also has been reported with the use of nasal packings, so it is suggested that appropriate antibiotic coverage be used; also, that a water-soluble carrier, rather than a petrolatum-based one, be used for topical application.

Major bleeding can occur in the postoperative period upon removal of the packing. Delayed bleeding can occur in the office up to 10 days or more postoperatively. At times hard-fixed crusts and clots cannot be removed without significant bleeding; therefore, it is often useful to soften these clots with saline sprays or irrigations prior to removal. If necessary, wait until later office visits to try to remove these, to give the mucosal membranes more chance to heal beneath the clots. Sometimes electrocautery or chemical cautery has been needed to control the bleeding in these situations.

If postoperative bleeding becomes severe, repacking the nose—with or without rehospitalization—may be in order.

EXTRAOCULAR MUSCLES

Injury to extraocular muscles has been known to occur with intranasal surgery as a result of extending the dissection beyond the accepted anatomic limits. There are two main reasons for this. First, the lamina papyracea is often quite thin and is very easy for the inexperienced surgeon to perforate during dissection. It is also easy for the novice surgeon or one who is not familiar with the anatomy to initiate the dissection too far anteriorly in the nose and go directly into the orbit rather than into the ethmoid sinus. Second, many individuals have dehiscent areas in the lamina papyracea, presenting no evidence of bone separation between the sinus and the orbit. This is a more significant problem in those who have had previous operation, where there actually may be scar formation between the contents of the sinus and the periosteum of the orbit. It is also a problem in individuals who have recurrent inflammatory disease that has produced a cicatrix between the mucosal membrane of the sinus and the periosteum of the orbit. When these diseased mucosal membranes are removed, they will pull the periosteum along with it, thereby exposing periorbital fat to the dissection. When the surgeon starts to remove this periorbital fat thinking that it is also diseased mucosa, it is very easy to snag one of the extraocular muscles, especially the medial rectus muscle or optic nerve.

The surgeon can do a few things to ascertain whether or not the orbit has been entered. First, be aware of the appearance of the tissues, with attention to their color and texture. Many times adipose tissue, as opposed to a polypoid mucosa, can be recognized. Second, palpate the globe constantly during the procedure. This maneuver will force orbital fat through the dehiscence and cause it to bulge with pressure. As one palpates the eye in a ballottement maneuver and examines the surgical site intranasally, one will see movement of the tissues. Sometimes, if the lamina papyracea is thin, even a movement of the not-yet-violated bone may be noted with a gentle ballottement of the globe. When this is seen, the surgeon should immediately be cautious of dissecting in this area.

Last, the scrub nurse should always place each piece of tissue removed into a medicine cup of water on the Mayo stand. If the tissue floats, the nurse immediately alerts the surgeon, for fat floats whereas other tissues sink to the bottom. If the surgeon has encountered fat, periorbital fat must be assumed, eliciting caution about any further dissection in this area. Postoperatively, the patient's extraocular movements and visual acuity should be examined as soon as possible. If any problems are noted, an immediate ophthalmologic consultation should be obtained.

BLINDNESS

Blindness will most commonly occur because of either an expanding orbital hematoma or direct injury to the optic nerve. To avoid the latter, it is important to stay within the anatomic limits of the sinus and to be aware at all times of where one is placing the instruments.

An expanding orbital hematoma may occur in spite of one's best efforts. It is important to discover the problem as early as possible, and to know what to do. The eye is never covered during intranasal surgery, so that evidence of proptosis and increased eye tension can be observed by repeated ballottement of the eye. If the patient is under intravenous sedation and local anesthesia, visual changes can be observed throughout the procedure. It is also important to note in the chart during the preoperative evaluation the patient's extraocular movements as well as visual acuity. These should be determined and recorded again postoperatively. If any eye changes occur under general anesthesia, immediate termination of the procedure is necessary so that the eye can be properly evaluated and treated. Emergency ophthalmologic consultation is necessary. In many cases, the loss in acuity or the blindness can be reversed if proper measures are taken immediately to reduce the eye pressure by redistributing either the intraocular pressure or the extraocular fluids or both.

Periorbital ecchymosis and chemosis can represent conjunctival hemorrhage alone. Proptosis usually occurs very slowly in such an instance. Lid edema, lid ecchymosis, chemosis, mydriasis, and proptosis are the hallmarks of retrobulbar hemorrhage. These changes will usually occur immediately. As the vision decreases, loss of pupillary reactivity and consensual pupillary reflexes follows, along with the appearance of a Marcus-Gunn pupil. If the patient is under a general anesthetic, many of these pupillary changes will not be noted. The mechanism for the blindness is unclear at this time, but it may result from pressure being exerted directly upon the globe or optic nerve that mechanically compresses the entire retinal vascular system, especially the venous outflow. The venous outflow will induce hypoxia within the optic nerve with the resultant death of the neural cells. If this complication occurs, the first step is to terminate the procedure. Next, eye massage should be carried out. This reduces the eye pressure directly and immediately by redistributing the intraocular and extraocular fluids. This can be repeated as necessary while waiting for other measures to work. A Schiotz tonometer should always be available in the operating room to measure intraocular pressures, and the surgeon should be familiar with its use.

Diuretics are useful in management of this complication. The two main diuretics used are acetazolamide and mannitol. Acetazolamide acts by lowering the intraocular pressure by decreasing production of aqueous humor. It is given intravenously, with an initial dose of 500 mg, which can be repeated every 2 to 4 hours. The electrolytes must be monitored closely during administration of this medication. The mannitol is also given intravenously; it works faster and is generally the preferred diuretic. The intraocular pressure is maximally reduced in 30 to 60 minutes, and the effect will last for 6 to 8 hours. If massive diuresis occurs, electrolytes must be monitored. A dose of 1 gm per kg of body weight is usually sufficient, in a 20 per cent infusion over 30 to 60 minutes.

Miotics, such as pilocarpine and carbachol, and epinephrine drops will also reduce the intraocular pressure; however, they interfere with pupillary response, which may mar subsequent evaluation of the patient. It is generally advisable to withhold these drugs until after ophthalmologic consultation has been obtained.

Steroids in megadose quantities (1 mg per kg of body weight of Decadron followed by 0.5 mg per kg body of weight every 6 hours) also has been recommended in the literature. They have been used for blindness following facial trauma; however, there is no evidence for or against use with retrobulbar hematoma. Ophthalmologists routinely do not use megadoses of steroids; therefore, use of them is left up to the surgeon. In most instances, massage and mannitol alone will control the pressure from orbital hematoma.

Anterior paracentesis has been performed to decrease orbital pressure by decreasing intraocular pressure. This is not a procedure to be performed by the otolaryngologist, and, in fact, most ophthalmologists do not perform this procedure for retrobulbar hemorrhage. Paracentesis itself may cause intraocular damage and lens prolapse.

Increased intraorbital pressure not adequately controlled by the aforementioned conservative measures can be reversed with a lateral canthotomy. This is performed by making a horizontal incision through all the tissues of the lateral canthus through the raphe. To clamp the lateral canthal commissure, a straight hemostat is used with one blade posterior to the lids as far laterally as possible and the other blade placed anteriorly. The structures are clamped for 1 minute, and the clamp is then removed. Scissors are then used, where the hemostat was clamped, to cut in a lateral and inferior direction and backward until the scissors' points contact the orbital rim. The skin and conjunctiva are then severed along with the inferior fibers of the lateral canthal tendon. If the patient's orbital pressure is not reduced by this maneuver, a medial decompression through a Lynch incision can be performed with the assistance of the ophthalmologist. The patient should then be admitted to the hospital for bed rest and sedation.

Both the surgeon and the nursing staff should be aware that even without intraoperative complications, postoperative problems can occur. If the periorbita has been entered, it is reasonable to admit the patient to the hospital for overnight. The hematoma in the orbit can form during the postoperative period; cases of gradual proptosis and blindness over 24 to 48 hours postoperatively have occurred. If the patient has had evidence of the orbit being entered and is to be released the next day, the nursing staff should be told what changes to look for and to report these immediately to the physician. Also, intranasal packing can provide enough pressure along a dehiscent lamina papyracea that visual changes can occur. In this instance, either the packing should be omitted if bleeding is minimal, or it should be placed rather loosely on that side.

CSF LEAK

Cerebrospinal fluid (CSF) leaks usually occur when the cribriform or foveal areas have been violated. In most instances, CSF leaks can be avoided if adequate attention is paid to a preoperative evaluation of intranasal anatomy using coronal computed tomography scans. By staying lateral to the attachment of the middle turbinate, the cribriform area is easily avoided. In many patients, the posterior ethmoid and fovea ethmoidalis are very thin or dehiscent and may be damaged by overly vigorous dissection. The surgeon should always use a gentle touch in these areas and may wish to be less aggressive than usual in stripping off the mucosa. CT scan may disclose that the level of the fovea is not always the same from one side to the other. CSF leaks also have occurred when working in the sphenoid and have resulted from damaging the posterior wall of the frontal nasal duct. If one uses the endoscopes to enlarge this duct, care should be taken not to curette the posterior aspect of it.

Most CSF leaks will be apparent to the observant surgeon during the procedure and are best dealt with immediately. Many CSF leaks will resolve spontaneously if they are low flow. Occasionally it is necessary to insert a spinal catheter to reduce the CSF pressure. If the leak is large, patching with postauricular fat and temporalis fascia will successfully control it.

LACRIMAL APPARATUS

The lacrimal apparatus may be damaged by dissection through the lamina papyracea, injuring either the duct or the lacrimal sac. Damage can also occur by extending the nasal antral window too far anteriorly and injuring the duct as it traverses the bone toward its opening into the nasal cavity in the inferior meatus. Should these injuries occur, the safest thing to do is an intranasal dacryocystorhinostomy using the endoscopes. If the injury is superior to the level of the lacrimal sac, this procedure may have to be combined with stenting the duct with a Silastic catheter to maintain its patency into the area of the sac. The opening of the os into the duct usually can be avoided when performing the nasal antrostomy by not extending the dissection beyond the very soft, thin bone. When the bone becomes thicker and more difficult to bite into, that is usually an indication that one should stop the dissection.

SYNECHIAE

Synechiae may occur after endoscopic sinus surgery. These seem to occur most commonly when the middle turbinate is preserved and there has been abrasion of either the lateral aspect of the middle turbinate or the medial aspect of the middle turbinate and septum. They usually occur anteriorly in the nose and have been known to occur between the inferior turbinate and the septum as well.

Postoperatively, the middle turbinate has a tendency to displace laterally and may become impacted against the lateral wall of the nose, increasing the possibility of synechiae formation. Partial removal of the anterior turbinate may avoid this problem, especially if the inlet is substantially narrowed by the turbinate, septum, or lateral wall of the nose. Occasionally, it is necessary to use either Surgicel, Telfa, or thin Silastic sheeting as a spacer between these structures to prevent postoperative synechiae. Recently it has been shown that suturing the middle turbinates to the septum during the postoperative period and then releasing them will prevent synechia formation.[14] If a synechia does form and surgical revision is needed to separate the scar, a spacer should always be used for at least a week until the mucosa has regrown.

If a spacer is placed in the nose, it is suggested that it be anchored in some way to the septum to prevent aspiration during the healing phase.[14] Reports in the literature describe using powdered sucralfate in the nose to coat the raw surfaces and prevent synechiae without the need for any physical barriers.[20] This may be a very useful modality.

NATURAL OSTIA CLOSURE

The natural ostia in the middle meatus can become stenotic during the healing process. One should remember that circumferential scars are being created in many instances, and there is a natural tendency for these to close down. If this is observed in the postoperative period, in many instances these ostia can be reopened in the office. Attempts should be made to leave the posterior and superior margins of mucosa intact to prevent this circumferential scar. A recent study has shown a strong correlation between closure of the os and poorly controlled or uncontrolled allergies, emphasizing the need for adequate medical as well as surgical care for these patients.[8]

SUBCUTANEOUS ORBITAL EMPHYSEMA

Subcutaneous orbital emphysema has been reported in some patients. It is not a serious complication and does not compromise the vision, unless it becomes extensive. The cause is air gaining an entrance into the orbit from an opening through the lamina papyracea. This usually can be prevented by instructing the patient not to increase the intranasal air pressure by nose blowing, using the Valsalva maneuver, and so on. In general, no specific control measure is needed for this, and it will resolve spontaneously over a 2- to 3-day period.

TOOTH PAIN

Tooth pain may occur in patients as a result of canine fossa antrotomy with a trocar and cannula. This usually can be avoided by placing the trocar laterally and superiorly over the face and sinus and aiming the trocar medially and inferiorly. The complication usually results from entering either too inferiorly and disrupting the innervation to the root of the tooth or too medially and opening into the nasal cavity, thereby disrupting the sensory innervation to the upper dental arch on the involved side. This also has occurred postoperatively in association with numbness of the palate after injection into the sphenopalatine fossa transorally. Reported tooth pain has been transient and has resolved spontaneously.

MENINGITIS

Meningitis has been reported to occur when the central nervous system has been entered. In general, this condition seems to be associated with failure to recognize a CSF leak and deal with it appropriately. This complication is usually managed by discovering the CSF leak, repairing it if necessary, and providing medical care for the meningitis to resolve.

PNEUMOCEPHALUS

Pneumocephalus also has been reported after CSF leaks. Usually, this has resolved spontaneously and has not been a serious patient problem.

ANOSMIA

If patients have severe disease, most often either total or partial anosmia is noted prior to the operation, which will improve postoperatively. The status of the olfactory nerve (CN I) should always be noted preoperatively. In some instances, anosmia has been known to occur after extensive resection, and, in many cases, it is a temporary result of edema of the nasal membranes with inability of air to pass toward the superior nasal vault. On occasion, this has persisted after resolution of all edema. Injury to the mucosa membranes and the superior aspect of the septum or injury in the cribriform area appears to be the cause. There is no specific treatment.

POSTOPERATIVE INFECTION

Postoperative infections, in general, have not been a significant problem. Toxic shock syndrome associated with nasal packing has already been discussed.

At least one instance of postoperative osteomyelitis of the lateral nasal wall following endoscopic sinus surgery has been reported. This appeared to be caused by desiccation of the bone of the lateral nasal wall after stripping of the mucosal membranes, which became infected in the postoperative period. This problem resolved with adequate debridement of the exposed bone back to healthy, mucosa-covered bone, and antibiotic coverage.

Postoperative infections have occurred because of inadequate debridement of crusts and clots within the nasal cavity, when the nasal cavity retained the packing material, or because of inadequate sinus drainage from the procedure or persistence of disease in unoperated sinuses. An example is a patient with frontal sinus disease that does not resolve after operation on the osteomeatal complex. Trephination and irrigation of the frontal sinus, along with opening the nasofrontal duct, have resulted in resolution of the intranasal inflammation and pain. Exenteration of ethmoid sinuses without sphenoidotomy has resulted in postoperative air fluid levels or infection of the sphenoid sinus, resolving by trephination of the sphenoid sinus. Placement of the nasal antral window away from the natural os, in either the inferior or middle meatus but without connecting the two, can result in a circular flow of mucus between the two openings and subsequent stasis and chronic inflammation or infection. Care in the placement of the new os and making sure that it connects with the natural os will prevent this problem.

ASSOCIATED DISEASES

Certain systemic diseases, such as uncontrolled allergy and cystic fibrosis, are associated with failure of endoscopic sinus surgery. Control of these conditions will improve outcomes; however, the word "failure" when used in the context of treating these diseases may be inappropriate. One should bear in mind that systemic disease is not being treated by these procedures, only a manifestation of the disease process. The more realistic goal may be to reduce the incidence of sinus disease and make the disease that will still occur more easily treated and less severe.

Studies by Freedman and Kern[9] and Friedman and associates[10] have indicated overall complication rates in endoscopic intranasal sinus surgery of 2.8 per cent and less than 3.7 per cent, respectively. Stankiewicz reported an initial complication rate in his first 80 patients of 31 per cent.[22] In his later series, his complication rate dropped remarkably. This indicates that there is definitely a learning phase with this operation and that, as with most complex surgical procedures, it is imperative that the surgeon gain experience and knowledge of the procedure in didactic courses that include hands-on laboratory work with cadaver dissections. Also, surgeons should start out with relatively simple cases and, as they gain experience and facility with the use of the instruments, progress to more complicated cases in a stepwise fashion to keep the complication rates to a minimum.

OTOSCOPY

Otoscopy could be considered the most common endoscopic procedure performed by physicians. In fact, it is so commonplace that most physicians do not look upon it as an endoscopic procedure. But whether one uses an ear speculum or short, rigid telescope, it is still an endoscopic procedure by definition and does carry with it some risks.

The complications of otoscopy relate to several factors: whether the procedure is for diagnosis or therapeutic intervention, selection of the appropriate instruments, physical and emotional condition of the patient and the patient's age.

The age of the patient is important not only from the standpoint of patient cooperation and possible psychologic trauma but also from an anatomic standpoint.[5] In the adult, the external auditory canal is about 2.5

cm long. The lateral one third is surrounded by cartilage, and the medial two thirds is surrounded by bone. From lateral to medial the canal has a "lazy S" shape through curving medially, anteriorly, and superiorly. Just medial to the bony-cartilaginous junction is a narrowed area of the bony canal referred to as the isthmus (Fig. 20–1*A*). Therefore, to examine the external auditory canal adequately, one must retract the adult ear superiorly and posteriorly to try to straighten the flexible cartilaginous canal in relation to the bony canal.

The anatomy in children is similar to that of an adult. But in neonates and young infants, the situation is different. The external auditory canal is composed of soft tissue and cartilage, with the tympanic ring representing the only bone (Fig. 20–1*B*). Redundant soft tissue of the inferior canal wall tends to be pushed over the end of the

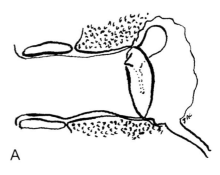

A

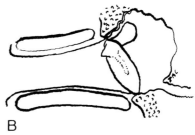

B

FIGURE 20–1. *A,* The adult ear canal in coronal section. Note the tympanomeatal angle and the relation of length of the bone canal *(stippled area)* to the cartilage canal. *B,* A neonate's ear canal in coronal section. Note the tympanomeatal angle (more acute relative to the canal) and the bony annulus with cartilaginous canal.

speculum and block adequate visualization of the tympanic membrane. To avoid this, the examiner must pull the pinna inferiorly and laterally to stretch the redundant skin before the speculum is inserted in the canal.

There is also an important difference in the tympanic membrane. In the neonate and infant, the tympanic membrane forms a much more acute angle with the external auditory canal than it does in the older individual (Fig. 20–1*A,B*). This can cause the lateral process of the malleus to be more prominent. This situation can also occur in retracted tympanic membranes. Such children are more prone to suffer soft tissue damage.

Common to both groups is the unique relationship of the skin of the ear canal to the underlying bone and cartilage. This skin is tightly bound to the perichondrium and periosteum of the external canal without the usual loose connective tissue in the subcutaneous layer. Because of this close association of the skin to the very sensitive periosteum, what would seem to be only mild pressure of a rigid speculum on the skin may cause severe discomfort. Many practitioners feel that a smaller speculum will be less uncomfortable to the patient. However, a speculum so small in diameter that it can be inserted to the junction of the cartilage and bone, where pressure against the hard bone not only would cause tremendous pain but also could lacerate the canal wall skin, must be avoided. In the infant, this junction is at the annulus, and an injury here could result in a perforation of the tympanic membrane or injury in the area of the protruding lateral process of the malleus. Lacerations in the canal also will tend to open and remain open and bleed more than one would expect, because normal wound contraction cannot take place with the adherent skin. This may also cause these wounds to require a longer healing time and make them prone to infection.

One must be careful during inspection through an ear speculum not to cause any soft tissue injury. It will be painful and, especially in a child, will result in a very uncooperative patient. It may also lead to bleeding, which can reduce the visibility of the ear being examined and reduce the patient's confidence in the physician. Whenever possible, instrumentation through the speculum should be performed with the aid of binocular microscopy to reduce the likelihood of injury to the canal and the tympanic membrane. If injury occurs, the ear should be thoroughly debrided and the patient instructed to keep the ear clean and dry. The patient should be followed until complete healing has occurred. If signs of infection are seen, appropriate antibiotic therapy should be started. If a perforation persists, it will need to be treated to stimulate healing.

Other structures in and around the ear should be noted. A high jugular vein or dehiscent jugular bulb may cause a reddish swelling in the inferior aspect of the medial canal. Manipulations in this area should be delicate. The same is true in the traumatized ear or the ear with a foreign body.

Of particular note in regard to the nerve supply to the external canal is the branch of the vagus nerve referred to as Arnold nerve. Stimulation of this nerve may cause sudden coughing; if the instrument in the ear is not stabilized to the patient, a severe laceration of the canal or perforation of the tympanic membrane may result. This seems to be a greater problem in older patients. An anecdotal account was related of a patient experiencing a vasovagal reaction and losing consciousness twice in the examining chair while having cerumen removed. Drops at home had to be used to remove the impaction.

A problem that all practitioners face in our mobile society is debridement of an ear that has had a prior mastoid procedure by another physician. One must watch for a possibly dehiscent facial nerve, reconstructed tympanic membrane, or in an older patient a previous fenestration of the horizontal semicircular canal. Injuries to these structures could leave the patient with severe impairments. Even with the most gentle of techniques, at times a patient may experience some vestibular stimulation and resultant vertigo. Rest and reassurance that this is temporary will see the patient through the episode, which usually lasts only minutes. Be sure the patient is fully recovered before leaving the office, especially if driving.

Most children hate to have their ears examined, much less cleaned, and may not be cooperative. Some gentle restraint may be in order. If the child is small enough, the parent is the best restraining system. A suggested method is as follows: If the right ear is to be examined, seat the child on the parent's right leg with the child's feet held between the parent's legs and the parent's right arm over the child's chest, with both arms of the child down to the sides. This will control the child's feet, legs, torso, and hands. The child's left ear is held against the parent's chest firmly by the parent's left hand over the child's right parietal scalp; this will stabilize the head. This is very effective and puts the parent in the position of being responsible for the child's holding still, not the nurse, reassuring the parent that the child is not being brutalized by the health care team. Microscopy can be carried out in this position. If examination with the child supine is needed or if the child is too large for the parent to hold in this manner, either a restraining board or sheet wrap is needed.[3] These methods were taught during my residency by the capable nurses in the Otolaryngology Clinic at the Children's Hospital of Pittsburgh. These methods will suffice in most cases for examination, debridement, tympanocentesis, and removal of simple foreign bodies. If absolute stillness is required, one should consider sedation or general anesthesia for the child.

DIRECT LARYNGOSCOPY AND SUBGLOTTOSCOPY

The procedures termed *laryngoscopy* and *subglottoscopy* also involve examination of the hypopharynx, esophageal introitus, and superior trachea, all with attendant complications.

Investigation of the airway carries with it the potential for disaster. The best way to avoid the hazards and complications is to anticipate them; a good preoperative evaluation of the patient by both the surgeon and anesthesiologist is important. Patient selection is a key factor. If the person is in a profession in which the voice is directly related to livelihood, such as a singer or an actor, one should consider referring the patient to a physician specially trained in this type of patient care. The surgeon must obtain and examine the appropriate preoperative radiographs. Pulmonary function tests may be in order, along with the other preoperative evaluations that are deemed necessary. Because of the potential for loss of control of the airway in these cases, it is my opinion that all patients, regardless of age, and their families should be warned about the possible need for a tracheotomy, and that this is documented. By approaching the subject of a possible tracheotomy as having the patient's best interests at heart, I have never had a patient or family refuse a procedure because of it. It cannot be overemphasized that the surgeon and the anesthesiologist must both have a clear understanding of the steps involved in the procedure, as well as concern about the status of the airway and the patient's general health. This requires talking to each other before the patient is on the table—simply reading each other's notes in the chart just will not do. If one follows this advice, one will find that these procedures cease to be harrowing experiences for both sides of the table but instead provide a sense of accomplishment for the well-coordinated surgical team.

One may be working with a compromised airway, and even if it is not the surgeon is going to proceed to compromise it with the passage of the instruments. It is imperative, therefore, that the operating room team do everything possible to minimize this compromise. The patient must be kept without food or drink for long enough prior to the procedure to allow for gastric emptying, in order to prevent reflux or regurgitation either during or after the procedure when the patient is unable to protect his or her own airway. This may not be possible in the emergency situation, so gastric sectioning as well as fast-acting H-2 antagonists should be used. A common cause of hypoventilation in patients is overpremedication and subsequent respiratory depression. No matter what type of anesthesia is used, a blood pressure cuff, electrocardiogram, and pulse oximeter should be considered the minimal monitoring devices for the patient.

Along with the usual problems and risks involved with a general anesthetic, there are also risks related to the use of local anesthetics that the endoscopist has direct control over and therefore must be especially aware of. Lidocaine is probably the most commonly used local anesthetic agent in endoscopy. While knowing the safe blood levels for the agent is important, it is also important to realize that very high, transient levels of anesthetic can be reached owing to the rapid absorption through the respiratory tract mucosa when these medications are used topically. Muscle fasciculation, nervousness, visual disturbance, weakness, or dizziness should alert the physician of toxicity that could result in seizure activity or cardiac toxicity.

Because the passage of instruments in and out of the airway can cause significant edema, the surgeon must always use a gentle, yet skillful, technique. This will help prevent such injuries as arytenoid dislocation. Should this occur, the arytenoid should be returned to its normal anatomic position and the patient followed closely in the postoperative period to ensure permanent reduction. A gentle technique will also help prevent distortion of the larynx, which could result in obscuring pathology. Steroid use as well as postoperative respiratory treatments with racemic epinephrine will help limit airway edema. Limiting the duration of the procedure is also important, and preoperative planning is the key here.

Even with the most gentle of techniques, there is still considerable stimulation of the patient's vagal nerve during these procedures. Most endoscopists have met with sudden drops in the patient's heart rate and blood pressure upon introduction of the endoscope, which sometimes will necessitate removing the instruments and medicating the patient. Dangerous arrhythmias can occur, especially in those patients who may be hypoxic.

Complications may ensue if the patient is not properly positioned on the table. Accidental extubation may occur while the surgeon is positioning the patient; then the surgeon stabilizes the endotracheal tube and informs the anesthetist of what is happening. The surgeon must insure that the head is adequately supported if a shoulder roll is used, not hanging so that the cervical spine could be injured. This precaution is especially important in elderly patients who may have degenerative disease of the cervical vertebrae and in children in whom the ligaments may be weak or lax, as Down syndrome. If atlantoaxial instability or dislocation is evident, one puts gentle pressure on the forehead with one hand, and, with the index finger of the opposite hand on the spinous process of the axis, moves the head backward in a gliding motion to reduce the subluxation. The procedure should be halted and cervical spine radiographs obtained with the patient on the table to confirm reduction. When reduction is confirmed, the neck is stabilized and neurologic evaluation carried out.[17] In elderly patients with cardiovascular disease, prolonged extension of the neck—especially under a general anesthetic—can increase the risk of stroke or compromise the cerebral blood flow, leading to hypoxia and hypotension in the central nervous system.

The possibility of injury to structures in and about the oral cavity must be kept in mind. It is all too easy to concentrate on the view through the laryngoscope and overlook the trauma being caused to lips that are caught between the endoscope and teeth or pressure injuries to unprotected gums. If electrocautery is to be used during the case, make sure that the cautery is not in contact with the endoscope so that the current will not be transmitted to the surrounding soft tissue structures.

The teeth must be evaluated closely before operation, and special attention paid to loose, capped, or carious teeth, especially the incisors, which usually take the brunt of the endoscope pressure. A tooth guard or padding for the gums always should be used. If a tooth should be chipped or knocked out of its socket, make sure that the entire dental unit is recovered, as a tooth could act as a foreign body and be aspirated. Any dentures or other appliance that can be removed before operation should be removed. Bear in mind that a loosened tooth often can be saved if returned to its normal anatomic position and stabilized. Let our dental colleagues lend a hand in such an instance. This also applies to children who may have loose deciduous teeth. On more than one occasion, I have removed a loose baby tooth before passing the endoscope rather than take a chance on its becoming dislodged in the postoperative period and being aspirated.

Another area that must be protected during the procedure is the eyes. Ocular injury usually occurs not because an instrument was inserted into the eye but rather because a careless finger was pushed into the eye as the endoscope was being manipulated. If the patient complains of something in the eye in the immediate postoperative period, one should suspect a corneal abrasion and rule it out.

One of the more serious complications that can occur in the immediate postoperative period is airway obstruction. All patients who have had instrumentation in and around the airway should be closely observed for obstruction. A retained foreign body, such as a sponge, is one reason for this, which can be prevented easily by counting all instruments and sponges at the beginning and end of the operation. Blood can accumulate in the airway, for which adequate hemostasis and suctioning are required.

Edema of the soft tissues also can block the airway; it could be in the glottis or immediate area but can also be in the tongue if the procedure has been long and a lot of pressure has been kept on it by the suspended laryngoscope. Judicious use of steroids and clocking the suspension time, as well as attention to technique, are the keys to prevention. Pulmonary edema is a well-recognized entity that occurs in both children and adults when a chronic obstruction of the upper airway is suddenly relieved. It presents as a frothy liquid from the patient's mouth or nose. Usually this will occur in the first couple of hours after surgery but has been seen as long as 12 hours later. The patient must be observed for an adequate length of time to guard against this complication. It is treated with positive end-expiratory pressure breathing from which the patient is slowly weaned.

Medialization of the vocal cords also can block the airway in the postoperative period. Two common mechanisms for this are laryngospasm and the operation itself. Laryngospasm is usually self-limited, but dangerously low blood oxygen levels can be reached before it breaks. This can be avoided by using a topical anesthetic in the airway at the end of the procedure and allowing enough time for it to work as well as waiting until the patient is more awake before extubation. If it happens despite this, positive pressure in the airway as well as intravenous lidocaine or short-term paralysis may be needed. Paralysis of the patient will probably mean reintubation and setting the scenario all over again.

Medialization of the vocal cords as a direct result of operation can be from vocal cord injection that overcorrects the problem. For this reason it is advisable to perform the procedure with the patient awake so that the airway can be continuously monitored. A late-onset complication is formation of a web from denuding the mucosa on both sides of the anterior commissure, circumferentially around the airway, or all the way across the posterior commissure. These are to be avoided even if it means staging the procedure and returning the patient to the operating room another day.

An unusual reason for the vocal cords to medialize is from paralysis of one or both cords at the end of the procedure, usually temporary. This may be due to pressure being applied to the recurrent nerve or nerves by the cricoid and thyroid cartilages approximating as the head is extended.

Complications with the voice may develop in the postoperative period. Because of the likelihood of some sort of voice alteration, whether temporary or permanent, it is important that the vocal cord appearance and function be documented both before and after operation. Ideally, this should include video-stroboscopy and a phonogram. To avoid complications, one should take care not to notch the vocal cord with resections and not to get into the vocal muscles. This may not be possible when dealing with a malignancy, so the patient should be forewarned of the possibility of permanent voice alteration.

DIRECT TRACHEOSCOPY AND BRONCHOSCOPY

The insertion of any instrument into the respiratory tract is traumatic to some degree and will be associated with some tissue injury and physiologic alteration. Because the instrument must be passed through the larynx, much of what appears in the previous section applies here.

Because it is so important, the risk of cardiac arrhythmias is reviewed again. The risk is increased if hypoxemia is allowed to occur, and the arrhythmias can be severe enough to cause cardiac arrest. It is advisable to avoid elective procedures on those individuals with a history of unstable angina, recent myocardial infarction, or hypoxia at rest. One should always check a preoperative electrocardiogram in those patients at risk, use lidocaine intraoperatively topically or intravenously or both, and avoid prolonged procedures.

Because the procedure often involves a biopsy or removal of tissue, hemorrhage in the lower airway is a complication that the surgeon sometimes will face. Sponges, topical adrenalin, adequate suction, cautery, and instruments to deliver these things through the endoscope to the bleeding site should be readily available. In the preoperative evaluation, a computed tomographic scan should be obtained if a lesion is suspected, in order to ascertain the surrounding anatomy before any tissue is removed. Immunosuppressed patients and renal failure patients are more likely to have bleeding problems. The surgeon also should have some idea of what he or she is looking at before biopsying a mass. Know what things might come across the trachea or bronchus that would cause a mass

effect but should not be biopsied (Fig. 20-2).[7] Some lesions will have a greater tendency to bleed, such as hemangiomas and some bronchial adenomas. If brisk bleeding does occur, try to keep the opposite lung from filling with blood. The patient should be put into Trendelenburg position with the bleeding side down while the bleeding is brought under control. Brisk bleeding may require tamponade; so an aortic balloon catheter should be at hand. If the bleeding cannot be brought under control, the patient may need an open procedure to stop it. Because of this possibility, it might be well to have a chest surgeon on standby should the need arise.

Occasionally, a vigorous biopsy will go all the way through the airway and a pneumothorax will result. This may not require treatment beyond observation, but early recognition is a key factor in this complication. All patients who undergo tracheoscopy or bronchoscopy should have a chest radiograph read in the recovery room. However, a pneumothorax may take some time to become manifest, so one must not ignore the later symptoms of a pneumothorax simply because the postoperative film was normal.

Mechanical stimulation of the tracheobronchial tree can result in spasm of the smooth muscle in the wall of the airway. Rare in the nonasthmatic patient, in the asthmatic it can be severe and lead to death if not recognized and treated promptly. The constriction of the muscle is partly mediated by the efferent vagal pathway after stimulation of the rapid receptors in the airway. A history of asthma will have been elicited during the preoperative evaluation of the patient and adequate preparations made by the anesthesiologist in the form of preoperative steroids and intraoperative atropine and aminophylline if needed. One should exercise caution in the use of topical anesthetics in these individuals. A topical anesthetic should be short acting so that the patient will be able to protect the airway when awake and prevent aspiration. Some local anesthetic agents, such as tetracaine, may contain preservatives like para-aminobenzoic acid that could cause anaphylaxis.

In the postoperative period, adequate ven-

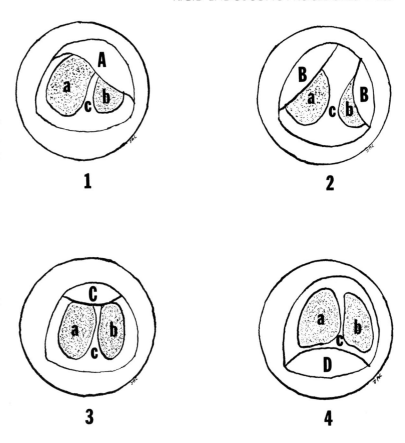

FIGURE 20–2. Diagrams of some extrinsic vascular compressions of the trachea that may be encountered on bronchoscopy. *1,* Innominate artery (A). *2,* Vascular ring (B). *3,* Pulmonary artery (C). *4,* Vascular sling (D). a, Left main stem bronchus; b, right main stem bronchus; c, carina. (Adapted from Desnos J, et al: Vascular strictures in the respiratory tract in children. Int J Pediatr Otorhinolaryngol 2: 269, 1980.)

tilatory effort and oxygenation should be documented. A pulse oximeter may be required. Because most of these procedures are now done on an outpatient basis, the patient must be educated prior to discharge and made aware of the need to report any signs of infection. Studies of fiberoptic bronchoscopies have shown that 1 in 50 patients will have some transient bacteremia.[6] Serious infections such as pneumonia and meningitis have occurred following endoscopies. Instruments must be properly cleaned and cared for. In spite of this, the lower airway is easily contaminated by organisms from the upper airway as the instrument is passed. Care must be taken if the lower airway is already infected, a condition associated with congestive heart failure, atelectasis, pulmonary embolism, and airway obstruction from a mass or foreign body.

The Pediatric Airway. With the advent of the rod lens systems for endoscopy, examination of the pediatric airway has become commonplace. The parameters of the child's airway and the size of the lumen; the small, delicate instruments; the fragility of the tissues; and the small respiratory reserve of the patient combine to present the surgeon with a system very unforgiving of mistakes. Most of the discussion about the pediatric airway will also apply to the adult patient.

Prior to beginning the procedure, all equipment should be in the room and checked. All pieces must be compatible, telescope optics checked; light sources functioning, instruments in good repair, and suction forceps and other instruments must be passed down the scope small enough and long enough. It is also suggested that a tracheotomy tray be available if needed. The surgeon should review the plan of the procedure with the anesthesiologist before the child is put to sleep. Removing the endotracheal tube, ventilation through the bronchoscope, jet ventilation, or apneic technique is reviewed and understood at the outset so that the proper anesthesia equipment can be ready and available.

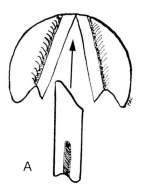

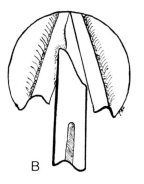

FIGURE 20–3. If one aims straight down the airway *(A)*, the tip of the bronchoscope could catch the vocal cord *(B)*.

As the bronchoscope is passed down to the glottis, there is a potential for injury to the vocal cords because of the small diameter of the airway. The surgeon has a tendency to aim down the center of the glottic chink. In the small airway this may cause the tip of the bronchoscope's bevel to catch on the superior aspect of the vocal cord. Increased pressure to pass the scope may result in a vocal cord hematoma (Fig. 20–3). To avoid this, one should aim the scope at the cord that the bevel opens toward so that the tip will slip through the chink without catching the vocal cord (Fig. 20–4). We use the Karl Storz system; with these bronchoscopes the ventilation port comes off in the same direction as the bevel opens. When the procedure is performed, the anesthesia equipment is to the right of the patient and the surgeon is at the head of the table. The bronchoscope is then passed with the ventilation port on the right, the bevel toward the right and aiming for the right vocal cord.

The tip of the telescope also may traumatize a vocal cord. If one looks closely at the aperture of the smaller bronchoscopes, one may sometimes note the tip of the telescope extending beyond the sheath (Fig. 20–5A,B). This could also catch the cord as the scope is passed. It is a useful practice to withdraw the telescope slightly until the bronchoscope is through the cords and then push the telescope all the way in (Fig. 20–6A,B).

At some time during the procedure the status of the vocal cords' movement must be assessed. Knowledge of this prior to awaking and extubating the patient may prevent serious postoperative airway obstruction. Also, any luxated arytenoid can be repaired at this time.

Below the level of the vocal cords, the subglottis may cause problems in the postoperative period because of edema and airway obstruction. Edema may occur because the bronchoscope selected may be too large for the airway. Outside diameters of bronchoscopes lack uniformity from one manufacturer to another even when the inside diameters are the same. Excessive manipulation of the airway also may result in edema. The experience of the surgeon is an important factor here, as well as adequate anesthesia techniques. Failure to use telescopes means not only increased manipulation but

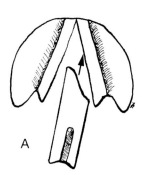

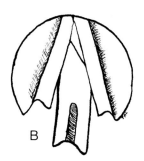

FIGURE 20–4. When the bevel is aimed toward the cord on the side of the bevel *(A)*, the tip of the bronchoscope will slip past the cords with ease *(B)*.

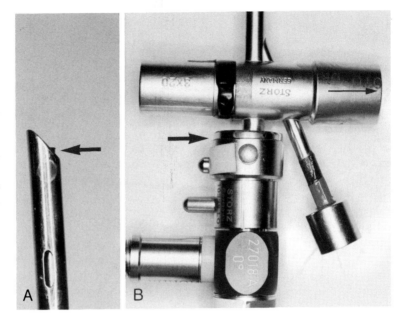

FIGURE 20–5. *A,* Note the tip of the telescope extending beyond the tip of the bronchoscope *(arrow). B,* The telescope is fully inserted into the bronchoscope *(large arrow).* The small arrow is on the ventilation port.

also may prolong the procedure. Lack of finesse when removing foreign bodies can result in damage to the membranes and postoperative swelling.

Decreased ventilation is always a concern when working within the airway. A complication with the ventilating bronchoscopes is that the telescope and sheath may cause significant obstruction to ventilation; at times the sheath or sheath and telescope may have to be removed to ventilate the patient. If a pulse oximeter is used, the oxygen saturation measured peripherally will lag behind changes in saturation of the blood. If the saturation drops below 90 per cent, one should be wary because the actual saturation of the blood will be somewhere in the 80s, and the oxygen saturation curve begins to drop off rapidly in the low 80s.

Foreign Body Removal. Foreign body removal from the airway presents complications frequently. Formerly this was the arena

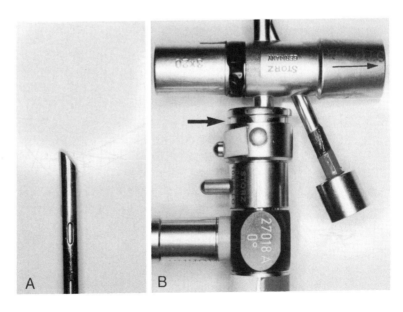

FIGURE 20–6. *A,* The tip of the telescope has been withdrawn into the lumen of the bronchoscope and is no longer visible. *B,* The telescope has been withdrawn slightly, but is still firmly seated in the bronchoscope *(large arrow).* The small arrow is on the ventilation port.

of a few very skilled endoscopists. As more people were trained and as endoscopy systems, both rigid and fiberoptic, became more readily available, more physicians in a variety of specialties began retrieving foreign bodies from the airways of children. The result is that today's endoscopist may not have the same wealth of experience to draw upon as his or her predecessors, and the level of expertise may not be as high in some cases. This may be partially compensated for by the use of superior equipment.

A major factor in the mismanagement of the foreign body patient is failing to include the possibility of a foreign body in the differential diagnosis. This will lead to an incorrect diagnosis based on an incomplete medical history. No radiographs or incomplete radiographs may be obtained, which may delay the correct diagnosis further.

Sometimes the history provided by the parent can be the physician's worst enemy. Many parents are poor historians, or they may dismiss their child's description of events or symptoms in favor of what they think. If the physician's suspicion is high, then the point must be pressed doggedly. At times it is prudent to go with what the child relates. If it turns out that there is no foreign body in the airway, one must not overlook the fact that a foreign body in the esophagus also can cause respiratory symptoms.

Once the diagnosis is established, proper treatment must be carried out without delay and with the proper instrumentation. Waiting for spontaneous extrusion of a foreign body from the airway is wrong. Avoid the pitfall of inappropriate use of fiberoptic endoscopes and Fogarty as well as Foley catheters, as these instruments do not allow one to maintain control of the object as it is extracted. Once an object has been removed, always go back and look for more. This is especially true of coins that may be stacked together, giving a radiographic appearance of a single coin.

A fiberoptic endoscope is not a good selection for foreign body removal in children.[4, 15] The visualization is not as good as with a rod lens system. In the smaller airway of a child it is difficult to ventilate the patient adequately either around or through the fiberscope. It is difficult to pass instruments to help in dislodging a foreign body that is impacted in the airway, nor are the available forceps heavy or varied enough to handle the types of foreign bodies encountered. The small lumen also does not provide adequate space to shield a sharp object for atraumatic extraction. Additionally, the instrument's inability to treat bleeding granulations, pus, and hemorrhage make it a less than adequate choice for foreign body work in children.

Of the complications reported in children, most are related to foreign bodies that have been present for some time. Such problems as bronchiectasis, bronchitis, and pneumonia are usually not acute events, nor is hemorrhage into the airway from an undiagnosed foreign body. Pneumothorax and mediastinitis from trauma to the airway due to overly aggressive technique or inadequate shielding of a sharp object also can occur. Occasionally the airway may be compromised if a foreign body is brought into the trachea and control of the object is lost. In this case the object should be pushed into either main stem bronchus so that ventilation to at least one lung may continue. Removal is attempted again after the patient is stabilized. If an emergency airway has been established because of an object in the larynx or trachea, severe laryngeal or subglottic stenosis can occur as a result of cricothyrotomy procedures.

In general, the complication rate in children can be reduced if the child with a suspected foreign body aspiration is referred to a center that has a well-equipped team to deal with these types of problems.

ESOPHAGOSCOPY

Esophagoscopy, like bronchoscopy, is a procedure that is practiced by several specialties using various types of instruments. The procedure is done for evaluation of dysphagia, odynophagia, assessment of malignancy both before and after treatment, reflux, hematemesis, and foreign body removal. The condition of the esophageal membranes can be just as varied as this list, and knowing when and how the mucosa of the esophagus will vary with different types of pathology is important to the safe execution of the procedure.

Of all the complications associated with esophagoscopy, the most dreaded and severe is perforation of the esophagus. According to Palmer, the incidence is 0.06 per cent.[18] This figure may be somewhat high as the sampling was among academic institutions where physicians in training may be performing the procedure on compromised patients. To avoid this complication, one should obtain a preoperative esophagogram to elucidate any anatomic irregularities. Never force the passage of the endoscope and always be able to visualize a lumen as the esophagoscope is advanced. If a perforation occurs, the surgeon almost always will see a tear and bleeding will be encountered. The key to treatment of the problem is prompt recognition of the complication.

Four general conditions of the esophagus can lead to a perforation during endoscopy. The first is the series of narrowings of the lumen, of the normal anatomy (Fig. 20–7). Next is when passing the scope over large anterior cervical osteophytes. This can cause erosion of the mucosa as it is pressed be-

tween the endoscope anteriorly and the bone posteriorly. A significant osteophyte should be visualized on the preoperative radiographs. When one is encountered, the scope should be lifted anteriorly and advanced through the well-visualized lumen without allowing too much posterior pressure. Third is in the area of a diverticulum, such as a Zenker diverticulum. This too should be seen on the preoperative films and should be examined with caution so that the endoscope is not pushed through the inferior aspect of the pouch. And last are strictures. These should be noted preoperatively; when encountered, a smaller scope may be needed. It may be necessary to dilate the stricture: the appropriate dilators should be used, not the endoscope.

In spite of one's best efforts perforations still occur, and one must know what to do when they happen. The problem that must be addressed is the possibility of infection starting in the soft tissues outside the lumen of the esophagus. In the cervical esophagus, this will be in the neck. In the thoracic esophagus, this will be in the mediastinum, where the danger is greatest, because the mortality rate for a severe mediastinitis can be as high as 90 per cent or more if it is not treated aggressively.

FIGURE 20–7. Locations of anatomic narrowings of the esophagus.

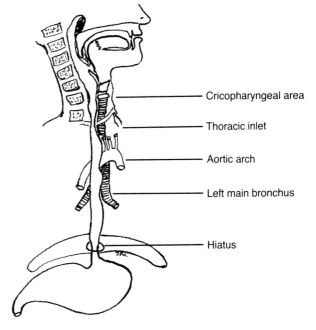

Cricopharyngeal area

Thoracic inlet

Aortic arch

Left main bronchus

Hiatus

Prior to the use of today's broad-spectrum antibiotics, a perforation of the esophagus committed the patient to an open exploration for repair and drainage. A perforation in the thoracic esophagus meant a major procedure. This is still required in some patients when a major rent is created or in those who do not respond to conservative measures. If the tear is small, sometimes one can be more conservative, but the procedure should be terminated immediately. Some surgeons place a nasogastric tube under endoscopic control: I do not believe one is needed. The patient should receive nothing by mouth, and a scopolamine patch is placed to reduce secretions. Saliva is suctioned or spit out by the patient, rather than swallowed. At the earliest opportunity in the postoperative period, a chest film and contrast swallow with a water-soluble contrast should be performed to document the amount of leakage and the appearance of the lungs, pleura, and mediastinum. The patient should be started on high doses of broad-spectrum antibiotics and the temperature, white blood cell count, and differential count followed closely. Some practitioners administer intravenous steroids. I see no reason to do this; in fact, the elevation of the white cell count from the steroids may confuse the picture. If the patient shows no sign of infection for 7 days, the contrast study is repeated. If there is still some leakage, therapy is continued for another week and the patient rechecked. If the leak is not apparent on the contrast study, clear liquids are started by mouth and the patient observed as before for 24 hours. If there is no sign of infection then, the antibiotics can be stopped and the diet advanced. If the patient does not respond to this therapy, open exploration is indicated. Perforations in the cervical esophagus require the same treatment plan.

If conservative treatment as described is to be followed, it should be started without delay, since mediastinitis can begin very rapidly. I treated a gunshot wound to the neck in which the cervical esophagus was penetrated by the bullet. The patient's neck was explored within 6 hours of the injury, and by that time a tract into the superior medias-

tinum had already formed and purulent material was recovered from the tract.

Bleeding can be another very significant complication of esophagoscopy. It is not unusual to encounter a small amount of bleeding during the procedure, especially if biopsies are performed. It is unusual to have to re-endoscope the patient to control the bleeding or prolong the patient's hospitalization to observe it. Significant bleeding can occur from erosions caused by either benign or malignant disease. One should be careful in removing the clots if a biopsy is needed. One must seriously consider whether it is prudent to continue the examination beyond this point to see what is distal to the clot or erosion, remembering that one may be risking a serious bleed or perforation. If the procedure is being performed to evaluate hemoptysis, coagulation studies should be done.

As with any invasive procedure, postoperative infections occur. The esophagoscopes should be properly cleaned and stored to prevent patient exposure. A protocol for this must be developed and adhered to by the persons responsible for the care and maintenance of the instruments.

Most infectious complications are due to respiratory tract contamination from aspiration. The patient receives nothing by mouth prior to the procedure for an adequate length of time to allow gastric emptying. In some patients who suffer from some type of abnormal motor function that either will not allow the stomach to empty properly or will cause insufficiency of the gastroesophageal junction; as in pyloric stenosis, stricture, achalasia, and gastroparesis, a nasogastric tube should be passed at the beginning and end of the procedure to suction the contents from the stomach. Preoperative use of glycopyrrolate and an H-2 blocker may be of benefit.

If aspiration occurs, one should administer intravenous steroids to reduce the chemical pneumonitis, suction the lungs to establish the pH of the liquid aspirated, and obtain a baseline postoperative film. Antibiotics should be started and the patient admitted and observed overnight. A chest film should be obtained the next day and compared with the previous film. The patient's clinical status will determine fitness for discharge.

In patients with rheumatic heart disease, prosthetic heart valves, or other indications for prophylactic antibiotics, the surgeon must decide the need for antibiotics in strictly diagnostic procedures. In invasive procedures, such as dilatations, biopsies, or sclerotherapy, prophylactic antibiotics are indicated. This is true for all endoscopic procedures.

Cardiopulmonary complications have been reported in association with esophagoscopy. Respiratory depression, hypotension, and arrhythmias can occur. Respiratory depression is one of the more common side effects, and most often is due to the effects of the medications used for sedation. Naloxone should be available for these cases; if it is needed, the patient should respond to it before the procedure is continued. Patients with liver disease may metabolize drugs more slowly, so the medications should be titrated accordingly. In patients with a history of atrial fibrillation or flutter, atropine should not be used as a drying agent preoperatively as it will decrease the refractory period of the nodal conduction system and cause serious tachycardia.

Foreign body removal from the esophagus can cause some severe complications if not done with adequate care and dexterity or if the object is sharp.[4] A sharp object can pierce the wall of the esophagus and cause abscess formation, pneumothorax, pneumomediastinum, mediastinitis, or the other complications of perforation already discussed. Perforation into the airway has been known to cause tracheoesophageal fistulas in children. If the wall of the esophagus is intact, it is very important to control the object by using instruments that will grip it firmly and bring any sharp portions into the lumen of the esophagoscope—something that cannot be done with fiberoptic scopes. Once the object is controlled and protected, the object, forceps, and endoscope should be removed as a unit while the foreign body is observed constantly. One does not want to have the object stripped from the grasp of the forceps at the pharyngoesophageal junction or hypopharynx, as this could lead to aspiration of the object. Once the foreign body has been removed, the esophagus should be re-examined to make sure no other object is present and to assess the esophageal wall.

Esophageal dilatation can result in perforation if a gentle touch is not used. For very tight strictures serial dilatations should be performed to avoid rupture of the wall. With benign strictures the perforation rate is 0.6 per cent , and with malignant strictures it is 5 per cent.[16, 19] This may represent disease involving only partial wall thickness as opposed to transmural disease.

In sclerotherapy, some ulcerations of the treated area have been reported, which have healed without specific therapy. If the therapy is performed circumferentially about the lumen of the esophagus, a stricture may form that could require dilatation.

COMPLICATIONS INVOLVING HEALTH CARE PERSONNEL

Just as important a consideration as what may befall the patient is what complication may befall persons rendering the patient's care. Before the advent of concern over the AIDS virus, little attention was paid to this issue, but in the current climate the precautions to prevent complications among ourselves as a result of treating patients should be mentioned.

Equipment needs to be disinfected between uses to prevent patient contamination. It is also important that instruments be handled in such a manner as to prevent contamination of others after the instruments are used but before they are disinfected. Gloves are worn at all times when handling the instruments. Care must be taken that the gloves are intact and confer adequate protection from any contaminants.

Sharp objects also should be handled with care, and protocols are available to do this in a safe manner. For the surgeon, not only are sharp instruments a potential hazard but unprotected teeth or partial plates also can be a problem—another good reason to use a tooth protector and have all dental appliances removed prior to surgery.

Light sources can generate considerable heat. This heat can be transmitted down the light cable to the endoscope. On at least two occasions in our institution, towels have been singed by the tip of an endoscope laid upon it with the light source at maximum illumination. I am not aware of any tissue injuries from this.

The entire operating room crew and especially the surgeon must protect themselves from the patient's secretions and possibly blood. This means not only gloves for the surgeon but also a gown that is water resistant, and face and eye protection. Eye protection is probably the most commonly overlooked precaution among surgeons, especially those surgeons who normally do not wear corrective lenses. If one wears contact lenses, it may be a useful habit not to wear them on operating days to force oneself to wear protective lenses.

Cautery may be used to control hemorrhage or ablate a lesion. Adequate room air suction must be available to remove the smoke plume and prevent airborne particulate matter from circulating about the room, since infective material potentially may be present in this suspended material.[11]

WHAT TO DO WHEN A COMPLICATION OCCURS

One of the most important things a surgeon can do when a complication occurs is to recognize it. The sooner it is recognized, the sooner appropriate treatment can be started and the more likely the sequelae will be less serious. Surgeons must do all in their power to correct the problem yet realize at what point their own abilities may not be sufficient. At this point surgeons must not be afraid to call for help from a colleague within or outside their own specialty.

At times the surgeon may not want to ask for help. This is not a time for one's ego to get in the way of good judgment and what is best for the patient. Fear may be another reason to delay in seeking help. Some of the more common fears that will cause a dilemma for the surgeon are fear of a law suit if the patient or family realizes that something has gone wrong, fear of losing stature among peers if they become aware of a problem, fear of losing patients if word gets out in a community of a serious complication, and fear that help is not available. Let us examine these one at a time.

One sure way to wind up in court is to have patients or families feel that you are withholding information or lying to them. If a complication occurs, the patient and family should be told and told so that they realize that everything was done to prevent it, that everything will be done to correct it, and together the problem will be solved. The surgeon should be kind, courteous, and sympathetic but not come across as feeling guilty. This may not always keep the surgeon from hearing from a lawyer later, but at least the surgeon's postoperative care of the patient will not be faulted. One should also let the hospital's risk management people know what happened as soon as possible—ideally before talking to patient and family—and follow their advice. The doctor's malpractice insurance carrier also should be informed early, as immediate depositions may be needed.

Loss of stature among one's peers is not a realistic concern. Most fellow physicians will have more respect for a person who is honest about complications than for those who try to cover them up. Those whose expertise is requested usually will feel honored that their talents are so highly regarded. Those who do not wish to be involved probably are not physicians one would want to have involved in the care of patients.

If, on the other hand, a surgeon is experiencing an inordinate number of complications, one's peers may become justifiably concerned, and some introspection on the surgeon's part may be in order to try to determine whether further training or turning these cases over to another might be warranted.

The possibility of people in a community losing faith in a physician is a real concern, especially in smaller communities. This may be directly proportional to the number of complications a surgeon experiences. Again, compassion for one's patients is probably the best solution to this problem.

Fear that help is not available is without foundation. It may not be available in one's own institution, but there is no reason why a patient cannot be transported to a referral center for more specialized care if needed.

References

1. Baltch AL, Buhac I, Agrawal A, et al: Bacteremia after upper gastrointestinal endoscopy. Arch Intern Med 137:594, 1977.
2. Barnes LE (ed): Surgical Pathology of the Head and Neck. New York, Marcel Dekker, 1985.
3. Bluestone D, Stool E: Pediatric Otolaryngology. Philadelphia, WB Saunders, 1983.
4. Cohen SR: Unusual presentations and problems created by mismanagement of foreign bodies in the aerodigestive tract of the pediatric patient. Ann Otol 90:316, 1981.
5. DeGowin EL, DeGowin RL: Bedside Diagnostic Examination. 2nd ed. London, Collier-Macmillan Ltd, 1969.
6. Dent TL, Strodel WE, Turcotte JG, Harper ML: Surgical Endoscopy. Chicago, Year Book Medical Publishers, 1985.
7. Desnos J, Andrieu-Guitrancourt J, Dehesdin D, Dubin J: Vascular strictures of the respiratory tract in children. Int J Pediatr Otorhinolaryngol 2:269, 1980.
8. Duncavage JA, Coleman JA Jr: Maxillary Sinus Antrostomy: Review of the Current Techniques and Why They Fail. Presented at the American Academy of Otolaryngoloic Allergy, Kansas City, MO, Sept 1991.
9. Freedman HM, Kern EB: Complications of intranasal ethmoidectomy: A review of 1000 consecutive operations (1957–1972). Laryngoscope 89:421, 1979.
10. Friedman WH, Katsantonis GP, et al: Sphenoethmoidectomy: The case for ethmoid marsupialization. Laryngoscope 96:473, 1986.
11. Hazards of Smoke Plume and Aerosols. Riverside, CA, Stackhouse Incorporated, 1990.
12. Holinger PH, Schild JA, Weprin TC: Pediatric Laryngology. Otolaryngol Clin North Am 3:625, 1970.
13. Jackson C, Jackson CL: Diseases of the Air and Food Passages of Foreign Body Origin. Philadelphia, WB Saunders, 1936.
14. Mair EA, Parsons DS, Bolger WE: Middle Meatal Splints in Pediatric Functional Endoscopic Sinus Surgery. Presented at American Academy of Otolaryngology–Head and Neck Surgery, Kansas City, MO, Sept 1991.
15. Marsh BR, Ravich WJ: Laryngoscopy, bronchoscopy and esophagoscopy. In Johns ME: Complications in Otolaryngology–Head and Neck Surgery. Philadelphia, BC Decker, 1986.
16. Moses FM, Peura DA, et al: Palliative dilations of esophageal carcinoma. Gastrointest Endosc 31:61, 1985.
17. Norton JD, Manhala G: Atlanto-axial instability revisited: An alert for endoscopists. Ann Oto Rhino Laryngol 91:567, 1982.
18. Palmer ED, Wirts CW: Survey of gastroscopic and esophagoscopic accidents: Report of Committee of Accidents of the American Gastroscopic Society. JAMA 164:2012, 1957.
19. Patterson DJ, Graham DY, Smith JL, et al: Natural history of benign esophageal stricture treated by dilatation. Gastroenterology 85:346, 1983.
20. Peterson RJ: Sucralfate and nasal synechiae. Ear Nose Throat J 69:660, 1990.
21. Slim MS, Yacoubian HD: Complications of foreign bodies in the tracheobronchial tree. Arch Surg 92:388, 1966.
22. Stankiewicz JA: Complications of endoscopic nasal surgery: Occurrence and treatment. Am J Rhinol 1:45, 1987.
23. Tucker GF Jr, Tucker JA: Complications of endoscopic procedures. In Conley JJ: Complications in Head and Neck Surgery. Philadelphia, WB Saunders, 1979.

CHAPTER 21

Complications of Chemotherapy

KIN LAM, MD
GREGORY J. SHYPULA, MD
A. PHILIPPE CHAHINIAN, MD

Systemic chemotherapy is now accepted as the standard treatment in recurrent or metastatic cancer of the head and neck. It is also being used with increased frequency in patients with previously untreated, locally advanced head and neck cancer. Trials are being conducted for evaluation of combined therapy (chemotherapy plus radiation therapy, chemotherapy plus surgery and radiation therapy), as well as primary neoadjuvant chemotherapy in these types of neoplasms. More active chemotherapeutic agents are being introduced, and new drug combinations replace old ones. The most commonly used single agents for head and neck cancer are methotrexate, bleomycin, cisplatinum, and 5-fluorouracil (5-FU). Others include mitomycin C, nitrosoureas, cyclophosphamide, doxorubicin, and vinca alkaloids. Most regimens use combinations of drugs.[1] Toxicity can be a significant cause of morbidity in patients with head and neck cancer malig-

nancies. These toxic reactions are frequently dose limiting, therefore one must be familiar with the spectrum of toxicity.

Clinical toxicology discovered new insights into the mechanisms of these adverse reactions and allowed development of techniques preventing them or diminishing their severity.

Toxicity related to chemotherapy is classified according to temporal occurrence: immediate, early, delayed, and late. Guidelines have been developed under the auspices of the World Health Organization for grading acute and subacute toxicity.[2] Frequently the major classes of toxicity are described listing the affected organ systems; which classification is used in this chapter.

HYPERSENSITIVITY

Some chemotherapeutic agents are capable of causing allergic reactions that may be serious and occasionally life-threatening. Hypersensitivity reactions range from Class I to IV, according to Gell and Coombs.[3]

The incidence of allergic reaction to cisplatin ranges from 1 per cent to 20 per cent.[4] They are mostly type I reactions, and they usually resolve with antihistamines and glucocorticoids. Patients who had reactions to previous cisplatin therapy may be able to receive further cisplatin administrations if premedication with antihistamine and corticosteroids is given. Hemolytic anemia secondary to cisplatin, a type II reaction, also has been described.[5] A positive direct Coombs' test is present.

In rare instances, severe allergic or anaphylactic reactions have been reported with the use of bleomycin. Bleomycin causes febrile reactions in 20 per cent to 25 per cent of patients treated. They appear to result from direct pyrogen release from leukocytes. A test dose of bleomycin prior to prescribing a therapeutic dose is recommended.

Type I reactions occasionally may occur with methotrexate, but they are severe only in high-dose administration.

Proper precautions should be taken when administering the antineoplastic agents. The medication should always be given by trained personnel and baseline vital signs should be obtained and monitored. Emergency equipment and medications should be available. In case of severe reaction, the infusion should be terminated immediately. Epinephrine administration is indicated for wheezing, laryngeal edema, and hypotension. Aminophylline is useful to relieve bronchospasm. For mild allergic reactions, such as urticaria, antihistamines can be given.

DRUG EXTRAVASATION

Extravasation of chemotherapy can cause pain, necrosis, and sloughing of tissue. Severe damage to nerves, tendons, and muscles can occur, especially in the dorsum of the hand and in the groin.

Antineoplastic agents that can cause severe tissue necrosis include doxorubicin, vincris-

tine, and vinblastine. Careful techniques can reduce the risk of extravasation:

1. A free-flowing intravenous line should be used.
2. The patency of the IV line should be verified by aspirating blood return or injecting normal saline before drug administration.
3. The dorsum of the hand and the antecubital fossa should be avoided as a site of injection, if possible.
4. The vesicant should be administered by a slow push. Continuous infusion should be administered through a central line.
5. Injection should be stopped if the patient complains of pain or burning at the infusion site.

Even with the most careful techniques, extravasation can occur. The site should be treated with an antidote if appropriate. Cold compresses may be used. If there is persistent pain or necrosis of skin, a plastic surgeon should be consulted.

ALOPECIA

Many chemotherapeutic agents can act on the rapidly dividing cells of the hair follicles (Table 21–1). Doxorubicin and cyclophosphamide are notoriously toxic to the hair follicles.[6, 7] Other agents include methotrexate, 5-FU and bleomycin. Leucovorin rescue in high-dose methotrexate can prevent alo-

TABLE 21–1. Alopecia from Chemotherapeutic Agents Used in Head and Neck Cancer

Bleomycin	Common
BCNU	Unusual
CCNU	Unusual
Cis-diamminedi-chloro-platinum	Unusual
Cyclophosphamide	Very frequent
Doxorubicin	Very frequent
5-Fluorouracil	Common
Methotrexate	Common
Mitomycin-C	Unusual
Vincristine	Common
Vinblastine	Occasional

pecia.[8] Scalp hypothermia—application of crushed ice in plastic bags for 10 minutes before and 20 minutes after administration of the drug—is frequently employed to minimize alopecia. This technique should not be used when tumor cells may be present in the scalp.

SKIN PIGMENTATION

Methotrexate and 5-FU can induce photosensitivity reactions, which may leave residual tanning.

Fluorouracil may cause a peculiar pigmentation over the veins into which the drug is given, termed *serpentine supravenous fluorouracil hyperpigmentation* (Fig. 21–1). The veins underlying the pigment remain patent and nonsclerosed. 5-FU may cause onycholysis and pigmentation of nails.[9]

Palmar-plantar erythrodysesthesia (the hand-foot syndrome) may be seen with use of 5-FU.[10] This reversible syndrome is uniquely associated with protracted infusion of 5-FU. It is never life-threatening and may require brief interruption of the infusion.

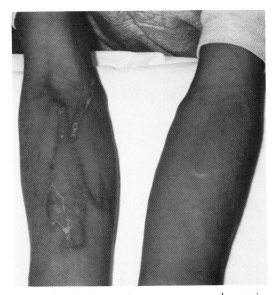

FIGURE 21–1. Serpentine supravenous hyperpigmentation of the veins of the right arm 3 weeks after one course of continuous, 24-hr infusion of fluorouracil for 5 days.

Cisplatin can produce a whitish line on the gingival mucosa similar to the blue-gray line in lead poisoning.

Bleomycin may cause pigmented banding of the nail.[11]

CARDIOTOXICITY

Antineoplastic agents can produce a number of cardiotoxic complications. These agents include doxorubicin, high-dose cyclophosphamide and fluorouracil (5-FU).

The cardiac lesions from doxorubicin may be caused by the formation of free radicals from cell membrane lipids, but the actual cause is unknown. Cardiotoxicity may manifest itself by acute effects with electrocardiographic abnormalities or a cumulative dose-dependent cardiomyopathy. The electrocardiographic abnormalities that have been described are nonspecific ST-T wave changes, sinus tachycardia, and premature ventricular and atrial beats. They appear to be reversible and transient. Their occurrence is usually not an indication to discontinue doxorubicin therapy. However, sudden death possibly due to doxorubicin-induced arrhythmia has been reported.[12] Low voltage of QRS in the electrocardiogram may be irreversible and may be related to the total dose of doxorubicin.[13] Rarely an acute syndrome of myopericarditis may also occur, which is often fatal.[14]

The second major form of cardiac toxicity by doxorubicin is delayed congestive heart failure. The histologic changes are characterized by fragmentation and dropout of myofibrils, mitochondrial swelling, and intracellular inclusions. The frequency of doxorubicin-induced cardiomyopathy ranges from 0.4 per cent to 9 per cent.[15, 16] The mortality from cardiomyopathy may be as high as 61 per cent. Cardiac complication may be prevented by limiting the total cumulative dose of doxorubicin to 450 mg per square meter. Serial measurement of left ventricular ejection fraction by radionuclide angiography scan is recommended. The drug should be discontinued if there is a fall greater than 15 per cent of cardiac ejection fraction from baseline values. Concomitant irradiation should be avoided.

Factors that may increase the risk of cardiotoxicity by doxorubicin and cause clinical problems at a lower total cumulative dosage are increasing age of the patient, concurrent administration of cyclophosphamide, and the existence of pre-existing cardiac diseases and radiation. A low-dose weekly schedule may prevent or decrease cardiotoxicity.[17] Although cardiotoxicity from doxorubicin appears to be irreversible, the associated congestive heart failure responds to digitalization and other standard treatment.

Fluorouracil may cause angina episodes and ECG changes with ST-segment deviation suggestive of ischemia.[18] Sudden death also has been reported, but its occurrence is very rare. The cardiotoxicity of 5-FU is probably secondary to coronary artery spasm.

PULMONARY TOXICITY

Pulmonary toxicity, usually in the form of fibrosis, has been associated with a number of chemotherapeutic agents. Bleomycin[19] and nitrosoureas[20] are the common agents that cause pulmonary toxicity. The histologic changes in the lung induced by these drugs are strikingly uniform. There is a marked decrease in Type I pneumocytes seen by electron microscopy, and the Type II pneumocytes proliferate and migrate into the pulmonary alveolar sacs with resulting thickened alveolar septa.

Symptoms of bleomycin pulmonary toxicity include dry cough, exertional dyspnea, orthopnea, fever, and cyanosis. Symptoms may occur as long as 1 to 3 months after discontinuance. Physical signs include fine bibasilar rales, rhonchi, and pleural rub.

Arterial blood gases show hypoxemia and hypocapnia when significant bleomycin toxicity develops. Radiographic manifestations include reticular infiltrates, lobar consolidation, and progressive pulmonary involvement.

Serial measurement of the diffusion capacity (DLCO) is helpful to detect early subclinical pulmonary toxicity.[21] Bleomycin therapy should be withheld if the DLCO falls to less than 40 per cent of the initial value or the FVC falls to less than 25 per cent of the initial value. Clinical evaluation, including symptoms, physical examination, and radiologic evidence, is also important to make an early diagnosis; therapy should be discontinued if there is a suspicion of bleomycin-induced pulmonary toxicity.

The incidence of nonlethal pulmonary fibrosis is 2 per cent to 3 per cent, whereas fatal bleomycin pulmonary toxicity occurs in 1 per cent to 2 per cent of patients. The incidence of bleomycin pulmonary toxicity increases significantly at cumulative doses of greater than 500 units. Other risk factors include patients over age 75 years, prior or concomitant chest radiotherapy, pre-existing pulmonary disease, and high-dose oxygen during anesthesia. The mortality from bleomycin pulmonary toxicity is 50 per cent. However, most patients with minimal radiologic changes or pulmonary function abnormalities will not progress to respiratory failure if bleomycin is stopped early. Intramuscular injection of bleomycin may decrease the incidence of overall pulmonary toxicity.[22]

Although steroid treatment such as prednisone has been suggested, there is no known effective treatment when bleomycin-pneumonitis progresses to pulmonary fibrosis. Bleomycin also can cause a hypersensitivity type of reaction with fever, pulmonary infiltrates, and eosinophilia. It responds favorably to prednisone administration.[23]

The predominant clinical features of BCNU-induced pulmonary toxicity are dyspnea and dry cough. As with bleomycin, the most effective way to manage BCNU pulmonary toxicity is to prevent it. Serial pulmonary function tests should be monitored.

Mitomycin also causes pulmonary toxicity in 5 per cent to 12 per cent of patients who receive the medication.[24] It causes dyspnea and unproductive cough. Chest radiograph is either normal or shows a fine, reticulonodular pattern. Symptoms and signs of disease resolve promptly (within weeks) after discontinuance of the drug and steroid therapy.

Methotrexate may have a direct toxicity in the lung, with alveolar and interstitial inflammation, and may assume a semigranulomatous configuration.[24] Affected patients often have malaise, dyspnea, and dry cough. Bilateral diffuse patchy infiltrates are seen on chest film. Toxicity usually resolves after discontinuation of methotrexate. Steroids may speed recovery, but leucovorin offers no protection.

The differential diagnosis of diffuse interstitial pneumonitis in a patient receiving antineoplastic drugs may include infection, drug-induced pulmonary toxicity, tumor involvement, and radiation injury. Sometimes an open lung biopsy is required to establish the correct etiology.

Physicians should be aware of the potential pulmonary toxicity and its associated clinical features. Early detection is the most important measure to prevent the development of fatal pulmonary fibrosis by prompt discontinuation of the offending agent.

NEUROTOXICITY

Neurologic impairment in cancer patients has diverse etiologies. The symptoms and signs may be attributable to the neoplastic disease process itself through involvement of the brain, peripheral nervous system, or meninges; metabolic or electrolyte imbalances (hypercalcemia, hyponatremia, hypo- or hyperkalemia); nutritional deficiencies; infectious complications; paraneoplastic syndromes; or drug toxicity.

NEUROPATHY

Peripheral. With the use of vigorous saline diuresis and other maneuvers, the incidence of nephrotoxicity secondary to cisplatin has decreased, and polyneuropathy has become the dose-limiting side effect.[25] Forty-five to one hundred per cent of patients will develop sensory impairment, predominantly in the upper and lower extremities, often in a stock-ing and glove distribution. Neurologic signs include loss of tendon reflexes and decrease in vibration perception and fine touch perception. Motor impairment is usually absent. Sensations of pain and temperature are well preserved. Cisplatin seem to affect large sensory fibers. Toxicity is dose-dependent, and it appears when total cumulative doses of 300 to 600 mg per square meter are reached. The neuropathy may be slowly reversible, and recovery may take a year. An adrenocorticotropic hormone analogue, Org 2766, recently has been used to prevent or delay cisplatin-induced neuropathy.[25] The results show that Org 2766 may exert a beneficial effect over neurotoxicity and does not adversely affect the cytotoxic effect of cisplatin. Another agent, ethiofos (WR-2721), is reported to have a potential protective effect against cisplatin neurotoxicity.

Vincristine affects large and small motor and sensory axons by impairing the axoplasmic transport. Peripheral neuropathy is asymptomatic in many patients. Sensory impairment includes paresthesias of extremities, loss of Achilles tendon reflex, gait disturbances, and muscle motor deficit, which may present as foot drop, or wrist drop. Paresthesia will disappear in a few weeks if vincristine is discontinued early. Recovery of motor weakness may take months and may be incomplete.

Autonomic. Vinblastine or vincristine can cause reversible paralytic ileus, urinary bladder atony, and orthostatic hypotension.

Cranial Nerve. Cisplatin-induced retrobulbar neuritis has been reported, and patients may have papilledema and increased intracranial pressure. Optic neuropathy and atrophy are rare but have been described with vincristine. Vincristine also can cause bilateral recurrent laryngeal nerve involvement with vocal cord paralysis.[26] Severe jaw pain may occur within a few hours after a first dose of vincristine or vinblastine. However, it is transient and does not recur with subsequent doses.

OTOTOXICITY

Cisplatin is known to cause ototoxicity. Tinnitus may occur in 9 per cent of patients treated and is usually reversible. Six per cent of patients may suffer symptomatic hearing loss. Twenty-four per cent of patients may have high-frequency pure tone hearing loss detected by audiogram, which may be irreversible. The mechanism of cisplatin ototoxicity is a progressive destruction of the outer hair cells of the organ of Corti. The only effective way to attenuate the ototoxicity is to limit the single and total cumulative dosages. At present, a baseline audiogram is recommended, but serial measurement are not indicated for asymptomatic patients.[27] If normal hearing is impaired, an audiogram should be obtained and further use of cisplatin evaluated. Ototoxicity is very rare with carboplatin.

CENTRAL NERVOUS SYSTEM

Ifosfamide can cause central nervous system (CNS) toxicity with somnolence, a reduced level of arousal, coma, and even death. Other CNS symptoms include confusion, incontinence, and seizures. The CNS toxicity usually starts within 2 hours of the bolus dose but will subside within 1 to 3 days after stopping ifosfamide. The only treatment available is discontinuation of the medication.

Intrathecal methotrexate can cause arachnoiditis, encephalopathy, somnolence, and cerebral atrophy. Methotrexate neurotoxicity may be decreased by reducing the dosage of chemotherapy. It can be achieved by administering the drug via an Ommaya reservoir.

HEMATOLOGIC TOXICITY

BONE MARROW

Bone marrow toxicity is the most frequent and the most important toxicity of the majority of anticancer agents. It is the bone marrow suppression that requires dose limitation. Leukopenia-related sepsis and bleeding secondary to thrombocytopenia are potentially lethal.

The bone marrow is the organ containing stem cell precursors for all blood components, red cells, white cells, and platelets. Hematopoietic elements as well as gastrointestinal epithelium are fast-growing tissues, and according to the principles introduced by Skipper and his colleagues,[28] chemotherapy is most active in tissues with high growth fraction. Hence, bone marrow precursor cells are the primary target for anticancer agents.

The kinetics of the particular cell line affected by a drug determines the severity of the depression of the given cell line. The development of leukopenia is much faster than that of anemia because of the tremendous difference in the half-lives of red and white blood cells.[29] Platelets with their half-life of 5 to 7 days fall between red and white cells. The time and severity of the bone marrow suppression depend also on the type of chemotherapeutic agent. Phase-specific agents, such as methotrexate or 5-FU, produce rapidly reversible bone marrow suppression.[30] Cycle-specific drugs, such as cyclophosphamide, present an intermediate pattern, and noncycle-specific chemotherapy agents or those acting on G zero phase, as for example nitrogen mustard, can cause delayed but also most protracted cytopenias.

The degree of cytopenia induced by a particular agent also will be affected by factors such as the degree of bone marrow cellularity, being more severe in patients with low marrow reserve than in those with normal cellularity. The nutritional status of the patient influences susceptibility of the bone marrow (the greater the negative nitrogen balance, the less tolerance).[31] Previous therapy always should be considered, since patients heavily pretreated with chemotherapy or radiation therapy will tolerate chemotherapy poorly.

Some drugs affect certain cell lines more selectively. Cyclophosphamide and ifosfamide traditionally have been considered as platelet-sparing agents. The impression conveyed by some reports may be artifactual, however, since the limit often used to define leukopenia (less than 4000 cells per cubic millimeter) may represent a smaller proportional reduction than in the case of thrombocytopenia with a limit of less than 100,000 per cubic millimeter.

Nitrosoureas are reported to produce severe late thrombocytopenia 4 to 6 weeks after administration of the agent.[32] Thrombocytopenia can occur even after recovery from leukopenia. Changes in schedule, such as a lower dose given more frequently, can decrease this side effect.

Few agents used in cancer treatment do not cause bone marrow toxicity. Several agents, however, such as cisplatin, vincristine and bleomycin in doses used clinically, generally do not cause bone marrow suppression. Exceptions to this may be situations when malfunction of the organ excreting the drug causes accumulation of the drug or its metabolites, such as cisplatin and renal failure, or cyclophosphamide and liver disease. It is important to mention the cisplatin analogue carboplatin, which shares a similar mechanism of action and to a certain point shares its activity. However, these drugs have quite different toxicities. Carboplatin is a myelosuppressive agent, especially for platelets, and its myelosuppressive action can be exacerbated in renal insufficiency since it is being excreted by the kidney.[33]

Although stem cells and red cell precursors are also affected by chemotherapeutic agents, anemia is usually not a significant problem.[34] The long half-life of red cells (120 days) makes a decrease in hematocrit less apparent. Nevertheless changes in the red cell line do occur and sometimes may be striking. The most frequent offenders are folic acid antagonists as well as purine and pyrimidine analogues.[35] Because these agents are cell cycle–nonspecific in inhibiting production of DNA, the nuclear development lags behind cytoplasmic maturation. This results in megaloblastic changes identical to those seen in vitamin B_{12} or folate deficiency. Levels of these two vitamins, however, are unaffected in such cases. Megaloblastic changes in bone marrow characterize patients treated with antimetabolites like methotrexate.[36]

Alkylating agents and cisplatin also can suppress red cell production. Anemia has been reported in up to 40 per cent of patients receiving cisplatin therapy.[37]

Hemolytic anemia has been described in association with several chemotherapeutic agents.[38] Cisplatin can be adsorbed to the red cell surface, and antibodies to cisplatin can mediate the destruction of the red blood cells.[39] Some cytotoxic drugs can destroy red cells by an oxidative mechanism. Doxorubicin, for example, can generate reactive oxygen compounds and cause oxidative hemolysis in patients with glucose-6-phosphate deficiency.[40]

HEMOSTASIS

A fairly frequent cause of morbidity in patients receiving chemotherapy for their head and neck tumors is altered coagulation.

Thrombocytopenia with subsequent bleeding episodes, described earlier, is secondary to myelotoxicity. Qualitative platelet abnormalities were encountered by Ahr and colleagues, who detected decreased platelet response to adenosine diphosphate (ADP), collagen, or epinephrine in patients treated with mithramycin.[41] Some of these patients developed bleeding diathesis despite lack of thrombocytopenia. Mithramycin also was associated with depression of clotting factors II, V, VII, and X. Some of these abnormalities may be explained by hepatic toxicity induced by mithramycin.

Increased circulating fibrinopeptide A levels can be caused by several anticancer agents. The most frequent offenders are 5-FU, vincristine, doxorubicin, and etoposide. The increase in fibrinopeptide levels was abolished by treatment with heparin.[42] This suggests activation of coagulation by certain chemotherapeutic agents. Thrombotic microangiopathic anemia was reported with a regimen containing cisplatin, bleomycin, and vinca alkaloids.[43] Vincristine is well known to elevate platelet counts. The mechanism is thought to be an inhibition of megakaryocytic endocytosis with compensatory stimulation of platelet production.[44, 45] The syndrome of microangiopathic hemolytic anemia, thrombocytopenia, renal failure, and pulmonary edema has been described in patients treated with mitomycin C.[46, 47] Chemotherapeutic regimens that included cyclophosphamide, methotrexate, and 5-FU (CMF) were reported to cause decreases in plasma protein C and protein S levels and lead to an increase in thrombotic events in patients with breast cancer.[48]

Indwelling catheters are a frequent source of venous thrombosis, and cancer patients on chemotherapy frequently experience this type of complication, as described by Haire and colleagues.[49]

PREVENTION AND TREATMENT OF HEMATOLOGIC COMPLICATIONS OF CHEMOTHERAPY

A new era has begun with the discovery and purification of colony-stimulating factors (CSF), a class of glycoprotein hormones that regulate production and function of blood cells.[50, 51] Several colony-stimulating factors were discovered and then molecularly cloned by recombinant technology: granulocyte macrophage colony-stimulating factor (GM-CSF), granulocyte colony-stimulating factor (G-CSF), macrophage colony-stimulating factor (M-CSF), and interleukin-3. The red cell growth hormone erythropoietin was also purified and approved for clinical use.[52]

The colony-stimulating factors increase production of granulocytes and monocytes by stimulating stem cell and precursor cell replication and maturation. Their precise level of action is still uncertain. They exert their biologic action by acting on specific cell surface receptors. GM-CSF receptors appear on neutrophils, eosinophils, and monocytes. The interleukin-3 receptor is expressed on monocytes, basophils, and eosinophils but not on neutrophils.

Growth factors not only stimulate proliferation and growth of precursors but also enhance neutrophil function by membrane changes, as well as having an indirect influence on oxidative mechanism.[53]

Several trials proved that colony-stimulating factors are useful in treatment of chemotherapy-induced cytopenias. Protection from the hematologic toxicity of cyclophosphamide with agent WR-2721 (ethyl phosphorothioic acid) was reported by Glover and associates.[54] These factors likely will become standard protection therapy in patients treated with chemotherapeutic agents. This should allow higher cytotoxic doses with better control of malignant tumors.[55]

Prompt recognition and treatment of chemotherapy-induced cytopenias can greatly reduce the morbidity and mortality of this complication.[56] Obtaining regular blood counts after chemotherapy to determine nadir values also can help determine the optimal dose of chemotherapy for a given patient. Rapid institution of treatment (vigorous antibiotic therapy for "nadir sepsis," blood transfusion, platelet transfusion) is mandatory for such complications.

GASTROINTESTINAL TOXICITY OF CHEMOTHERAPEUTIC AGENTS

MUCOSITIS

Gastrointestinal side effects of chemotherapeutic agents are frequent. At times they may be severe and dose-limiting.

The susceptibility of the gastrointestinal system is explained by the rapid proliferation of its epithelium, similar to that of bone marrow elements and the reproductive system. The fastest-dividing cells of the mucosa lining the gastrointestinal tract are the undifferentiated and goblet cells of the small intestine, which form the majority of the crypts. The resulting effect of chemotherapy is mucositis, including stomatitis, cheilosis, glossitis, esophagitis, and diarrhea associated with colitis or enteritis. Drugs most commonly causing mucositis are methotrexate, 5-FU, vinca alkaloids, and doxorubicin. The toxicity of the drug appears to depend on the duration of the exposure rather than on the peak levels achieved, as is the case for methotrexate.[57]

Prior or concurrent irradiation increases the risk, especially when using chemotherapeutic agents known for their "recall" reaction, such as doxorubicin

Scheduling and mode of administration (continuous infusion versus intermittent bolus) also was proved to affect the severity of the gastrointestinal reaction. Doxorubicin was shown to cause more severe stomatitis when given as a prolonged infusion compared with intermittent bolus therapy. 5-Fluorouracil is well known for its gastrointestinal toxicity. It causes diarrhea, stomatitis, and esophagitis.[58] These effects are also increased when given by continuous IV infusion, whereas an IV bolus schedule is more marrow-toxic.

Malabsorption in association with chemotherapy has been described. Xylose malabsorption in patients receiving methotrexate was reported. Shaw and associates reported villous blunting, swelling, dilatation of mitochondria and endoplasmic reticulum, and shortening of microvilli.[59] Malignant neoplasms are frequently associated with weight loss and nutritional dificiency. The reasons range from anatomic, as in head and neck cancer, to metabolic. Antineoplastic therapy additionally may exacerbate the already poor nutritional and metabolic status of patients with cancer. Anorexia, vomiting, and nausea further complicate this problem and are discussed later.

Nutritional complications (hypoproteinemia, thiamine deficiency) are frequently experienced. Alcoholic patients with head and neck cancer often have liver disease and poor nutrition with hypovitaminosis. As a result, tolerance of chemotherapy can be poor; such patients may not even qualify for treatment.

Nutritional support is particularly crucial in patients with head and neck cancer.

NAUSEA AND VOMITING

The most frequent nonhematologic toxicity, and one of the most disturbing as well, is chemotherapy-induced nausea and emesis. Often used agents in head and neck neoplasms, such as cisplatin, particularly doxorubicin, and even 5-FU, are well known for their emetogenic effects. The physiology of emesis is still not completely understood. The vomiting control centers are in two topographically and functionally distinct units of the medulla oblongata: the emetic center and the chemoreceptor trigger zone. The emetic center is the final control pathway that mediates all vomiting, and it is located

in the lateral reticular formation. It is activated by electrical stimuli. The chemoreceptor trigger zone is located in the area postrema and is accessible both from blood and cerebrospinal fluid. It appears to be activated by chemical stimuli only. In addition to chemoreceptor trigger zone input from the vestibular apparatus, the peripheral (gastrointestinal tract), cortex, and higher brain stem can induce emesis through the emetic center. A multiafferent neuroreflex arc is thus formed with several pathways.

The humoral pathway consists of chemical mediators affecting the chemoreceptor trigger zone. Activation of peripheral nerve endings in the gastrointestinal tract stimulates the peripheral pathway. Higher parts of the brain stimulated by odors, sights, and memory form a cerebral cortical pathway. Different chemotherapeutic agents act on different emetogenic centers through different neuroreflex arc pathways. One of the most potent emetogenic drugs, mechlorethamine (nitrogen mustard), appears to induce vomiting through the chemoreceptor trigger zone, whereas cisplatin with its poor blood-brain barrier penetration appears to act through a peripheral mechanism. Quite frequent (74 per cent in some reports), yet unexplained, is delayed emesis in patients treated with high doses of cisplatin.[60]

Several agents are in use to prevent and treat chemotherapy-associated nausea and vomiting. Antihistamines, anticholinergics, phenothiazines, butyrophenones, and cannabinoids have been used.[61] The discovery of dopamine receptors in the chemoreceptor trigger zone and gastrointestinal tract led to introduction of metoclopramide, a procainamide derivative and antidopaminergic agent. Metoclopramide, often in combination with phenothiazines, lorazepam, and/or steroids, was highly effective in prevention and treatment of chemotherapy-induced nausea and vomiting. The mechanism behind steroid usefulness in prevention of chemotherapy-induced nausea and vomiting is still not elucidated.

More recently a serotonin receptor (5'HT3) was discovered in the chemoreceptor trigger zone and within the gastrointestinal tract.

The serotonin receptor was proved to mediate the emetic reflex. Metoclopramide is also known to act as a serotonin antagonist in high doses. This causes frequent extrapyramidal side effects, especially in younger patients. A newly developed antiemetic agent, ondansetron, a highly selective 5-hydroxy-4-tryptamine receptor antagonist, proved to be significantly more effective than metoclopromide in preventing acute nausea and vomiting. However, it was inferior to metoclopromide in treatment of delayed emesis.[62, 63]

Vinca alkaloids and especially vincristine were associated with an interesting syndrome of vomiting and constipation. Neurotoxicity to autonomic nerves within the gastrointestinal tract causes paralytic ileus and gastric distention. Metoclopromide appears to be useful in this syndrome as well.

HEPATOTOXICITY

The liver plays a central role in drug metabolism. Several chemotherapeutic agents are excreted by the liver; others, even though cleared by other mechanisms, undergo hepatic transformation. Liver injury has been described during and after the course of several therapeutic drugs. Elevation of serum transaminase, alkaline phosphatase, and bilirubin levels was induced by nitrosoureas. Methotrexate was proved to cause liver damage.[30] In 1972, Vestfrid and associates described a fatal case of 5-FU-induced hepatitis,[68] and Sotaniemi and colleagues reported an association of hepatotoxicity with exposure to bleomycin, vincristine, cyclophosphamide (Cytoxan), doxorubicin (Adriamycin), dacarbazine, 5-FU, and methotrexate.[69]

It is important that in patients with pre-existing hepatic disease different agents should be considered or the dose of the drug should be modified according to results of a liver function test and bilirubin study, as is done with doxorubicin or vinca alkaloids.

RENAL TOXICITY

Renal failure and associated metabolic and electrolyte disturbances may develop in patients receiving cancer treatment.

Injury to renal tissue may be due to release of intracellular ions and especially urate after the destruction of a large amount of cells—the so-called tumor lysis syndrome—occurring most often in hematologic and small cell cancers. Pretreatment with allopurinol and good hydration prevent hyperuricemia in most instances.

Solid tumors, such as those of head and neck cancer, rarely if ever are associated with the tumor lysis syndrome. However, one must anticipate nephrotoxicity due to the antitumor agents. Cisplatin nephrotoxicity has proved to be dose-limiting. Lower doses of 50 mg per square meter can cause azotemia, which is usually reversible. More severe and irreversible renal damage follows higher doses. Patients with pre-existing renal disease are at increased risk for renal failure when taking cisplatin. The mechanism of the toxicity is ascribed to renal tubular necrosis, found in damaged kidneys of patients treated with cisplatin.

Of great concern is the syndrome of magnesium wasting occurring in association with cisplatin therapy.[64] Life-threatening hypomagnesemia and secondary hypocalcemia and tetany occur. Patients who are to receive cisplatin chemotherapy for their tumors should have determinations of 24-hour creatinine clearance and magnesium levels before treatment. Vigorous saline hydration decreases the risk of renal toxicity. Renal function and magnesium levels should be followed throughout and after the treatment.

Renal excretion is the primary route of elimination of methotrexate. Therapy with this drug, especially when higher doses (50 to 250 mg/kg) are applied, resulted in renal failure in some patients.[65] Renal injury is due to precipitation of the drug within the renal tubular and collecting systems.

Cyclophosphamide and vincristine were found to cause hyponatremia, and sodium-wasting was described in some patients treated with these agents.[66, 67]

Other chemotherapeutic drugs, such as streptozotocin, nitrosoureas, and mithramycin, were also found to cause injury to the kidney.

Careful monitoring of renal function, appropriate hydration, and aggressive treatment if nephrotoxicity occurs is required for safe administration of all cancer chemotherapy.

References

1. Al-Sarraf M: Head and neck cancer: Chemotherapy concepts. Semin Oncol 15:70–85, 1988.
2. Miler AB, Hoogstrate B, Staquet M, Winkler A: Reporting results of cancer treatment. Cancer 47:207–214, 1981.
3. Gell PGH, Coombs RRA: Clinical Aspects of Immunology. Oxford, Blackwell Scientific Publications, 1975.
4. Weiss RB, Bruno S: Hypersensitivity reactions to cancer therapeutic agents. Ann Intern Med 94:66–72, 1981.
5. Getaz EP, Beckley S, Fitzpatrick J, et al: Cis-platin-induced hemolysis. N Engl J Med 302:334–335, 1980.
6. Dean JC, Salmon SE, Griffith KS: Prevention of doxorubicin-induced hair loss with scalp hypothermia. N Engl J Med 301:1427–1429, 1979.
7. Jessen RT, Straight M, Smith EB: Cutaneous and other complications of cyclophosphamide: A brief review. Rocky Mount Med J 75:204–206, 1978.
8. Cadman E: Toxicity of chemotherapeutic agents. In Becker FF: Cancer: A Comprehensive Treatise. Vol 5. New York, Plenum Press, 1977, pp 59–111.
9. Katz ME, Hansen TW: A nail plate–nail bed separation: An unusual side effect of systemic fluorouracil administration. Arch Dermatol 115:860–861, 1979.
10. Lokich JJ, Ahlgren JD: A prospective randomized comparison of continuous infusion fluorouracil with a bolus schedule in metastatic colorectal carcinoma. J Clin Oncol 7:425–432, 1989.
11. Shetty MR: Case of pigmented banding of the nail caused by bleomycin. Cancer Treat Rep 61:501–502, 1977.
12. Worthman JR, Lucas VS, Schuster E, et al: Sudden death during doxorubicin administration. Cancer 44:1588–1591, 1979.
13. Minow RA, Benjamin RS, Lee ET, et al: QRS voltage change with Adriamycin administration. Cancer Treat Rep 62:931–934, 1978.
14. Bristow MR, Thompson PD, Martin RP, et al: Early anthracycline cardiotoxicity. Am J Med 65:823–832, 1978.
15. Blum RH, Carter SK: Adriamycin, a new anticancer drug with significant clinical activity. Ann Intern Med 80:249–259, 1974.
16. Von Hoff DD, Layard MW, Basa P, et al: Risk factors for doxorubicin-induced congestive heart failure. Ann Intern Med 91:710–717, 1979.
17. Chlebowski R, Pugh R, Parohy W, et al: Adriamycin on a weekly schedule: Clinically effective with low incidence of cardiotoxicity. Clin Res 27:53A, 1979.
18. Rezkalla S, Kloner RA, Enslen J: Continuous ambulatory ECG monitoring during fluorouracil therapy: A prospective study. J Oncol 7:509–514, 1989.
19. Comis RL: Bleomycin: Pulmonary toxicity. In Crooke ST, Umezawa H (eds): Bleomycin: Current Status and New Developments. New York, Academic Press, 1978, pp 279–291.
20. Aronin PA, Mahaley MS, Rudnick SA, et al: Prediction of BCNU pulmonary toxicity in patients with malignant gliomas. An assessment of risk factor. N Engl J Med 303:183–191, 1980.
21. Comis RL, Kuppinger MS, Ginsberg SJ, et al: Role of single carbon monoxide diffusing capacity in monitoring the pulmonary effects of bleomycin in germ tumor patients. Cancer Res 39:5076–5080, 1979.
22. Haas CD, Coltman CA, Gottlieb AJ, et al: Phase II evaluation of bleomycin. A Southwest Oncology Group Study. Cancer 38:8–12, 1976.
23. Holoye PY, Luna MA, MacKay B, et al: Bleomycin hypersensitivity pneumonitis Ann Intern Med 88:47–49, 1978.
24. Batist G, Andrews JL, Jr: Pulmonary toxicity of antineoplastic drugs. JAMA 246:1449–1453, 1981.
25. Van Der Hoop RG, Vecht CJ, Van Der Burg ME: Prevention of cisplatin neurotoxicity with ACTH (4–9) analogue in patients with ovarian cancer. N Engl J Med 322: 89–94, 1990.
26. Holland JF, Scharlav C, Gailani S, et al: Vincristine treatment of advanced cancer: A cooperative study of 392 cases. Cancer Res 33:1258–1264, 1973.
27. Von Goff DD, Schilsky R, Reichert CM, et al: Toxic effects of cis-dichlorodiammineplatinum (II) in man. Cancer Treat Rep 63:157–1531, 1979.
28. Skipper HE: Biochemical, biological, pharmacologic, toxicologic, kinetic and clinical (subhuman and human) relationships. Cancer 21:600–610, 1968.
29. Israel L, Chiahinian P: Comparative toxicity of leucocytes and platelets of two regimens of CCNU: The relationhip between maximum dose and optimum dose. Eur J Cancer 9:799–802, 1973.
30. Weinstein GD: Methotrexate. Ann Intern Med 86:199–204, 1977.
31. Nixon DW, Heymsfield SB, Cohen AE, et al: Protein-calorie undernutrition in hospitalized cancer patients. Am J Med 68:683–690, 1980.
32. Wasserman TH, Slavik M, Carter SK: Clinical comparison of the nitrosoureas. Cancer 36:1258–1268, 1975.
33. Marsh JC: The effect of cancer therapeutic agents on normal hematopoietic precursor cells: A review. Cancer Res 36:1853–1882, 1976.
34. Doll DC, Weiss RB: Chemotherapeutic agents and erythron. Cancer Treat Rev 10:185–200, 1983.
35. Berlin NI, Rall D, Mead JAR, et al: Folic acid antagonists: Effects on the cell and the patient. Ann Intern Med 59:931–956, 1963.
36. Frei E III, Jaffe N, Tattersall MHN, et al: New approaches to cancer chemotherapy with methotrexate. N Engl J Med 292:846–851, 1975.
37. Von Hoff DD, Schilsky R, Reichert CM, et al: Toxic effects of cis-dichlorodiammineplatinum (II) in man. Cancer Treat Rep 63:1527–1531, 1979.
38. Doll DC, Weiss RB: Hemolytic anemia asociated with antineoplastic agents. Cancer Treat Rep 69:777–782, 1985.
39. Getaz EP, Beckley S, Fitzpatrick J, Dozier A: Cisplatin-induced hemolysis. N Engl J Med 302:334–335, 1980.
40. Henderson CA, Metz EN, Balcerzak SP, Sagone AL

Jr: Adriamycin and daunomycin generate oxygen compounds in erythrocytes. Blood 52:878–885, 1978.

41. Ahr DJ, Scialla SJ, Kimball DB Jr: Acquired platelet dysfunction following mithramycin therapy. Cancer 41:448–454, 1978.

42. Edwards RL, Klaus M, Matthews E, et al: Heparin abolishes the chemotherapy-induced increase in plasma fibrinopeptide A levels. Am J Med 89:25–28, 1990.

43. Jackson AM, Rose BD, Graff LG, et al: Thrombotic microangiopathy and renal failure associated with antineoplastic chemotherapy. Ann Intern Med 101:41–44, 1984.

44. Robertson JH, Crozier EH, Woodend BE: The effect of vincristine on the platelet count in rats. Br J Haematol 19:331–337, 1970.

45. Carbone PP, Bono V, Frei E III, Brindley CO: Clinical studies with vincristine. Blood 21:640–647, 1963.

46. Sheldon R, Slaughter D: A syndrome of microangiopathic hemolytic anemia, renal impairment and pulmonary edema in chemotherapy-treated patients with adenocarcinoma. Cancer 58:1428–1436, 1986.

47. Cantrell Jr JE, Phillips TM, Schein PS: Carcinoma-asociated hemolytic uremic syndrome: A complication of mitomycin C chemotherapy. J Clin Oncol 3:723–734, 1985.

48. Rogers JS II, Murgo AJ, Fontana JA, Raich PC: Chemotherapy for breast cancer decreases plasma protein C and protein S. J Clin Oncol 6:276–281, 1988.

49. Haire WD, Lieberman RP, Edney J, et al: Hickman catheter–induced thoracic vein thrombosis. Cancer 66:900–908, 1990.

50. Gabrilove JL: Introduction and overview of hematopoietic growth factors. Semin Hematol 26(Suppl2):1–4, 1989.

51. Glaspy JA, Golde DW: The colony-stimulating factors: Biology and clinical use. Oncology 4:25–32, 1990.

52. Zanjani ED, Ascensao JL: Erythropoietin. Transfusion 29:46–57, 1989.

53. Gabrilove JL, Jakubowski A, Fain K, et al: Phase I study of granulocyte colony-stimulating factor in patients with transitional cell carcinoma of the urothelium. J Clin Invest 82:1454–1461, 1988.

54. Glover D, Glick JH, Weiler C, et al: WR-2721 protects against the hematologic toxicity of cyclophosphamide: A controlled phase II trial. J Clin Oncol 4:584–588, 1986.

55. Groopman JE, Molina JM, Scadden DT: Hematopoietic growth factors: Biology and clinical applications. N Engl J Med 321:1449–1459, 1989.

56. Herrmann F, Schultz G, Wieser M, et al: Effect of granulocyte-macrophage colony-stimulating factor on neutropenia and related morbidity induced by myelotoxic chemotherapy. Am J Med 88:619–624, 1990.

57. Bleyer WA: The clinical pharmacology of methotrexate. Cancer 41:36–51, 1978.

58. Horton J, Olson KB, Sullivan J, et al: 5-Fluorouracil in cancer. An improved regimen. Ann Intern Med 73:897–900, 1970.

59. Shaw MT, Spector MH, Ladman AJ: Effect of cancer radiotherapy and cytotoxic drugs on intestinal structure and function. Cancer Treat Rev 6:141–151, 1979.

60. Kris MG, Gralla RJ, Clark RA, et al: Incidence, course and severity of delayed nausea and vomiting following the administration of high-dose cisplatin. J Clin Oncol 3:1379–1384, 1985.

61. Seigel LJ, Longo DL: The control of chemotherapy-induced emesis. Ann Intern Med 95:352–359, 1981.

62. Einhorn LH, Nagy C, Werner K, Finn AL: Ondansetron: A new antiemetic for patients receiving cisplatin chemotherapy. J Clin Oncol 8:731–735, 1990.

63. De Mulder PHM, Seynaeve C, Vermorken JB, et al: Ondansetron compared with high dose metoclopramide in prophylaxis of acute and delayed cisplatin-induced nausea and vomiting. Ann Intern Med 113:834–840, 1990.

64. Schilsky RL, Anderson T: Hypomagnesemia and renal magnesium wasting in patients receiving cisplatinum. Ann Intern Med 90:929–931, 1979.

65. Pitman SW, Parker LM, Tattersall MHN, et al: Clinical trial of high dose of methotrexate (NSC 740) with citrovorum factor (NSC3590)—toxicologic and therapeutic observations. Cancer Chemother Rep 6:43–49, 1975.

66. De Fronzo RA, Colvin OM, Braine H, et al: Cyclophosphamide and the kidney. Cancer 33:483–491, 1974.

67. Cutting HO: Inappropriate secretion of antidiuretic hormone secondary to vincristine therapy. Am J Med 51:269–271, 1971.

68. Vestfrid MA, Castelleto L, Gimenez PO: Diffuse liver necrosis in treatment with 5-fluorouracil. Rev Clin Esp 125:549–550, 1972.

69. Sotaniemi EA, Sutinen S, Arranto AJ, et al: Liver damage in nurses handling cytostatic agents. Acta Med Scand 214.181–189, 1983.

Complications of Radiation Therapy

BHADRASAIN VIKRAM, MD

Radiation therapy, like all medical treatments, carries inherent risks. Any living cell can be injured if exposed to ionizing radiation. The injuries can range from trivial to lethal, however, depending upon the dose and the kind of irradiation. A considerable amount of radiation injury can be repaired by individual normal cells. Furthermore, many tissues can compensate for cell loss by repopulation. These factors are taken into account during radiation therapy planning in order to determine the largest dose that can be safely delivered to a cancer. Clearly, some normal tissues are more important than others, and some are even dispensable. For instance, the lens of the eye might develop a cataract with a dose of only a few hundred centigray (cGy or rad), and the lens is frequently sacrificed in order to adequately irradiate a tumor in the periorbital region. On the other hand, extreme care is taken to prevent radiation injury to the optic chiasm, so as not to risk permanent bilateral blindness.

Radiation injury, in clinical practice, is rarely an all-or-none phenomenon. During irradiation, billions of radiation particles (photons, electrons, and so on) interact with billions of molecules in the body. The clinical end result is governed by probability. Occasionally, serious injury might result even at low doses. As the dose increases, the probability of injury increases, but even at high doses not all patients manifest serious injury. Prediction of complications for an individual patient is therefore not possible, but, based upon cumulative experience with similar patients treated by similar techniques in the past, a reasonable prediction of the probability of complications might be made. Whether this probability is regarded as acceptable or prohibitive for an individual patient depends upon:

(1) the danger to life or function from the neoplasm,

(2) the availability of safer treatment alternatives, if any,

(3) the availability of effective treatment

311

for the complication (for example, extraction for cataract, myringotomy for otitis media), and

(4) the understanding by and acceptability to the patient of the risk-benefit ratio.

Several patient factors influence the risk of complications. The ability to repair radiation injury is strongly influenced by the patient's performance status and nutritional status. Poor performance status increases the likelihood of complications. Other factors that increase the risk of complications include pre-existing tissue damage from extensive tumor, infection, surgical procedures, chemotherapy, or prior radiation therapy. Vascular insufficiency due to diabetes, arteriosclerosis, or smoking also increases the likelihood of complications. Certain genetic disorders, such as ataxia-telengiectasia, markedly increase the susceptibility of cells to radiation injury. Similar increases in susceptibility also have been observed recently in patients with the acquired immunodeficiency syndrome (AIDS). In general, however, the influence of the immunologic status on radiation complications, if any, is not clear.

Several treatment-related factors are now also known to influence the likelihood of radiation-related complications. In addition to the actual dose of radiation therapy, the volume of normal tissue exposed to that dose is very important. Clearly, patients often can tolerate and repair injury to a small portion of a normal tissue much better than injury to a larger portion of the same tissue. Efforts to minimize the volume of normal tissue exposed to radiation therapy, by techniques such as multiple fields, shaped beam blocks, brachytherapy, and particle beams, are very worthwhile.

In addition to the total dose and the volume, the rate of delivery of irradiation is now recognized as an important factor. Clinically, radiation reactions are divided into early and late. The former appear during, or shortly after, a course of radiation therapy, whereas the latter might not become manifest until months or years later. Early reactions result from radiation injury to rapidly proliferating tissues (for example, mucous membranes and the bone marrow) with short cell cycle times measured in hours or days. The faster radiation therapy is delivered, the more severe are these reactions. In clinical practice, external radiation therapy is typically delivered at the rate of 200 cGy per day, 5 days per week for several weeks. During this time frame, acute reactions (mucositis, myelosuppression, and so on) generally can be monitored closely, and, if a severe reaction appears to be developing, the rate of delivery of radiation therapy can be decreased or interrupted, to allow repopulation of the depleted stem cell pool in the affected tissues by uninjured stem cells. In theory, such maneuvers also risk repopulation in the neoplasm, but in practice an interruption of a few days, after several weeks of treatment, generally does not appear to affect the therapeutic ratio. Long or frequent interruptions, however, do compromise tumor control and must be avoided.[1, 2]

Late effects result from radiation injury to slowly proliferating or nonproliferating tissues (for example, connective tissues, microvasculature, and nervous tissue) with long cell cycle times measured in months or years. The entire course of radiation therapy is usually over long before such effects appear; therefore, little can be done to alter their severity once they do develop. Late effects can include such serious complications as myelopathy, blindness, and osteonecrosis. The dose delivered to the tumor is frequently limited by the fear of such complications.

An important discovery in recent decades has been the recognition that the fraction size can profoundly influence the incidence and the severity of late complications.[3] For instance, myelopathy rarely results when the spinal cord is irradiated to a dose of 5000 cGy at the rate of 200 cGy per fraction. However, if the fraction size were increased to 800 cGy, myelopathy would frequently result at doses as low as 1600 cGy. To minimize late complications, large fraction sizes are rarely used in contemporary radiation oncology, except in patients for whom the intent of treatment is clearly palliative, and whose life expectancy is so limited that they are not likely to survive long enough to manifest late injury. For most other patients, "conventional" fraction sizes of 180 to 200 cGy each day are utilized. A large body of data is available to the radiation oncologist for estimating the probability of complications when irradiation is delivered to the head and neck region at these fraction sizes.

The realization that fraction sizes larger than the "conventional" 200 cGy can decrease the tolerance of critical late-reacting tissues to radiation therapy has also raised the intriguing possibility that, by employing fraction sizes smaller than 200 cGy, the radiation tolerance of such tissues might be improved, thus permitting delivery of higher total doses to the tumor safely. Too small a daily dose facilitates tumor repopulation, however; therefore, a popular contemporary strategy is to deliver multiple fractions of less than 200 cGy each day, with a 6- to 12-hour interval between fractions to allow cellular repair. Several recent studies suggest that this is indeed a fruitful area for research that might decrease the rate of complications, increase the tumor control rates, or both.[4–6]

SKIN

Skin erythema is commonly observed during radiation therapy after doses of 2000 to 3000 cGy in 2 to 3 weeks. With higher doses pigmentation and dry desquamation are seen. At doses in excess of 4000 cGy in 4 weeks, moist desquamation may be encountered. The latter is uncommonly seen today because megavoltage photon beams used in contemporary practice have a "surface-sparing" property, which means that even when the tumor dose is 6000 to 7000 cGy the skin dose is generally under 4000 cGy. In patients whose skin is infiltrated by cancer, the radiation oncologist might employ techniques such as bolus placement or electron beams, to deliberately increase the dose to the skin; this, of course, will result in moist desquamation.

Temporary loss of hair in the treatment field is a common occurrence after 2000 to 3000 cGy to the skin. At higher doses, alopecia can be permanent. Sometimes alopecia can occur in unexpected places; for instance, a patient receiving radiation therapy to the ethmoid sinuses from a high-energy anterior photon field might develop alopecia in the occipital region because of the exit dose from the anterior beam.

Late effects include atrophic skin, telangiectasia, and ulceration. Ulcers are rarely seen today unless the skin was infiltrated by cancer or large fraction sizes were used.

FIBROSIS AND TRISMUS

Subcutaneous fibrosis is a common late effect after megavoltage radiation therapy. The severity of the fibrosis is worst with large fraction sizes and high total doses. Recent reports suggest that the fibrosis may be decreased if a fraction size smaller than 200 cGy is employed.[4]

Patients who receive radiation therapy to their pterygoid muscles may develop trismus owing to fibrosis of these muscles. This is seen after radical radiation therapy for nasopharyngeal carcinoma, tonsillar carcinoma, soft palate carcinoma, and so on. Jaw exercises should be prescribed for all such patients at the outset to prevent the development of trismus. Once trismus develops, it can be difficult to reverse.

SALIVARY GLANDS

A transient sialadenitis develops in about 10 per cent of patients during the first few days of radiation therapy, often within the first 24 hours, but it subsides within 2 to 3 days. Salivary acinar cells are exquisitely sensitive to radiation therapy. In fact they, along with lymphocytes, are the only kinds of cells in the body known to undergo interphase death at doses of a few hundred centigray.[7] Alteration in the character of saliva is noticed by most patients after 1000 to 2000 cGy have been delivered. Long-term xerostomia is frequently seen in patients who receive doses in excess of 4000 cGy to all the major salivary glands. Chencharick and Mossman observed that xerostomia was present in 20 per cent of patients with head and neck cancer even before any radiation therapy was delivered, however.[8]

It is usually not possible to irradiate the pharynx or the upper jugular nodes without irradiating the submandibular salivary glands. However, parts of the parotid glands and the sublingual glands can and should be shielded during radiation therapy for early-stage disease, and this can considerably reduce the severity of xerostomia that might develop subsequently.

TASTE

Chencharick and Mossman studied the effects of radiation therapy on taste in patients with head and neck cancer and observed that 25 per cent of patients exhibited significant impairment of taste even prior to the start of radiation therapy.[8] After 4 to 5 weeks of irradiation, almost all patients demonstrate diminished taste sensation. Taste sensation returns to normal or near-normal 8 to 12 weeks after completion of radiation therapy in most patients, but approximately 10 per cent suffer long-term impairment.

MUCOUS MEMBRANES

Mucosal surfaces have rapid cell turnover. They manifest erythema after doses of 1000 to 2000 cGy, patchy mucositis with accompanying sore throat or odynophagia after 2000 to 3000 cGy, and confluent mucositis after 3000 to 4000 cGy. Frequent irrigations with a saline and bicarbonate solution are recommended to remove debris and loosen the thick, tenacious mucus. Coexistent infection with *Candida*, bacteria, or the herpes simplex virus might be present and should be treated appropriately. Recently the prophylactic use of triple antibiotics has been reported to be effective in reducing the symptomatology associated with oral and pharyn-

geal mucositis.[9] Trauma to the inflamed mucous membranes should be minimized by a soft diet and by avoiding dentures, smoking, and alcohol.

These acute mucosal reactions usually heal within 2 to 4 weeks after the completion of radiation therapy. In some patients, however, mucosal ulceration or necrosis might develop. This is usually associated with extensive tumor, trauma, and the use of high doses of irradiation or of large fraction sizes. Management includes antibiotics, analgesics, meticulous oral hygiene by irrigations and sprays, avoidance of denture trauma, and a soft diet. Surgical resection of the ulcerated or necrotic area is rarely required, although gentle debridement might help. If the ulcerated area overlies the mandible, bone might be exposed. The risk of osteoradionecrosis is small, however, unless the exposed area is greater than 1 cm across. If the ulcerated or necrotic area overlies the laryngeal cartilages, there is the risk of laryngeal cartilage necrosis. Management is similar to that outlined previously, but a tracheostomy might also be necessary in this instance.

TEETH AND BONES

Teeth and the jaw bones, especially the mandible, can be profoundly affected by radiation therapy. There are few early effects of radiation therapy on these structures but over the long term (principally as a result of xerostomia) the teeth exhibit great susceptibility to decay, especially perigingival caries, which can lead to loss of the teeth and entry of infection into the mandible, culminating in osteoradionecrosis. Similar changes can occur in the maxilla, but, clinically, osteoradionecrosis of the mandible is much more troublesome and symptomatic.

Xerostomia is often unavoidable in order to cure cancer but the aforementioned consequences are not. A systematic program of prophylactic dental care can drastically reduce or eliminate the risk of osteoradionecrosis and the loss of teeth.[10] The essentials of such a program include:

1. Preradiotherapy evaluation, cleaning, and restoration of the dentition by an experienced dentist.
2. Institution of lifelong good dental hygiene practices, such as flossing, brushing, and regular professional dental care.
3. Topical application of fluoride to the teeth on a regular basis.

The goal of treatment is to eliminate the need for performing invasive dental procedures, such as extractions, on an irradiated mandible. Inappropriate dental extractions by unwary dentists often precipitate osteoradionecrosis. The decision to perform an invasive procedure on an irradiated mandible must not be made lightly and only if no reasonable alternative is available, and the procedure should be performed by a dentist with some experience in handling irradiated tissues, using meticulous technique to minimize trauma and infection.

In addition to extractions, disruption of the mucosal lining of the mandible from other causes also can permit infection and cause osteoradionecrosis. For this reason, cancers that invade bone are rarely suitable for radical treatment by radiation therapy only. Resection of tumor and the diseased mandible, with restoration of the soft tissue cover over the bone, is preferred prior to radiation therapy. However, if the suture line does not heal, the risk of infection and osteoradionecrosis remains high. Ulceration or necrosis of the mucosa overlying the mandible, particularly after high doses of brachytherapy, also can predispose to osteoradionecrosis if the area of ulceration is larger than 1 cm across.

Management of osteoradionecrosis generally should be conservative. It consists of antibiotics, analgesics, meticulous oral hygiene by irrigations and sprays, avoidance of denture trauma, a soft diet, and a great deal of patience. Local debridement and gentle removal of sequestra should be undertaken as necessary. It is unclear whether hyperbaric oxygen adds anything except cost to this conservative management. Curettage or mandibulectomy is rarely necessary. If these are undertaken, careful treatment planning jointly by the radiation oncologist and the surgeon is mandatory to determine the radiation dose distribution to the various parts of the mandible.

LARYNX

Laryngeal cartilage covered by normal mucous membrane tolerates radiation therapy well unless very high doses (in excess of 7000 cGy in 7 weeks) are delivered or large fraction sizes (in excess of 200 cGy) are employed. If the laryngeal mucosa is impaired by extensive tumor, infection, or surgery, the risk of cartilage radionecrosis is greater; the risk might still be acceptable to the patient if the only alternative is a total laryngectomy. At present it is not clear whether doses in excess of 7000 cGy might be better tolerated by the larynx if fraction sizes smaller than 200 cGy are employed.

Biopsies in an irradiated larynx should be performed cautiously and only when indicated, because disruption of the overlying mucosa by biopsy can facilitate infection of the laryngeal cartilages that might culminate in chondronecrosis. Conservative treatment for chondronecrosis may be successful as outlined in the previous section. If the larynx is essentially useless, however, a total laryngectomy is sometimes necessary and also rules out persistent or recurrent cancer definitively.

EAR

Otitis externa can develop after doses of 3000 to 4000 cGy in 3 to 4 weeks to the skin of the external ear canal. Symptomatic treatment is usually helpful. Long-term effects include dryness and increased scaling of the skin of the external ear canal.

A sterile otitis media can develop secondary to edema and inflammation during irradiation of the nasopharynx. In a minority of patients myringotomy is necessary.

Chondritis or chondronecrosis of the ear cartilage is rarely seen with megavoltage photon beams, partly because surface sparing by megavoltage photons also spares the cartilage. Painful chondritis can develop, however, with orthovoltage or even electron beams if the cartilage is heavily damaged by cancer or if large fractions or doses are delivered to most of the cartilage.

CENTRAL NERVOUS SYSTEM

Usually no acute effects on the central nervous system (CNS) are seen during radiation therapy for head and neck cancer. Late effects caused by parenchymal injury or compromised vasculature can occur and are frequently the dose-limiting factor in clinical practice. When radiation therapy is delivered at 200 cGy per fraction or less, CNS injury is rarely seen at doses of up to 5000 cGy. Injury might be produced by lower doses in children, however, or if large volumes or whole brain radiation therapy is necessary (this is rarely the case during treatment of head and neck cancer), or if large dose fractions are employed.

Parts of the brain close to the base of the skull are at the highest risk during radiation therapy for cancers of the ethmoid, nasopharynx, or parotid regions. Use of custom shielding, compensators, and electron beams can drastically reduce the volume of central nervous system exposed to high-dose irradiation and thereby reduce the risk of injury.

It is far from certain at the present time whether hyperfractionation using fraction sizes significantly less than 200 cGy improves the radiation tolerance of central nervous system tissues. Recent animal studies suggest that while fraction sizes larger than 200 cGy produced disproportionately more radiation injury, fraction sizes less than 200 cGy might not offer meaningful protection.[11]

In selected patients, the addition of surgery before or after irradiation can reduce the need for high doses of radiation therapy by substantially reducing the tumor burden. Chemotherapy also can reduce the tumor burden sometimes, especially in patients with lymphoma or embryonal rhabdomyosarcoma. It is not clear at the present time, however, whether chemotherapy also might decrease tolerance of normal brain tissue to radiation therapy, thereby increasing the risk of late injury.

Most instances of spinal cord injury following radiation therapy can be attributed to overlapping radiation fields that can result in doubling the dose the spinal cord was supposed to receive.[12] This is of particular concern in head and neck oncology due to the popularity of techniques in which the upper and the lower parts of the neck are treated by separate fields, which produces significant potential for overlap. Careful shielding and treatment planning are mandatory to prevent the catastrophe of radiation myelopathy.

A mild, self-limiting form of myelopathy called Lhermitte syndrome is seen in 10 per cent to 20 per cent of patients who receive radiation therapy to the cervical spinal cord. This can occur after doses as low as 3000 cGy in 4 weeks. Characteristically, the patient experiences a sensation like an electric shock spreading down the spine and into the back of the thighs upon suddenly flexing the neck. Lhermitte syndrome typically appears 1 to 4 months after irradiation and lasts for 2 to 6 months. The pathogenesis is unclear, and it does not progress to permanent myelopathy. Reassurance and avoidance of sudden neck flexion are all the treatment that is usually necessary. In some cases a cervical collar might be helpful.

THE VISUAL APPARATUS

The lacrimal glands, like the salivary glands, can be injured by radiation therapy. Fortunately, it is possible to shield the major lacrimal gland as well as the accessory lacrimal glands in the upper eyelid in most instances when treating neoplasms arising from the paranasal sinuses. If tumor is present within the orbit, however, it might be unwise to shield the lacrimal gland. In such patients xerophthalmia might develop, which is treated by the use of artificial tears and ointments. Epilation of eyelashes can occur while treating neoplasms of the eyelid, such as basal cell carcinoma, but this produces no symptoms in most patients.

Acute conjunctivitis and punctate keratitis develop after doses of 2000 to 4000 cGy in 2 to 4 weeks to the conjunctiva and cornea. With doses in excess of 4000 cGy, corneal ulceration can develop. Fortunately, by using megavoltage photon beams with their surface-sparing property from an anterior approach, and custom shielding from the lateral approach, the dose to the cornea and the exposed bulbar conjunctiva can be kept well below 4000 cGy in almost all patients. It is important to instruct the patient to keep the eye open during treatment of the anterior field, otherwise the closed eyelid would cause loss of surface sparing, substantially increasing the corneal dose. For the same reason, the palpebral conjunctiva usually does manifest conjunctivitis, which is treated symptomatically. Uveitis or closed-angle glaucoma are rarely caused by radiation therapy but can occur as a late effect due to neovascularization.

A baseline opthalmologic evaluation is recommended in all patients prior to initiating radiation therapy to the orbit.

Premature cataract formation in the lens is promoted by radiation therapy even at modest doses. Most patients whose lens receives a dose of 1500 cGy and some patients with doses of as little as 200 cGy develop a cataract visible on slit lamp examination during the subsequent 6 months to 5 years. Not all patients with radiation-induced cataracts require extraction of the cataract, especially if vision in the contralateral eye is good. The decision to operate must be individualized, based upon not only vision in the contralateral eye but also the likelihood of retinopathy or optic neuropathy in the ipsilateral eye, the degree of xerophthalmia, and the ability of the patient to tolerate a contact lens or intraocular lens implant. In general, the treatment of radiation-induced cataracts is similar to the usual treatment of other cataracts. It is not worthwhile to risk death from persistent tumor in or around the orbit due to misguided attempts at minimizing the radiation dose to the lens; the only exception is in the treatment of small retinoblastomas located in the posterior part of the globe.

The retina, the optic nerve, and the optic chiasm usually manifest no early effects from radiation therapy. Late injury, however, can become manifest, sometimes years later, as retinopathy or optic neuropathy with progressive and permanent loss of vision. Injury to the optic chiasm can produce bilateral blindness and is obviously the most devastating.

Our understanding of the time-dose volume relationships of radiation injury to the retina and optic nerve has been greatly enhanced by the painstaking studies of investigators at the University of Florida.[13] When fraction sizes of 180 to 200 cGy are employed, injury to the retina, optic nerve, or optic chiasm is distinctly uncommon with total doses of less than 5000 cGy. The use of fraction sizes larger than 200 cGy markedly increases the likelihood of radiation injury. As yet, convincing evidence is lacking that a fraction size significantly smaller than 200 cGy (hyperfractionation) offers any particular advantage in this regard. With total doses in excess of 6000 cGy, the incidence of radiation injury can be quite high, and with doses in excess of 7000 cGy most patients will manifest severe injury. Efforts to restrict the dose to the retina, optic nerve, and chiasm to 5000 cGy in 5 weeks or less are worthwhile. In selected patients, the addition of surgery before or after radiation therapy can reduce the need for high doses of radiation therapy by substantially reducing the tumor burden. Chemotherapy also can reduce the tumor burden sometimes, especially in patients with lymphoma or embryonal rhabdomyosarcoma. It is also possible, however, that chemotherapy might reduce the tolerance of the visual structures to radiation therapy and thereby increase the risk of blindness.

An important practical observation made by Parsons and colleagues is that, during treatment of paranasal sinus tumors, the area of the retina receiving a high dose of radiation therapy can be minimized by having the patient look straight ahead during treatment with the anterior photon beam, with a shield skirting the medial limbus of the cornea.[14] In the past it was customary to ask the patient to look away from the beam. In the orthovoltage era this maneuver presumably reduced the dose to the cornea, which was important since orthovoltage beams had no surface-sparing property. With megavoltage beams, however, this maneuver succeeds only in increasing the area of the retina in the high-dose region, thereby increasing the risk of retinopathy.

Careful shielding and treatment planning can minimize the risk of radiation injury to the retina and the optic nerve. Little can be done, however, to reverse the loss of vision once radiation injury does become manifest. It is possible in many cases to prevent the blind eye from turning into a painful blind eye by treating radiation-induced retinopathy by such modalities as the laser. If a painful blind eye does develop, enucleation may be the only solution.

THYROID AND PITUITARY GLANDS

No acute effects from radiation therapy are seen on either the thyroid or the pituitary gland, as a rule. Over the long term, clinical hypothyroidism is seen in 5 per cent to 10 per cent of the patients irradiated to the lower neck and responds readily to administration of thyroid hormone. Biochemical hypothyroidism might be more common, although the exact incidence is uncertain.[15] Overt hypopituitarism is uncommon in adults except after treatment of pituitary adenomas, but biochemical hypopituitarism might be more common. Pituitary hypofunction is common in children after irradiation. All children irradiated to the pituitary region should be followed by an endocrinologist, and replacement therapy for growth hormone, ACTH, thyrotropin, and so on should be instituted as appropriate.

PERIPHERAL NERVES AND CAROTID ARTERY

Radiation injury to the peripheral nerves is very uncommon in clinical practice. Rare instances of 12th nerve injury have been reported after doses in excess of 7000 cGy.[16] I have also seen one instance of progressive and chronic bulbar cranial nerve paralysis in a patient who had received 6000 cGy to the brain stem 3 years earlier with no shielding employed. Recent animal studies suggest that intraoperative external beam radiation therapy with single acute doses in excess of 2000 cGy to the lumbosacral plexus produced a high incidence of hind limb paralysis.[17] This has not been observed in clinical practice, in which fractionated external beam radiation therapy or low-dose rate brachytherapy is employed. In fact, a recent experimental study evaluating the tolerance of the carotid sheath contents to low-dose rate brachytherapy in rabbits found that doses as high as 13,000 cGy produced no measurable injury to the vagus nerve up to 1 year after radiation therapy.[18] Nor were any carotid blowouts encountered with doses of up to 13,000 cGy to healthy rabbit carotids. Carotid patency, as evaluated by ultrasound, was also found to be within normal limits up to 1 year after radiation therapy. Kumar recently reported on a patient who received a dose of 20,000 cGy to the internal carotid artery by iodine-125 brachytherapy.[19] At autopsy 5 months later the arterial wall showed normal thickness without fibrosis.

The high tolerance of major blood vessels such as the carotid artery is in striking contrast to what occurs in small arterioles and capillaries, where changes include microaneurysm formation, thickening and hyalinization of the vessel walls, and occlusion of the lumen by a fine fibrillary material. These changes are most dramatically seen in the retinal blood vessels, as discussed previously, and are probably responsible for a significant component of late radiation injury not only to the retina but also perhaps to many other late-reacting structures, such as the central nervous system.

References

1. Vikram B, Mishra UB, Strong EW, Manolatos S: Patterns of failure in carcinoma of the nasopharynx. I. Failure at the primary site. Int J Radiat Oncol Biol Phys 11:1455–1459, 1985.

2. Parsons JT, Bova FJ, Million RR: A reevaluation of split course technique for squamous cell carcinoma of the head and neck. Int J Radiat Oncol Biol Phys 6:1645–1652, 1980.

3. Thames HD Jr, Withers HR, Peters LJ, et al: Changes in early and late radiation responses with altered dose fractionation. Int J Radiat Oncol Biol Phys 8:219, 1982.

4. Parsons JT, Mendenhall W, Cassisi N, et al: Accelerated hyperfractionation for head and neck cancer. Int J Radiat Oncol Biol Phys 14:649–658, 1988.

5. Wang CC: Local control of oropharyngeal cancer after two hyperfractionation radiation therapy schemes. Int J Radiat Oncol Biol Phys 14:1143–1146, 1988.

6. Horiot JC, Lefur R, Nguyen T, et al: Two fractions per day versus a single fraction per day in the radiotherapy of oropharynx trial. Int J Radiat Oncol Biol Phys 15(Suppl 1):178, 1988.

7. Stephens LC, King GK, Peters LJ, et al: Acute and late radiation injury in rhesus monkey parotid glands: Evidence of interphase cell death. Am J Pathol 124:469, 1986.

8. Chencharick JD, Mossman KL: Nutritional consequences of the radiotherapy of head and neck cancer. Cancer 51(5):811–815, 1983.

9. Spijkervet F, Vermey A, Panders A, et al: Prevention of irradiation mucositis in head-neck cancer patients. Proc ASCO 9(673):174, 1990.

10. Levendag PC, Vikram B, Wright R, Schweiger JW: Dental problems following surgery and external radiation in patients with advanced carcinomas of the oral cavity and oropharynx. Acta Oncol 28(4):550–552, 1989.

11. Ang KK, Van-der-Kogel AJ, Van-der-Schueren E: Lack of evidence for increased tolerance of rat spinal cord with decreasing fraction doses below 2 Gy. Int J Radiat Oncol Biol Phys 11:105, 1985.

12. Kim YH, Fayos JV: Radiation tolerance of the cervical spinal cord. Radiology 139(2):473–478, 1981.

13. Parsons JT: The effect of radiation on normal tissues of the head and neck. In Million RR, Cassisi NJ (eds): Management of Head and Neck Cancer. Philadelphia, JB Lippincott, 1984, pp 185–198.

14. Parsons JT, Fitzgerald CR, Hood CI, et al: The effects of irradiation on the eye and optic nerve. Int J Radiat Oncol Biol Phys 9:609–622, 1983.

15. Kim YH, Fayos JV, Sisson JC: Thyroid function following neck irradiation for malignant lymphoma. Radiology 134(1):205–208, 1980.

16. Berger PS, Bataini JP: Radiation-induced cranial nerve palsy. Cancer 40:152–155, 1977.

17. Kinsella TJ, Deluca AM, Barnes M, et al: Threshold dose for peripheral neuropathy following intraoperative radiotherapy (IORT) in a large animal model. Int J Radiat Oncol Biol Phys 20:697–701, 1991.

18. Werber JL, Sood BM, Alfieri A, et al: Tolerance of the carotid-sheath contents to brachytherapy: An experimental study. Laryngoscope 101(6):587–591, June 1991.

19. Kumar PP, Good RR, Leibrock LG, et al: Tissue tolerance to continuous low dose rate iodine-125 irradiation. Endocurietherapy/Hyperthermia Oncology 6:53–63, 1990.

CHAPTER 23

Maxillofacial Trauma

ROBERT M. KELLMAN, MD
EDWIN F. WILLIAMS, III, MD

The complications of maxillofacial trauma result from injuries, treatment of these injuries, normal and aberrant healing processes, and those resulting from a failure to diagnose or treat injuries in this area. This is a complex subject; it is obviously impossible to include every possibility that may occur. In this chapter, complications are classified by the anatomic area affected. The incidence of these complications as well as their prevention and management are discussed. Since similar complications can sometimes affect various anatomic areas in the head and neck, a certain amount of redundancy is to be anticipated.

AIRWAY/ASPIRATION

As in any major injury, airway access and stabilization are of primary importance in patient management and survival. The airway represents the "A" in the A,B,Cs of emergency patient care. Thompson and associates reviewed 117 consecutive LeFort fractures.[126] Thirty-one (26.5 per cent) required emergency airway intervention for airway obstruction or decreased respiration. There were no deaths. However, occasional reports of death due to airway obstruction exist—1 in 45 in one series[1] and 1 in 300 in another.[2]

Bleeding is a common cause of airway obstruction in the traumatized face. Skull base trauma can result in damage to the internal carotid artery, which can cause an exsanguinating bleed in the nasopharynx. Less severe bleeding, of course, can occur as a result of vessels torn in midfacial fractures, and this can result in aspiration of blood and inability of the patient to maintain adequate ventilation via the normal pathways. A reduced level of consciousness will further aggravate this situation, making the possibility of hypoxemia secondary to massive aspiration more likely. Blood in the pharynx interferes with efforts at mask ventilation and also makes intubation technically more difficult. Stabilization of the airway becomes critically important so that ventilation can be accomplished, and bleeding can then be controlled.

If bleeding from the nasopharynx and pharynx is too brisk to allow for direct airway visualization via the transoral route, then tracheotomy should be considered. In the adult patient, in the emergency situation, a cricothyrotomy is usually the preferred technique for establishing an emergency transtracheal airway. Care should be taken not to extend the neck if the cervical spine has not been cleared.

If the decision has been made that an emergency transtracheal airway needs to be established, this should be performed. However, the presence of free air in the neck should alert the surgeon to the possibility of a cricotracheal separation that would mandate tracheotomy rather than cricothyrotomy. Otherwise, cricothyrotomy should be carried out at this time. A cricothyrotomy is performed by digitally identifying the cricothyroid space and then making an incision right down over this space. With the cricothyroid under direct visualization, an incision is made into the tracheal lumen and the space spread open, giving the surgeon immediate airway access. A 6-mm endotracheal tube is generally passed into the tracheal lumen at this point. If passage of this tube does not immediately result in ventilation, then cricotracheal separation and thus intubation of the soft tissues of the neck rather than the trachea is possible. If this is suspected, the incision is taken down through the tissues of the midneck and the trachea identified and cannulated. Further difficulty of ventilation at this point should alert the physician to the possibility of foreign body aspiration and obstruction. Once the airway has been established, attention can be turned to controlling bleeding and other related problems.

Other problems related to facial injuries that can lead to airway difficulties include foreign body aspirations and aspiration of vomitus. The most common foreign body encountered in facial trauma is a tooth that has been dislodged and aspirated. When an initial attempt at mask ventilation proves difficult or impossible, the possibility of a laryngeal foreign body should be ruled out. Frequently, a pharyngeal or hypopharyngeal foreign body can be cleared from the patient's mouth manually. Suction also can be used to help clear the patient's pharynx. In the partially conscious or unconscious patient, the posterior position of the tongue may result in airway obstruction; this usually can be corrected by elevating the mandible or by passing an instrument through the tongue and pulling it forward. An oral airway often will help improve the status of the airway for mask ventilation as well.

Bilateral mandibular body or angle fractures can result in a loss of hyomandibular support and result in retropositioning of the tongue. If this compromises the airway, it often can be improved by anterior traction on the tongue or mandible or the placement of an oral or nasopharyngeal airway. If a nasopharyngeal airway is utilized, a shortened nasotracheal tube will provide better support than a soft rubber nasopharyngeal airway.

Evidence of bruising of the anterior neck or subcutaneous air in the neck should alert the evaluating physician to the possibility of an airway injury. Laryngeal fractures can be easily missed. A laryngeal fracture may result in progressive airway obstruction from swelling or hematoma formation within the larynx. Failure to recognize this injury can result in an unanticipated airway obstruction after the patient is thought to have been stabilized. If the possibility of an airway injury has been recognized, appropriate precautions include constant observation, monitoring of arterial oxygenation such as by percutaneous oximetry, and maintaining availability of emergency airway equipment at all times.

Any patient with blunt maxillofacial trauma should be considered as having a possible cervical spine injury as well. The reported incidence of associated cervical spine injuries with maxillofacial trauma varies from extremely rare[3] to as high as 5 or 6 per cent when injury occurred in a motor vehicle accident.[4–6] Clearly, a missed cervical spine (c-spine) fracture can result in a devastating complication such as quadriplegia. The evaluating physician must have a high index of suspicion and treat patients as though they may indeed have a cervical spine injury until proved otherwise.[7, 8] The possibility of a c-spine injury also affects the selection of emergency airway management technique.

A patient may be brought in from the field with an esophageal obturator airway (EOA) already in place. This device is designed to obstruct the esophagus and blow air into the pharynx so that airway ventilation can be carried out via the pharynx, without requiring endotracheal intubation. Since many of these patients have full stomachs, it is critical that the patient be endotracheally intubated prior to removal of the esophageal obturator airway. Otherwise, vomiting and aspirating at the time of decompression of the EOA are possible. The EOA should not be used as an emergency airway management tool in the hospital setting. If a patient with an EOA in place is not ventilating adequately, the possibility of mispositioning of this device in the trachea should be considered.

Complications of Airway Management

An awareness of the complications of an artificial airway helps avoid these problems and also makes it more likely that a problem will be recognized if it occurs. The most common means for establishing an airway is endotracheal intubation. The use of a laryngoscope and an endotracheal tube in the presence of a possible c-spine injury is quite controversial. Some have advocated the use of axial stabilization by an assistant,[9] and others, the use of axial traction.[10–12] Several studies have been carried out to assess the amount of cervical spine movement created by these maneuvers.[9, 13] The safety of endotracheal intubation in the presence of these maneuvers when a cervical spine injury is possible is far from established. When in doubt, several other techniques for airway management are possible. The complications of each of these techniques will be briefly mentioned.

ENDOTRACHEAL INTUBATION

Besides the direct orotracheal intubation risk if the c-spine is at all unstable, other complications include esophageal intubation, particularly dangerous if this goes unrecognized and the stomach is ventilated instead of the airway; damaging the hypopharynx or creating an esophageal or hypopharyngeal tear; and arytenoid dislocation from endotracheal intubation.[14]

NASOTRACHEAL INTUBATION

Nasotracheal intubation has been advocated as a means of avoiding movement of the cervical spine.[15, 16] However, it is generally not advocated in the presence of midfacial and possible skull base fractures.[16] Aggravating or restarting a significant nasal hemorrhage is certainly a risk. The possibility of passing the endotracheal tube through the cribriform plate or through the skull base into the brain also exists. As in orotracheal intubation, hypopharyngeal or esophageal tears or arytenoid injuries can occur. Finally, it is a blind technique and is thus difficult and undependable.

RETROGRADE INTUBATION

This technique involves the passage of a wire through the cricothyroid membrane or first tracheal interspace up through the larynx and out the mouth, followed by the passage of the tube over this wire. This technique is tricky and does not guarantee passage of the tube into the airway. The tube may pass through the cords over the wire and then still slip out and end up being passed into the esophagus. This technique should be performed only by those who have skill and experience with it. If one can pass the guide wire into the airway and up and out the mouth, it is also likely that the guide wire could be passed downward and be used to perform percutaneous tracheotomy, probably a wiser approach.

THE PERCUTANEOUS TRACHEOTOMY

This is certainly a reasonable technique to utilize so long as the landmarks can be palpated. However, if the landmarks are not obvious, or if there is swelling or injury in the neck itself, this technique could easily result in the creation of a false passageway.

USE OF THE LIGHTED STYLET

As in the retrograde passage of an endotracheal tube, this technique seems to be reasonably effective in skilled and experienced hands.[17] A tube with a lighted stylet is passed down toward the larynx in a darkened room. Visualization of the light percutaneously over the trachea signals that the tube has in fact passed into the airway. However, this blind technique runs the risk of creating airway trauma and injury. It also requires a patient who is not combative and who is stable enough to allow for darkening of the room. Such optimal circumstances are not typical.

PASSAGE OVER A FLEXIBLE BRONCHOSCOPE OR LARYNGOSCOPE

This technique provides for direct visualization of the larynx and trachea and passage of the endotracheal tube over the scope when it has been passed through the vocal cords into the airway.[18, 19] This is an excellent technique in the hands of a skilled practitioner. Direct passage into the airway allows the physician to recognize an airway disruption by direct visualization. This technique is difficult in the presence of blood and vomitus.

All these techniques become more difficult when the patient is combative.

Direct Airway Exposure

In an emergency situation when time is critical and the preceding techniques are either precluded or difficult, direct airway exposure and placement of a tracheotomy tube remains the procedure of choice. Cricothyrotomy or direct tracheotomy can be quickly performed by the skilled surgeon. However, certain pitfalls may still occur. Failure to properly identify the landmarks of the neck may result in mispositioning the inci-

sion and therefore lead the surgeon away from the trachea or cricothyroid membrane. Missing the midline can result in injury to the recurrent laryngeal nerve, which would worsen the patient's airway. Injury to the carotid artery or jugular vein can occur. Such complications are certainly more likely in younger patients, particularly the very young. Hemorrhage during emergency tracheotomy also can result from transection of the thyroid isthmus. If this occurs, the trachea should be controlled and entered, the tube positioned, and the cuff inflated. Hemostasis can be established once the patient is being adequately ventilated.

Rapid and aggressive attempts at "slash" tracheotomy also can result in through-and-through penetration of the trachea and damage to the cervical esophagus. If this occurs, establishment and maintenance of the patient's airway and stabilization of other injuries are done. Repair of the cervical esophagus can then be carried out, once the patient is stable, by directly repairing the esophageal injury and draining the neck to prevent development of neck infection or mediastinitis.

DELAYED AIRWAY COMPLICATIONS

Late sequelae of airway injury can be the result of the initial trauma or of an iatrogenic injury at the time of resuscitation or later medical management. A hurried intubation, particularly in the semiawake, combative patient, easily can result in damage to the vocal cords, such as tearing of the membranous cord or dislocation of an arytenoid cartilage. Most vocal cord tears heal uneventfully without any long-term sequelae. A dislocated arytenoid, on the other hand, can result in permanent vocal cord dysfunction. This can occur from external trauma[20] or can be secondary to the intubation itself.[14]

It is most important to identify and diagnose an arytenoid dislocation early, so that correction can be made in a timely fashion. It is generally believed that it is possible to relocate a dislocated arytenoid cartilage acutely during only 7 to 14 days. Although fixation is reported to be a risk in as little as 24 to 48 hours,[21] it is still reasonable to attempt endoscopic relocation for up to 1 month after injury.[22] A case has been reported of a successful outcome with reduction 5 weeks after dislocation.[21] The possibility of an arytenoid dislocation should be evaluated early via direct laryngoscopy. The finding of an edematous, mispositioned arytenoid with decreased cord mobility at endoscopy should be confirmed with computed tomography (CT) scanning.[21] The arytenoid is manually relocated endoscopically, preferably under local anesthesia, by manipulating it back into its proper position.

Prolonged or traumatic intubation can result in trauma to the glottis and subglottis, which is likely to lead to voice and airway problems. If a laryngeal fracture has been overlooked, the patient is at great risk for developing laryngeal dysfunction and stenosis that may well be irreversible. When the suspicion of a possible laryngeal injury is present, the larynx must be aggressively evaluated via flexible and rigid endoscopy as well as CT scanning of the airway.[23] If a laryngeal injury is identified, particularly if there is any cartilaginous disruption, an artificial airway through the larynx should be avoided, or, if already present, it should be converted to a tracheotomy that bypasses the endolarynx as soon as possible. Attention should then be turned to early restoration of normal laryngeal anatomy via surgical intervention.[24] If the larynx heals in an abnormal position after significant injury, the likelihood of being able to restore normal laryngeal shape, size, and function will be greatly decreased.

Limited laryngeal function includes problems with the voice, the adequacy of the airway for breathing, and airway protection, which may result in swallowing problems.

Small webs and localized areas of stenosis sometimes can be effectively managed via endoscopic laser excision. More severe areas of stenosis often require open surgical procedures and graft reconstruction. This is most common when the posterior commissure is involved with severe stenosis.

Injuries at the cricoid level frequently result in subglottic stenosis, which also may result from prolonged intubation, particularly if the intubation was traumatic or if denuded cartilage from high-pressure cuffs, multiple intubations, or infection is present. It is emphasized that early recognition and, whenever possible, early conversion to tracheotomy can minimize the occurrence of such stenoses.

Tracheal stenosis can be mild or severe, depending on the percentage of narrowing of the tracheal air column. A mild stenosis commonly occurs at the level of a tracheotomy; however, any airway limitation that does not result in a loss of function for the patient is generally considered insignificant. If the airway stenosis results in a loss of exercise tolerance, or in more severe cases the necessity for maintenance of an artificial airway, then this is a serious problem that requires surgical intervention. As in the area of the glottis, a mild stenosis may sometimes be effectively handled by either laser excision or bronchoscopic dilatation. According to some reports,[25] most any tracheal stenosis can be handled via aggressive dilatation and prolonged stenting with a silicone T-tube. Others have advocated tracheal resection with end-to-end anastomosis.[26, 27] When this is not feasible, tracheal reconstruction using various grafts such as rib cartilage have been successfully employed.

MISCELLANEOUS COMPLICATIONS OF AIRWAY MANAGEMENT

Complications can occur in any setting but certainly are more likely to occur in the emergency setting during resuscitation of the polytraumatized patient. The incidence may be underestimated, since injuries that could be iatrogenic might also under these circumstances be attributed to the source of injury that brought the patient to the hospital.

Attempts at intubation in the field have resulted in pharyngeal and esophageal lacerations. These also could result from attempts at passage of an esophageal obturator airway. Use of a rigid stylet is a likely source of injury. Esophageal tears have been reported during intubation attempts, and the likelihood of esophageal tear is increased in the older patient with anterior cervical osteophytes. It is important to identify and recognize an esophageal or significant pharyngeal tear, since this can result in severe, deep neck infection as well as mediastinitis. Unrecognized mediastinitis has a high mortality rate. A through-and-through tear of the pharynx or esophagus necessitates drainage of the neck. The presence of free air in the neck should alert the examining physician to the possibility of a tear.

Nasal injuries, such as septal deflections or lacerations or lacerations of both the septum and lateral nasal walls that result in synechia formation, can occur as a result of nasotracheal intubation, even without a pre-existing nasal injury. When a nasal or nasoseptal injury has occurred, the likelihood of further disruption of the nasal, septal, and lateral nasal wall tissue secondary to nasotracheal intubation is greatly increased. If a nasotracheal tube has been used, the head and neck surgeon addresses the nasal tissues as soon as possible and corrects any injuries that are identified. Disruptions of the lateral and medial nasal mucosa are repaired or stented, and care is taken to position mucosal tissues so as to increase the likelihood of healing in the correct position. Trauma to the nasopharynx from an endotracheal tube, particularly when it is combined with pre-existing trauma from the injury, can also result in nasopharyngeal stenosis.

Of course, manipulation of the cervical spine in the presence of an injury can result in spinal cord damage. This has already been discussed.

BLEEDING/VASCULAR

Bleeding into the airway, of course, will result in problems with aspiration and loss of adequate airway. When bleeding is profuse, it may prove impossible to establish a safe airway through the normal routes. An artificial airway should be established either via cricothyrotomy or tracheotomy as appropriate, and then intraluminal pressure can be applied with packing to gain control of massive bleeding. More direct control can be obtained after the patient is resuscitated.

When pharyngeal or hypopharyngeal bleeding has diminished, great care should be taken with instrumentation of the pharynx and larynx, since a clot can be knocked loose and an exsanguinating hemorrhage result.

Excessive blood loss can result in hypotension and shock. The volume of bleeding from the nose and nasopharynx in facial injuries can be underestimated when large amounts of blood have been swallowed or lost at the scene of the injury. It is important to recognize that exsanguination from the nose and nasopharynx is possible. Often valuable time in the emergency department is spent searching the hypotensive patient with massive facial trauma for a source of bleeding, when in fact the hemorrhage has been primarily from the head and neck region.

First a safe airway is established, and then tamponade is used to control bleeding. In skull base fractures, great care must be taken not to penetrate into the sphenoid and skull base when tamponading bleeding in the nasopharynx. Emergency intervention can include extensive packing, including vaginal packing in the pharynx. Sometimes a 30-cc Foley balloon placed into the nasopharynx, combined with anterior nasal packing, will help tamponade an anterior and posterior nasal bleed.

Intratractable bleeding must be stopped. Ligation of the external carotid artery in the neck usually can be performed expeditiously and results in a decreased flow of blood to the area involved. An alternative is acute reduction of the fractures. While this is not guaranteed to stop the bleeding, typically it will decrease the flow and allow bleeding to be controlled via aforementioned techniques. When feasible, interventional radiography can be used to identify and approach the bleeding sites through an intra-arterial catheter. Once the bleeding sites have been identified, vascular sources can be occluded using intra-arterial coils or particulate embolization.[28] This technique has been successfully used in our institution in severe bleeding after trauma, including internal carotid transection at the skull base. However, safe and rapid performance of this procedure usually requires the skills of an experienced interventional radiologist.

Both blunt and penetrating neck trauma can result in injuries to the carotid circulation. The possibility of cerebrovascular accident secondary to traumatic dislodgment of an intra-arterial plaque or clot should be considered when neurologic findings are present. Dissection of the carotid artery also can occur secondary to blunt or penetrating neck trauma. Angiographic evaluation of the carotid circulation becomes extremely important in these situations for the proper evaluation of the carotid and cerebral circulation. An injury to the internal carotid artery generally necessitates exploration and repair.

A complication sometimes seen after blunt head trauma is carotid cavernous fistula. This can be missed easily unless there is an index of suspicion. It can result in pulsatile proptosis on the involved side, though this may not be present. The telltale finding is a bruit over the involved eye. Failure to recognize this problem can have devastating consequences.

Complications of Management

Aggressive resuscitation is fraught with risk, which of course, is far outweighed by the benefits of a successful resuscitation. Early resuscitation usually includes large volumes of crystalloid as well as some colloid transfusions. Also frequently used are packed cells and whole blood transfusions. Use of type-specific or uncross-matched blood is sometimes necessary to save a life but frequently results in significant transfusion reactions. While most are managed by the resuscitation itself, sometimes severe reactions such as further vascular collapse or renal failure may result. A less well-understood but frequently deadly process is adult respiratory distress syndrome. At times, this seems to result from aggressive hemodynamic resuscitation. The exact mechanism by which this occurs is unclear, but it can have devastating consequences. Patients may go on to severe diffuse pulmonary infiltrates, poor oxygenation, and ultimately complete respiratory failure.

Nasal packing used to control hemorrhage also can be a source of complications. Toxic shock syndrome caused by exotoxins produced by *Staphylococcus aureus* can lead to shock and even death.[29] Breda and associates found a 32 per cent asymptomatic carrier rate for *S. aureus* in 119 patients studied; in 9 patients (7.5 per cent), isolates were capable of producing toxic shock exotoxin in vitro.[30] Even in the absence of toxic shock syndrome, bacterial colonization of packing can be a source of infection and with a dural leak may increase the risk of meningitis.

Late Sequelae

A patient who has been successfully resuscitated, including restoration of normal hemodynamic and respiratory function, may still suffer the consequences of injuries that were caused by stabilization efforts during the initial period. Despite great efforts at providing a healthy and safe blood supply, the possibility of bloodborne disease is still a concern, and these diseases do continue to occur. Acquired immunodeficiency syndrome (AIDS) can be the result of a tainted blood transfusion. However, this occurrence right now is believed to be extremely low. Hepatitis B has been virtually eliminated from the blood supply by careful testing. However, non-B hepatitis continues to be a concern.

Aggressive packing also can result in damage to soft tissue and scar formation. Posterior packing necessitates stabilization of the posterior pack at the anterior naris. When the clamp or tie holding the posterior pack in place is not well insulated from the nasal ala, injury can result in a late nasal alar stenosis. This also can result from overaggressive anterior packing of the nasal vestibule and alar region (Fig. 23–1). Repair generally requires either a Z-plasty of the nasal alar base or a local flap. Other nasal injuries include stenosis of the nasal vestibule and nasal valve and significant deviation of the septum with formation of synechiae between the nasal septum and lateral nasal wall.

Chronic sinus disease may result from scarring in the areas of the sinus ostia. Recurrent

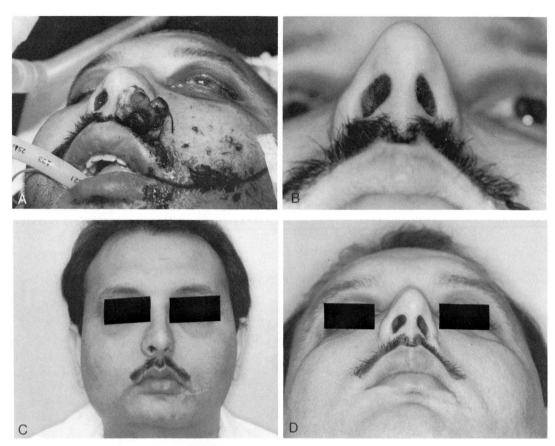

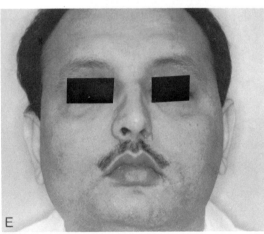

FIGURE 23–1. *A,* A patient with panfacial trauma, including bilateral Le Fort III (including II and I) and mandible fractures. Severe epistaxis necessitated anterior and posterior nasal packing in the emergency department. *B,* Basal view, and *C,* frontal view of patient several months later. Packing resulted in injury to the left nasal ala, with tissue loss, scar formation, and ultimate stenosis. Note the narrowing of the left nares on both views. *D,* Basal view, and *E,* frontal view after Z-plasty repositioning of the alar base. Note the improved symmetry of the nares and the width of the nasal base, both of which result in better function. However, the nasal sill is depressed, which is a distinct limitation of the Z-plasty technique.

sinusitis after trauma should alert the physician to this possibility, and radiologic CT evaluation of this area should be done. Modern techniques of endoscopic sinus surgery allow for effective surgical correction and drainage of the involved sinuses. However, great care should be taken when endoscopic repair is carried out. Traumatic disruption of the naso-orbital area can result in unexpected anatomic position of orbital contents. This can lead the unwary surgeon to create an orbital injury.

Cervical Spine. The sequelae of cervical spinal cord damage are without question among the most devastating seen in modern medicine. Great care and attention must

Cervical Spine. The sequelae of cervical spinal cord damage are without question among the most devastating seen in modern medicine. Great care and attention must therefore be given to preventing movement of the cervical spine during any manipulations of the patient. Sandbags should be placed on either side of the patient's neck at the accident scene, and any movement of the patient should be carried out on a spine board. If airway intervention is necessary, a technique that avoids neck extension should be utilized.

A patient with a high cervical spinal cord injury likely will be apneic owing to paralysis of the muscles of respiration. Failure to provide assisted ventilation may result in hypoxic brain damage prior to the arrival of emergency personnel at the scene. Assisted ventilation must be started as soon as possible, generally via face mask prior to establishing an artificial airway. Once the patient has been resuscitated, the cervical spine is stabilized by the orthopedic or neurosurgical physicians.

Cervical spinal cord injuries, of course, have other complications than complete quadriplegia and death. A cervical cord injury can result in an incomplete paralysis, confining a patient to a wheelchair, with limited arm function. Patients frequently require the assistance of skilled personnel for the rest of their lives and sometimes are limited to nursing home existences.

Tissue Management

Although an in-depth discussion of soft tissue principles and closure techniques is beyond the scope of this text, the importance of proper management of soft tissue injuries in maxillofacial trauma cannot be overemphasized. When possible, a careful history should be taken, including details of the event, medical problems, immunizations, and allergies.

The best approach to tetanus is prevention. Immunization records are important, and a booster of tetanus toxoid should be given intramuscularly if the most recent immunization was greater than 10 years ago (some say 5 years[31]). Following the initial dose of tetanus toxoid, nonimmunized individuals require 30 days to acquire a safe antibody level; therefore, the nonimmunized patient should receive human hyperimmune globulin (250 units) simultaneously with the toxoid. The effectiveness of the hyperimmune globulin lasts for approximately 4 weeks, allowing time for active immunization to take effect. In the patient who has had two or more previous toxoid injections, passive immunization is not recommended since a booster will rapidly recall complete active protection. In addition, regardless of immunization status of the patient, meticulous surgical care, including removal of all devitalized tissue and foreign bodies, should be accomplished. This minimizes the anaerobic conditions that promote growth of and exotoxin production by *Clostridium tetani* in a wound that has been inoculated with the organism. Finally, a high index of suspicion can be lifesaving, as demonstrated by an unexpected case of tetanus seen after zygomatic trauma.[32]

In the patient at high risk for infection, careful cleansing of the wound is most important. The pulse irrigation system may help decrease the amount of contamination (Fig. 23–2). Aggressive cleansing is best carried out after local or general anesthesia has been obtained. Foreign bodies in the wound increase the risk of infection, and a retained foreign body may be noticeable and quite bothersome to the patient. In addition, retained pigmented foreign material will cause tattooing when trapped in the dermis and subcutaneous tissue. This should be prevented by aggressive cleansing and scrubbing at the time of initial care.

Complex lacerations often give the deceptive appearance of tissue loss. Proper tissue alignment becomes apparent only during a careful unhurried repair. It is generally accepted that facial debridement should be limited to devitalized tissue, if any. This is particularly true around the eyes and nose where tissue loss may place the patient at high risk for cosmetic and functional problems.

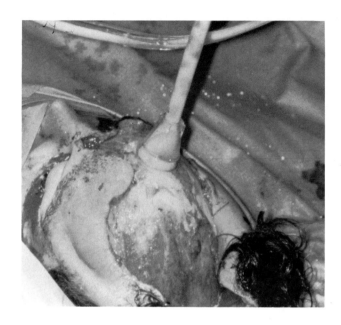

FIGURE 23–2. A severe scalping injury. The pulse irrigation system depicted here is used to cleanse the wound mechanically. This helps remove foreign particles as well as decrease the overall bacterial count, which decreases the risk of infection.

scar of the same thickness. One exception, however, is the trap-door laceration that often has a beveled edge. Since delayed edema and fullness of the flap often occur, this type of flap is often best managed by creating a perpendicular edge to the flap surface and undermining the surrounding tissue, so that a careful multilayer closure is possible. When the pedicle of the trap-door flap is in a nondependent position, the edema of the flap in addition to scar formation often gives the tissue a fullness that may be improved only by a secondary revision procedure (Fig. 23–3).

When true tissue loss occurs, the decision whether to reconstruct acutely depends on the nature of the tissue loss. Clean wounds with sufficient local tissue are best reconstructed with local flaps. One must be very careful in the perioral and periorbital areas when transposing tissue, since scar contracture in these regions may result in functional and cosmetic problems. Acute tissue expansion enjoyed early enthusiasm and is advocated by some.[33] However, recent studies suggest that the amount of tissue gained is only a small amount more than is gained by undermining and there is a risk of further tissue injury.[34] For this reason, we do not advocate acute tissue expansion in the trauma patient. When massive tissue loss occurs, such as in a gunshot wound to the face, regional pedicle flaps should be employed after debridement and irrigation, or delayed repair with slow tissue expansion performed.

Secondary intent healing also has a role in the trauma patient. When a small-to-moderate amount of tissue loss has occurred in a contaminated wound, aggressive local wound care may result in an acceptable outcome. In some cases, while awaiting a secondary repair, patients have healed satisfactorily on their own, thereby obviating the need for surgical reconstruction.

Human and animal bites are considered contaminated; these have a higher risk of infection when closed primarily. Injuries on the extremities are best managed by allowing secondary healing to proceed after aggressive local care. On the face, this practice is discouraged. If the wound is less than 8 hours old, closure over a drain is recommended after vigorous cleansing with a high-power jet, since cosmesis is a factor and the excellent blood supply in the head and neck region is believed to reduce the incidence of infection.[35, 36] Broad-spectrum systemic antibiotics should be given in the contaminated wound in an attempt to avoid infection. If infection develops, the wound should be opened quickly. According to Stucker and

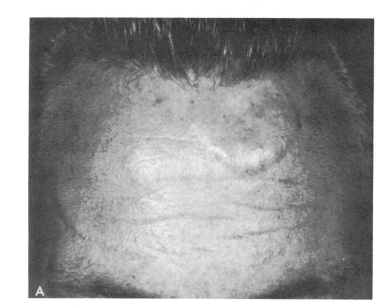

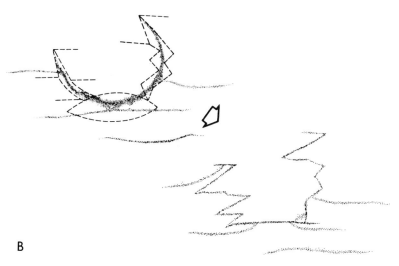

FIGURE 23–3. *A,* A trap-door scar deformity. *B,* Diagram of surgical treatment of trap-door deformities: partial simple excision in conjunction with multiple W- and Z-plasties. (From Dingman RO, Izenberg PH: Complications of facial trauma. *In* Conley J: Complications of Head and Neck Surgery. Philadelphia, WB Saunders, 1979, p 357.)

B

associates, reattachment of soft tissue (auricle, nose, skin) that has been avulsed by an animal or human bite is doomed to failure and should not be attempted.[36] Rather, local wound care with late reconstruction is preferred.

Delayed Complications

Delayed complications may be the result of the initial injury, the healing process, or the treatment that was provided.

The hypertrophic scar or one that may be improved upon by revision is described as either greater than 2 mm in width or 2 cm in length, or is a facial scar that crosses the relaxed skin tension lines. The details of scar revision are beyond the scope of this text; however, prevention by minimal debridement of devitalized tissue only (if any), use of aseptic technique, and meticulous multilayer closure at the time of initial repair cannot be overemphasized. Some are now advocating a feathering dermabrasion of the wound at 4 to 6 weeks to improve the overall long-term result. Avoidance of direct sunlight for at least one full year must be stressed to the patient, with liberal use of sun block for a period of several years to minimize scar formation and skin discoloration. In the early postinjury period, prevention of crust formation on the wound by frequent cleansing with hydrogen peroxide and application of antibiotic ointment should be stressed to the patient, since scab formation may result in a wider scar.

Bothersome hyperpigmentation may occur in traumatized tissue, especially when it is exposed to sunlight; however, a conservative approach with reassurance is the prudent method for managing these patients.

Tattooing of the traumatized skin is best prevented by rigorous scrubbing of the wound at the time of initial closure. When the material is in the deep epidermis or superficial dermis, dermabrasion may be used. However, an excision of the tattooed area may be necessary when the deep dermis or subcutaneous tissue is involved. Serial excision or use of tissue expansion may be required if the area involved is large and requires the sacrifice of a large amount of tissue.

A soft tissue complication that appears to be directly related to surgical exposure is an antimongoloid slant of the lateral canthi after use of the coronal incision (Fig. 23–4). This is a result of failure to resuspend the upper face and lateral canthi when closing the incision. It can be prevented by wiring the lateral canthi into position in the upper lateral orbit, along with use of heavy nonabsorbable or slowly absorbable suture material to suspend the fascia and soft tissue of the face prior to closure of the galea. Using the coronal incision, we have also witnessed temporal wasting, which may occur as the result of edema and direct trauma to the temporalis

muscle. This may be minimized by careful, nontraumatic technique; minimal cauterization; and proper resuspension of soft tissues.

Special Considerations

NERVES

Cranial Nerve VII. A variety of nerve injuries can occur in the face. Both motor and sensory nerves can be injured, and, depending upon the importance of the individual nerves or branches, more or less attention will be paid to efforts at nerve repair. The facial nerve (cranial nerve VII) is the most important nerve in the face, and great attention therefore is directed to repair of a facial nerve injury.

The facial nerve traverses the lateral face and is therefore vulnerable to penetrating wounds to this area. The facial nerve subtends the muscles of facial expression, and loss of function is thus cosmetically very deforming. Injury to the zygomatic branches that supply the orbicularis oculi muscle results in damage to eyelid function and the potential for corneal abrasion and exposure keratitis, which can result in blindness. Of all the facial nerve branches, the branches to the upper eyelid are the most important and the ones to which most attention must be paid when planning the repair of a facial injury.

Failure to identify an existing facial paralysis and take the appropriate precautions may result in avoidable eye injury. In the unconscious patient, it is crucial to protect the cornea by temporary tarsorrhaphy or

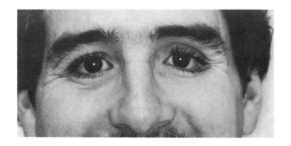

FIGURE 23–4. This patient was referred for secondary repair of panfacial fractures, after a prior attempt resulted in a less than satisfactory outcome. Bicoronal exposure allowed for proper repositioning of the facial bones in three dimensions. However, a mild antimongoloid slant is seen because of healing of lateral canthi in a slightly lowered position. Note also some minimal thinning in the temporal regions.

frequent lubrication and taping until such time as facial nerve function has improved or recovered. Failure to protect the cornea can result in complete loss, necessitating corneal transplantation.

When a facial paralysis has been identified, the surgeon's first concern is to localize the injury. The presence of forehead function in the absence of function of the lower division nerves usually suggests a central facial paralysis. When a peripheral paralysis has been identified, the next priority is to identify the level at which the facial nerve has been injured. In head trauma, a temporal bone fracture may result in trauma to or transection of the facial nerve within the temporal bone. If an area of actual facial nerve disruption or penetration by a bony spicule can be identified on a high resolution CT scan of the temporal bone, then surgical exploration and repair are warranted. In the absence of this finding, most surgeons today have become less aggressive in the management of intratemporal facial nerve injuries.

Facial nerve disruption within the extratemporal portion of the facial nerve is explored and directly repaired. When an injury can be localized to the area of the main trunk or just beyond the main trunk at the area of the pes anserinus, the surgeon must identify the proximal and distal branches to create continuity. If nerve tissue is intact, this can be done by direct end-to-end anastomosis, which generally provides the best long-term result. Damaged edges should be freshened. There has been a lot of controversy in the literature about the timing of facial nerve repair; however, most surgeons now generally believe that repair should be carried out acutely, as soon as possible after the injury.

If any nerve continuity has been lost and tissue is missing, then a sensory nerve is generally sacrificed and used as an interposition graft to gain direct repair of the facial nerve. This should be accomplished by taking an appropriate-sized piece of nerve (commonly the great auricular nerve can be harvested in the neck or the sural nerve from the leg), and this cable graft is sutured without tension to the freshened proximal nerve and distal identified portions.

Surgical repair should be attempted whenever distal branches can be identified. When this is not possible, the use of a sling procedure can be considered. When the injury is quite distal, the sling is not likely to prevent possible spontaneous regeneration. Great care must be taken not to injure the intact proximal nerve.

The nerve muscle pedicle concept has been advocated by Tucker,[37] but this is possible only for the lowermost portions of the facial nerve musculature. Tucker suggests that this approach will allow active nerve firing into the muscles, particularly around the mouth, without preventing any possible regeneration of facial nerve fibers. This may maintain tone and function in these muscles while one waits to see whether facial regeneration will take place.

When the injury is severe and facial nerve loss has been significant, greatest attention should be paid to efforts at reconstructing continuity between the main nerve trunk and the branches to the orbicularis oculi, particularly in the area of the upper lid. When it proves impossible to find branches of the nerve to repair, protection of the eye is most important, as noted earlier.

Other alternatives for facial nerve function include static and dynamic slings. A static sling is generally a fascial sling created from temporalis fascia or fascia lata. It provides static facial tone, offering cosmetic but minimal if any functional improvement.

The dynamic sling is certainly a more popular technique and generally involves muscles that are innervated by the trigeminal nerve (cranial nerve V). The two most commonly used muscles for dynamic slings are the temporalis and masseter muscles.[38, 39] The temporalis muscle can provide support for the lower lid as well as the oral commissure region. The masseter muscle is available for use for the oral commissure, though it is too inferior to be used for the eyelid region. In using these techniques, it is most important to make certain that fascia is used with muscle, not muscle alone, since muscle fibers tend to give over time and the repair will be lost.

Recent developments for repair of facial

paralysis are the microneurovascular free muscle transfer,[40, 41] cross-face seventh nerve grafting,[42] and the combined use of free muscle transfer with the use of the cross-face facial nerve graft.[43] These techniques provide the possibility for mimetic function because the natural facial nerve pathways are being utilized to gain muscle function. However, cross-face grafting also sacrifices some of the function of the normal side in order to supply a donor nerve. This technique is technically difficult and controversial.

A technique for protection of the eye is gold weight implantation. Implantation of a weight or even a spring into the upper eyelid tends to keep the upper lid closed. Since the levator palpebrae muscle is supplied not by the facial nerve (VII) but by the oculomotor nerve (III), eyelid opening remains intact in a facial paralysis. The patient can still open the eye voluntarily, so this does not interfere with function. Recent literature suggests that early intervention of this nature not only provides corneal protection but also does not interfere with facial nerve regeneration or proper function after regeneration has taken place.[44, 45] Finally, a wide variety of procedures exist for improving cosmesis and function in the patient with a facial paralysis, such as face lift, brow lift, lower eyelid shortening procedures, and lower lip excision. It is important to select the appropriate procedure for the individual patient's needs and avoid procedures that may aggravate the patient's condition.[46]

Cranial Nerves III, IV, and VI. Injuries to cranial nerves III, IV, and VI are generally the result of intracranial or orbital trauma. These injuries can result in immobility of the globe and diplopia in various fields. Injuries to the oculomotor nerve (III) also often result in upper lid ptosis secondary to loss of innervation of the levator palpebrae muscle. Although the head and neck surgeon generally will not be intervening for any of these nerve injuries, it is important to differentiate between a nerve injury and a limitation of extraocular motions that would be secondary to entrapment of any of the extraocular muscles in periorbital bone fractures or impingement upon any of these muscles by bone

fragments in the orbit. These nerve injuries are generally treated conservatively. It is important to wait at least 6 to 12 months before considering levator shortening operations and extraocular muscle adjustment procedures, since it is not uncommon for this problem to resolve on its own over time.

Vagus (Cranial Nerve X). High vagal injuries may result from penetrating neck trauma. A high vagal paralysis usually results in a breathy voice and aspiration. Bilateral high vagal injury can result in a loss of the airway, necessitating airway intervention. We treated a patient who sustained a gun shot injury that entered the neck laterally on one side and exited on the opposite side. The vascular compartments were penetrated but not damaged. However, the patient did sustain bilateral high vagal paralysis, resulting in the need for a tracheotomy. This patient's airway problem was not of acute onset but seemed to develop slowly over several days. If a high vagal paralysis fails to recover, typically the problem is a breathy voice that is weak rather than an airway problem. Teflon cord injection or thyroplasty may result in improvement in voice and airway protection.

Recurrent laryngeal nerve injury is most likely iatrogenic secondary to tracheotomy, though it also can be secondary to a penetrating neck wound. Although recurrent laryngeal nerve paralysis has been described secondary to prolonged intubation, this is still a rather controversial finding.[47]

Accessory Nerve (Cranial Nerve XI). Injury to the accessory nerve from neck trauma is uncommon, but it can occur from penetrating neck wounds and from injuries such as when a snowmobile or motorcycle rider hits some type of line. Diagnosis of this injury requires an awareness of its possibility and then noticing the weakness of shoulder function, particularly shoulder shrugging. Failure to recognize and repair this injury will result in a winged scapula. The accessory nerve is a fairly large nerve and usually can be repaired directly if a transection is identified. An avulsion injury is less likely to respond to repair, though one still should be attempted.

Hypoglossal Nerve (Cranial Nerve XII). Like those of the accessory nerve, hypoglossal nerve injuries generally result from directly penetrating trauma to the area of the hypoglossal nerve. We have seen bilateral hypoglossal nerve transection from the "clothes line" type of injury incurred by a snowmobiler. Although they are uncommon, it is important to recognize these injuries to attempt direct neural anastomosis. An index of suspicion will lead to identification by noticing the limited mobility of the tongue and the difficulty that the patient may have with articulation. The tongue will protrude to the side of a hypoglossal weakness. If both hypoglossal nerves have been injured, tongue mobility will be extremely minimal. Direct exploration and repair should be carried out.

Sensory Nerves. Although sensory innervation is considered less critical than motor innervation, patients often find areas of numbness annoying and do seek repair. The most common sensory nerve injury seen in maxillofacial trauma is injury to the infraorbital nerve (V_2) which occurs secondary to fractures in the area of the infraorbital foramen.[48] Injuries to the first division of the trigeminal nerve (V_1) may result from fractures in the area of the superior orbital rim and frontal region. Injuries to the third division of the trigeminal nerve are also commonly seen in grossly displaced fractures of the mandibular body and angle region, since this nerve can be disrupted within the bone.

Repair of the first division should be carried out when disrupted portions of the nerve are visualized within a wound in the frontal region. However, if the nerve is not obvious in the wound, it is generally not considered a high priority concern. Unlike the case with the motor nerves, repair of the surrounding soft tissues usually will allow for spontaneous delayed return of the sensory nerve function over time. For injuries of the second division, the most common cause is trauma and compression as the nerve traverses the orbital floor and infraorbital foramen. Reduction and repair of orbital floor and zygomatic fractures will often decompress these injuries, allowing for either immediate or delayed return of function. As with the first division of the trigeminal nerve, transection of the second division does not necessarily result in a permanent sensory deficit. It is quite common for the nerve to regenerate and ultimately provide partial, if not complete, sensory function over time. In the series of Steidler and associates, 40 per cent of 240 patients with LeFort II and III fractures had disturbances of V_2 at presentation, and only 22 per cent had residual deficits at the time of review.[48] Others report higher persistence rates of up to 46 per cent to 60 per cent.[49] Secondary and delayed decompression of the infraorbital foramen region for persistent numbness is of questionable value, and Nordgaard suggests that surgical technique plays little or no significant role in outcome.[49] However, proper reduction and fixation of zygomatic fractures may minimize the persistence of numbness.[50] Injuries of the third division of the trigeminal nerve are best treated by proper anatomic realignment of the mandible in the area where the nerve has been injured. If the nerve has been stretched, great care is taken to avoid compression of a portion of the nerve within the fracture as it is repositioned.

Another common cause of injury to the trigeminal nerve is iatrogenic injury. Such damage will generally take place during efforts to repair facial injuries. The first division of the trigeminal (V_1) can be injured easily during the coronal approach for exposure and repair of facial fractures. To avoid this, great care is taken to dissect the supraorbital and supratrochlear nerves out of their bony foramina in the superior orbital rim (Fig. 23–5). If these nerves are inadvertently transected during this procedure, direct surgical repair can easily be carried out immediately. The second division of the trigeminal nerve (V_2) can be injured or further traumatized during exposure of the front face of the maxilla from a sublabial approach, as well as the infraorbital rim from above. It is also possible to damage this nerve further during manipulation of fractured fragments in this area. Great care is therefore taken by the operating surgeon to avoid injuring an already traumatized nerve. Finally, and most

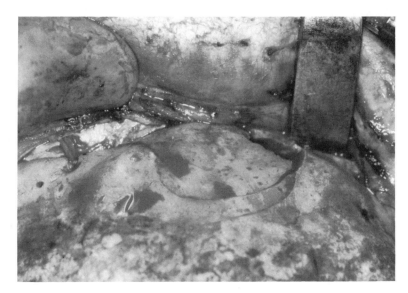

FIGURE 23–5. A bicoronal flap has been elevated for exposure and repair of a depressed frontal fracture. Note that the supraorbital nerves have been freed from their bony foramina so that their function can be preserved.

commonly, the mental nerve is at great risk during open reduction of parasymphyseal and body fractures of the mandible, particularly via the intraoral approach. The surgeon must be careful to visualize this nerve and to provide adequate exposure and dissection around it so as to minimize stretch and tearing during bony repair. If the nerve is in fact transected, reanastomosis is advocated. Great care must be taken not to catch the nerve in the drill when drilling holes in the bone.

Great Auricular Nerve. Although this nerve is generally considered to be less important, injuries here sometimes provoke annoying areas of numbness on the cheek and auricle. The nerve is sometimes sacrificed intentionally (particularly for the repair of motor nerves), but inadvertent injury should be carefully avoided. This nerve also may be injured from a penetrating neck injury; spontaneous regeneration is the most likely outcome.

LIPS

Lacerations

When repairing lip lacerations, the most important aspect of the closure is exact reapproximation of the vermilion border. Failure to do this will result in quite noticeable unevenness of the border. This complication may be corrected using a simple Z-plasty or wedge excision technique. The philtrum also should be carefully approximated.

Full-thickness lacerations should undergo a three-layer (mucosal, orbicularis, epidermis) closure, or notching or depression of the lip will result. Careful approximation of the vermilion and muscle are essential to minimize complications during the healing period. Defects are best repaired using a wedge excision with exacting technique.

Soft Tissue Loss

Some traumatic injuries to the lip involve tissue loss. One must be certain that tissue loss has indeed occurred, since at first appearance complex lacerations may thus appear until the "jigsaw puzzle" has been carefully assessed. Failure to recognize this may result in poor approximation, excessive scarring, and unnecessary sacrifice of healthy tissue. Full-thickness skin loss (not full thickness of lip) may be repaired by a local nasolabial flap when lateral, or a full-thickness skin graft when the loss is more medial. Split-thickness grafts should be avoided, since contracture will occur that may cause foreshortening of the lip. Full-thickness grafts are best harvested from the postauricular or supraclavicular regions for color match. Grafts also should be bolstered carefully, since motion in the lip (which is unavoidable) may result in decreased graft survival. Healing by secondary intent should be avoided when full-thickness loss is greater than 1 square centimeter, since contracture and foreshortening may occur.

Full-thickness tissue loss of the upper or lower lip is repaired with an approach similar to that used for reconstruction after removal of epidermal carcinomas.[51, 52] Soft tissue defects of up to one half of the lip width may be closed primarily. If necessary, edges of the wound may be trimmed and extended to make a straight scar; however, care must be taken not to extend into the mental crease, which results in a more noticeable repair. When the tissue defect is more significant, one must consider employing a lip switch technique, Karapandzic flap, or advancement or distant flaps.[51, 53–55] Great care should be taken to advance enough tissue to avoid the development of microstomia, a complication that will certainly result in an unhappy patient.

AURICLE

Blunt Trauma

Blunt trauma may occur to the auricle in association with other facial trauma, but it is more commonly seen as an isolated injury in wrestlers, boxers, and profoundly retarded patients who exhibit head-banging behavior. The pathophysiology of the injury involves a shearing force between pinna cartilage and perichondrium, resulting in a separation and hematoma formation in this potential space. With time, if allowed to organize, this will result in the formation of new cartilage.[56] The resulting deformity is known as a "cauliflower ear," and it has been noted with some degree of deformity in approximately 39 per cent of WCAA Division 1 wrestlers.[57] Since the perichondrium is the sole blood supply to the pinna cartilage, hematoma formation in the subperichondrial space may also result

in cartilage necrosis with resultant deformity, although this is much less common. Prevention of auricular hematoma is important, and its occurrence can be minimized with the strict use of headgear by wrestlers and boxers. Early recognition, drainage, and prevention of subsequent hematoma are advocated. After drainage, a through-and-through mattress-stitch dressing sutured to dental rolls, as described by Schuller and associates will allow for a rapid return to training.[58]

Lacerations

Lacerations of the auricle can range from simple skin lacerations to a subtotal avulsion with complex through-and-through lacerations of the skin and cartilage. As with all soft tissue lacerations of the face, tetanus prophylaxis should be addressed. Tissue should be irrigated profusely and minimally debrided of skin and cartilage in areas where the tissue is obviously devitalized, to minimize ultimate loss of tissue and support. Wound edges should be approximated meticulously on the pinna to minimize the notching that is commonly seen at the helical rim. When cartilage is involved, attempts to approximate perichondrium separately are often unsuccessful, resulting in denuding the cartilage at the wound edge. We advocate the use of a stitch through both layers of perichondrium and cartilage, with a separate meticulous skin closure, in an attempt to preserve cartilage viability and minimize notching at the helical rim.

Hypertrophic scarring and keloid formation may occur as a complication in patients who have a predilection for this, even with only minor lacerations. Injection with triamcinolone at the time of surgical excision as well as postoperatively may help prevent keloid formation.[59] Some surgeons suggest removal of keloids with the CO_2 laser to minimize recurrence, though the benefits over scalpel removal remain equivocal.

Chondritis is a dreaded complication more commonly occurring after thermal injury. It should be suspected when there is a progressive increase in pain several days into the postinjury period.[60] Early recognition is essential, since extension into abscess formation will result in cartilage loss and significant subsequent deformity. Upon diagnosis, patients should be treated medically with prolonged intravenous antibiotics with gram-negative and gram-positive coverage. Early workers advocated surgical debridement, bivalving the pinna, and complete removal of cartilage, allowing healing by secondary intent.[61] This method is effective; however, total cartilage removal is quite deforming, and recent workers advocate removal only of necrotic cartilage on a daily basis, coupled with continuous irrigation via polyethylene catheters and antibiotic solutions.[62, 63] This method, although labor intensive, is effective and well worth the effort when the sequelae of total cartilage removal and difficulty in total reconstruction are considered.

Avulsions

Avulsion injuries that extend into the external auditory canal may result in canal stenosis. In addition to meticulous soft tissue technique, stenting of the canal for several weeks is recommended in an attempt to avoid this complication. Meatoplasty and canalplasty with skin grafting may be necessary should stenosis occur.

When partial or subtotal avulsion occurs, reattachment with meticulous attention to detail is often a timely yet rewarding procedure, since a rather small intact pedicle may result in no loss of viability. Small, avulsed pieces of less than 2 to 3 cm should be cleansed and reattached as composite grafts.[64] When an avulsion is due to a bite-related injury, Stucker and associates suggested that reattachment as a composite graft will almost uniformly result in failure.[36] These injuries should undergo a delayed reconstruction using an autograft composite from the contralateral ear. When small, a defect of the anthelix and helix may be closed primarily by employing Burrow triangles at the base (similar to a wedge excision), to prevent anterior malpositioning (cupping) of the pinna.

The total avulsion injury is a very difficult and challenging problem that often results in a significant deformity regardless of the reconstructive technique employed. Disagreement among workers regarding the method of choice indicates the limited successes achieved. Some advocate simple reattachment using multiple stab incisions to relieve venous congestion, surface cooling to reduce metabolic requirements, and anticoagulants to prevent clotting.[64, 65] Others report successful results using microsurgical reimplantation,[66, 67] though reports remain anecdotal. When an experienced microvascular surgeon is not available, or when no obvious vessels are present, salvage by dermabrading the skin and reattaching or burying the auricle in a subcutaneous pocket may provide the greatest chance of success.[68] Residual post-traumatic deformities of the auricle are difficult to repair. Skin damage and scar make repair more difficult than primary congenital reconstructions.[69] Modern techniques of tissue expansion and costochondral graft sculpting, along with the creative use of local skin flaps, should provide better results than were previously possible.

EYELID

Lacerations

Only after the patient has had a thorough eye examination should eyelid lacerations be addressed. Wounds are irrigated profusely with normal saline and closed primarily when possible, even when theoretically contaminated. Contaminated wounds are defined as those having a probability of more than 10^6 bacteria per cubic centimeter of tissue. Organism counts generally exceed these numbers in wounds more than 12 hours old or human or animal bite injuries. The standard practice of allowing contaminated wounds to close by secondary intention on the trunk or extremities does not apply to eyelid injuries. Fortunately, the blood supply to this area is excellent, resulting in a very low incidence of infection. Furthermore, scarring associated with healing by secondary intention around the eye is unsightly and often results in a functional problem as well. As with other facial skin wound edges, only nonviable tissue should be removed, and edges of lacerations should not be trimmed routinely. However, when a full-thickness laceration involves the lid margin, a poor closure will result if the skin edges are not freshened (a No. 11 scalpel blade works well for this). The lid margin should be closed with three sutures of 6–0 silk to avoid a corneal abrasion. Sutures are placed at (1) the posterior lid margin, (2) the meibomian gland ducts on the tarsal plate, and (3) the gray line that corresponds to the anterior aspect of the tarsal plate. The remainder of the tarsal plate is approximated in an interrupted fashion with an absorbable suture. Failure to freshen the edges of the lid prior to suture or poor suturing technique likely will result in notching of the eyelid margin. If this occurs, repair is excision of the notched portion of the eyelid with a correct closure. Deep sutures in the orbicularis muscle should be avoided as they may result in scarring, retraction, and ectropion when there is a full-thickness eyelid injury.

Full-thickness skin loss of the eyelid, especially in an elderly patient with excessive skin laxity, sometimes may be closed primarily, with or without a small amount of undermining. If the defect is too large to close without risk of ectropion, the contralateral lid is an ideal donor site for skin. In the younger patient with minimal or no excess skin, a full thickness graft from the postauricular region is an excellent alternative. When full-thickness eyelid loss is less than 25 per cent of the lid, it often can be closed primarily; however, when the loss is 25 per cent to 50 per cent of the lid, a canthotomy and cantholysis may be required to relieve tension and allow closure. When the loss is more than 50 per cent, full-thickness eyelid from the contralateral side should be used as a composite graft to minimize both the cosmetic and functional deficit. When the lid has been avulsed, it should be irrigated and reattached. It has even been suggested that a free piece of eyelid that has been bitten off

should be replaced, since there have been case reports of survival of the retrieved eyelid tissue even after a 24-hour delay in reattachment.

Common sequelae from eyelid lacerations include hypertrophic scarring and cicatricial entropion and ectropion. Conservative measures are employed during the first 6 to 12 months, including massage and triamcinolone injection, along with measures to prevent exposure keratitis. After this time, it is appropriate to consider scar revision. For minor cicatricial deformities, a V- to Y-plasty may be successful; moderate scarring with vertical contracture and entropion or ectropion usually is best treated with Z-plasty.

Lacerations of the upper eyelid, particularly horizontal ones, require careful evaluation. Often edema makes examination and assessment of upper lid ptosis difficult. However, asymmetry of upper eyelid position with greater than 1-mm coverage of the limbus by the upper eyelid may represent a laceration of the levator palpebrae aponeurosis, which, if left unrepaired at the time of closure of the lid laceration, could result in permanent upper lid ptosis. If this occurs, a levator shortening procedure may be required after an appropriate delay (6 to 12 months).

Lacerations in the medial and lateral canthal regions also deserve special attention. On physical examination, the presence of asymmetric lid laxity or a positive "bowstring" test suggests disruption of the canthal tendon. Careful inspection of the wound will reveal the presence of a lacerated tendon. Evaluation and repair are best performed using magnification (loupes or microscope), and a nonabsorbable suture should be utilized for repair. If the tendon is shredded, sutures may be anchored from the periosteum of the orbital rim to the tendon remnant or even to the tarsal plate when no usable tendon remains. When reapproximating medial or lateral canthal tendon injuries, it is important to overcorrect, since not doing so increases the risk of subsequent scleral show and persistent epiphora.

Lacerations in the medial canthal region also can involve the lacrimal system. This often can be suggested by unilateral epiphora, though epiphora may result from edema or tendon disruption without actual lacrimal injury. Careful exploration and cannulation of the lacrimal canaliculi will identify the specific injury. Such injuries should be closed over silicone stents, which should be left in place for several months. Failure to recognize and repair an injury to the lacrimal system often results in stenosis and subsequent recurrent dacryocystitis and epiphora.

NASAL

Soft Tissue Loss

It is particularly important not to sacrifice skin unnecessarily on the nose. Repairing skin loss with local flaps can be difficult, both technically as well as cosmetically, in terms of achieving an optimal outcome. Skin over the nose drapes fairly tightly, and it can be difficult to advance skin to make up for any tissue loss. Therefore, as a first step, any salvageable skin at the time of the initial repair should be saved. Unfortunately, however, sometimes nose skin is either completely nonviable or missing.

When the nasal tissues have been severely torn and disrupted, it may be difficult initially to determine whether or not tissue loss has indeed occurred. First, of course, all attempts should be made to reapproximate the tissues that are present. If it is not clear whether or not tissue loss has occurred, then the tissues should be allowed to heal in position; a decision generally can be made within 7 to 21 days about the developing result. If it appears that cicatrization is resulting in deformities of the nasal contour, then early intervention to release the scar and fill in any skin defects should be considered or progressive changes in the nasal contour and progressive scar tissue deformities may result. This may make later repair more difficult, particularly when there is loss of cartilaginous support with resultant distraction of the nasal cartilage positions. This can be particularly deforming when the nasal ala is involved, and notching of the anterior or lateral ala can be very difficult to repair.

Reconstruction acutely should be aimed at first trying to re-establish the foundation elements of nasal support. One can either immediately replace missing skin or can leave the defect to allow some granulation tissue to heal in before repairing the skin loss. For small defects of the nasal dorsum or lateral nose, healing by secondary intention can sometimes provide surprisingly good cosmetic outcomes. This is also sometimes true in the area of the nasal tip. The alternative is to proceed with immediate repair, which could be performed using either a skin graft or a local skin flap. Loss of the nasal alar margin is a more complex problem and will always require some type of reconstructive procedure. A traumatic loss of alar soft tissue that is not due to a bite wound can be reconstructed immediately. Options include the use of a composite skin and cartilage graft from the auricle or local reconstruction with inferiorly or superiorly based nasolabial flaps. More extensive defects, including the nasal tip and columella, generally are repaired using a forehead flap. Baker suggests that when there is extensive, full-thickness loss of the nasal tip, the forehead flap is the only satisfactory reconstructive technique available (Fig. 23–6).[70] However, when the tissue loss is due to a bite injury, particularly a human bite, most surgeons recommend waiting 7 to 10 days to eliminate any infection risk before going ahead with graft or flap reconstruction of the defect. Nasal tip defects sometimes can be repaired with full-thickness skin grafts from behind the ear or the supraclavicular region. Despite careful attempts at reconstruction of these defects, sometimes scar tissue and unpredictable healing can result in less than completely satisfactory outcomes. Repair of the nasal alar crease can be very challenging and may require Z-plasties and repositioning to try to recreate the normal nasal contour. Lacerations that transect the nasal vestibules are likely to result in nasal stenosis (Fig. 23–7). Careful reapproximation of nasal tissue and use of minimal packing may prevent this complication. It is best treated using intranasal Z-plasties.

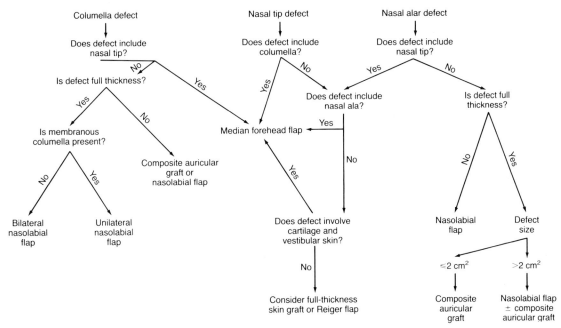

FIGURE 23–6. Algorithm for the repair of defects of the nasal tip, columella, and/or ala, as advocated by Shan Baker. (From Baker SR: Regional flaps in facial reconstruction. Otolaryngol Clin North Am 23:931, 1990.)

Cartilaginous Framework

The cartilaginous framework of the nose is very important to both its structure and function. The most common complication that results from missed diagnosis in nasal trauma is damage to the nasal septum from a septal hematoma or a septal abscess. Whenever a patient presents with nasal trauma, the nasal septum should be carefully examined. This is often done by the emergency department personnel, and it is important that they be educated in how to evaluate the nasal septum. The patient may complain of worsening inability to breathe through the nose or of pain or intermittent drainage, which should alert the physician to evaluate the nasal septum carefully. If it appears swollen or boggy or an area does not appear straight or symmetric, it should be palpated with a cotton-tipped applicator. When in doubt, needle aspiration may reveal the presence of a hematoma. Failure to recognize a septal hematoma can result in devascularization of the septal cartilage owing to elevation of its perichondrium and therefore its blood supply. This in itself can lead to absorption of the

cartilage, or it could lead to the delayed outcome of increased calcification with widening and thickening of the cartilage. If a hematoma becomes infected, then the likelihood of complete degeneration of the septal cartilage, with ultimate loss of dorsal support and saddle deformity, is quite high.

When a septal hematoma has been identified, two alternatives exist. The first is to drain the hematoma in the outpatient setting and then to either suture the mucosa in place with mattress sutures or pack it in place with bilateral nasal packing. Reaccumulation usually will be drained again the next day; a drain and tight packing can be placed and left for several days. The second is the so-called "acute" septoplasty. This is actually a desirable procedure, since it is technically quite easy. The hematoma has elevated the planes so that the surgery is facilitated.

Failure to recognize disruptions of the nasal septum can result in the development of septal perforations. Small perforations are usually asymptomatic, though they may sometimes result in whistling. Larger perforations are more likely to result in crusting and recurrent epistaxis. Large perforations

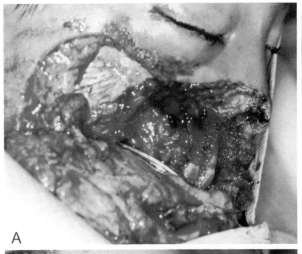

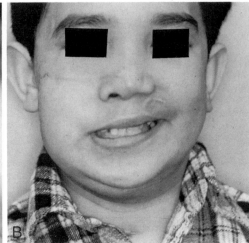

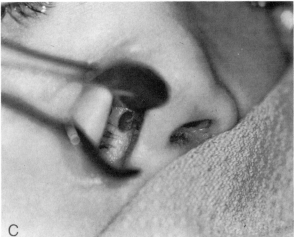

FIGURE 23–7. *A,* A severe degloving injury of the lower face, which included a complete transection of the right nose through the vestibule. *B,* The result after meticulous repair, including primary repair of the multiple facial nerve branches. *C,* Note the dramatic right nasal stenosis that resulted, despite meticulous reapproximation of mucosa. Approximately 60 per cent of the normal airway was ultimately obtained after intranasal Z-plasty.

can be difficult to repair, and they provide much annoyance to both patient and physician.

A loss of septal cartilage results in a saddle nose deformity. The saddle deformity is cosmetically very displeasing and often has been referred to as the pugilist's nose. Repair generally requires bone grafting of the nasal dorsum, though many surgeons advocate the use of various plastic material, including Supramid and Proplast among others. Despite evidence of high resorption rates, irradiated homograft cartilage remains popular as a graft material.[71]

Some of the most difficult problems encountered relate to damage and loss of the upper and lower lateral cartilages. A common problem is the loss of attachment of the upper lateral cartilage to the nasal bone. This happens frequently after nasal trauma and results in valvular collapse, leading to significant valvular stenosis and loss of adequate nasal airway. It also creates the appearance of some cosmetic collapse on that side of the nose, though this tends to be less a problem than the airway obstruction. This complication of nasal trauma is easily missed, underdiagnosed, and also a difficult problem to repair. Valvular stenosis can be repaired most effectively via an external approach using a mattress suture across the top of the upper lateral cartilages. This suture crosses the nasal dorsum from one to the other upper lateral cartilage so that by tying it into position the valves are pulled open. However, this tends to open the nasal valves at the expense of the cosmetic appearance, and it is therefore not a commonly practiced approach. Another approach is to excise the distal edge of the upper lateral cartilage submucosally from an intranasal approach. It is important to make sure that the excision is parallel to the normal direction of the upper lateral cartilage so that the angle of the valve is not altered. Because of the complications of valvular stenosis that occur when there is either mucosal loss or mucosal stenosis in the valve area from communication between intercartilaginous and hemitransfixion incisions, it is probably safest to perform the valveplasty either in isolation or via an external approach septorhinoplasty.

Tip asymmetries are common after trauma to the nasal tip region, particularly if there has been damage to or loss of lower lateral cartilage. Great care should be taken to reapproximate and reposition the upper and lower lateral cartilages in their normal anatomic positions. It is also important to reestablish the relationship between the lower lateral cartilages and the nasal septum. When tip asymmetries result from trauma, the wisest and most successful approach to their repair is the external approach septorhinoplasty. This allows direct visualization of these complex cartilages and therefore allows for optimal repair.

Bone

Probably the most common complication of a nasal fracture is the failure to obtain adequate reduction. One of the commonest causes is delay in treatment. Often by the time the patient is seen the bones have frozen in position, and acute reduction has become difficult, if not impossible. If it is more than a week since the injury, general anesthesia may allow the surgeon to assert greater force in the attempt at reduction of the fracture. Another common cause of inability to reduce the fracture is a pre-existing injury or preexisting nasal deformity. The surgeon may not always be aware of this, in which case it will be difficult to know the reason for the persisting asymmetry. If elevation of the nasal bones and the exertion of reasonable force fail to permit central positioning of the nasal

bones, it is wise to stop and consider open reduction with osteotomies, either acutely or at a later time. In either case, the rhinoplasty allows the surgeon to perform controlled osteotomies and to reposition the bones as desired.

The choice of immediate versus delayed rhinoplasty for the deviated nasal bone that cannot be perfectly repositioned by closed reduction is made by the surgeon and patient. Many surgeons still prefer the more conventional approach of allowing at least 6 months for bony healing and calcification, proceeding with a rhinoplasty at that time. However, the disrupted periosteum may not provide adequate support for osteotomies, which can result in inadequate support of the bony fragments and may compromise the outcome. Furthermore, hairline fractures that are not grossly unstable can be further destabilized by attempts at osteotomy, and this may result in multiple fractures rather than a single clean osteotomy line. Illum has pointed out that of 106 patients with nasal fractures treated by closed reduction, 90 per cent remained fully satisfied 3 years later.[72] Those who prefer the acute approach believe that they are giving the patient a better outcome more immediately and are more likely to have a satisfactory long-term outcome.

Another complication sometimes seen is the open sky deformity, which results from a loss of nasal dorsal bone with a space now existing between the nasal bones. This can be diagnosed by recognizing that the dorsal contour is broad: the individual nasal bones can be palpated instead of meeting a smooth dorsal surface. When adequate dorsal height is present, this can be corrected by performing lateral osteotomies and bringing the nasal bones into position. When adequate dorsal height is not present, a wiser approach is to graft the nasal dorsum. The choice of autograft versus homograft or alloplastic material is up to the surgeon.

When a loss of nasal dorsal bone has occurred, the persistent septum may protrude between the nasal bones and create a sharp ridge along the nasal dorsum. Like the open sky deformity, with adequate dorsal height this can be corrected by excision of the overriding bone and the performance of lateral osteotomies. If the dorsal height is inadequate, it is wiser to graft the dorsum to obtain the proper dorsal contour and height.

A frequently missed injury is the fractured nasal spine. In many cases, this may indeed be an insignificant injury with no instability or airway or cosmetic problem. However, in the patient with a well-developed nasal spine, this injury may result in a loss of tip projection. How serious and important a problem this really is requires research and assessment.

FRONTAL SINUS FRACTURES

Frontal sinus fractures engender a lot of controversy in the literature. Schultz claims that in a large series of frontal sinus fractures over many years, careful reapproximation and reconstruction of the anatomic contour of the fractured frontal sinus will result in normal function; he claims never to have had a complication such as chronic sinusitis or mucocele develop despite the fact that he has never obliterated a sinus.[73] Luce reports a similar experience and conclusion.[74] Others have advocated the routine obliteration of the frontal sinus for any fracture in which the duct is either clearly or possibly involved.[75–76a] This is felt to eliminate the possibility of later frontal sinus disease or mucocele formation. This is a particular concern in fractures through the posterior table in which a mucocele and particularly a mucopyocele can extend into the anterior cranial fossa and result in meningitis. The incidence of such complications is difficult to determine, particularly prospectively, since it is very low.

Alternatives for acute repair include exact bony repositioning without obliteration, obliteration with fat or bone after drilling away all mucosa, or cranialization. Cranialization has been advocated by Donald and Bernstein, who suggested that it is technically easier to remove the back wall when it is severely damaged and allow the brain to fill in that space.[77, 78] However, the brain may

not fill this space, and a dead space may remain in the intracranial cavity. Duvall and associates found a lower complication rate when the posterior wall was reconstructed and the sinus obliterated with fat than with cranialization.[79] Stanley has suggested that the presence of the posterior table provides an additional boundary between the brain, meninges, and nasal cavity, and it is therefore worthwhile to reconstruct it when possible.[76]

When a nondisplaced fracture has occurred, particularly of the posterior table, and the surgeon is uncertain whether exploration and obliteration are necessary, we have used endoscopic exploration via a trephine incision below the brow. The telescope can be used to visualize any disruption in the posterior wall, particularly brain herniation, that may necessitate further exploration. We saw a patient in whom a fracture of the posterior table was believed to be nondisplaced and exploration discouraged by the neurosurgeons. We chose to perform an endoscopy in the intensive care unit by way of a small incision and trephine opening. Brain tissue was seen herniating through this posterior table fracture, and further surgery was therefore mandated.

Frontal sinus mucosa can be trapped in a posterior table fracture, and the potential for an intracranial mucocele is present. Missed fractures can result in communication between the intracranial cavity and the frontal sinus as well as cosmetic defects when an anterior wall fracture is missed. Complications can include CSF leak, which may be associated with meningitis and certainly requires repair. A CSF leak can be repaired via a subfrontal craniotomy or directly through the frontal sinus if it is a small enough tear. With a smaller tear, the osteoplastic flap can be elevated anteriorly, the back wall elevated, and the dural tear repaired directly. The back wall then can be reconstituted, the sinus obliterated, and the osteoplastic flap replaced or reconstructed as needed. Other complications can include epidural and subdural abscess. The worst is cerebritis or brain abscess, often complicated by death.

Late complications include mucocele and

mucopyocele. The incidence is uncertain, but they represent a more serious problem in the presence of a dural communication than when limited to the frontal sinus. Once a mucocele or mucopyocele has occurred, it is best handled via osteoplastic obliteration of the frontal sinus. A CSF leak that occurs or is recognized late is treated primarily via the subfrontal craniotomy approach.

A cosmetic deformity in the frontal area is usually the result of a failure or inability to reconstruct the anterior wall defect primarily. The defects can be easily repaired with either acrylic or bone grafts. Bone grafts in the frontal area are easily positioned and stabilized using either wires or miniplates. The miniplates increase the rigidity of fixation and therefore increase the likelihood of success.

ORBIT

Injuries to the eye and adnexa are common in maxillofacial trauma, and they can be missed easily by the casual observer. In a series of 777 midfacial fractures reported by Holt and associates the incidence of ocular injury (including minimal injuries) was 67 per cent.[80] Eighteen per cent of patients sustained serious visual or adnexal injuries, with 3 per cent resulting in total loss of vision. When total loss of vision occurred, 80 per cent to 90 per cent resulted from injuries to the globe and 10 per cent to 20 per cent occurred as a result of optic nerve injury.[81]

The initial evaluation begins with careful history taking. Families or friends of mute patients should be questioned when a problem with visual acuity exists, since this may have predated the injury. Next comes careful inspection for asymmetry from globe ptosis, enophthalmos, exophthalmos, or asymmetry in the medial canthal region. The orbital region is gently palpated for subcutaneous emphysema, orbital rim stepoff deformities suggesting a fracture, and hypesthesia in the infraorbital distribution of V_2. The anterior aspect of the eye is inspected very carefully for a conjunctival laceration or puncture that may herald an intraorbital foreign body.

A high index of suspicion for an orbital foreign body and confirmation on plain radiograph or CT scan will confirm diagnosis. Materials such as glass, plastic, or lead are best treated conservatively; however, copper and iron must be removed surgically because they are likely to cause a toxic reaction, placing the globe at risk. The anterior aspect of the eye is also inspected for evidence of corneal abrasions, lacerations, or hyphema. A corneal abrasion, one of the most common injuries to the eye, is a partial-thickness loss that is usually suspected in the conscious patient who reports a foreign body sensation in the eye where no foreign body is found, and the examined eye is found to be injected and lacrimating. Diagnosis is made by examining the eye with a Wood lamp after application of fluorescein, which has an affinity for intercellular bridges. Management includes application of an antibiotic ointment or solution, patching the eye, and daily examination until it resolves. Usually no long-term sequelae occur. A corneal laceration should be noted early and urgent ophthalmologic consultation obtained, as edema of the cornea can make closure difficult. Larger lacerations must be sutured, although smaller lacerations may be treated with splinting. Very large stellate lacerations may require an immediate corneal transplantation. The late sequalae of corneal lacerations may include scarring with varying degrees of opacification, sometimes necessitating a corneal transplant.

Hyphema is also a relatively common ophthalmologic complication after penetrating or blunt trauma and is defined as the presence of blood in the anterior chamber of the eye, which layers out when the patient is in the upright position. Bleeding comes from the ciliary vessels of the iris and may account for loss of vision. Treatment is aimed at minimizing increases in intraocular pressure by placing the patient on strict bed rest. The use of carbonic anhydrase and steroids is controversial. When the hyphema is less than 30 per cent, it will generally resolve; however, in hyphemas filling two thirds of the anterior chamber, approximately 70 per cent of patients will have traumatic filtration angle abnormalities and 20 per cent will eventually develop glaucoma.

After examination of the anterior aspects of the eye, the cooperative patient is tested for extraocular movement in all ranges of gaze with any diplopia documented. Although diplopia upon upward gaze often occurs without orbital blowout fractures, diplopia in neutral gaze usually indicates a significant one (or neurologic injury).

Visual acuity is tested next for each eye. With an ambulatory patient the 20-fact Snellen chart should be used; use of the hand-held cards in the immobilized patient is acceptable. Both tests should take into account the patient's refraction, and the patient's glasses should be worn, if possible, when testing visual acuity. When glasses are broken or lost, use of a pinhole card will eliminate the refractive error. If the patient cannot see the letters, documentation should be done with a progression to counting fingers at a distance, to identifying the direction of light, to light perception. When a penetrating injury is suspected, at this point a metal shield should be placed over the eye, with no further manipulation.

The unconscious patient is tested for the presence or absence of a Marcus Gunn pupil. This test is sensitive to an afferent injury of the optic nerve and is done by noting the consensual response when a bright light is shone in the eye. When moving a light back and forth between the eyes, an appropriate response is constriction of the ipsilateral and contralateral pupils. When the flashlight is moved to the suspected eye, dilation of the contralateral pupil indicates a significant afferent injury.

After a thorough examination of the eye and adnexa, any patient sustaining significant maxillofacial trauma should undergo a bilateral dilated fundoscopic examination, provided the patient is neurologically stable. This must be done prior to manipulation of soft tissue during closure of eyelid lacerations or bony tissue in the operating room, since manipulation of an eye with an undetected posterior globe injury or retinal detachment could result in blindness.

Optic Nerve

Penetrating injuries of the orbit often involve the apex, and transection of the optic nerve may occur, since the bony orbit directs the object in this direction. However, most injuries to the optic nerve are the result of closed head trauma. Although fractures at the base of the skull were previously seen in only 50 per cent to 60 per cent of optic nerve injuries, with improved radiologic techniques and routine CT scanning it is becoming evident that these fractures are probably present in all cases of optic nerve injury associated with closed head injuries. The pathophysiology is probably a combination of several factors, including nerve stretching with deceleration, impingement by a bony spicule, hemorrhage, and edema. Regardless of the exact cause in each case, the common pathway is thought to be ischemic necrosis of the nerve by compression.

Evaluation of the patient in whom optic nerve injury is suspected consists of serial visual acuity examinations in the conscious patient. In the unconscious patient or the patient with no perception of light, a Marcus Gunn pupil indicates an afferent injury; however, it is useful in documenting integrity of the optic nerve. Visual evoked responses (VER) are necessary to assess and follow potential decreases or loss in perception. When a documented decrease in visual acuity has occurred (or decreased VER in the unconscious patient), high resolution CT scanning must be done to rule out the presence of an intraorbital hemorrhage that would be treated via canthotomy and anterior decompression of the orbit rather than addressing the optic canal directly. When total visual loss occurs at the time of injury, it is likely irreversible. Medical therapy may be attempted, but surgery is probably not warranted.

When gradual or progressive visual loss occurs, medical therapy should be initiated. Appropriate medical therapy for optic nerve compression consists of megadose steroids (dexamethasone, 0.75 mg/kg load with 0.3 mg/kg every 6 hours) and an osmotic diuretic (mannitol). If response occurs with stabilization or improvement over the subsequent 12 hours, steroids should be continued for a total of 5 days with a rapid taper. In Strohm and Jahnke's literature review, as cited by Osguthorpe and Sofferman, amelioration of amaurosis with medical therapy occurred in 46 per cent, and improvement after operation was seen in 58 per cent.[82, 83] Whenever progression of visual loss is noted, one should consider extracranial optic nerve decompression. Using the transethmoid or sphenoethmoid approaches avoids the risks and complications associated with a transfrontal craniotomy. The low reported morbidity from operation justifies an aggressive approach to optic nerve decompression when medical therapy fails.[84] It has been reported recently that intraorbital (as opposed to intracanalicular) compression of the optic nerve can occur when the orbital plate of the greater wing of the sphenoid presses into the orbital apex after fracture.[85] Repair of the posterolateral orbit via the temporal approach resulted in improvement in visual and ocular function.

Superior Orbital Fissure Syndrome

The superior orbital fissure syndrome is characterized by ophthalmoplegia, lid ptosis, proptosis, and a fixed, dilated pupil, along with sensory disturbance of V_1, due to involvement of cranial nerves III, IV, VI, and V_1. This can occur secondary to orbital/zygomatic trauma and is usually due to edema.[86] When orbital hematoma is the cause, drainage should be instituted immediately. When the optic nerve is involved also, this constitutes the orbital apex syndrome. As noted, this can be due to direct bony impaction, and, in this case, surgical repair with decompression is indicated.[85]

Orbital Fractures

Orbital fractures are common injuries that occur in isolation or in association with other bony facial trauma. Physical findings suggestive of an orbital fracture include gross asymmetry, enophthalmos, dystopia or more commonly periorbital ecchymosis, edema, crepitus, and frequently a stepoff when the orbital rim is involved; subconjunctival hemorrhage, a common finding, generally appears 24 to 36 hours postinjury. The neutral and cardinal positions of gaze should be tested for the presence of diplopia. In the unconscious patient, a forced duction test should be done to examine for entrapment. This is done by gently grasping the conjunctiva with a small pair of toothed forceps at the scleral conjunctival junction and actively moving the eye through the cardinal positions of gaze while noting the resistance to movement in each position.

Blowout Fractures

Fractures involving the orbital floor are commonly referred to as "blowout" fractures. However, one should make the distinction between "pure" and "impure" blowout fractures, since the pathophysiology and management are different. Impure blowout fracture refers to a fracture of the orbital walls in which the orbital rim is also fractured, whereas "pure" blowout fractures are fractures of the orbital wall(s) without orbital rim fractures. The exact pathophysiology of a "pure" blowout fracture is still debated; it may be due to a rapid increase in intraorbital pressure that occurs with a blow to the globe and rims[87]; or it could be a direct compressive or buckling force transmitted through the infraorbital rim.[88] Most likely it is a combination of both, since not only does the floor fracture, but also the weak medial wall frequently gives way.

Recognition and accurate assessment are important to minimize late sequelae. In the early postinjury period, the extent of injury may be difficult to assess due to edema. As edema resolves, the larger floor fractures with significant herniation of orbital fat will result in globe retropositioning and ptosis and resultant cosmetic and functional deformities. Converse and colleagues have indicated that delayed repair of significant blowout fractures is more difficult and is associated with a higher incidence of poor results, including persistent diplopia and enophthalmos, and a higher risk of surgically caused infraorbital and optic nerve injury.[89] Many workers agree that the increased technical difficulty and risk associated with delayed orbital exploration, including the higher risk of failure, mandate earlier surgical intervention for optimal results.[89–91]

However, orbital exploration and repair are not risk-free. Converse and colleagues note a blindness due to posterior placement of an implant,[89] and Nicholson and Guzak reported visual loss in 6 of 72 patients after orbital floor repair.[92] With this in mind, the aggressive approach to blowout fractures has been questioned by Putterman and coworkers.[93] They followed 57 patients with blowout fractures (28 retrospectively and 29 prospectively). Approximately 70 per cent of the patients had diplopia on initial examination; however, only one patient had persistent diplopia in primary gaze. Enophthalmos, generally considered minor when less than 3 mm, occurred in only one patient. These workers discredit the initial physical finding of diplopia on upward gaze and a positive forced duction test and suggest that these findings are due to edema and hemorrhage in the posterior inferior orbital fat pad. They feel all blowout fractures should be managed conservatively for 6 to 8 months, and surgical treatment considered only when significant sequelae have developed after this time period. Furthermore, Putterman argues that the cosmetic and functional deficits associated with blowout fractures can be more safely managed by less invasive procedures than direct repair (e.g., lid shortening, muscle adjustment, contralateral fat excision, discussed later), thereby avoiding the risk of iatrogenic blindness.[94]

In a review of 597 orbital floor fractures, Koutroupas and Meyerhoff[95] showed that complications can be minimized for all groups by carefully selecting patients. Since blowout fractures that need no surgical treatment usually will be asymptomatic within 10 to 14 days postinjury, we support an intermediate approach. After an ophthalmologic consultation to rule out globe injury or retinal detachment, the patient is followed very closely for 10 to 14 days. Exploration and repair are done then for muscle entrapment with diplopia on upward gaze with a positive forced duction test; enophthalmos greater than 2 mm; and large blowout fractures, in which ultimate enophthalmos is likely, as recommended by Manson and Iliff.[96] Coronal CT scanning has been helpful in evaluating large blowout fractures at risk for these complications, based on the degree of orbital expansion and the position of the inferior rectus muscle.[97]

Surgical approaches to the orbit with an isolated floor fracture include the infraorbital (rim), subciliary, and transconjunctival incisions. The infraorbital incision, although technically less demanding and once popular, is currently believed less favorable as it is associated with a poor overall cosmetic result caused by persistent lower lid edema and scarring of the incision and skin to the infraorbital rim. The subciliary incision, in conjunction with a skin muscle flap stepwise through the orbicularis muscle and periosteum, is essentially a blepharoplasty incision; the major advantage is a more acceptable scar. Complications include scleral show and ectropion in approximately 10 per cent of patients in the early postoperative period. This incidence can be decreased by the routine use of a Frost stitch, a suture from the lower lid that is taped to the forehead for 1 to 2 postoperative days, stretching the lower lid. These ectropions often resolve with conservative measures, including massage and warm compresses. The tranconjunctival approach for isolated blowout fractures is probably the most satisfactory cosmetically when performed correctly, particularly in younger patients without excess skin and rhytids.[98] Disadvantages include limited medial and lateral exposure (without canthotomy) and potential injury to the inferior oblique muscle. When a lateral canthotomy is performed, great care must be taken to reapproximate the margins precisely or an unsightly outcome can be anticipated. It is also important to try to stay anterior to the orbital septum when dissecting down to the bone.

Repair of the blowout fracture begins with

elevation of the orbital floor periosteum with good visualization of the floor defect. Care is taken to avoid injury to the infraorbital nerve, which may be damaged as it traverses the orbital floor. Once the orbital contents have been carefully elevated, a graft is designed not only to support the contents and keep them from entering the defect but also to replace the orbital volume as closely as possible.

An approach through the maxillary sinus is acceptable when done in conjunction with a superior approach exposing the floor; however, a sinus approach should never be used alone, since blind manipulation of bony floor fragments creates undue risk for globe injury. Occasionally, such a combined approach is best for a large, comminuted orbital floor fracture, using the subperiosteal dissection along the floor from above together with a transantral exposure of the floor from below. One may manipulate the orbital floor and contents through the maxillary sinus; but this must be done under direct vision from above, since elevation of the orbital contents, including bony fragments, may result in rupture of the globe if done blindly.

A technique advocated in the past is use of a Foley catheter balloon or packing in the maxillary sinus to keep the orbital floor and contents elevated in an extensive blowout fracture.[99] Although this may be helpful in elevating the orbital contents and floor, it does not provide any long-term reconstruction of the orbital floor. Therefore, when the packing or balloon is ultimately removed, there will be no support for the orbital contents, and enophthalmos, diplopia, and globe ptosis likely will recur. In a provocative study by Tovi and associates, antral balloons effectively supported the orbital periosteum in dogs while bone grew across the defect in as little as 3 weeks.[100] However, there is no evidence that the same result occurs in humans. Another complication of this technique is the higher incidence of extrusion and infection when antral packing is used in association with an alloplastic implant for orbital floor repair.[101]

Graft extrusion has been a problem in some series, even when antral packing is not used.[95] However, more recent studies advocating the use of alloplastic materials, including Teflon, Silastic, and Gelfilm, have reported minimal incidences of extrusion and infection, with good long-term results.[102] When using alloplastic materials, some anchoring method, such as a slip of material placed into a bony crevice, will decrease the likelihood of extrusion.

With autologous grafts, many options are available. When a small blowout fracture occurs, a small piece of the anterior wall of the maxillary sinus can be used to prevent entrapment. Advantages of this technique are limited donor site morbidity, easy accessibility, and possibly longevity of the graft. A disadvantage is that with significant trauma, the anterior maxilla may be shattered and unavailable. It also provides only limited amounts of bone for minimal defects. Calvarial bone provides membranous bone with minimal donor site morbidity, particularly when a coronal incision is already being used for reconstruction of the upper face. Animal and clinical studies indicate significantly less resorption over time with membranous bone grafts compared with enchondral bone.[103, 104] However, a disadvantage of calvarial bone is its non-malleability. Grafts from the frontal region leave an unsightly defect, so grafts should be harvested from the parietal region. Care must be taken not to go through the inner table, which can result in a dural tear. A dural tear is repaired with watertight closure, using nonabsorbable sutures. If the calvarial bone graft is harvested too close to the midline, a sagittal sinus tear may ensue that can result in an exsanguinating hemorrhage. Thus it is imperative that the most medial aspect of the graft site be at least 2 cm from the midline.

Other autologous grafting materials that may be used in reconstructing the orbital floor include rib, tibia, and iliac crest. However, harvesting these bone grafts can result in significant donor site morbidities, including pneumothorax and pain on ambulation. A major advantage of rib grafts is their abundance. Furthermore, since split rib is very malleable it can be readily fashioned for complex orbital reconstructions. Mathog[105] and

Tessier[107] favor iliac crest for orbital reconstruction. Mathog and associates advocate the use of carefully designed and strategically placed iliac crest corticocancellous grafts inferiorly, medially and superolaterally.[106] These are meticulously and laboriously positioned around the orbit, since, if enophthalmos is to be corrected, it is important to reconstruct the orbital volume as closely as possible. It is also important to fix the graft in place to minimize the risks of displacement, absorption, and extrusion, as well as the feared risk of posterior displacement and optic nerve injury.

As noted, the operation can result in complications, including decreased visual acuity and even blindness, scarring, ectropion, corneal abrasion, infection, and aggravation or creation of infraorbital nerve injury. Over- and undercorrection of enophthalmos are not rare, and the patient should be warned in advance that revison occasionally may be necessary. Diplopia can be aggravated or created by trauma to extraocular muscles or their impingement by a graft. This latter complication is avoidable by performing duction testing after graft placement. Finally, careful and frequent postoperative evaluation for the first 12 to 24 hours minimizes the chance of missing a postoperative hematoma, which would require emergency drainage to prevent visual loss.

Revision and Adjunctive Procedures

Late post-traumatic enophthalmos and diplopia may result in significant deformity and

dysfunction and may prove difficult to repair. Enophthalmos may occur alone, but it is commonly associated with hypophthalmos and motility problems. Hypophthalmos is commonly more significant when injury to the orbital floor occurs in association with a trimalar fracture with inferior and lateral displacement. Late repair of a significant blowout fracture, or secondary revision operation when a poor result has been obtained initially, is extremely difficult, and results are frequently suboptimal with higher complication rates. Globe traction testing should be carried out to see whether the globe is indeed free to move outward. Tessier reports 15 per cent permanent diplopia after all orbital fractures, and the incidence is 25 per cent if only orbital floor fractures are considered.[107] He suggests that much of the diplopia is due to shrinkage of herniated tissues and retraction of tissues with anchorage to the edges of the defects. This can be improved by freeing these areas of fixation (and sometimes excision of scar along the muscles may be necessary). Enophthalmos is due to an increase in orbital volume and a decrease in volume of the orbital contents.

Delayed repair requires complete freeing of herniated orbital contents, replacing them into the orbital cavity, and grafting of the orbital walls to recreate the original anatomy as closely as possible. For secondary repair, Mathog and associates describe a technique involving the strategic implantation of autologous bone grafts around the orbit (Fig. 23–8). These are placed behind the equator of the globe to push the globe forward and

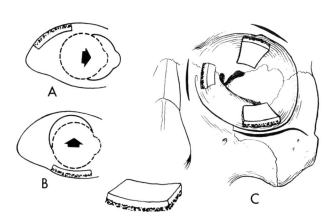

FIGURE 23–8. Placement of incisions and bone grafts, and the forces needed for correction of enophthalmos. Note that in A, insertion of grafts to the superior wall pushes the eye outward, whereas B, insertion into the floor raises the eye upward. C, All grafts contract the intraorbital volume. (From Mathog RH: Reconstruction of the orbit following trauma. Otolaryngol Clin North Am 16:600, 1983.)

reconstitute the normal orbital shape and contour with very good success.[108]

When deep prolapse of orbital contents into the antrum, a very posterior floor fracture, or a previously placed graft interfere with access to the posterior orbital floor, Tessier recommends an inferior orbitotomy.[107] The lateral inferior orbital rim is cut and elevated, keeping the infraorbital nerve and orbital contents superior and the mucosa of the maxillary sinus inferior. This allows wide access to the orbital floor medially, laterally, and posteriorly. Intraoperative duction testing indicates when all adhesions have been freed. Like Mathog's group, Tessier prefers iliac grafts for reconstruction of the orbital walls.

Some patients with significant enophthalmos, measuring greater than 3 mm, have no functional problems but complain of the cosmetic asymmetry. In some of these patients, the cosmetic deformity appears mostly as a narrowed, vertical palpebral fissure height and upper lid ptosis. This can be effectively treated surgically with a Müller muscle–conjunctival resection ptosis repair to create the illusion of exophthalmos and improve the overall cosmetic result as advocated by Putterman and Urist.[109, 110] This will even the palpebral fissures and lid positions. An asymmetric appearance of the upper eyelid resulting from a deep supratarsal fold may be improved by resection of contralateral upper eyelid skin and orbital fat with elevation of the supratarsal crease.[111] Thus, without surgically invading the orbit, the cosmetic benefit of repair can be obtained. Diplopia often can be successfully repaired by appropriate adjustments of the extraocular muscles.

MIDFACIAL FRACTURES

Repair of midfacial fractures can be challenging, particularly when they are complex and comminuted. Initial difficulties may be associated with diagnosis and assessment. Even classification can be challenging, since few fractures fit into classic categories. The most commonly accepted classification of midfacial fractures was first described by René LeFort in 1900.[112, 113] LeFort created midfacial fractures by inflicting trauma on cadaver heads.[114] When the soft tissue was dissected off the bony skeleton, three reproducible basic patterns of fracture were identified (Fig. 23–9).

1. LeFort I fracture traverses the midface above the maxillary alveoli, passes through the piriform apertures, and crosses the pterygoid plates.
2. LeFort II fracture, the most common of maxillary fractures,[115] crosses the nasal dorsum and extends across the medial and inferior orbits, across the anterior and lateral maxillae, and through the pterygoid plates, effectively mobilizing the nasomaxillary areas as a pyramidal segment.
3. LeFort III fracture separates the facial bones from the cranium and is often referred to as craniofacial separation. This fracture crosses the nasofrontal region, enters the orbit medially across the nasomaxillary buttress, involves the orbital floor, then passes laterally through the lateral orbital rim through the frontozygomatic region and involves the zygomatic arch and pterygoid plates.

Most fractures do not follow these exact patterns, and most LeFort fractures indeed represent mixed patterns.[115-117] Klotch and Gilliland noted that this time-honored classification does not address areas of comminution of the facial skeleton, and it fails to consider palatal fractures, fractures of the lower dental arch, cranial injuries, nasoethmoid complex fractures, and orbital injuries.[116] Unfortunately, other proposed classification schemes seem cumbersome. Therefore, despite its limitations, the simplicity of the LeFort classification system has resulted in its continued use. However, the anatomic locations of additional fractures, including cranial, nasoethmoid complex, orbital, palatal, and alveolar, should be identified, along with the degrees of comminution and displacement. In addition, we advocate the use of a trauma work sheet for meticulous

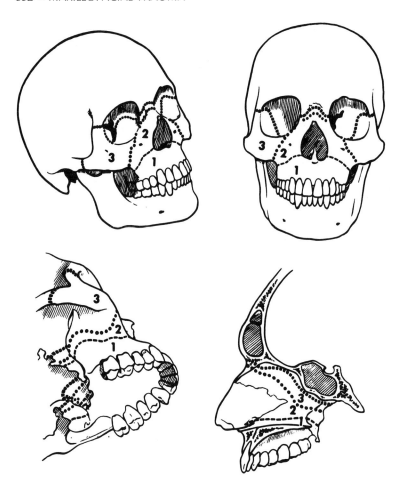

FIGURE 23–9. The classic patterns of fractures of the midface as described by Le Fort. (1) The Le Fort I fracture is considered a transverse fracture of the lower midface. It functions to mobilize the maxillary dentition. (2) The Le Fort II, or pyramidal, fracture includes the nasal root (rather than the piriform apertures). (3) The Le Fort III fracture includes most of the zygomas and traverses the orbits. It thus separates the facial skeleton from the skull base, which is why it is described as craniofacial separation.

Note that most fractures seen today are generally combinations of the three fractures and rarely follow the precise classic pattern as described by Le Fort. (From Dingman RO, Natvig P: Surgery of Facial Features. Philadelphia, WB Saunders, 1964, p 248.)

record-keeping as well as to facilitate any revision that may be necessary later.

The most common complication associated with midfacial fractures is malposition of the fractured fragments resulting from misdiagnosis or nondiagnosis. Unless severe hemorrhage or airway compromise necessitates early involvement of the head and neck surgeon, it is common for facial injuries to be completely disregarded in favor of stabilization of severe neurosurgical and general surgical injuries. Delay in diagnosis leads to delay in treatment; furthermore, repair of facial fractures is sometimes viewed as an elective procedure that should not be performed in the neurologically unstable patient. This failure to address midfacial fractures can lead to permanent malocclusions, cosmetic deformities, and nasal airway obstruction. Orbital deformities and ocular dysfunction may persist as well. Even in the neurologically impaired patient, such deformities and dysfunctions may contribute to patient and family dissatisfaction. Furthermore, chronic malocclusion, trismus, and difficulty with mastication can lead to difficulty with nutritional intake, even in the neurologically impaired and nursing home–bound patient.

To minimize the missed diagnosis, the brain CT should be extended to include at least cursory views of the face. This scan can identify fractures, so that the need for further evaluation will be recognized.

Severe deformity and malocclusion often can be prevented by early use of intermaxillary fixation (IMF). Even in patients too unstable to undergo extensive and thorough fracture repair, the placement of arch bars and sometimes Ivy loops or Ernst ligatures may provide enough stabilization to result in a more reasonable occlusal relation, and sometimes even reduce the fractures. Early disimpaction of midfacial fractures with placement of IMF may simplify later repair, when a delay in such repair is necessary.

When a CT scan cannot be obtained, certain signs of facial injury should alert the examining physician to the possibility of midfacial fractures. Facial edema, ecchymosis, mobile or broken teeth, and malocclusion when it can be recognized are suggestive. These may be difficult to identify in the intubated patient. Palpation of the facial bones may indicate gross asymmetries and stepoffs. The patient should be examined for midfacial mobility by placing the nondominant hand firmly over the frontal region and grasping the lower midface with the dominant hand and gently rocking the midface. If midface mobility is equivocal, the diagnosis will be made on CT scan. The area of mobility will help identify the level of the fracture. In LeFort I injuries, the palate and maxillary alveoli will move; with LeFort II (pyramidal) fractures, the nasomaxillary regions will move while the zygomatic areas will remain stable; mobility of the entire facial region separately from the cranial vault indicates a LeFort III type of fracture. Although the clinical examination provides an indication of the fractures, these should be confirmed on CT scan before planning repair.

The quality and technique of CT scanning can be a problem source. Fractures can be missed easily for technical reasons. In some centers, 5-mm CT cuts are utilized. Gross fractures can be visualized with this technique, but many will be missed; at least 3-mm slices should be obtained, and preferably 1.5-mm high-resolution scanning should be performed if maximal information is to be obtained.[118] Furthermore, high-frequency artifacts from dental fillings and metal appliances can interfere with fracture visualization, as can fracture lines parallel to the scanning plane.[119] The coronal scan direction is of great importance for visualizing fractures of the orbital floor and palatal fractures. Unfortunately, however, direct coronal scanning may be impossible in the multiply injured patient, particularly in the presence of a potential c-spine injury. Finally, three-di-

mensional (3-D) CT scanning can enhance the surgeon's sense of the injuries and thereby aid in planning surgical repair.[120–122] However, it is important to keep in mind that the 3-D scan is a reconstruction and thus implies the potential for added and subtracted information by the computer as the 3-D view is created. Again, narrow slices are critical for gaining adequate information, and at least 1.5-mm sections are recommended.[123, 124] Just as the coronal and axial scans may contain different information, so will reconstructions from each of these scanning angles, and different amounts of information will be lost as well. From the work of Levy and associates, it appears that for the best 3-D reconstructions axial scans should be used for zygomatic fractures and coronal scans for LeFort fractures.[118, 125] However, due to artifact and information loss, a 3-D CT scan should not replace careful review of the two-dimensional scan; and both axial and coronal scans should be obtained if needed.

Associated Complications

AIRWAY OBSTRUCTION

In an excellent review by Thompson and coworkers, 117 consecutive patients suffering LeFort fractures were studied.[126] Of these, 26.5 per cent required emergency airway intervention. Airway compromise was seen in 17 of 39 patients with LeFort III fractures.

BLEEDING

Severe and potentially exsanguinating hemorrhage may indicate skull base fracture or potential internal carotid injury. One must also consider the possibility of major vessel laceration with bleeding into the pharynx or hypopharynx. Bleeding from fractured facial bones usually will tamponade. Proper management consists of establishment of an artificial airway, followed by initial tamponade of the bleeding with packing of the mouth and pharynx. Further evaluation and management can then be carried out. In extreme cases, angiography may prove helpful.[28]

CSF LEAK

CSF rhinorrhea in association with midfacial fractures is most likely secondary to a fracture of the cribriform plate. However, other sources of leakage should be ruled out. A fracture of the posterior table of the frontal sinus can result in CSF drainage into the frontal sinus and nose. Fractures through the roof of the ethmoid sinuses can produce the same phenomenon. Skull base fractures, including fractures in the sphenoid and temporal bones, also can be the source. CSF otorhinorrhea through the ear and eustachian tube into the nose will be missed unless it is suspected.

CSF leakage is quite common with LeFort II and III fractures. In their series of 240 midfacial fractures, Steidler and colleagues reported a 47 per cent incidence in LeFort III and a 33 per cent incidence in LeFort II fractures.[48] Fortunately, 60 per cent of these resolved within 3 days of diagnosis, and dural repair was needed only in 14 per cent. Diagnosis, however, requires a high index of suspicion.

The approach to CSF rhinorrhea remains controversial. Early reduction of the fractures is advocated, which may be enough to stop the leak, though whether this is adequate treatment still remains controversial. Some neurosurgeons advocate the repair of all CSF leaks via a craniotomy approach. On the other hand, the repair of ethmoid and cribriform leaks using nasal mucosal flaps, as advocated by Montgomery, has proved successful in many cases.[127] Posterior frontal sinus leaks can be repaired during the frontal sinus repair,[74, 76, 76a] and temporal bone leaks sometimes can be repaired via mastoidectomy.

The use of prophylactic antibiotics is controversial as well, though most clinicians favor them. It has been argued that broad-spectrum antibiotics can put the patient at risk for a resistant meningitis. This risk could be balanced by a decreased risk of meningitis. Unfortunately, adequate prospective data to answer this question are not available.

CSF rhinorrhea may present as a delayed complication. In this instance, it is most important to proceed with a careful diagnostic evaluation to identify the location of the leak specifically. Gamma cysternography or metrizamide scanning is generally necessary. When an extracranial approach to repair is planned, a preoperative injection of fluorescein via lumbar puncture will help identify the leak at the time of surgery. Cribriform leaks now can be successfully closed using endoscopic surgical techniques.

CRANIAL NERVE INJURY

The most common cranial nerve injury is to the second division of the trigeminal, V_2. In the review of 240 midfacial fractures by Steidler and group, approximately 40 per cent of patients with LeFort II and III injuries had an infraorbital sensory defect on initial examination, and approximately 22 per cent of these persisted.[48] Although repair of this nerve is rarely advocated, documentation of injury is warranted. When a crushed nerve is identified at surgery, decompression is appropriate. Care must be taken during elevation of the tissues from the front face of the maxilla and the orbital floor so as not to create or aggravate an injury.

Anosmia occurred in 2 per cent of patients in Steidler's series, but this number increased to 5 per cent when the effects of surgical treatment (i.e., craniotomy) were included.[48] If it does persist, there is no specific treatment unless it is due to obstruction of the olfactory groove in the nose, in which case surgical repair of the airway may result in improvement. If the olfactory nerves have been damaged, no improvement should be anticipated, though it is believed to be possible.[128]

Cranial nerves III, IV, and VI can be injured in the orbit, the so-called superior orbital fissure syndrome. This may occur in up to 2 per cent of facial fractures. Management is conservative (unless it is due to compression of the posterolateral orbit by a depressed fracture, as described by Funk and colleagues[85]), and improvement is generally anticipated. With diplopia, it is important to distinguish between neuromuscular injury and rectus muscle entrapment.

INTRACRANIAL COMPLICATIONS

Intracranial complications generally result from associated injuries rather than facial trauma. However, iatrogenic injury at the time of facial fracture repair can occur. As noted, intracranial complications can occur when harvesting calvarial bone for grafting purposes. Proper and careful techniques should avoid such complications.

SINUSITIS

Despite the involvement of the maxillary sinus in all these fractures, sinusitis is not the rule. However, when it occurs in the multiply injured, critically ill patient, it can be a source of sepsis and even death.[129] It can be related to nasal instrumentation as well as trauma, and an indwelling nasogastric or nasotracheal tube can be the source.

Since prophylactic antibiotics are used routinely in these fractures, it is hard to determine what the infection rate would be otherwise. In a prospective study by Chole and Yee of 101 facial fractures, cefazolin given in two single doses, one pre- and one postoperatively, resulted in a reduction in the infection rate from 42 per cent to 9 per cent; however, this series involved primarily mandibular fractures, and all infections occurred in the mandible.[130] When an infection does occur, drainage followed by culture and specific antibiotic treatment is advocated. Nasal tubes, of course, should be removed.

POOR OUTCOME

Outcome analysis for midfacial fractures is difficult since no uniformly accepted standards for analyzing results exist. While an obviously excellent result would imply precise reconstruction of the preinjury cosmetic appearance along with a normal preinjury functional status, such a perfect outcome is rare. However, "normal" facies without obvious asymmetry with normal ocular, nasal, and occlusal function should define an excellent outcome. Analysis of results in the literature is difficult, since an excellent outcome may be defined as a satisfied patient or no gross dysfunction or asymmetry. A truly un-satisfactory outcome, however, implies a significant cosmetic or functional deformity, and great efforts should be made to avoid this result. It is important to keep in mind that as techniques improve, expectations will change as well. Manson[131] cites four advances that have revolutionized the treatment of facial fractures in recent years:

1. better CT scanning;
2. the frequent use of bone grafts to recreate facial skeletal support;
3. extended exposure allowing for better repositioning of fractured fragments; and
4. earlier treatment.

In addition, we believe that the addition of rigid skeletal fixation has allowed for more precise and stable repositioning of the fractured fragments. These advances must also be viewed in historical prospective. Not only do better techniques imply better treatment outcomes, there is also the elimination of techniques that may have contributed to poorer outcomes in the past.

CRANIOFACIAL SUSPENSION WIRING

This technique was introduced by Adams in 1942, and it has been until recently the mainstay for repair of midfacial fractures.[132] A problem in untreated midfacial fractures was facial elongation, and craniofacial suspension wiring was developed to prevent this complication. Unfortunately, many surgeons neglected to perform further open reduction along with it. Tightening of the suspension wires, particularly in severely comminuted facial fractures, often produced facial foreshortening and rotation with a loss of dorsal nasal height and an ultimate anterior open bite.[115, 133–135] Ferarro and Berggren found late posterosuperior maxillary displacement in 62 per cent of LeFort fractures that had been treated using craniofacial suspension.[136] To counteract these effects, Kufner suggested frontal cranial suspension wiring as an improvement in technique.[137] Ultimately, however, the best approach has been wide surgical exposure and direct repair. Craniofacial suspension wiring, when used in combination with meticulous direct bony repair, may indeed add stability.[135, 138] However, the use of rigid skeletal fixation combined with the judicious use of bone grafts will obviate the need for suspension altogether.[50, 115, 133]

MALUNION/MALOCCLUSION

A malocclusion as a result of a midfacial fracture indicates the presence of a malunion. A severe malocclusion can be a significant functional problem and may even make chewing impossible. Clearly, as noted, a failure to treat due to patient instability often can lead to devastating malocclusions that may prove exceedingly difficult to correct later. Early intermaxillary fixation, even in the absence of total facial fracture repair, is strongly advocated to minimize the occurrence of this complication.

Malocclusion also can result from failure to recognize or maintain the proper occlusal relationship at the time of repair. For example, proper intermaxillary fixation (IMF) may be applied, followed by craniofacial suspension wiring. As the suspension wires are tightened, the midface may be foreshortened and rotated. Since the patient is in IMF, the surgeon may believe that the appropriate occlusal relationship is being maintained. However, it is possible to pull the mandible forward as the craniofacial suspension wires are being tightened. The patient may seem to be in excellent occlusion during the healing period. However, when the intermaxillary fixation wires are released, the mandible will revert to its proper position, and an anterior open bite results. Again, this complication is best avoided by direct open reduction of the midfacial fractures, taking care not to foreshorten the midface when maxillary bone is missing. Recognition of bone loss and repair with calvarial or rib grafts will increase the likelihood of a good result. Care also should be taken to see that the mandible is in a neutral position during repair.

In palatal or split alveolar fractures, application of intermaxillary fixation using arch bars can inadvertently result in lingual displacement of the segments. Since the arch bars sit above the level of the maxillary dentition, it should be apparent that the downward pull exerted on the arch bar by wires or rubber bands can also create a lingual version of free-floating alveolar fragments. When this potential problem is recognized preoperatively, an occlusal splint can be manufactured to help avoid it. Rigid fixation also may help decrease the likelihood.

Of course, the presence of mandibular fractures in combination with maxillary fractures adds to the technical difficulty of identifying the proper position and thereby increases the likelihood of a malocclusion postoperatively. Technical skill, experience, preoperative planning, and the use of dental models, articulators, and splints, along with meticulous attention to detail, will minimize postoperative occlusal discrepancies.

Failure to recognize the proper occlusal relationship at operation will increase the likelihood of an unsatisfactory outcome. We believe that in some cases even the most skilled and careful surgeon will not always be able to obtain the desired outcome. Then revisional surgery combined with appropriate orthodontic and prosthodontic intervention should provide the best result possible. Finally, when rigid fixation has been used to repair fractures of the midface or mandible, a helpful hint is to release the intermaxillary fixation at the end of the procedure and allow the mandible to go through passive opening and closing maneuvers. With the patient relaxed, the mandible should close easily into a normal occlusal relationship if the repair has been accomplished effectively with proper positioning of bone fragments. Any significant discrepancies seen should be addressed at this time rather than allowing healing to occur with the bones in an improper position. Note that no matter how good the bony position seems during direct exposure, visualization, and repair, it is still imperative that intermaxillary fixation be used during the surgical repair, even when it is to be released at the end of the procedure. If this is not done, the likelihood of iatrogenic malocclusion is extremely high.

Facial Elongation and Dish Face Deformity. As noted, concerns for facial elongation after LeFort fractures prompted the use of craniofacial suspension. In fact, facial elongation is more likely to be the result of an unrepaired or grossly malpositioned fracture.

The dish face deformity is a result of inadequate repositioning of the midfacial bones. With loss of posterior support in the sphenoid and pterygoid regions, the midface can be pulled posteriorly, and there are no natural anatomic stops in such fractures to prevent this.

Most important in prevention is an adequate preoperative evaluation, including clinical and CT evaluations, allowing for proper planning of the surgical repair. When necessary and feasible, the operation can be planned on dental models and splints devised as needed. The extended exposure provided by the coronal flap, combined with the sublabial degloving incision, allows for excellent direct exposure of the fractures to be repaired. This technique, advanced by the early work in craniofacial reconstructive surgery,[139] has been advocated by many as the ideal approach to craniomaxillofacial trauma.[131, 138, 140–143] Once the bones have been exposed, attention is given to reconstruction of the normal anatomic relationship. Repair is carried out from the stable bones to the unstable[141] or, as described by Champy and colleagues,[144] from the periphery toward the center. The facial buttresses are re-established as described by Manson and colleagues[115] and Stanley.[135] Midfacial position must be re-established in all three dimensions, using the zygomatic arches to define anteroposterior dimension, the frontozygomatic and zygomaticomaxillary buttresses for posterior vertical dimension, the frontonasomaxillary buttresses for anterior vertical dimension, and the palate and anterior maxillae inferiorly and the malar eminence buttress across the midline to define the lateral dimension. Wherever the critical buttress bone is deficient, it should be replaced with bone grafts that are rigidly fixed in place.[145, 146] A bone graft fixed in place at either end with lag screws will serve the dual purpose of providing a means of rigid fixation while also providing bone substance to heal across the defect. Furthermore, it has been demonstrated that rigid fixation

via lag screws will decrease ultimate resorption of the bone graft.[147] Finally, proper attention to bone fixation technique will create maximal stabilization of the fractures and decrease the likelihood of delayed malposition of the bony segments after release of intermaxillary fixation.

When less stable techniques are utilized, such as intermaxillary fixation and craniofacial suspension or external fixation, particularly with a head cap or halo device, maxillary retrusion after release of the fixation can occur. It is unclear how rapidly maxillary fractures heal completely. Until recently, many have accepted the belief that the maxilla heals by fibrous union only and not by bony union; however, recent data suggest that solid bony union occurs.[148] In 10 consecutive patients who underwent biopsy during secondary repair of maxillary fractures, Thaller and Kawamoto found evidence of solid bony union.[148] However, the shortest time interval before secondary repair was 9 months, so it is certainly possible that bony union in the midfacial region takes longer than the traditional 6- to 8-week fixation period. This would explain why secondary deformities may develop after removal of intermaxillary fixation or head cap devices. Rigid fixation and bone graft techniques should minimize the occurrence of this late complication.

When a severely comminuted midfacial fracture is combined with bilateral subcondylar fractures of the mandible, there is no template to help define the vertical dimension of facial height. In this situation, the likelihood of facial foreshortening is dramatically increased, and great care must be taken to avoid this complication. It becomes imperative that at least one, if not both, of the subcondylar fractures be directly opened and repaired so that the vertical mandibular height may provide a template to define the proper midfacial position. The maxillary buttresses must then be bone grafted to make certain that the proper result not only will be obtained but also persist long term.

NONUNION

Depending on how nonunion is defined, it may or may not occur frequently in the midface. As noted, the maxilla frequently may heal in a slow fashion with fibrous union persisting for a lengthy period of time. If biopsied during this time period, the fibrous union could be interpreted to be a nonunion. However, long-term persistent mobility after midfacial fracture is extremely rare. When it occurs, the best approach is direct periosteal exposure via the sublabial approach, followed by debridement of the area, primary bone grafting, and rigid fixation. When rigid fixation techniques are properly utilized initially, along with usc of bone grafts when necessary, nonunion should be a very rare problem indeed.

DELAYED MAXILLARY HYPOPLASIA

Fortunately, midfacial fractures are relatively uncommon in the pediatric age group, especially in the younger child.[149] The specific effects of trauma on facial bone growth are not well known; however, case reports of impaired midfacial bone growth resulting in maxillary hypoplasia in patients who had midfacial fractures repaired as children suggest that this problem occurs.[150] The results of craniofacial surgery for congenital anomalies suggest that patients should do well after proper bony repair. It is thus unclear whether delayed problems are due to the specific nature of the trauma involved, or whether they may relate to subtleties in the repair process. Delayed repair will, of course, entail carefully planned osteotomies and repositioning.

MISCELLANEOUS COMPLICATIONS

Other complications associated with LeFort fractures include orbital and nasal complications, malar malpositioning, dental complications, lacrimal problems, and problems related to bone graft resorption and infection. These are discussed elsewhere in the chapter.

Certain problems may be directly related to the surgical repair itself. Infections can be seen along the route of passage of percutaneously placed suspension wires. These can occur at the time of initial passage or when the wires are removed. Oral antibiotics will

usually resolve this problem, though we have seen one parotid space abscess. If care is not taken to saw through the tissues when suspension wires are placed, dimpling of the skin may occur in the area over the zygomatic arch. Facial nerve injury to the zygomatic branch is also theoretically possible, though this has not been described. The bicoronal approach to the upper face has some unique complications. Failure to resuspend the soft tissues of the cheek at closure can result in drooping of the cheek prominence. This can be mistaken for inadequate repair of the malar eminence, when it is in fact a soft tissue problem. Excessive trauma to the temporalis muscle can result in temporalis wasting. It is recommended that the lateral canthal ligament be resuspended within the upper lateral orbit after complete detachment and bony repair via the coronal approach. Failure to do so can result in an antimongoloid slant to the palpebral fissures postoperatively (see Fig. 23–4). Finally, injury to the temporal branch of the facial nerve can be caused by elevation of the coronal flap in too superficial a plane over the temporalis fascia. This nerve runs just superficial to the superficial layer of the temporalis fascia. If great care is taken to elevate this layer with the flap, nerve injury should not occur.

DELAYED REPAIR

When an unsatisfactory outcome has resulted due to nonrepair or unsatisfactory repair of midfacial fractures, each case must be carefully individualized and an appropriate repair planned. Minor facial asymmetries can sometimes be repaired using simple augmentation grafts for the apparently deficient area. Grafts can be autografts or alloplastic implants, according to the surgeon's preference. More significant discrepancies will generally require osteotomy and repositioning of the malpositioned bones. A marked occlusal discrepancy due to loss of maxillary bone may require LeFort osteotomy, along with bone grafting of the defective area, to assure long-term healing and a permanent result. With gross malpositioning of LeFort II and LeFort III fractures, carefully planned osteotomies can be carried out, as done in congenital craniofacial anomalies.[107] As with the primary surgery, careful attention to preoperative planning is critical. Dental models should be prepared, and the osteotomies should be planned and tested on an articulator. CT scanning (including 3-D scanning when indicated) helps in the surgical planning. As in the initial repair, bone grafting to any defective areas will be necessary, and grafts should be used as needed to replace orbital volume. The patient must be advised of the potential risks before the decision to proceed with this operation is made. Ocular injuries are of course possible, as is the reactivation of an already previously sealed CSF leak.

ZYGOMATIC ARCH/TRIMALAR FRACTURE

The trimalar (tripod) fracture can vary from the most mild requiring no repair whatsoever to the most severe with associated significant disruption of the orbit and interference with mastication. Other than orbital injuries (which are discussed in detail elsewhere), complications generally will be due to inadequate repair. This can be the result of delayed presentation of the patient for medical help, inadequate assessment of the severity of the injury, or inadequate repair. The availability of high-resolution CT scanning has made the underdiagnosis of associated orbital injuries or even the presence of displacement of a trimalar fracture less likely.

The following complications may be encountered.

Trismus. This most often results from pressure of a depressed zygomatic arch into the temporalis muscle. Some patients experience pain on closing, owing to inability of the coronoid process to fit comfortably under the fractured arch. This usually can be relieved by elevating the zygomatic arch into its proper position. Delayed repair may necessitate wide exposure and osteotomy of the bone for proper repositioning. Chronic fibrosis or calcium deposition in the muscle may

require surgical relief. The coronoid actually can fibrose to the zygomatic arch, causing ankylosis, which can be repaired via intraoral coronoidectomy.

Flattening of the Malar Eminence. This may be due to nontreatment, inadequate repositioning of the zygoma, or even perhaps delayed displacement over time because of failure to properly fix the zygoma in place after reduction. The incidence of facial asymmetry after zygomatic and midfacial repair has been reported to be as high as 24 per cent.[151] A mild deformity may require no intervention. A moderate deformity can be handled either via onlay grafting with autograft bone or alloplastic augmentation; in a more severe case, osteotomy and repositioning of the zygoma may provide the best results.

Widening of the Lateral Dimension. Like flattening of the malar eminence, widening of the lateral dimension is due to malposition of the zygomatic tripod that has been retrodisplaced. Failure to re-establish the anteroposterior dimension along the zygomatic arch can produce this problem, along with flattening of the malar eminence. A disturbing orbital dystopia may be seen as well (Fig. 23–10). Gruss attributes this classic asymmetry—malar flattening, inadequate AP projection of the malar eminence (seen in tripod and LeFort III fractures), and facial widening in the horizontal dimension—to inadequate surgical exposure and fixation.[152] Since many fractures are repaired using minimal surgical exposure and even one-point fixation,[153] some are bound to be undertreated. The keys to good results are proper preoperative assessment, adequate exposure, including the coronal flap when necessary, and adequate fixation, generally at least two-point rigid fixation for an unstable fracture.[154]

When this problem is seen in the secondary case, the surgical approach is the same. Careful preoperative assessment, combined with wide exposure, osteotomies, adequate fixation, and the judicious use of bone grafts, should provide optimal long-term results.

Caveat. All the aforementioned complications have been seen in patients after seemingly adequate repair of displaced zygomatic

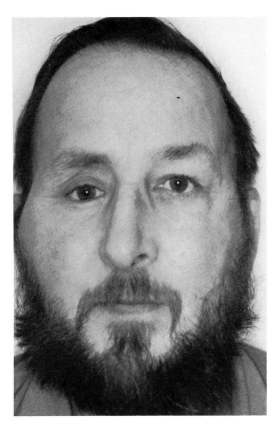

FIGURE 23–10. The extent of this patient's original injuries are uncertain, but it is believed to have included a complex Le Fort III. Analysis of his present appearance reveals widening of the lateral dimension, right orbital dystopia, and malposition of the right malar prominence. This result can be attributed primarily to failure to achieve proper repositioning of the zygomatico-orbital complex, presumably owing to moderate exposure, three-dimensional analysis, and possibly fixation.

tripod fractures. Prior to routine CT scanning, complete and adequate assessment of the extent of injury was difficult. Routine use of CT scans in evaluation of these injuries allows identification of orbital components as well as aiding the surgeon to identify a loss of AP projection. Attempts to utilize shortcuts, including minimal surgical exposure and fixation, increases the risk of unsatisfactory results. (The idea that antral packing can be used to stabilize a tripod fracture is mentioned only to be condemned.) The surgeon repairing the zygomatic tripod fracture must be willing to provide wide exposure, particularly of the zygomatic arch, when necessary;

there must also be a willingness to explore the orbit whenever needed. In addition to exposure of the lateral orbital rim and zygomatic arch, sublabial exposure of the zygomaticomaxillary region aids in the proper three-dimensional positioning of the zygomatic bone. A compression plate at the frontozygomatic area generally provides reasonably rigid fixation, and this can be significantly enhanced by fixation of the zygomaxillary buttress as well.[154]

Infraorbital Nerve Paresthesia/Anesthesia. Infraorbital nerve injury is commonly seen in association with the zygomatic tripod fracture. Persistent anesthesia is a questionable indication for open reduction and decompression, though it makes sense when there is CT evidence of a fracture that is directly impinging upon the nerve. Proper realignment of the zygomatic bone with rigid fixation seems to provide the highest likelihood of recovery of infraorbital nerve function.[50] Persistent paresthesia and anesthesia, while sometimes annoying, is generally well tolerated by patients. Care must be taken not to injure an intact or bruised nerve during repair of the zygomatic tripod fracture. In addition to possible injury when elevating the mucoperiosteum off the front face of the maxilla, the nerve is at risk during repair of the orbital floor. When the orbital floor has been disrupted by trauma, the nerve is frequently exposed and can be injured during orbital floor exploration and grafting.

Orbital Complications. The zygoma contributes anatomically to the floor and lateral wall of the orbit as well as to the inferior and lateral orbital rims. The orbit is therefore involved in all zygomatic tripod fractures. Due to the risk of globe injury, an ophthalmology consultation is recommended prior to repair. In some instances (e.g., retinal detachment or ruptured globe), the fracture repair may need to be delayed until the ocular injuries have stabilized. The appropriate secondary repair can then be carried out.

When there has been significant disruption of the orbital floor, globe ptosis and enophthalmos may ensue. Diplopia may occur owing to entrapment of the inferior rectus muscle in a crack in the orbital floor or secondary to a change in globe position. Globe ptosis and enophthalmos generally respond to reconstitution of the orbital shape and volume via grafting, using either autogenous bone (which we prefer) or an alloplastic implant. Diplopia sometimes is the result of direct neuromuscular injury and may not respond to orbital reconstruction. It is wise to inform the patient of this possibility preoperatively, since this can avoid patient dissatisfaction and complaints.

Another deformity sometimes seen is depression of the lateral canthus, due to depression of the lateral orbital rim bone to which the canthal ligament is attached. Proper repositioning of the bone generally solves this problem. Sometimes this is the result of extensive surgical exposure via the coronal approach, with complete detachment of the soft tissues from the bone. This can be improved by wiring in its proper position the lateral canthus to the inner portion of the upper lateral orbital rim.

Mild enophthalmos sometimes can be disguised by performing an upper lid shortening to create a symmetric, vertical palpebral fissure distance bilaterally. This may obviate the need for a more aggressive orbital exploration and grafting procedure.

Finally, lower lid ectropion can occur from failure to rebuild a depressed infraorbital rim, or from unsatisfactory healing of a lower lid incision used for approaching the orbital rim or cavity. This complication seems to be most common with the subciliary incision, and more common when the infraorbital rim has been inadequately repositioned. It can be repaired by lower lid shortening and lateral canthopexy, with suspension of the tarsus to the lateral rim periosteum. Full-thickness skin grafting from another eyelid sometimes may be necessary when skin loss has occurred. The incidence of this problem should be diminished by using the transconjunctival approach.

NASOETHMOID INJURIES

Early

The most common problem with nasoethmoid fractures is failure to diagnose the injury. The nasoethmoid complex fracture can vary from a fairly minimal injury to the most dramatic with complete loss of the nasal dorsum and telecanthus. Subtle injuries can be overlooked easily and underdiagnosis, of course, leads to undertreatment. High-resolution CT scanning has made the diagnosis of the nasoethmoid complex fracture easier and more likely. Clinically, however, it remains important to test for a laxity of the lower lid attachment medially;[155] or one can place an instrument into the nose and directly palpate bimanually the mobility of the lacrimal bone and medial canthal tendon attachments.[96]

Once diagnosed, certain treatments, most notably the percutaneous transnasal wiring technique, have led to inadequate reconstitution and stabilization of the nasoethmoid complex fracture. For the less severe injuries, the early appearance may belie the severity of the problem, and, particularly, the later outcome. The medial canthal region may sometimes lateralize slowly, so the severity of the deformity may not be appreciated initially. Furthermore, when stabilization is indicated, the direction of tension needed to properly position the medial canthal tendon (and, thereby, obtain an adequate cosmetic and functional repair of the medial canthal region), must be directed superiorly, posteriorly, and medially to counteract the natural tension that pulls inferiorly, laterally, and anteriorly. If one analyzes the position of percutaneously placed wires, it should be immediately apparent that, while medial pull may be possible, posterior and superior pull will be very difficult to obtain, and, in fact, proper posterior positioning will be virtually impossible (Fig. 23–11).

It is not surprising that misdiagnosis and undertreatment of these fractures occur, since this area represents the most complex and challenging area in facial trauma. The anatomy is complex, and classification of injuries has proved to be complicated as well.[90] Even after diagnosis and surgical exposure, repair remains challenging. This results in an all too high frequency of suboptimal outcomes, as evidenced by the frequency of secondary and subsequent re-

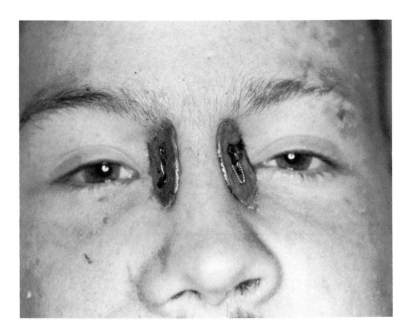

FIGURE 23–11. An example of an attempt to repair a nasoethmoid complex fracture using percutaneously placed wires fixed over lead plates. Even while the wires are in place, there is an apparent asymmetry of the medial canthi, with rounding and inferior displacement of the right canthus. It appears to be more anterior than the left as well, but this is difficult to appreciate in this view.

pair and the large body of literature on it. Several workers have indicated that secondary repair of the deformities that result from these fractures will rarely be fully satisfactory, either cosmetically or functionally.[156–158] Therefore, an aggressive approach to the initial repair as propounded by Gruss is advocated, to minimize the complications and the number of secondary procedures required.[90]

The best approach to the nasoethmoid complex fracture is direct open exposure, either via a coronal flap or through bilateral ethmoidectomy incisions, typically with an open sky communication across the nasal dorsum.[159] Even with this exposure, adequate repair can sometimes prove technically challenging. Failure to properly reposition the medial canthal ligaments generally results in a significant deformity, including lateralization of the medial canthus with the appearance of pseudohypertelorism (traumatic telecanthus). The medial canthus will be rounded and the horizontal palpebral fissure will be narrowed, creating an unsightly appearance. Epicanthal folds may develop, and this deformity is exaggerated by a loss of dorsal nasal height (Fig. 23–12). Furthermore, there will be a functional deficit in the lacrimal collecting system, which also de-

pends upon the proper positioning of the medial canthus.

Assuming proper exposure and direct transnasal wiring, the difficulties encountered include:

1. Difficulty identifying the medial canthal ligament. If it has been badly macerated, it may be hard to identify. Usually, placing a mosquito clamp into the medial canthus and pushing medially will help identify the area of the ligament, which can then be identified by the horizontal fibers crossing from the medial canthal area toward the lacrimal bone.

2. Separation of the ligament from the bone. When the ligament is attached to the bone, the bone usually can be more easily medialized by passing a wire through two holes in the bone and pulling it medially from the opposite side of the nose. If the ligament has completely detached from the bone, it may be more difficult to identify as well as more difficult to grasp. This is best overcome by placing a permanent suture such as a white merseline suture through the ligament, using several loops that can go around the wire to allow more even distribution of the pull through the ligaments rather than a single pass of the

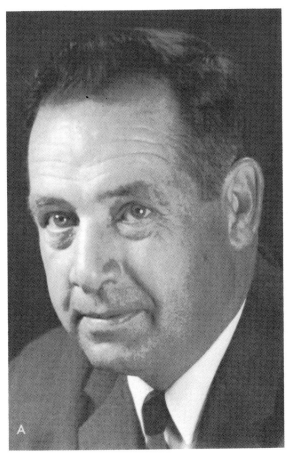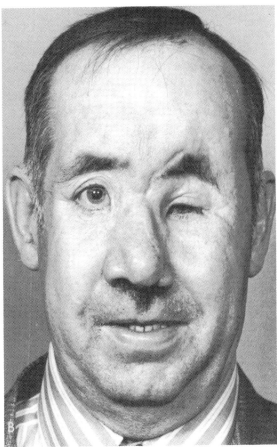

FIGURE 23–12. *A,* Portrait of the patient prior to his injuries, which were sustained in an automobile accident. *B,* Photograph of the patient with malunited fractures. Malunion of the naso-orbital-ethmoid complex and midfacial region has resulted in a tragic alteration in the patient's appearance. (From Converse JM, et al: Deformities of the eyelids and adnexa, orbit, and the zygoma. *In* Converse JM: Reconstructive Plastic Surgery. Vol 2. Philadelphia, WB Saunders, 1977, p 1008.)

wire through the ligament. When attempting to pass the wire directly through the ligament, it can be further macerated and torn, making repair even more difficult.

3. Fragmentation of the thin lacrimal bone. In this situation, even though the ligament remains attached to the bone, it may prove difficult to grasp. In this case, it sometimes proves necessary to directly attach the ligament to the wire as mentioned in paragraph 2.

4. Inadequate positioning of the transnasal wiring. It is important to make sure that the transnasal wire is placed high enough and posterior enough to position the canthus properly. This can be accomplished visually after the wire is passed; if the positioning of the medial canthus does not appear to be either superior or posterior enough, then the wire should be repositioned. Because of the difficulty in drilling the thin bones in this area, particularly when they are in their natural position, Manson and Iliff advocated the actual delivery of the bone up away from the nasal area to facilitate drilling and passage of the wire; then this bone with the attached ligament is repositioned and the wire tightened.[96]

In severe disruption of the medial orbit, sometimes better stabilization is accomplished by bone grafting of the medial orbital area and passage of the transnasal wires through these bone grafts; these grafts provide better support for fixation of the wires.

Finally, attention must be paid to the loss of nasal dorsal height. In a severely comminuted nasoethmoid complex fracture, there is usually inadequate bone to reconstitute the nasal dorsum. A flattened nasal dorsum exaggerates an appearance of telecanthus and worsens the cosmetic deformity. It is therefore important to bone graft the nasal dorsum to recreate the proper anatomic position.

Lacrimal System

The lacrimal system is frequently injured in complex nasoethmoid fractures. The best time for repair is generally at the initial procedure, though sometimes this is not done for various reasons. Probing of the lacrimal system via the canaliculi sometimes reveals the system to be intact and merely malpositioned. In this case, great care should be taken not to injure it, and it should return to normal function once the reconstruction is completed. If it is discontinuous, then passage of silicone or polyethylene tubing in a loop through both canaliculi and tying it in the nose after passage through the nasal lacrimal duct are recommended. This is generally considered a reasonable first step, and it is hoped that recanalization of the system will take place along the tract created by the tubing. When this fails, other procedures are needed, depending on the location of the discontinuity. If both proximal canaliculi are damaged, a conjunctivodacryocystorhinostomy with placement of a tube is needed.[160] When only one canaliculus is injured, there is a reasonable chance that adequate function will develop, though the patient may still be symptomatic. When damage is to the lacrimal sac or distal to it, a dacryocystorhinostomy should be performed. If flaps from the lacrimal sac are sutured to nasal mucosa, an excellent chance of success is anticipated.

Delayed Repair

The incidence of traumatic telecanthus is between 12 per cent and 20 per cent in series of facial fractures.[155] Failure to diagnose or treat nasoethmoid complex fractures properly results in unsightly cosmetic deformities, and, as noted, delayed repair is difficult and often less than completely satisfactory. As in the primary repair, meticulous attention to detail and proper repositioning of the medial canthal ligaments, along with proper reconstruction of the dorsal nasal height, provides optimal results. If, along with flattening of the nasal dorsum, there has been broadening with excessive bone formation, then this bone needs to be drilled down to allow adequate medialization of the medial canthal ligaments. Sometimes the amount of scar that has formed and the foreshortening of the horizontal palpebrae make it impossible to re-create the normal medial canthal position without performing a lateral release via a lateral canthotomy. This is done by making a lateral canthal incision, exposing the lateral canthal ligament, putting a clamp under it, and severing it sharply. This allows some relaxation and, therefore, better repositioning of the medial canthus.

A common problem seen with delayed repair is the development of an epicanthal fold. This generally requires repair via a double Z-plasty[161] (Fig. 23–13) or the rectangular four-flap approach of Mustardé[162] (Fig. 23–14).

Other complications are lacrimal system dysfunction, which requires surgical repair, and anosmia, presumably due to disruption of the cribriform area and the olfactory nerve endings. Persistent anosmia is believed to be unlikely to recover.

MANDIBULAR FRACTURES

Treating fractures of the mandible is fraught with many risks and complications. Complications may result from a failure to treat, as when patients who sustain mandibular fractures do not seek treatment, or treatment is delayed because of associated injuries. Complications may also result from treatment. For many mandibular fractures, the treatment is indeed controversial, and a variety of options are available. The mandible

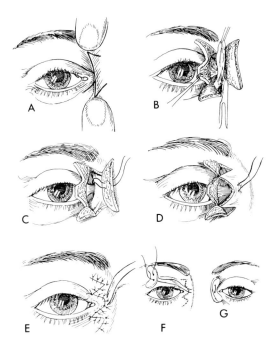

FIGURE 23–13. Double opposing Z-plasties. Two Z-plasties done in opposing directions constitute an excellent technique for relaxing tension and releasing contracture of a linear scar. This technique is of particular usefulness in areas where only small flaps may be designed. The limited amount of tissue in the confined naso-orbital valley limits the size of the Z-flaps. *A*, Design of the opposing Z-plasties. *B*, Flaps are raised, and deep scar tissue is excised. *C*, Transosseous wires have been placed through the bony skeleton of the nose for fixation of the canthal buttons (see *F* and *G*). *D*, The flaps have been transposed. *E*, Double opposing Z-plasties completed. *F* and *G*, The canthal buttons are maintained by through-and-through wiring, assuring the coaptation of the flaps to the underlying skeleton and preventing hematoma. (From Converse JM, Smith B: Naso-orbital fractures and traumatic deformities of the medial Canthus. Plast Reconstr Surg 38:147, 1966.)

dental structures, further increases the occurrence of infection and nonunion. Furthermore, the location of the mandible in the oral cavity can lead to problems with the airway and nutrition, particularly when a severe fracture is present. The basic approach to treatment and a few of the controversies will be discussed.

First, the key to proper repair of mandibular (as well as maxillary) fractures is reestablishment of the patient's occlusal relationship. Failure to do so can result in a significant malocclusion that may require refracturing via osteotomy to repair the damage and get a good functional result. With a minimal, greenstick, or otherwise nondis-

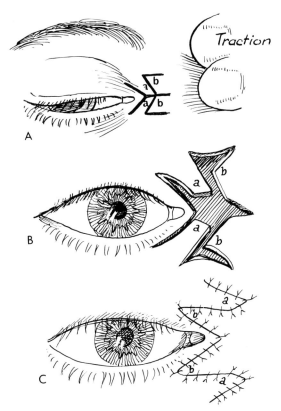

FIGURE 23–14. Four-flap technique for correction of the epicanthus. *A*, The incision lines are drawn. *B*, The flaps have been incised and raised and are ready for transposition. *C*, The flaps have been transposed and sutured. (From Converse JM, et al: Deformities of the eyelids and adnexa, orbit, and the zygoma. *In* Converse JM: Reconstructive Plastic Surgery. Vol 2. Philadelphia, WB Saunders, 1977, p 941.)

is a bone under significant stress in function, and, therefore, it can be anticipated that there will be a greater risk of interfragmentary mobility after fixation compared with other facial bone fractures. Therefore, the incidence of malunion and nonunion would be expected to be higher. The functional stress to which the mandible is subjected, combined with the high degree of contamination encountered from the oral cavity and the frequent presence of infected or compromised placed or nonmobile fracture, when the occlusal relationship is normal, sometimes no intervention is required and the patient will heal in proper position if a soft diet is maintained. However, when this decision is made, the surgeon must follow the patient's progress closely so that a problem does not go unnoticed and untreated. If the bone is shifting, early intervention, generally requiring only intermaxillary fixation (IMF), will prevent complications.

With adequate dentition, a relatively stable fracture can often be splinted merely by the use of intermaxillary fixation (using one of many techniques with which this can be accomplished). Although the duration of IMF remains controversial, typical treatment via this technique will range from 2 to 6 weeks. Proper results depend upon proper patient and fracture selection and careful follow-up, so that developing problems are recognized early and an alternative treatment method can be selected before either a malunion or a nonunion develops. Intermaxillary fixation can be associated with complications, particularly in the brain-injured patient. A patient with severe neurologic compromise, particularly in coma, is at risk of aspiration when treated with IMF. This risk can be minimized by adding a tracheotomy or by considering an alternative repair technique that does not require IMF.

In some cases, inadequate dentition makes the establishment of the occlusal relationship difficult. If the patient has dentures, then these should be modified so they can be utilized for the IMF. When this is not possible, a splint of some type should be created to allow the proper occlusal relationship to be redefined and fixed. If this is not done, a malocclusion and its associated problems likely will result.

Once a decision has been made that an open reduction is necessary, a common controversy involved wire fixation versus more rigid fixation with various types of plates and screws. Previously rigid fixation was considered a controversial technique, but in 1992 it is considered "state of the art."[163] When performed properly, rigid fixation improves the likelihood of a successful outcome and

seems to provide greater resistance to infection. A more common controversy today is whether the mandible should be repaired using miniplates or compression plates. When the surgeon pays proper attention to the biomechanical principles involved in the particular anatomic area to be repaired, good results are to be anticipated with either technique. Most complications associated with plate fixation can be attributed to either problems with patient compliance or improper utilization of the technique. That is not to say that complications will not occur under optimal circumstances with optimal utilization of the technique; however, the chances of a good outcome can certainly be maximized.

Finally, a lack of compliance by patients with mandibular fractures can be implicated in many complications. It is quite common for patients to remove their IMF appliances frequently and prematurely, which often leads to malunion and even nonunion. When appropriate, rigid fixation can sometimes avoid this problem.

Infection

Infection/Cellulitis. Infection is a common problem in mandibular fractures, presumably due to their contaminated nature. Aside from isolated subcondylar fractures, most mandibular fractures involve tears of the gingiva, which result in contamination of the fracture site with oral flora. Most mandibular fractures, therefore, should be considered "compound fractures." Some also may be combined with lacerations of the external skin, resulting in further contamination. Patients may have pre-existing gingivitis or severe dental caries. It is therefore recommended that antibiotic prophylaxis be initiated when the patient is first seen. Generally speaking, penicillin, a first-generation cephalosporin, or clindamycin will provide good coverage for the common oral contaminants. A decreased infection rate of from 42 per cent to 9 per cent has in fact been seen with one preoperative and one postoperative dose of cefazolin in a prospective study.[130] Oral cleansing and frequent mouth rinses are beneficial.

Once clinical infection develops, it is important to treat it aggressively to avoid the development of osteomyelitis. Initially, infections begin in the soft tissues; they involve the bone only after infection has been present for some time, generally weeks. It is therefore recommended that cultures be obtained and intravenous antibiotics be used to treat the early infection. Rigid fixation, particularly with compression or reconstruction plates, provides maximal stability of the bone fragments and thereby minimizes the chance of infection involving the bone and leading to osteomyelitis.[164]

Osteomyelitis. Osteomyelitis usually develops in a bone that has either been inadequately repaired or not treated at all. This can occur when the patient has failed to come in for treatment or has not complied with antibiotic therapy. It may also be seen with an infected tooth in a fracture line, with the dental infection becoming the source of persistent bone infection. Finally, failure to recognize an early infection after initial fracture treatment may result in progression of this infection to osteomyelitis. Osteomyelitis is a serious complication, since it results in loss of bone structure. It requires prolonged treatment with intravenous antibiotics and frequently results in the need for additional surgery, with obvious increased patient morbidity and health care expense. This can be best avoided by early recognition of infection and proper treatment of the causative factors. Noncompliance cannot be avoided. If the problem was due to infection in the presence of a fixation device, then early management with aggressive therapy for a local wound infection may allow progression to normal healing. When a question of the stability of the fixation device exists, the patient should be surgically explored and the tightness of the screws tested. If they are indeed tight, then intravenous antibiotic therapy should lead to good healing. If there is instability, the device should be removed and replaced with a more stable fixation. If the problem is due to an unstable or infected tooth, this should be removed. When tooth removal will

lead to further instability at the fracture site, rigid fixation is mandatory to impart the stability to the bone necessary to insure healing.

Once osteomyelitis has developed, the mainstay of treatment is the removal of any unstable hardware and treatment with specific antibiotic therapy via the intravenous route. Surgical debridement of osteitic bone should be accompanied by the placement of a fixation device. This can include intermaxillary or external fixation, or, as we prefer, bridging of the area with a reconstruction plate. When a reconstruction plate is used, screws should be placed at a distance from the osteitic area and only into solid, healthy, noninflamed bone. At least three and preferably four screws on either side should be used, treating the area as a defect area. Intravenous antibiotic therapy should be continued for 6 weeks. If pretreatment with IV antibiotics has been possible and no gross infection is present at the time of exploration, then bone grafting can be performed at the same procedure, once all osteitic bone has been removed. Otherwise, rigid fixation can be employed at the initial procedure and bone grafting delayed until completion of IV antibiotic therapy.

Malocclusion/Malunion

If the mandible heals with the bones in a position different from their original position, a malunion has resulted. When teeth are present, this will result in a malocclusion. Small degrees of malocclusion often can be improved by simple grinding of the dental surfaces to arrange for a better interaction of the occlusal surfaces of the teeth. However, significant malunions will generally not respond to this. If orthodontic movement of the teeth in the bone can result in a good functional occlusion without significant weakening of the teeth, then this is the recommended approach. However, when this is not reasonable, mandibular osteotomy and repositioning, followed by refixation in a proper occlusal relationship, are generally necessary. This is a significant complication and essentially results in the need to recreate the fracture. In the absence of teeth, sometimes dentures can be redeveloped so that they can compensate for a malunion. However, the dentures must be able to function so that they do not put undue stress on the bone and so that a good functional occlusion can be created. Otherwise, again, osteotomy will be necessary. When considering osteotomy and refixation, study models and careful analysis and planning are essential.

Delayed Union

The definition of delayed union is not universal, though most people will consider a failure to achieve solid bony union by 2 to 3 months to be a delayed union. The difference between a delayed union and a nonunion is that continued fixation such as by prolonged IMF will result in the conversion of a delayed union to a solid union.[165] Although this means additional morbidity and sometimes time lost from work for the patient, it will often go on to a bony fusion.

Nonunion

A nonunion occurs when healing does not ensue. This can result from osteomyelitis, or it can mean that a fibrous union has developed precluding healing by bony union. When continued fixation beyond 6 months fails to result in healing, most will agree that this is a nonunion, though some will consider it a delayed union until 1 year. Whether a nonunion can be converted to bony union by rigid fixation without debridement and bone grafting is not clear.

A nonunion also may result from bone loss at the initial injury. In this case, intermaxillary fixation may have been used to define the occlusal relationship, and the defective area may have been bridged by a reconstruction plate or via external fixation. Primary bone grafting is possible, although most surgeons favor having a clean, noncontaminated field for placement of a bone graft. A free bone flap would be more logical as a primary technique, since the blood supply allows delivery of antibiotics to this contaminated area. Rigid fixation appliances, such as the mandibular reconstruction plate, maintain the proper bony relationships while soft tissue healing takes place, so that secondary bone grafting can be performed. The success of secondary bone grafting with a traumatic defect approaches 90 per cent to 94 per cent.[166, 167]

Rigid fixation techniques are a great advance for the management of traumatic bone loss in the mandible. Traditionally, initial attention was directed at establishing soft tissue coverage, so that bone reconstruction could be carried out later. Unfortunately, significant soft tissue contracture over the defective area frequently precluded satisfactory bony reconstruction. The advent of rigid fixation techniques has shifted the initial emphasis from soft tissue to hard tissue repair. Properly utilized, rigid fixation allows for the recreation of the architecture of the defective area, even in the absence of immediate soft tissue coverage. A solid repair seems to impart resistance to infection,[164] and secondary soft and hard tissue repair can be completed over time as the tissue heals and is ready for surgical manipulation and grafting. Long-term results are thereby dramatically improved.

Inferior Alveolar Nerve Paresthesia/Anesthesia

The inferior alveolar nerve can be traumatized by marked displacement of the bony canal through which it travels when the fracture occurs. It can also be injured during repair, by aggressive cleaning of the fracture site with damage to the nerve and its canal or the penetration through the nerve of a drill or screw when fixing the fracture. Injury to this nerve will cause desensitization of teeth distal to the injury as well as numbness of the lower lip and chin on the ipsilateral side. This is an annoying and frustrating problem, and great care should be taken to avoid iatrogenic injury.

Facial Nerve Paresis/Paralysis

Injury to the facial nerve can occur due to a major traumatic injury, but it is more likely the result of damage during surgical repair in two areas. First, the ramus mandibularis of the facial nerve may be injured during the approach to the submandibular region, where the nerve travels deep to the platysma muscle and overlies the submaxillary gland. This will cause loss of function of the depressors of the lower lip on that side and can lead to drooling. Although an annoying problem, it is generally well tolerated. Second, the main trunk of the facial nerve can be injured during open reduction of subcondylar and ramus fractures of the mandible. Great care should be taken to avoid facial nerve injury in this area, because a complete facial paralysis is a very significant morbidity both cosmetically and functionally. When injury has occurred, the nerve should be explored and direct anastomosis performed when necessary.

Tooth Loss/Tooth Abscess

Tooth loss is a frequent result of the injury, though sometimes it can occur during attempts at repair. An acutely loose or avulsed tooth should be replaced whenever possible, as it may hold. A root canal should be performed as soon as possible to decrease the likelihood of abscess. When an abscess does form, generally the tooth must be extracted to avoid infection of the bone.

Temporomandibular Joint (TMJ) Dysfunction

TMJ dysfunction, unfortunately, is not a rare occurrence after trauma to the mandible. Any trauma significant enough to fracture the mandible is likely to transmit significant force to one or both temporomandibular joints, even without obvious TMJ trauma or patient complaints. Some patients will develop a traumatic arthritis with subsequent problems in the joint region; others may experience an immediate disruption in the joint. Damage to the articular cartilage or ligamentous tears generally results in various forms of TMJ discomfort and/or pain. At this time, it is not generally advocated that the joint be routinely explored and repaired; though in a preliminary report of 10 fractures in nine patients Chuong and Piper suggest that it may well be beneficial.[168] Patients who develop severe TMJ dysfunction likely will require joint repair at a later time. Most importantly, the occurrence of TMJ dysfunction after trauma is not trivial, and it would be wise for all surgeons treating this problem to inform patients that the joint(s) may be a source of discomfort or trouble for them for an indefinite time.

TEMPOROMANDIBULAR JOINT ANKYLOSIS

TMJ ankylosis is a serious complication compromising all normal oral functions. A true ankylosis implies a fibro-osseous union between the mandible and the glenoid fossa. Although some limitation of mandibular mobility is not uncommon, true ankylosis is rare. It is seen primarily in fractures involving the TMJ, particularly intracapsular fractures.[169] This risk is significantly increased in children.[170] Intracapsular hemorrhage has been implicated as an etiologic factor in joint ankylosis, but this has not been proved in the experimental model.[171]

No specific preventive measures have been found, though some have suggested that early mobilization may decrease its occurrence. It has even been implied that IMF may be a causative factor. However, no scientific evidence supports this contention, and Markey,[172] as cited by Bradley,[173] was unable to produce ankylosis experimentally in primates via prolonged immobilization.

Treatment is most successful using condylectomy and soft tissue interposition.[174, 175] Various options are used for interposition, including various soft tissues and alloplasts, and an artificial implant or costochondral graft may be used if needed to restore ramus height.

Miscellaneous

Other complications that can occur include malnutrition, which is more likely in the elderly patient who is unable to eat due to prolonged IMF or discomfort secondary to the injury. Patients in IMF can sometimes aspirate, particularly if there is an associated neurologic injury. Airway obstruction can occur from loss of hyomandibular support, with retrodisplacement of the tongue. A nasopharyngeal airway usually protects the patient in this situation, though sometimes intubation may be necessary. Of course, early repair of the mandible will solve this problem. An unusual complication is Ludwig's angina, which also can result in airway compromise. Surgical drainage and airway protection are mandatory for this. Finally, unsightly scars can result not only from a laceration at injury but also from the repair. A hypertrophic scar, or keloid, is unattractive and is an unpleasant experience for both patient and physician. Great care and attention to surgical wound closure can at least minimize the occurrence of unsatisfactory scarring.

Mandibular Fracture Complications by Anatomic Location

ANGLE

Fractures of the mandibular angle appear to have the highest incidence of complications after repair.[163] First, the angle fracture is behind the dentition, so IMF adds little stabilization. The mandible is also very thin in this area, so the amount of bone-to-bone contact is less than in other areas, and fixation devices have less bone to grip. The forces in this area tend to vary more during function,[176] so absolute fixation in this area is more difficult to obtain. In addition, the masseter muscle inserts laterally and the medial pterygoid inserts medially in this area, which may contribute to instability after fracture as well. Finally, the presence of unerupted and partially erupted third molars in the area of fractures also may contribute to infection,

though the management of this remains controversial.

To minimize complications when repairing fractures in this area, it is recommended that the surgeon attempt to achieve maximum stability and fixation. For miniplate fixation, Levy and associates recommend two miniplates in repair.[163] When using compression plates, two plates may be wise as well. We prefer the reconstruction plate to bridge this area for maximum stability.

SYMPHYSIS/PARASYMPHYSIS

The main complications that we have seen in this area have been due to inadequate fixation. During function, rotational forces as well as axial distracting forces operate in this area. It is therefore wise, except in the most stable situations, to proceed with some form of open reduction and direct interosseous fixation.

BODY

With proper fixation, fractures in the body region generally heal well. The key is establishment of the proper occlusal relationship, along with careful fixation. A fracture in this area may disrupt the inferior alveolar nerve; care should be taken not to injure it surgically.

SUBCONDYLAR/CONDYLAR

Unfortunately, the best treatment and therefore the best method for prevention of complications of the subcondylar area is controversial and not defined. Complications occur regardless of the treatment method utilized, making it impossible at this time to make a recommendation. Complications include malocclusion, TMJ dysfunction, and trismus. Trismus can vary from mild to complete ankylosis with the inability to open the mouth for speech and eating of solid foods, ultimately necessitating secondary surgery if normal function is to be regained.

A major controversy is whether subcondylar fractures should be treated by closed or open reduction. When a subcondylar fracture is treated with closed reduction, sometimes a normal anatomic repositioning develops, and, at other times, a pseudoarthrosis develops with persistent displacement of the condyle and formation of a false joint between the upper portion of the ramus and the surrounding tissue. This frequently results in normal function with normal occlusion. When an abnormality of function develops, some will then attribute this abnormality to the anatomic nonalignment of the fracture. However, the frequent good outcome in the presence of such nonalignment makes this a dubious conclusion. Furthermore, the same abnormalities of function, including occlusal and functional abnormalities, occur after open reduction with normal alignment of the fracture fragments. It is possible, though not proved, that in fact the joint is so disrupted that fixation of the fracture could result in an increased incidence of limited opening, since a pseudoarthrosis cannot be obtained to bypass the ankylosis or limitation that may develop in the joint. The fact that patients can function well after condylectomy as a treatment of ankylosis, without reconstruction of the joints with a prosthesis, adds to this question. Further clinical and laboratory studies may prove helpful in determining the answers to some of these difficult and important issues.

Treatment. An isolated subcondylar fracture may respond to minimal treatment using a soft diet and exercises if the patient is able, on his or her own, to open and close into proper occlusion. The patient should be followed closely when no active intervention is planned. Jaw exercise, trying to get maximal excursion, particularly laterally to the side opposite the fracture, is important, as are protrusion, opening, and closing. When a malocclusion persists, intermaxillary fixation is indicated. This generally can be utilized initially by using intermaxillary fixation in proper occlusion; after 1 to 2 weeks, this can be replaced with rubber bands used as "training elastics." The effort here is to try to train the muscles to overcome the pull that is working against the proper occlusal relationship. If persistent foreshortening on the side of the fracture results in prematurity of clo-

sure on that side, an open reduction may be necessary.

Sometimes associated fractures or difficulty maintaining occlusion requires maintenance of intermaxillary fixation for 3 to 6 weeks. In these instances, one should aggressively encourage the patient to perform mouth opening and stretching and excursion exercises once the IMF has been released. Patient cooperation is important here, since an uncooperative patient who does not exercise his or her mandible may well end up with severe restriction of opening. Despite the best efforts, sometimes the joint injury and fibrosis that develop secondary to the injury will result in trismus or ankylosis. Condylectomy with or without joint replacement generally is necessary then to regain function.

The bilateral subcondylar fracture creates a more difficult situation. Foreshortening posteriorly is fairly common, with development of posterior premature contact with an anterior open bite. Sometimes this can be improved with IMF; at other times, an open reduction of at least one side will be necessary. When this is associated with midfacial LeFort fractures, it may prove necessary to open at least one subcondylar fracture to use the vertical height of the mandible as an indicator of facial height.

Finally, as noted, it may be reasonable to repair acutely the disrupted disk at open reduction.[168] This may decrease the incidence of later TMJ dysfunction.

Intracapsular Fractures

Intracapsular fractures represent a particularly difficult situation, since they indicate the presence of a fracture within the joint. The likelihood of complications in the joint as a result is quite high.[177] Re-establishment of the occlusal relationship with IMF, combined with early mobilization and exercise, provides the best results. It is not yet clear whether early intervention via joint surgery will improve ultimate long-term results.

Fractures into the External Auditory Canal/Middle Cranial Fossa

Direct anterior trauma to the mandible may force the condylar heads into and sometimes through the posterior wall of the glenoid fossa, which is the anterior wall of the external auditory canal. This is generally approached via repair of the mandible under anesthesia, combined with repositioning of the external canal structures, including bone and skin. The external ear canal is packed for a period of several weeks to allow reformation of the normal bony contour. External canal stenosis may occur. When significant, this will require secondary repair, including canalplasty and meatoplasty. Fracture displacement through the glenoid fossa into the middle cranial fossa can occur, but fortunately it is a rare complication.[178]

TMJ Syndrome/Myofascial Pain– Dysfunction Syndrome

The so-called TMJ syndrome is a syndrome of pain of neuromuscular origin. It seems to be the result of any stress on the temporomandibular joint or its associated musculature. The stress could be related to occlusal discrepancies, even as mild as those related to occlusal wear, and muscle tension due to stress and bruxism. Certainly, the disruption due to fracture and joint injury can cause significant stress on this region and lead to discomfort. Early treatment includes muscle relaxants, topical anesthetics such as ethyl chloride, and physical therapy, including tension-relieving and range of motion exercises. Occlusal splinting and occlusal adjustments by orthodontia sometimes relieve some of the pressure on the joint(s). When conservative measures fail, surgical treatment to reconstruct the joint may prove helpful. The MRI scan has added an excellent modality for evaluation of the TMJ structurally, and this has frequently replaced the arthrogram for TMJ evaluation.

Special Considerations

ATROPHIC EDENTULOUS MANDIBLE

This represents a special situation because of the combination of the lack of dentition as a guide to repair, the thin small bone available for repair, and, probably most importantly, the poor blood supply to the thin atrophic mandible. Studies by Bradley have indicated that the inferior alveolar artery is one of the early arteries affected by atherosclerosis.[179] This results in poor blood supply from the inferior alveolar canal and the replacement of this with the periosteal blood supply as the only remaining source for the aged, atrophic mandible. Bradley has called this the change from centrifugal to centripetal blood supply. The small bone volume means a small area of contact as well as little support for functional stresses.

Failure rates for repair of fractures in the pencil-thin mandible range from 20 per cent to 60 per cent, and the highest complication rate seems to be associated with open reduction and interosseous wire fixation.[180] Some have advocated the routine acceptance of less than anatomic reduction and even nonunion, because of the risks of infection and further bone loss with aggressive intervention.[181, 182] Repair using circumandibular wiring of dentures or splints, while sometimes successful and frequently advocated, provides little stabilization and support and may be inadequate. Some surgeons advocate routine primary bone grafting,[183, 184] external fixation, and even the immediate use of rigid reconstruction plating techniques such as the mandibular reconstruction plate.[185] When an open technique is used, it is wise not to strip the periosteum from the bone but to place any fixation appliances directly through the periosteum, so as to limit any devascularization that is carried out at the time of fixation. Once a failure of primary repair has occurred, the liberal use of bone grafts should be considered.

MANDIBULAR FRACTURES IN CHILDREN

As noted, children under the age of 10 bear a higher incidence of ankylosis in fractures. The exact mechanism of this is uncertain, though it may be due to more rapid bone growth allowing bone fixation between the damaged condyle and the glenoid fossa.

Clearly, as in adults, this is more likely to occur with an intracapsular fracture.

Another concern in children is the possibility of abnormal growth of the mandible after a fracture has occurred. The theoretic explanations and concerns for growth impairment are beyond the scope of this chapter, yet it should be noted that in young children, a growth disturbance can be anticipated on the side of a mandible fracture.[186] In a recent review of long-term outcomes in 28 patients who had suffered mandibular fractures in childhood, two thirds had radiographic abnormalities, and about one third had abnormal occlusion. Almost half had clinically notable asymmetry, though only 5 of the 28 patients were bothered by this.[186] Asymmetric growth is more likely to occur after a condylar fracture, and it is possible that a decrease in mobility and function may in fact contribute to decreased growth. When the deformity is significant, treatment will require vertical ramus osteotomy and bone grafting for lengthening as needed for the individual case.

DENTAL

The most significant dental complication of mandible and maxillary fractures (discussed in more detail earlier) is an occlusal discrepancy due to failure to obtain healing with the exact proper occlusion. A minor occlusal discrepancy may sometimes be reparable by grinding of selected dental surfaces. More commonly, some orthodontic readjustment will be needed. In the more severe cases, refracture via osteotomy after careful planning may be the method of choice. In the edentulous or partially dentulous patient, repairs sometimes can be carried out on the dentures or partials.

Another common problem is gingival injury due to the combination of the injury and the repair. Arch bars, while helpful in the repair of these fractures, do injure the gingiva. Many trauma patients present in a state of poor oral hygiene and already have gingival disease. These patients will be particularly prone to aggravation of this problem from treatment. Every attempt should be made to have the patient exercise meticulous oral hygiene during the course of therapy. Once therapy is completed, referral to the dentist or periodontist for further treatment should be considered as needed.

TOOTH INJURIES

Associated tooth injuries are often seen when a bony fracture has occurred. These may vary from a minor chip to a lost facet to devitalization, cracking, or complete avulsion. Avulsed teeth should be reimplanted whenever possible and stabilized to surrounding teeth, as should loosened teeth. The advent of light-curing acrylics has assisted in the stabilization of loose or avulsed teeth. Early root canal should be practiced for devitalized teeth to decrease the risk of infection. When a tooth is fractured above the crown, it becomes a source of instability and infection and should be removed. When a tooth that needs to be removed is contributing to the anatomic alignment of a fracture, the fracture can be first repaired using a rigid technique, such as a compression plate or a reconstruction plate, and the tooth can be removed once the plating procedure has been completed.

TECHNICAL COMPLICATIONS/TECHNIQUE FAILURE

As technology advances, so do the demands upon the surgeon. Surgeons may fail to recognize the new technical complexities involved and inadvertently misuse techniques; the results at times can be most unsatisfying. Furthermore, even experienced surgeons may sometimes choose shortcuts, and this may lead to complications as well.

Technique Selection

A potential pitfall when a surgeon is familiar with too few techniques is the selection of an inappropriate technique for the particular fracture. For example, intermaxillary fixation may be adequate for the majority of mandibular fractures; however, it behooves the surgeon to closely follow a patient with an unstable fracture and perform an appropriate interosseous fixation when IMF is failing to maintain the occlusal relationship, or interfragmentary motion is persisting. Although miniplates may prove very effective in selected fractures, they will generally not be satisfactory when marked comminution or bone loss is present. Similarly, failing to choose an appropriate reconstructive technique likely will lead to failure of the procedure.

ARCH BARS

Arch bars provide excellent stabilization of many mandibular fractures, but risks are involved as well. When mobile alveolar fragments are present, or when numerous teeth are loose, arch bars alone may not produce satisfactory results. Injudicious application of arch bars and wires can lead to tooth movement and even tooth extraction.

A particular problem exists when segments of the mandibular body are separated from the remainder of the mandible or when the palate is split, creating a similar problem in the maxilla. Intermaxillary fixation will tend to pull the lateral bony portions downward, causing some rotation of the fragments and diverting the occlusal portions of the teeth in a lingual direction. Prevention of this may require rigid fixation or the use of dental splints.

In children, arch bars are a problem because they do not hold well on deciduous dentition and there is a greater likelihood of dental extraction. It is therefore recommended that mandibular fractures in children be repaired with dental splints.

DENTAL SPLINTS

With dental splints, the repair can be only as good as the splints themselves. Improper splint fabrication can lead to the iatrogenic creation of a malunion. When uncertainty about the proper position exists, splints can be designed so that they are incomplete prior to operation and completed intraoperatively.

As noted, circumandibular wiring can result in infection and skin dimpling when not properly applied. Injury to the facial artery can result in hematoma formation. When significant bleeding occurs intraoperatively, great care should be taken to apply pressure long enough to make certain that bleeding has completely stopped.

INTEROSSEOUS WIRE FIXATION

Interosseus wire fixation, along with intermaxillary fixation, has been one of the mainstays of surgical repair of mandibular fractures for many years. However, since the onset of rigid fixation techniques, the relative instability of various wire fixation techniques has been clearly demonstrated.[187] When a fracture has been reasonably well stabilized with IMF, interosseous wires may provide enough additional stabilization to insure healing in a borderline situation, but not when significant instability exists. In the latter situation, the wire may act as a foreign body and increase the risk of infection. When it is used and an infection appears to be developing, it is recommended that the wound be re-explored, the wire removed, and a more rigid fixation applied.

KIRSCHNER WIRES

Kirschner wires are not commonly used today for mandibular fixation. Although they may hold fragments together, the fixation is unstable and therefore a significant risk of infection and subsequent osteomyelitis exists.

EXTERNAL FIXATION

External fixation continues to provide a "fall-back" technique for difficult fractures and osteomyelitis. The most commonly used system is the Joe Hall Morris.[188] For this technique to work successfully, it is wise to have at least two fixation points on either side of an unstable area, though three may be better. The pins provide a source of infection from the skin into the bone. Skin infection alone is more common; unsightly scars may develop at the pin sites. When applying the acrylic to the pins, care must be taken to keep the skin area cooled, since the heat generated as the acrylic hardens can cause a tissue burn.

RIGID FIXATION TECHNIQUES

Rigid fixation, the most recent technical advance, can provide the highest success rates in the most complicated cases. However, such good results are very technique-sensitive, and lack of familiarity with some of the specific biomechanical requirements of the mandible in general and of the particular plating system being used in particular, can lead to a surprising array of complications. (Spiessl provides a complete review of biomechanical principles.[189]) Certain common areas of error are noted:

Occlusion. As in any technique for mandibular fracture repair, a proper occlusion must be re-established. However, maintaining this throughout operation is more critical in rigid fixation. If the rigid fixation shifts the occlusal relationship, no amount of traction with arch bars, rubber bands, or even halo fixation will re-establish the proper relationship. If an occlusal shift occurs as a result of application of a plate or lag screw, the device should be removed and reapplied to avoid an unsatisfactory outcome.

Screw Application. Screws must be placed properly or failure and even osteomyelitis may result. In general, the drill will be the size of the shaft of the screw, not the thread. The appropriate drill from the appropriate system should be utilized, and it should be sharp. Drilling should be performed with constant cooling and without force so as to minimize bone damage. The drill must not wobble, or a funnel-shaped hole will be created. Careful depth measurement is important, so that the proper length screw is selected. When tapping is necessary, great care should be taken to tap in the same direction as the hole. Finally, screw application should be atraumatic, and the screw should be snug. If a screw has stripped and cannot be tight-

ened, it should be removed. A loose screw adds nothing to the stability of the fixation, but it does provide a foreign body that can increase the risk of infection.

Plate Bending. Plate bending can be difficult and frustrating. However, failure to achieve the proper shape over the fracture area will likely lead to malposition of the fragments. It is wiser to not use a plate at all than to leave an improperly positioned plate. Frequent rebending of the plate will weaken it and decrease the likelihood of a stable fixation; plate fracture may even occur. If excessive bending was necessary, it is wise to discard the plate and select another.

Selection of Materials. It is critical that materials be compatible when metals are being used. Metals should never be mixed! When different metals are used together, the likelihood of an ionic gradient occurring that may lead to corrosion and tissue damage becomes a significant concern.[190] It is therefore wise to use only one system at a time when approaching rigid fixation of facial fractures.

Adherence to Biomechanical Principles. The biomechanical requirements must be addressed when repairing mandibular fractures. When rigid fixation is utilized, generally no intermaxillary fixation is used and the patient is allowed to eat postoperatively. If inadequate fixation for the fractured area has been applied, interfragmentary motion becomes likely, and the possibility of infection and nonunion becomes significant.

Miniplates. It is imperative that miniplates be applied along the proper tension line, the so-called "ideal line of osteosynthesis" as described by Champy and coworkers.[191] This requires two miniplates, one above the other, from parasymphysis to parasymphysis. According to some, two plates are required at the angle as well to avoid mobility and failure.[163, 176]

Compression Plates. A common mistake when using compression plates for mandibular fracture repair is to apply one along the inferior mandibular border without first performing the critical step of establishing a tension band across the alveolar border. Placing the compression plate inferiorly in this fashion will lead to gapping at the alveolar border with significant instability.[192] A tension band can be an arch bar, an interosseus wire, a miniplate, or even a compression plate. However, complete neglect of the tension band principle risks failure.

When a tension band cannot be used, an eccentric dynamic compression plate (EDCP) can be used. This plate is somewhat more technically difficult to apply. Figure 23–15 is a radiograph of an EDCP that was applied upside down. The patient developed osteomyelitis; ultimately, repair using a reconstruction plate along with a cancellous bone graft provided a satisfactory result.

Reconstruction Plates. Reconstruction plates provide maximal stability in areas of bone loss or severe comminution. However, it is important that enough screws be utilized to insure such stability. In bridging a defective or severely comminuted area, it is generally recommended that at least three screws be placed on either side in the stable bone. If four or more screws are used, stability is assured. To repair a defect created by osteomyelitis, the screws must be placed in healthy bone at a significant distance from the defect.

Finally, it cannot be overemphasized how important it is to be familiar with the techniques being utilized. An example of random plate placement leading to severe tissue damage with ultimate osteomyelitis and bone loss is shown in Figure 23–16.

Lag Screws. Lag screws are used to repair oblique fractures or in any situation where bone is overlapping. Failure to use a lag screw when the bones overlap will lead to separation of the fracture fragments. This separation cannot be decreased by further tightening of the screw. A lag screw should not grasp the first fragment, so that it can compress the fragments together when it is tightened into the second fragment.

Inferior Alveolar Nerve/Tooth Root Injury. Injudicious placement of a screw can result in direct injury to the inferior alveolar nerve or a tooth root. In addition to annoying numbness and devitalization of teeth, nerve injury can lead to drooling and lip biting.

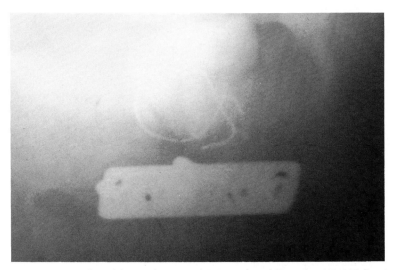

FIGURE 23–15. A patient was referred for evaluation of pain and mobility after "rigid" fixation of a posterior body mandible fracture. The radiograph revealed a wire used as a tension band and an eccentric dynamic compression plate (EDCP) along the basal border of the mandible. Careful inspection revealed that the outer compression holes are angled away from the fracture, preventing the EDCP from compressing the alveolar border of the mandible as it does when properly directed. An unstable fixation resulted, explaining the unsatisfactory outcome.

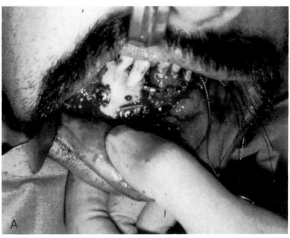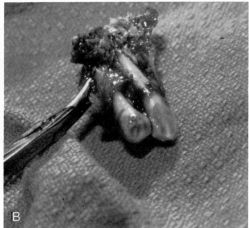

FIGURE 23–16. A patient was referred with osteomyelitis of the mandible "due to plate failure." *A,* At exploration, inadequate plate fixation and a poor position were noted. *B,* A segment of osteitic bone was recovered, including teeth needing to be debrided. This fragment was covered with greenish bacterial growth.

Tooth root injury leads to devitalization of the involved tooth; of greater concern might be an increased risk of infection at the fracture site.

MISCELLANEOUS COMPLICATIONS

Pain

Pain may be related to a nerve injury or persistent infection. When due to nerve injury, it is difficult to treat and often requires patient adjustment and education. A neuralgia can sometimes be improved by injection of the nerve with anesthetics or steroids and sometimes alcohol to deaden the nerve. One should look for signs of infection, particularly sinusitis, which may occur after disruption of the sinuses. Bone grafts and implants may increase the risk of infection and make infection more difficult to eradicate once it develops. Infected implants may need to be removed. Patients in cold climates will sometimes complain of pain in an area that has been plated. Removal of the plate often relieves this problem.

Donor Site Complications

With the frequent use of bone and skin grafting, the surgeon must be aware of the potential for donor site complications. Bone grafting is now advocated routinely for the repair of many midfacial and orbital fractures.[145, 146] Grafts are also particularly useful for treating bony defects and nonunions and for most secondary repairs.

The use of split calvarial grafts introduces new risks because of possible intracranial penetration. Dural tears can occur, particularly when an osteotome is used to free the bone graft. The midline must be avoided, since injury to the sagittal sinus may result in an exsanguinating hemorrhage. On the other hand, when a coronal approach is already in use, an additional donor site incision is avoided. Furthermore, there is the theoretical advantage that membranous bone is less likely to be resorbed.

When harvesting rib grafts, great care should be taken to avoid penetration of the pleura. Although not a serious complication, pneumothorax does necessitate the use of a chest tube, and it will prolong the hospital stay. Gruss reports an incidence of 5 per cent in 212 rib grafts.[145]

In an iliac crest graft, avoiding the use of the lateral cortex will diminish the postoperative morbidity. Penetration or excision of the lateral cortex results in muscular pain upon walking. It also increases the risks of leg numbness. If cancellous bone is harvested through unroofing of the top of the crest, or if corticocancellous bone is taken from the superior crest, the likelihood of such a complication is significantly diminished. Avoid penetration medially into the peritoneal cavity.

Unrealistic Expectations

Modern surgical and technologic advances combined with wide media publicity about new surgical techniques have led to the common misconception that a "perfect" or "near-perfect" outcome can be anticipated in most situations. Failure properly to prepare patients and their families for a realistic outcome, particularly after severe trauma, often leads to dissatisfaction and, unfortunately, to litigation. This has become an all-too-frequent complication of modern medicine, and the facial trauma surgeon is at great risk. Competitive medical practice and interspecialty rivalry have further increased the occurrence of this complication.

The surgeon should be familiar with the latest techniques available and apply them properly. The advent of new technology often mandates supplemental education, so that these technologic advances are utilized appropriately; this increases the likelihood that the best possible results will be obtained.

A good cooperative relationship between the different specialties will enhance patient care as well as decrease the likelihood of poor communication, particularly when a patient seeks a second opinion. Chuong and colleagues have emphasized the multiple benefits available to patients and staff that a true interdisciplinary approach can offer.[193]

Most importantly, the physician must make certain that the patient and the family understand the severity of the injuries as well as the anticipated long-term sequelae. Unrealistic expectations by the patient or family ensure dissatisfaction with the ultimate outcome. Despite all the recent technologic and surgical advances, we still remain the prisoners of the healing process.

References

1. Heimgartner-Candinas B, Heimgartner M, Jonutis A: Results of treatment of midfacial fractures. Indications for exploration and drainage of the maxillary sinuses. J Maxillofac Surg 6:293–301, 1978.
2. Morgan BDG, Madan DK, Begerot JPC: Fractures of the middle third of the face—a review of 300 cases. Br J Plast Surg 25:147–151, 1972.
3. Gwynn PP, Carroway JN, Horton CE, et al: Facial fractures; Associated injuries and complications. Plast Reconstr Surg 47:225–230, 1971.
4. Davidson JS, Birdsell DC: Cervical spine injury in patients with facial skeletal trauma. J Trauma 29:1276–1278, 1989.
5. Luce EA, Tubb TD, Moore AM: Review of 1000 major facial fractures and associated injuries. Plast Reconstr Surg 63:26–30, 1979.
6. Schultz RC: Facial injuries from automobile accidents: A study of 400 consecutive cases. Plast Reconstr Surg 40:415–425, 1967.
7. Foster CA, Maisel RH, Meyerhoff WL: Head and neck trauma: Initial evaluation, diagnosis and management. Minn Med 64:85–90, 1981.
8. Kellman RM: The cervical spine in maxillofacial trauma: Assessment and airway management. Otolaryngol Clin North Am 24:1–13, 1991.
9. Majernik TG, Bienick R, Houston JB, et al: Cervical spine movement during orotracheal intubation. Ann Emerg Med 15:417–420, 1986.
10. Allo MD, Miller CF: Airway management. In Zuidema GD, Rutherford RB, Bellinger WF (eds): The Management of Trauma. 4th ed. Philadelphia, WB Saunders, 1985, pp 379–390.
11. Dula DJ: Trauma to the cervical spine. J Am Coll Emerg Phy8:504–507, 1979.
12. Pepe PE, Joyce TH, Copass MK: Prehospital endotracheal intubation: Rationale for training emergency medical personnel. Ann Emerg Med 14:1085–1092, 1985.
13. Aprahamian C, Thompson BM, Finger WA, et al: Experimental cervical spine injury model: Evaluation of airway management and splinting techniques. Ann Emerg Med 13:584–587, 1984.
14. Quick CA, Merwin GE: Arytenoid dislocation. Arch Otolaryngol 104:267–270, 1978.
15. Iserson KV: Blind nasotracheal intubation. Ann Emerg Med 10:468–471, 1981.
16. Jorden RC, Rosen P: Airway management in the acutely injured. In Moore EE, Eiseman B, VanWay EW III (eds): Critical Decisions in Trauma. St. Louis, CV Mosby, 1984, pp 30–35.
17. Ellis DG, Stewart RD, Kaplan RM, et al: Success rates of blind orotracheal intubation using a trans-illumination technique with a lighted stylet. Ann Emerg Med 15:138–142, 1986.
18. Rucker RW, Silva W, Worchester CC: Fiberoptic bronchoscope nasotracheal intubation in children. Chest 76:56–58, 1979.
19. Taylor PA, Towey RM: The bronchofiberscope as an aid to endotracheal intubation. Br J Anaesth 44:611–612, 1976.

20. Stanley RB, Colman MF: Unilateral degloving injuries of the arytenoid cartilage. Arch Otolaryngol Head Neck Surg 112:516–518, 1986.
21. Close LG, Merkel M, Watson B, Schaefer SD: Cricoarytenoid subluxation, computed tomography, and electromyography findings. Head Neck Surg 9:341–348, 1987.
22. Hoffman HT, Brunberg JA, Winter P, et al: Arytenoid subluxation: Diagnosis and treatment. Ann Otol Rhinol Laryngol 100:1–9, 1991.
23. Schild JA, Denneny EC: Evaluation and treatment of acute laryngeal fractures. Head Neck Surg 11:491–496, 1989.
24. Leopold DA: Laryngeal trauma: A historical comparison of treatment methods. Arch Otolaryngol 109:106–111, 1983.
25. Maniglia AJ: Tracheal stenosis: Conservative surgery as a primary mode of management. Otolaryngol Clin North Am 12:877–892, 1979.
26. Grillo HC: Tracheal reconstruction: Indications and techniques. Arch Otolaryngol 6:31–39, 1972.
27. Grillo HC: Primary reconstruction of the airway after resection of subglottic laryngeal and upper tracheal stenosis. Ann Thorac Surg 33:3–18, 1982.
28. Mehrotra ON, Brown GED, Widdowson WP, Wilson JP: Arteriography and selective embolization in the control of life-threatening haemorrhage following facial fractures. Br J Plast Surg 37:482–485, 1984.
29. Jacobson JA, Kasworm EM: Toxic shock syndrome after nasal surgery. Arch Otolaryngol Head Neck Surg 112:329–332, 1986.
30. Breda SD, Jacobs JB, Lebowitz AS, Tierno PM: Toxic shock syndrome in nasal surgery: A physiochemical and microbiologic evaluation of Merocel and NuGAUZE nasal packing. Laryngoscope 97:1388–1391, 1987.
31. Holt GR: Concepts of soft-tissue trauma repair. Otolaryngol Clin North Am 23:1019–1030, 1990.
32. Robson MC, Frank DH, Heggers JP: Tetanus resulting from osteomyelitis of the zygoma. Plast Reconstr Surg 65:679–681, 1980.
33. Sasaki GH: Intraoperative expansion as an immediate reconstructive technique. Facial Plast Surg 5:362–378, 1988.
34. Baker SR: Fundamentals of expanded tissue. Head Neck Surg 13:327–333, 1991.
35. Baker MD, Moore SE: Human bites in children: A six-year experience. Am J Dis Child 141:1285–1290, 1987.
36. Stucker FJ, Shaw GY, Boyd S, Shockley WW: Management of animal and human bites in the head and neck. Arch Otolaryngol Head Neck Surg 116:789–793, 1990.
37. Tucker HM: Restoration of selective facial nerve function by the nerve-muscle pedicle technique. Clin Plast Surg 6:293–300, 1979.
38. Baker DC, Conley J: Regional muscle transposition for rehabilitation of the paralyzed face. Clin Plast Surg 6:317–333, 1979.
39. Rubin LR: Temporalis and masseter muscle transposition. In May M (ed): The Facial Nerve. New York, Thieme Inc., 1980, pp 665–679.
40. Harii K, Ohmori K, Torii S: Free gracilis muscle transplantation with neurovascular anastomoses for the treatment of facial paralysis. Plast Reconstr Surg 57:133–143, 1976.
41. Harii K: Microneurovascular free muscle transplantation for reanimation of facial paralysis. Clin Plast Surg 6:361–375, 1979.
42. Anderl H: Cross-face nerve transplant. Clin Plast Surg 6:433–449, 1979.
43. Verdung S, Hakelius L, Stalberg E: Cross-face nerve grafting followed by free muscle transplantation in young patients with long-standing facial paralysis. Scand J Plast Reconstr Surg 18:201–208, 1984.
44. Freeman MS, Thomas JR, Spector JG, et al: Surgical therapy of the eyelids in patients with facial paralysis. Laryngoscope 100:1086–1096, 1990.
45. Sobol SM, Alward PD: Early gold weight lid implant for rehabilitation of faulty eyelid closure with facial paralysis: An alternative to tarsorrhaphy. Head Neck Surg 12:149–153, 1990.
46. May M: Surgical rehabilitation of facial palsy: Total approach. In May M (ed): The Facial Nerve. New York, Thieme Inc, 1986, pp 695–777.
47. Cavo JW: True vocal cord paralysis following intubation. Laryngoscope 95:1352–1359, 1985.
48. Steidler NE, Cook RM, Reade PC: Residual complications in patients with major middle third facial fractures. Int J Oral Surg 9:259–266, 1980.
49. Nordgaard JO: Persistent sensory disturbances and diplopia following fractures of the zygoma. Arch Otolaryngol 102:80–182, 1976.
50. Kellman RH, Schilli W: Plate fixation of fractures of the mid and upper face. Otolaryngol Clin North Am 20:559–572, 1987.
51. Baker SR, Krause CJ: Pedicle flaps in reconstruction of the lip. Facial Plast Surg 1:61–68, 1983.
52. Renner GJ, Zitsch R: Reconstruction of the lip. Otolaryngol Clin North Am 23:975–990, 1990.
53. Karapandzic M: Reconstruction of the lip defects by local arterial flaps. Br J Plast Surg 27:93–97, 1974.
54. Webster JP: Crescentic peri-alar cheek excision for upper lip flap advancement with a short history of upper lip repair. Plast Reconstr Surg 16:434–464, 1955.
55. Webster RC, Coffey RJ, Kelleher RE: Total and partial reconstruction of the lower lip with innervated muscle-bearing flaps. Plast Reconstr Surg 25:360–371, 1960.
56. Kellerher JC, Sullivan JG, Baibak GJ, Dean RK: The wrestler's ear. Plast Reconstr Surg 40:540–546, 1967.
57. Schuller DE, Dankle SK, Martin M, Strauss RH: Auricular injury and the use of headgear in wrestlers. Arch Otolaryngol Head Neck Surg 115:714–717, 1989.
58. Schuller DE, Dankle SD, Strauss RH: A technique to treat wrestlers' auricular hematoma without interrupting training or competition. Arch Otolaryngol Head Neck Surg 115:202–206, 1989.
59. Liston SL: Injury of the external ear. In Gates G (ed): Current Therapy in Otolaryngology–Head and Neck Surgery. 3rd ed. Toronto, BC Decker, 1987, pp 93–95.
60. Dowling JA, Foley FD, Moncrief JA: Chondritis in the burned ear. Plast Reconstr Surg 42:115–122, 1968.
61. Stroud MH: A simple treatment for suppurative perichondritis. Laryngoscope 73:556–563, 1963.
62. Apfelberg DB, Waisbren BA, Masters FW, Robinson DW: Treatment of chondritis in the burned ear

by the local instillation of antibiotics. Plast Reconstr Surg 53:179–183, 1974.

63. Wanamaker HH: Suppurative perichondritis of the auricle. Trans Am Acad Ophthalmol Otol 76:1289–1291, 1972.

64. Bernstein L, Nelson RH: Replanting the severed auricle. An update. Arch Otolaryngol 108:587–590, 1982.

65. Clemons JE, Connelly MV: Reattachment of a totally amputated auricle. Arch Otolaryngol 97:269–272, 1973.

66. Nahai F, Hayhurst JW, Salibian AH: Microvascular surgery in avulsive trauma to the external ear. Clin Plast Surg 5:423–426, 1978.

67. Turpin IM: Microsurgical replantation of the external ear. Clin Plast Surg 17:397–404, 1990.

68. Mladick RA: Salvage of the ear in acute trauma. Clin Plast Surg 5:427–435, 1978.

69. Brent B: Reconstruction of traumatic ear deformities. Clin Plast Surg 5:437–445, 1978.

70. Baker SR: Regional flaps in facial reconstruction. Otolaryngol Clin North Am 23:925–946, 1990.

71. Welling DB, Maves MD, Schuller DE, Bardach J: Irradiated homologous cartilage grafts. Long-term results. Arch Otolaryngol Head Neck Surg 114:291–295, 1988.

72. Illum P: Long-term results after treatment of nasal fractures. J Laryngol Otol 100:273–277, 1986.

73. Schultz RC: Frontal sinus and supraorbital fractures from vehicle accidents. Clin Plast Surg 2:93–106, 1975.

74. Luce EA: Frontal sinus fractures: Guidelines to management. Plast Reconstr Surg 80:500–510, 1987.

75. Hybels RL, Newman MH: Posterior table fractures of the frontal sinus. I. An experimental study. Laryngoscope 87:171–179, 1977.

76. Stanley RB: Management of frontal sinus fractures. Facial Plast Surg 5:231–235, 1988.

76a. Stanley RB, Becker TS: Injuries of the nasofrontal orifices in frontal sinus fractures. Laryngoscope 97:728–731, 1987.

77. Donald PJ, Bernstein L: Compound frontal sinus injuries with intracranial penetration. Laryngoscope 88:225–232, 1978.

78. Donald PJ: Frontal sinus ablation by cranialization: Report of 21 cases. Arch Otolaryngol 108:142–146, 1982.

79. Duvall AJ III, Porto DP, Lyons D, Boies LR: Frontal sinus fractures: Analysis of treatment results. Arch Otolaryngol Head Neck Surg 113:933–935, 1987.

80. Holt JE, Holt GR, Blodgett J: Ocular injuries sustained after blunt facial trauma. Ophthalmology 90:14–18, 1983.

81. Ketchum LD, Ferris B, Masters FW: Blindness without direct injury to the globe: A complication of facial fractures. Plast Reconstr Surg 58:187–191, 1976.

82. Strohm M, Jahnke K: Decompression du nerf optique par un transethmoidale. J Fr Oto Rhin Laryngol 31:363–368, 1982.

83. Osguthorpe JD, Sofferman RA: Optic nerve decompression. Otolaryngol Clin North Am 21:155–169, 1988.

84. Sofferman RA: Sphenoethmoid approach to the optic nerve. Laryngoscope 91:184–196, 1981.

85. Funk GF, Stanley RB, Becker TS: Reversible visual loss due to impacted lateral orbital wall fractures. Head Neck Surg 11:295–300, 1989.

86. Kurzer A, Patel MP: Superior orbital fissure syndrome associated with fractures of the zygoma and orbit. Plast Reconstr Surg 64:715–719, 1979.

87. Smith B, Regan WF: Blowout fracture of the orbit: Mechanism and correction of internal orbital fractures. Am J Ophthalmol 44:733–739, 1957.

88. Fujino T: Experimental "blowout" fracture of the orbit. Plast Reconstr Surg 54:81–82, 1974.

89. Converse JM, Smith B, Obear MF, Wood-Smith D: Orbital blowout fractures: A ten year survey. Plast Reconstr Surg 39:20–36, 1967.

90. Gruss JS: Naso-ethmoid-orbital fractures: Classification and role of primary bone grafting. Plast Reconstr Surg 75:303–315, 1985.

91. Manson PN, Grivas A, Rosenbaum A, et al: Studies on enophthalmos. II: The measurement of orbital injuries and their treatment by quantitative computed tomography. Plast Reconstr Surg 77:203–214, 1986.

92. Nicholson DH, Guzak SV: Visual loss complicating repair of orbital floor fractures. Arch Ophthalmol 86:369–375, 1971.

93. Putterman AM, Stevens T, Urist MJ: Nonsurgical management of blowout fractures of the orbital floor. Am J Ophthalmol 77:232–239, 1974.

94. Putterman AM: Late management of blowout fractures of the orbital floor. Trans Am Acad Ophthalmol Otol 83:650–659, 1977.

95. Koutroupas S, Meyerhoff WL: Surgical treatment of orbital floor fractures. Arch Otolaryngol 108:184–186, 1982.

96. Manson PN, Iliff NT: Orbital fractures. Facial Plast Surg 5:243–259, 1988.

97. Gilbard SM, Mafee MF, Lagouros PA, Langer BG: Orbital blowout fractures: The prognostic significance of computed tomography. Ophthalmology 92:1523–1528, 1985.

98. Maniglia AJ: Conjunctival approach for the repair of pure orbital blowout fractures. Otolaryngol Clin North Am 16:575–583, 1983.

99. Walter WL: Early surgical repair of blowout fracture of the orbital floor by using the transantral approach. South Med J 65:1229–1243, 1972.

100. Tovi F, Pitchazade N, Sidi J, Winer T: Healing of experimentally induced orbital floor defects. J Oral Maxillofac Surg 41:385–388, 1983.

101. Aronowitz JA, Freeman BS, Spira M: Long-term stability of Teflon orbital implants. Plast Reconstr Surg 78:166–173, 1986.

102. Polley JW, Ringler SL: The use of Teflon in orbital floor reconstruction following blunt facial trauma: A 20-year experience. Plast Reconstr Surg 79:39–43, 1987.

103. Smith JD, Abramson M: Membranous versus endochondral bone autografts. Arch Otolaryngol 99:203–205, 1974.

104. Zins JE, Whitaker LA: Membranous versus endochondral bone: Implications for craniofacial reconstruction. Plast Reconstr Surg 72:778–785, 1983.

105. Mathog RH: Reconstruction of the orbit following trauma. Otolaryngol Clin North Am 16:585–607, 1983.

106. Mathog RH, Nesi FA, Smith B: Post-traumatic enophthalmos and diplopia. In Mathog RH (ed):

Maxillofacial Trauma. Baltimore, Williams & Wilkins, 1984, pp 329–339.

107. Tessier P: Complications of facial trauma: Principles of late reconstruction. Ann Plast Surg 17:411–420, 1986.

108. Mathog RH, Archer KF, Nesi FA: Post-traumatic enophthalmos and diplopia. Otolaryngol Head Neck Surg 94:69–77, 1986.

109. Putterman AM, Urist MJ: Müller muscle–conjunctiva resection: Technique for treatment of blepharoptosis. Arch Ophthalmol 93:619–623, 1975.

110. Putterman AM, Urist MJ: Treatment of enophthalmic narrow palpebral fissure after blowout fracture. Ophthalmic Surg 6:45–49, 1975.

111. Putterman AM, Urist MJ: Reconstruction of the upper eyelid crease and fold. Arch Ophthalmol 94:1941–1954, 1976.

112. LeFort R: Fractures de la machoire superieure. Intern Med (Paris) Sect de Chir Gen, 1900, p 175.

113. Helfrick J: Pathogenesis and evaluation of maxillary fractures. In Mathog RH (ed): Maxillofacial Trauma. Baltimore, Williams and Wilkins, 1984, pp 223–228.

114. LeFort R: Étude expérimental sur les fractures de la machoire supérieure, parts I, II, III. Rev Chir Paris 23:208–227, 360–379, 479–507, 1901. Translated and reprinted as Experimental study of fractures of the upper jaw. Plast Reconstr Surg 50:497–506, 600–607, 1972.

115. Manson PN, Hoopes JE, Su CT: Structural pillars of the facial skeleton: An approach to the management of LeFort fractures. Plast Reconstr Surg 66:54–61, 1980.

116. Klotch DW, Gilliland R: Internal fixation vs. conventional therapy in midface fractures. J Trauma 27:1136–1145, 1987.

117. McCoy FJ, Chandler RA, Magnan CG, et al: An analysis of facial fractures and their complications. Plast Reconstr Surg 29:381–391, 1962.

118. Levy RA, Rosenbaum AE, Kellman RM, et al: Assessing whether the plane of section on CT affects accuracy in demonstrating facial fractures in 3-D reconstruction using a dried skull. Am J Neuroradiol 12:861–866, 1991.

119. Finkle DR, Ringler SL, Luttenton CR, et al: Comparison of the diagnostic methods used in maxillofacial trauma. Plast Reconstr Surg 75:32–38, 1985.

120. DeMarino DP, Steiner E, Poster RB, et al: Trauma: Three-dimensional computed tomography in maxillofacial trauma. Arch Otolaryngol Head Neck Surg 112:146–150, 1986.

121. Marsh JL, Vannier MW, Stevens WG, et al: Computerized imaging for soft tissue and osseous reconstruction in the head and neck. Clin Plast Surg 12:279–291, 1985.

122. Marsh JL, Vannier MW, Gado M, Stevens WG: In vivo delineation of facial fractures: The application of advanced medical imaging technology. Ann Plast Surg 17:364–376, 1986.

123. Hemmy DC, Tessier PL: CT of dry skulls with craniofacial deformities: Accuracy of three-dimensional reconstruction. Radiology 157:113–116, 1985.

124. Tessier P, Hemmy D: Three-dimensional imaging in medicine. Scand J Plast Reconstr Surg 20:3–11, 1986.

125. Levy RA, Kellman RM, Rosenbaum AE: The effect of computed tomographic scan orientation on information loss in the three-dimensional reconstruc-

tion of tripod zygomatic fractures. Invest Radiol 26:427–431, 1991.

126. Thompson JN, Gibson B, Kohut RI: Airway obstruction in LeFort fractures. Laryngoscope 97:275–279, 1987.

127. Montgomery WW: Surgery for cerebrospinal fluid rhinorrhea and otorrhea. Arch Otolaryngol 84:538–550, 1966.

128. Leopold DA: Personal communication, 1991.

129. Bell RM, Page GV, Bynoe RP, et al: Post-traumatic sinusitis. J Trauma 28:923–930, 1988.

130. Chole RA, Yee J: Antibiotic prophylaxis for facial fractures: A prospective, randomized clinical trial. Arch Otolaryngol Head Neck Surg 113:1055–1057, 1987.

131. Manson PN: Some thoughts on the classification and treatment of LeFort fractures. Ann Plast Surg 17:356–361, 1986.

132. Adams WM: Internal wiring fixation of facial fractures. Surgery 12:523–540, 1942.

133. Gruss JS, Mackinnon SE: Complex maxillary fractures: Role of buttress reconstruction and immediate bone grafts. Plast Reconstr Surg 78:9–22, 1986.

134. Sofferman RA, Danielson PA, Quatela V, Reed RR: Retrospective analysis of surgically treated LeFort fractures: Is suspension necessary? Arch Otolaryngol 109:446–448, 1983.

135. Stanley RB: Reconstruction of the midfacial vertical dimension following LeFort fractures. Arch Otolaryngol 100:571–575, 1984.

136. Ferraro JW, Berggren RB: Treatment of complex facial fractures. J Trauma 13:783–787, 1973.

137. Kufner J: A method of craniofacial suspension. J Oral Surg 28:260–262, 1970.

138. Stanley RB, Toffel PH: The extended access approach for treatment of maxillary fractures. Facial Plastic Surg 5:213–219, 1988.

139. Tessier P: Total osteotomy of the middle third of the face for faciostenosis or for sequelae of LeFort III fractures. Plast Reconstr Surg 48:533–541, 1971.

140. Gruss JS: Complex nasoethmoid orbital and midfacial fractures: Role of craniofacial surgical techniques and immediate bone grafting. Ann Plast Surg 17:377–390, 1986.

141. Kellman RM: Midfacial fractures. In Gates GA (ed): Current Therapy in Otolaryngology–Head and Neck Surgery. 4th ed. Toronto, BC Decker, 1990, pp 114–118.

142. Lauritzen C, Lilja J, Vällfors B: The craniofacial approach to trauma. Ann Plast Surg 17:503–512, 1986.

143. Marschall MA, Cohen M, Garcia J, Schafer ME: Craniofacial approach for the reconstruction of severe facial injuries. J Oral Maxillofac Surg 46:305–310, 1988.

144. Champy M, Lodde JP, Muster D, et al: Osteosynthesis using miniaturized screw-on plates in facial and cranial surgery. Ann Chir Plast Esthet 22:261–264, 1977.

145. Gruss JS, Mackinnon SE, Kassel EE, Cooper PW: The role of primary bone grafting in complex craniomaxillofacial trauma. Plast Reconstr Surg 75:17–24, 1985.

146. Manson PN, Crawley WA, Yaremchuk MJ, et al: Midface fractures: Advantages of immediate extended open reduction and bone grafting. Plast Reconstr Surg 76:1–12, 1985.

147. Phillips JH, Rahn BA: Fixation effects on membranous and endochondral only bone-graft resorption. Plast Reconstr Surg 82:872–877, 1988.

148. Thaller SR, Kawamoto HK: A histologic evaluation of fracture repair in the midface. Plast Reconstr Surg 85:196–201, 1990.

149. Gussack GS, Luterman A, Powell RW, et al: Pediatric maxillofacial trauma: Unique features in diagnosis and treatment. Laryngoscope 97:925–930, 1987.

150. Ousterhout DK, Vargervik K: Maxillary hypoplasia secondary to midfacial trauma in childhood. Plast Reconstr Surg 80:491–497, 1987.

151. Thaller SR, Zarem HA, Kawamoto HK: Surgical correction of late sequelae from facial bone fractures. Am J Surg 154:149–152, 1987.

152. Gruss JS, VanWyck L, Phillips JH, Antonyshyn O: The importance of the zygomatic arch in complex midfacial fracture repair and correction of posttraumatic orbitozygomatic deformities. Plast Reconstr Surg 85:878–890, 1990.

153. Eisele DW, Duckert LG: Single-point stabilization of zygomatic fractures with the minicompression plate. Arch Otolaryngol Head Neck Surg 113:267–270, 1987.

154. Davidson J, Nickerson D, Nickerson B: Zygomatic fractures: Comparison of methods of internal fixation. Plast Reconstr Surg 86:25–32, 1990.

155. Mathog RH: Posttraumatic telecanthus. In Mathog RH (ed): Maxillofacial Trauma. Baltimore, Williams & Wilkins, 1984, pp 303–318.

156. Converse JM, Smith B, Wood-Smith D: Malunited fractures of the orbit. In Converse JM (ed): Reconstructive Plastic Surgery. Vol 2. Philadelphia, WB Saunders, 1977, pp 989–1039.

157. Mathog RH, Bauer W: Post-traumatic pseudohypertelorism (telecanthus). Arch Otolaryngol 105:81–85, 1979.

158. Stranc MF: Primary treatment of naso-ethmoid injuries with increased intercanthal distance. Br J Plast Surg 23:3–25, 1970.

159. Converse JM, Hogan VM: Open-sky approach for reduction of naso-orbital fractures. Plast Reconstr Surg 46:396–398, 1970.

160. Jones LT: The cure of epiphora due to canalicular disorders, trauma and surgical failures on the lacrimal passages. Trans Am Acad Ophthalmol Otol 66:506–521, 1962.

161. Converse JM, Smith B: Naso-orbital fractures and traumatic deformities of the medial canthus. Plast Reconstr Surg 38:147–162, 1966.

162. Mustardé JC: Epicanthus and telecanthus. Br J Plast Surg 16:346–356, 1963.

163. Levy RA, Smith RW, Odland RM, Marentette LJ: Monocortical miniplate fixation of mandibular angle fractures. Arch Otolaryngol Head Neck Surg 117:149–154, 1991.

164. Beckers HL: Treatment of initially infected mandibular fractures with bone plates. J Oral Surg 37:310–313, 1979.

165. Mathog RH: Nonunion of the mandible. Otolaryngol Clin North Am 16:533–547, 1983.

166. Adekeye EO: Reconstruction of mandibular defects by autogenous bone grafts: A review of 37 cases. J Oral Surg 36:125–128, 1978.

167. Boyne PJ, Zarem H: Osseous reconstruction of the resected mandible. Am J Surg 132:49–53, 1976.

168. Chuong R, Piper MA: Open reduction of condylar fractures of the mandible in conjunction with repair of discal injury: A preliminary report. J Oral Maxillofac Surg 46:257–263, 1988.

169. Rowe NL: Ankylosis of the temporomandibular joint. Parts I, II, and III. J R Coll Surg Edinb 27:67–79, 167–173, 209–218, 1982.

170. Topazian RG: Etiology of ankylosis of temporomandibular joint: Analysis of 44 cases. J Oral Surg 22:227–233, 1964.

171. Hoaglund FT: Experimental haemarthrosis: The response of canine knees to injections of autologous blood. J Bone Joint Surg 49:285–298, 1967.

172. Markey RG: Condylar trauma and facial asymmetry: An experimental study. Thesis, University of Washington, 1974, pp 1–32.

173. Bradley P: Injuries of the condylar and coronoid process. In Rowe NL, Williams JL (eds): Maxillofacial Injuries. Vol 1. Edinburgh, Churchill Livingstone, 1985, pp 337–362.

174. Dingman RO, Grabb WC: Reconstruction of both mandibular condyles with metatarsal bone grafts. Plast Reconstr Surg 34:441–451, 1964.

175. Dingman RO: Ankylosis of the temporomandibular joint. In Mathog RH (ed): Maxillofacial Trauma. Baltimore, Williams and Wilkins, 1984, pp 208–222.

176. Kroon F: Effects of three-dimensional loading on stability of internal fixation of mandible fractures. In preparation, as cited by Spiessl B: Internal Fixation of the Mandible. Berlin, Springer-Verlag, 1989, pp 26–27.

177. Leopard P: Complications. In Rowe NL, Williams J (eds): Maxillofacial Injuries. Vol 2. Edinburgh, Churchill Livingstone, 1985, pp 724–763.

178. Zide MF, Kent JN: Indications for open reduction of mandibular condyle fractures. J Oral Maxillofac Surg 41:89–98, 1983.

179. Bradley JC: Age changes in the vascular supply of the mandible. Br Dent J 132:142–144, 1972.

180. Bruce RA, Strachen DS: Fractures of the edentulous mandible: Chalmers J. Lyons academy study. J Oral Surg 34:973–979, 1976.

181. Cope MR: Spontaneous fracture of an atrophic edentulous mandible treated without fixation. Br J Oral Surg 20:22–30, 1982.

182. Degnan EJ: Mandibular fracture in the geriatric patient: Problems in treatment planning: Report of case. J Oral Surg 28:438–442, 1970.

183. Obwegeser HL, Sailer HF: Another way of treating fractures of the atrophic edentulous mandible. J Maxillofac Surg 1:213–221, 1973.

184. Woods WR, Hiatt WR, Brooks RL: A technique for simultaneous fracture repair and augmentation of the atrophic edentulous mandible. J Oral Surg 37:131–135, 1979.

185. Kellman RM: Maxillofacial trauma. In Pillsbury HC III, Goldsmith MM III (eds): Operative Challenges in Otolaryngology–Head and Neck Surgery. Chicago, Year Book Medical Publishers, Inc, 1990, pp 471–481.

186. McGuirt WF, Salisbury PL: Mandibular fractures: Their effect on growth and dentition. Arch Otolaryngol Head Neck Surg 113:257–261, 1987.

187. Luhr HG: Compression plate osteosynthesis through the Luhr system. In Kruger E, Schilli W (eds): Oral and Maxillofacial Traumatology. Vol 1.

Chicago, Quintessence Publishing Company, 1982, pp 319–348.

188. Morris JH: Biphase connector, external skeletal splint for reduction and fixation of mandibular fractures. Oral Surg 2:1382–1398, 1949.

189. Spiessl B: Internal Fixation of the Mandible. Berlin, Springer-Verlag, 1989.

190. Steiner M, von Fraunhofer JA, Mascaro J: The possible role of corrosion in inhibiting the healing of a mandibular fracture: Report of case. J Oral Surg 39:140–143, 1981.

191. Champy M, Pepe HD, Gerlach KL, et al: The Strasbourg miniplate osteosynthesis. In Kruger E, Schilli W, Worthington P (eds): Oral and Maxillofacial Traumatology. Vol 2. Chicago, Quintessence Publishing Company, 1986, pp 19–43.

192. Kellman RM: Repair of mandibular fractures via compression plating and more traditional techniques: A comparison of results. Laryngoscope 94:1560–1570, 1984.

193. Chuong R, Mulliken JB, Kaban LB, Strome M: Fragmented care of facial fractures. J Trauma 27:477–482, 1987.

Aesthetic Facial Surgery

VITO C. QUATELA, MD
W. RUSSELL RIES, MD

In the past two decades the number of aesthetic facial procedures performed has increased dramatically. As the population ages, the demand will undoubtedly continue to increase. In elective surgery, a physiologically well patient decides to undergo a procedure advised by the surgeon after the alternatives, limitations and risks have been thoroughly discussed. Therefore, the surgeon must be knowledgeable about all possible complications including their etiologies, manifestations, and treatments.

A preoperative discussion regarding possible complications associated with aesthetic facial procedures is essential for several reasons. Perhaps most importantly, this consultation establishes a foundation for prevention, the first line of defense against complications. Preoperatively, a review of complications assists the surgeon in the patient selection and patient assessment process; for example, a patient's compliance with postoperative routines can be assessed. This discussion orients the patient to the limitations of the surgeon and the operation, and helps define patient motivation, expectation, and commitment. Reviewing routine symptoms such as pain, edema, and ecchymosis sets the stage preoperatively for reassurance following the procedure; clarifying a benign postoperative course from a predetermined misconception of a "complication" by the patient. Sharing a review of the medical literature promotes trust between the patient and surgeon and helps create an alliance toward a common goal of an uncomplicated postoperative course.

Preoperative assessment should include an appropriate physical examination and an adequate history. The surgeon should have an understanding of the patient's overall medical status. Preoperative consultations should be obtained when appropriate. If the preoperative assessment turns up any abnormalities, then the operation should be postponed until these abnormalities have been resolved.

Patient selection and timing are equally as important as surgical technique in the attempt to avoid complications. Patient satisfaction is the measure by which to judge the success of the procedure. Unrealistic patient expectations can detract from an otherwise excellent result. The patient should understand clearly that the goal of aesthetic surgery is improvement and not perfection. This is a critical part of the initial consultation and preoperative process. We prefer to utilize a second preoperative consultation at no cost to the patient to achieve a greater level of understanding by the patient.

The patient's motivation for seeking aesthetic surgery should be carefully reviewed. The best patient is self-motivated, has realistic expectations, and has contemplated an operation for an appropriate period of time. Be wary of the well-adjusted young patient who is being coerced by a well-intended parent, or a person seeking aging-face operation with the idea that it may save a relationship. The staff should alert the physician to the problem patient, i.e., missing multiple appointments, scheduling difficulties, or excessive rudeness toward staff while being pleasant to the physician. The patient's response to complications postoperatively is, in part, indicated by the commitment to the operation. The financial arrangements for aesthetic facial surgery should be clearly outlined and understood prior to the procedure. Prepayment in advance of the operation date forces the patient to understand the finances and indicates a commitment as well as compliance with routines.

Aesthetic facial surgery may constitute the whole or a part of a head and neck surgeon's practice. If a surgeon rarely performs a certain aesthetic procedure, then it may be in the patient's and the surgeon's best interest to refer the patient to a colleague with greater expertise. Patients always have respect for a physician who admits his or her limitations.

All surgeons will encounter complications, but it should be one's goal to continually refine techniques in order to perform surgery as safely as possible. As humbling as it may be, more is learned from the discussion of complications than from a presentation of satisfactory uncomplicated cases. To that end, we share our ever-evolving knowledge of complications of aesthetic facial surgery.

RHINOPLASTY COMPLICATIONS

Preventive Measures

Many factors are at odds with the surgeon performing rhinoplasty, making it one of the most challenging aesthetic procedures through which to obtain consistently predictable results. M. Eugene Tardy, MD, has described rhinoplasty as an "easy operation to perform but difficult to obtain good results." Multiple variables, such as healing characteristics, anatomic differences of skin and cartilage, patient selection, and surgical proficiency, combine to determine success or failure. The ability to successfully predict a surgical result at 1 year demonstrates one level of rhinoplasty comprehension; the ability to predict good results consistently 10 years postoperatively is the sign of a rhinoplasty master.

Due to factors beyond the surgeon's control, such as patient noncompliance contributing to complication, or because of an unavoidable complication, a certain percentage of patients will require revision surgery. It is acceptable for a skilled surgeon with a large rhinoplasty practice to have 5 to 10 per cent of patients require revision surgery.

Providing the patient preoperatively with information concerning the occasional need for revision surgery helps avoid patient dissatisfaction postoperatively. This emphasizes the realities of the procedure and that the surgeon is not infallible. Since the patient will request revision surgery as soon as a deformity is appreciated, it should be stressed preoperatively that the timing of a second operation is 6 months postoperatively for simple revisions and 1 year postoperatively for more complicated interventions.

Rhinoplasty performed on the patient with inappropriate motives will result in failure. Thorough preoperative evaluation and consultation are required to assess properly the patient's motives, desires, and realistic possibilities within the individual's unique set of anatomic variables. The neuroses associated with one's nose can represent a nightmare for the surgeon who delves into them for the wrong reasons. Thorough evaluation can be made with questionnaires or multiple consultations. The patient's understanding and expectations of surgery need to be assessed. It is best to avoid operation in those patients with unrealistic expectations. In addition to a complete psychiatric assessment, a thorough medical history is required. Knowledge of nasal obstruction, bleeding diathesis, hypertension, drug abuse, and previous anesthetic complication will help direct the course of management to avoid untoward results.

Accurate analysis and diagnosis of the nasal deformity is essential to properly execute correction. Failure to correct a deviated nasal septum may result in nasal obstruction postrhinoplasty. Further, lowering a dorsum with a low radix may result in an undesirable contour. Proper analysis of a tip and understanding of tip dynamics can assure successful tip rhinoplasty.

Early Complications

BLEEDING

It should be stressed to the patient that it is normal to expect some postoperative bleeding for 48 hours following a rhinoplasty. When bleeding persists beyond this period or is excessive, further evaluation is required. The incidence of hemorrhage postrhinoplasty is about 3 per cent.[23, 44, 75] It usually occurs within 48 hours of the procedure or at 10 days. The incidence is the same even if septoplasty is not performed.[23]

Simple measures should be attempted prior to repacking the nose. Cocaine pledgets will stop most bleeding to allow for a light packing of Surgicel. If the patient has had a septoplasty or a turbinate procedure, a specific bleeding site may be identified and cauterized. The bleeding site, although most commonly anterior, may require a posterior pack as well.[23] It is always distressing to place an anterior and posterior pack in a postoperative rhinoplasty patient because of the disturbance of the nasal bones that occurs. This temporary widening usually can be managed through nasal molding exercises. When epistaxis persists despite a full packing, the usual measure of anterior ethmoid artery and internal maxillary artery ligation must be instituted.[48]

Prevention is the best course of action. Coagulopathy history should be elicited and, if suggestive, followed by a coagulation profile and bleeding time study. Patients should refrain from aspirin, nonsteroidal anti-inflammatory agents, and vitamin E for 2 weeks prior to surgery.[12] Nose blowing and intranasal manipulation is not allowed. Patients are cautioned to avoid aerobic exercise for 3 weeks.

INFECTION

The overall incidence of infection in rhinoplasty is between 1 and 3 per cent.[3, 44, 54] This is a surprisingly low incidence of infection for a procedure that is performed in a nonsterile field. The manifestation of infection can range from a simple cellulitis or abscess (Fig. 24–1) to septic shock, cavernous sinus thrombosis, cerebritis, and death.[34, 48, 51] The most common offending organisms are *Staphylococcus aureus*, anaerobic streptococci, *Haemophilus influenzae* and *Klebsiella pneumoniae*. More rarely reported are *Pseudomonas*[40, 41] and *Actinomyces*.[56, 76] Cellulitis will manifest by pain, erythema, and fever. Intranasal drainage should be established to avoid external scar. In the event of cartilage grafting or poor initial response to oral antibiotics, hospital admission and intravenous broad-spectrum antibiotics may be required. Septicemia can be a complication, and staphylococcal endocarditis secondary to rhinoplasty has occurred.[14]

Toxic shock syndrome following rhinoplasty has been reported.[35, 80] This entity is more commonly associated with nasal packing, but it has occurred with septal splinting

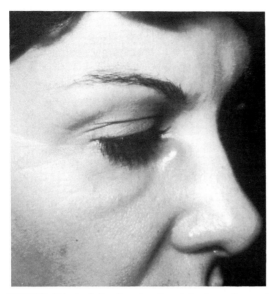

FIGURE 24–1. Infection in the right lateral nasal wall resulting in abscess over lateral osteotomy.

alone.[81] Onset is usually within 24 hours, with unusual nausea and vomiting, high fever, tachycardia, hypotension, and diffuse rash. Removal of splints or packing, culture, check for TSS Toxin 1, and hospital admission and hydration with antistaphylococcal antibiotics is the usual course of therapy. *Staphylococcus aureus* may not grow because of previous antibiotic ointment or prophylaxis.[80]

Postrhinoplasty intracranial infection can manifest as meningitis, cerebritis, and cavernous sinus thrombosis. Lacy and Conway described meningitis following septorhinoplasty.[46] Levin and associates described a postrhinoplasty patient who developed a medial canthal abscess that rapidly progressed to focal cerebritis with abscess.[49] Several surgeons have described cavernous sinus thrombosis leading to death.[9, 18, 51] The cavernous sinus drains the nose through the ophthalmic veins and also emissary veins in the pterygoid plexus. Septal emboli can easily seed the cavernous sinus. Even with the most aggressive management, mortality is about 20 per cent.[51]

Speculated modes of intracranial spread are through the following routes: (1) natural bony dehiscences in the cribriform plate, (2) iatrogenic fractures of the cribriform plate and the intracranial fossa, (3) retrograde thrombophlebitis, (4) extension via the olfactory perineural sheath, (5) acute sinusitis secondary to nasal packing, and (6) bacteremia secondary to nasal packing or splints.[51, 63]

Prophylactic antibiotics are controversial and of questionable value. It has been demonstrated that bacteremia during septorhinoplasty does not occur.[61, 66] Eschelman and associates, using a double-blind study, concluded that prophylactic antibiotics were not necessary for septonasal procedures.[17] Herzon demonstrated that bacteremia occurred in 12 per cent of the patients requiring packing.[32] We use prophylactic cephalosporin antibiotics perioperatively in patients requiring packing or in those who have multiple cartilage grafts or alloplastic implants.[37–39] All patients are instructed to notify the doctor if they develop an upper respiratory or skin infection in the immediate preoperative period as it is best to postpone operation until these potentially seeding sites of infection are controlled.

HEMATOMA

Hematoma can occur in the septum or between the plane of skin elevation and bony cartilagenous vault. The latter is usually prevented if adequate pressure taping and cast dressing are applied immediately following rhinoplasty. With a cast in place, hematoma is usually limited to the glabellar area where it resorbs without intervention. A hematoma of the dorsal nasal skin should be evacuated internally and nasal dressing applied.

Septal hematoma manifests with complaints of nasal congestion. The septum is found to be widened and boggy in appearance. Drainage is performed with a 16-gauge needle or stab incision and suctioning. When the diagnosis of septal hematoma is established, prophylactic antibiotics should be instituted to prevent septal abscess. Failure to diagnose and treat septal hematoma will lead to loss of cartilage and subsequent dorsal support.[6, 69] The use of continuous mattress suture following septoplasty has reduced the incidence of septal hematoma and limited the need for septal splints.[64]

OPHTHALMOLOGIC

In the preoperative consultation patients should be forewarned that they may experience a transient period of epiphora.[57, 77] This is presumably due to edema secondary to lateral osteotomies creating a functional blockage of tears.[13] Injury to the well-protected lacrimal duct ostium in the interior meatus or the lacrimal sac could occur with an excessively low and careless osteotomy.[1] Thomas and Griner have demonstrated that the lacrimal duct and sac are protected below the course of a conventional lateral osteotomy.[77] Epiphora following rhinoplasty is self-limiting and usually resolves within a week. Persistent epiphora beyond 1 month needs ophthalmologic evaluation and may require dacrocystorhinostomy. Occasionally epiphora will be accompanied by irritation of the eye, and this may alert the surgeon to the presence of a corneal abrasion. In particular, during a procedure employing local anesthesia with sedation, a patient may inadvertently open the eyes; it is advisable to protect the patient's eyes with moist gauze. This will prevent unwanted suture materials, instruments, or gauze sponges from causing corneal abrasions.

A rarer ophthalmologic complication following rhinoplasty and its aftercare is visual acuity disturbances, including blindness.[11] Well documented is the relationship of steroid injection of the turbinate and retinal artery embolization.[50] Retinal artery ischemia and unilateral blindness have occurred after routine rhinoplasty, but the mechanism of injury is unknown.

EDEMA AND ECCHYMOSIS

A patient must always be forewarned of a transient period of edema and periorbital ecchymosis following rhinoplasty. The surgeon should make clear to the patient that the intent of many of the preoperative instructions is to minimize edema and ecchymosis.[71]

Edema of the nose and especially the nasal tip can take up to 12 months to completely resolve. Most patients will have some degree of swelling or discoloration that lasts 1 to 2 weeks. Occasionally periorbital pigmentation can persist for 3 to 12 months. Patients with pigmentation persisting beyond 1 month should be alerted that the resolution of the pigment will be slow. Patients with pre-existing pigmentation or of Mediterranean descent are more predisposed to this.

Patients with thick, sebaceous skin and revision rhinoplasty patients take longest to resolve the edema. Even within the same skin type there is tremendous variation in the amount and resolution time of the edema. Judicious use of intralesional steroids, triamcinolone acetonide (Kenalog), 10 mg/ml in the supratip area can help reduce edema.[2, 38]

Regardless of how excessive the degree of edema and ecchymosis, the final outcome will not be affected. Since swelling and bruising are perceived as pain and discomfort by friends, family, and sometimes the patient, all measures should be employed to attempt to minimize their occurrence. Aspirin, nonsteroidal anti-inflammatory agents, and vitamin E should be stopped 2 weeks in advance of operation because of their ability to prolong bleeding.[12] Patients are placed on supplemental vitamin C 2 weeks prior to operation. Attention to management of nausea and hypertension can diminish edema and ecchymosis. Patients are instructed to elevate the head of the bed 30 to 45 degrees for 1 week following operation. Patients also receive intravenous steroids (Decadron, 8 mg) as well as oral steroids (Medrol Dosepak) the week following surgery.[27, 33] Occlusive types of nasal packing contribute to edema and do not allow for drainage, and so are avoided. Meticulous attention to surgical technique, which begins with avoidance of the angular vessels during anesthetic infiltration, is important. Suction and bipolar electrocautery are used on visible bleeding sites. Nasal osteotomies are appropriately performed toward the end of the operation so that a nasal dressing can be applied before the ecchymosis and edema ensue.[78] Patients are discharged with cold compresses for their eyes.

SKIN COMPLICATIONS

Most complications of the skin are directly related to the nasal dressing. The exception to this is the genetic predisposition to form telangiectasias. Some patients will form telangiectasias of the entire nose, known as "red nose syndrome."[16, 55] Treatment of these larger areas of telangiectasias is best performed with a yellow wavelength dye laser. If a laser is not available, the smaller areas can be treated with a depilatory (32-gauge) electrocautery needle passed into the lumen of the capillary.

Complications of the nasal dressing are related to its occlusive nature. Contact dermatitis from the skin adhesive and tape can occur. Ointments with neomycin should be avoided because of its high incidence of contact dermatitis.

Pustules of the skin as a result of the occlusive dressing are fairly common. Unlike impetigo, these do not require treatment and do not spread. Although these pustules resolve with simple cleansing, patients may be afraid to touch their nose and so must be encouraged to do so. The nasal skin also may demonstrate wrinkling, and the patient must be reassured that this will resolve spontaneously. Taping placed on the nose excessively tight can cause necrosis of the skin. Likewise, quick-setting nasal cast materials, such as Aquaplast, can be placed on the nose in such a way that it causes constant pressure and therefore leads to necrosis. Skin slough of nasal skin is initially managed conservatively with watchful waiting and reassurance. When wound healing and contracture are complete, flap reconstruction is performed if needed. Skin slough can also be caused by excessive dissection and thinning of the skin, especially in the revision case (Fig. 24–2).

Cautery when used during rhinoplasty should be employed judiciously. Unipolar cautery, because of its heat dissipation, should never be used on the nasal flaps. Bipolar cautery has been shown to be safe and effective on nasal flaps during open rhinoplasty.[38] Skin slough is a devastating complication but fortunately rare and routinely avoidable with the aforementioned preventive measures.

Most patients complain of sensory disturbances in the nasal tip, especially after open rhinoplasty.[8, 79] This usually resolves in 3

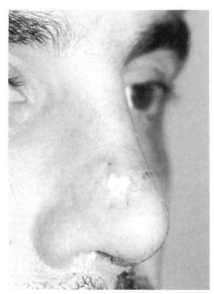

FIGURE 24–2. Full-thickness slough in a revision rhinoplasty.

months. A permanent infraorbital nerve injury following the saw osteotomy technique has been reported.[53] Occasionally, following septal surgery, patients will complain of numbness of the upper palate and incisors which resolves within several weeks. A devitalized tooth secondary to septorhinoplasty has been reported. Injury to the anterior-superior alveolar nerves during nasal spine reduction was the probable cause.[72]

Dorsal nasal cyst formation following rhinoplasty has been reported by several workers.[28, 31, 48] The presumed mechanism is via entrapment of the nasal mucosa through reductive osteotomies. Complete excision is usually curative (Fig. 24–3). Anderson and associates reported a recurrent dorsal nasal mass of trapped respiratory epithelium that ultimately had a tentative diagnosis of mucoepidermoid carcinoma.[4] Formation of mucosal tunnels and keeping mucosa intact, as described by Johnson and Anderson,[36] may help avoid this complication (Fig. 24–4). Arteriovenous malformation in the skin has been described postrhinoplasty and is treated by electrocautery and excision if necessary.[29, 59]

SEPTAL PERFORATION

Septal perforation as a complication of rhinoplasty is the result of an improperly exe-

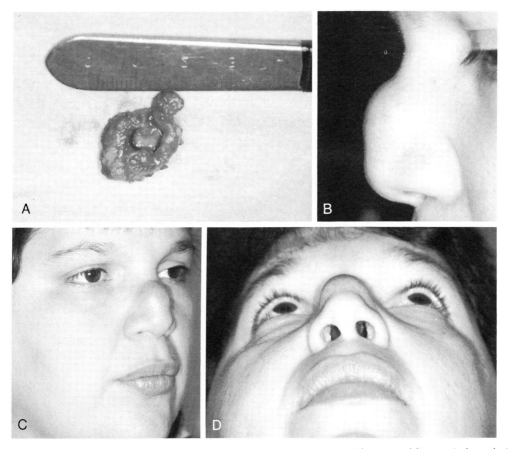

FIGURE 24–3. Intranasal mucous cyst one year postrhinoplasty. *A,* Cyst with mucosal lining; *B,* lateral view; *C,* three quarter view; *D,* basal view.

cuted septoplasty. Elevation of mucoperichondral flaps in the correct plane is key in avoiding perforation. Unilateral tears in mucoperichondrium are of little consequence. When tears in the mucoperichondral flap occur intraoperatively, repair should be instituted and will usually avoid a septal perforation. Unrecognized septal hematoma may lead to infection and subsequent perforation. Other predisposing factors include previous septal surgery, cocaine abuse, infection, excessive nasal packing, and necrosis from mattressing sutures or septal splinting.

Perforation manifests as crusting and bleeding. Small perforations that are limited posteriorly rarely require repair and may close spontaneously with saline cleansing and topical antibiotic ointment.[19, 26] Perforations located in the anterior septum tend to whistle with inspiration. The larger perforations and those located anteriorly will require repair using tissue grafts or flaps of nasal floor and turbinate as well as buccal mucosa.[19, 26, 45] Romo and colleagues described a midfacial degloving technique utilizing posteriorly based mucosal flaps of nasal septum, floor, and inferior turbinate[62] (Fig. 24–5).

INTRACRANIAL COMPLICATIONS

Fortunately, these life-threatening complications are exceedingly rare.[48] Cerebrospinal fluid (CSF) rhinorrhea, pneumocephalus, laceration of the frontal lobe, carotid cavernous sinus fistula, and the fatal infectious sequelae of these have all been reported.[30, 48, 51] The mechanism of injury in cases at autopsy was fracture of the cribriform plate. Song and Bromberg reported a carotid cavernous sinus fistula with proptosis, chemosis, and

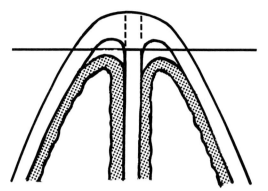

FIGURE 24–4. Hump removal is performed external to the mucosa. The solid line represents the line of resection. The mucosa is represented by the dotted area. (From Johnson CM, Toriumi DM: Open Structure Rhinoplasty. Philadelphia, WB Saunders, 1990, p 188.)

ophthalmoplegia.[70] Diagnosis was made by angiography, and treatment was by ligation of the common carotid artery.

Late Complications

NASAL OBSTRUCTIONS

All patients will experience some degree of transient nasal obstruction from mucosal edema and crusting for 2 weeks following a rhinoplasty. Most of this will improve spontaneously without treatment.[5] Postoperative steroids and beclomethasone nasal sprays have been beneficial and frequently will improve the congestion. Patients are routinely encouraged to use saline nasal spray frequently for up to 6 weeks postoperatively, especially with the congestion and crusting associated with turbinate surgery.

Permanent nasal obstruction results from either a pathogenic cause or a failure to recognize a pre-existing condition. A septal deflection that may not be a functional problem becomes one following bony vault narrowing.[24] Persistent septal deflection, especially caudal, is a common cause of nasal obstruction postoperatively[42] (Fig. 24–6). Cocaine abusers and the post-traumatic twisted nose present special problems in persistent septal deflection.[36, 67] In the immediate postoperative period, mild nasal trauma can result in a septal deflection. Management is

early revision septoplasty. Some septal deflections appear as late manifestations 6 to 9 months postoperatively.[34] These require re-evaluation of the original plan and use of innovative revision septoplasty techniques.

Turbinate hypertrophy can be missed as a preoperative diagnosis only to present a problem postoperatively.[58] However, excessive turbinate resection will result in crusting, oozing, and patient dissatisfaction.[25] Many patients will have a combination of anatomic obstruction and physiologic obstruction secondary to allergic or vasomotor rhinitis. Patients should be maximized on medical therapy prior to operation and forewarned that allergic symptoms will persist postoperatively.[34] In addition, 10 per cent of the patients will experience persistent turbinate hypertrophy resulting in an obstructive vasomotor rhinitis.[5] The use of topical steroid sprays, such as beclomethasone, improves this type of obstruction. Vasomotor rhinitis can manifest postoperatively to the extent

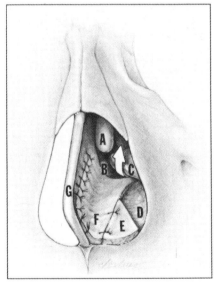

FIGURE 24–5. Completion of flap elevation, rotation, and repair of perforation. *A* indicates the middle turbinate; *B*, posterior nare; *C*, inferior turbinate infractured; *D*, raw surface area left by flap rotation; *E*, full-thickness skin graft on floor of nose; *F*, rotated flap; and *G*, septal angle. (From Romo T, Foster CA, Korovin GS, Sachs ME: Repair of nasal septal perforation utilizing the midface degloving technique. Arch Otolaryngol Head Neck Surg 114:739–742, 1988. Copyright 1988, American Medical Association.)

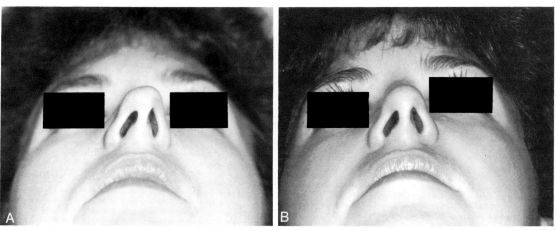

FIGURE 24–6. Caudal septal deflection. *A,* Preoperative, *B* postoperative.

that it may become an embarrassing persistent problematic rhinorrhea. Topical steroid inhalers are of some benefit. Patients also should be reassured that the exacerbation is self-limiting and will revert to baseline.

Intranasal synechiae, which are more common following turbinate surgery, can contribute to nasal obstruction.[5, 24] These synechiae form because of trauma to the mucous membrane of the nasal vault. Juxtaposing deepithelialized surfaces then develop into synechiae, often between the turbinate and septum, and warrant the use of septal splinting until appropriate healing occurs. Treatment of synechiae includes Z-plasty, flaps, tissue-grafts, intralesional steroids and, when indicated, septal splinting.[24]

Several investigators have demonstrated no decrease in nasal air flow following uneventful cosmetic rhinoplasty.[3, 15] This occurs despite a decreased cross-sectional area of the valve region. However, inappropriately high intercartilaginous incisions,[1, 65] synechiae, over-resection of the lower lateral cartilages[7] (Fig. 24–7), avulsion of the upper lateral cartilage[58, 60] (Fig. 24–8), overaggressive infracture of nasal bones,[21] and loss of tip support all can lead to nasal valve compromise and contribute to nasal obstruction. Patients will be seen in the office with a positive Cottle sign (Fig. 24–9). Proper diagnosis and restoration lead to successful outcome. Goode recommended replacement of vestibular lining with skin graft and, if carti-

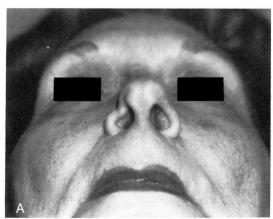
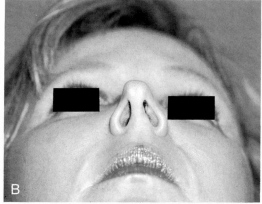

FIGURE 24–7. *A,* Right-sided nasal valve collapse, with soft tissue triangle deformity secondary to over-resection of lower lateral cartilage. *B,* Bilateral nasal valve collapse; correction with bilateral spreader grafts.

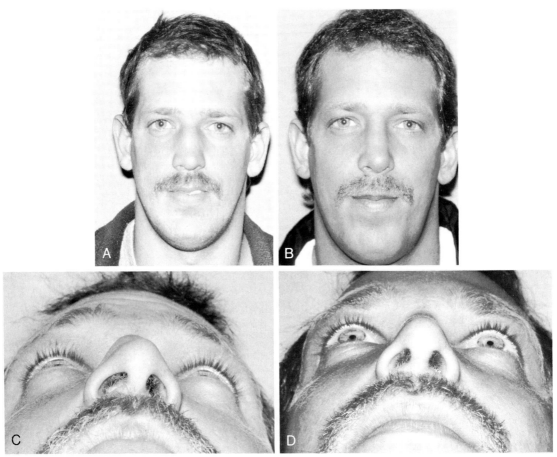

FIGURE 24–8. Right upper lateral cartilage discoloration with caudal septal deflection. *A*, Preoperative frontal view; *B*, postoperative frontal view; *C*, preoperative basal view; *D*, postoperative basal view. Tip grafting, dorsal onlay graft, and unilateral spreader grafts were used.

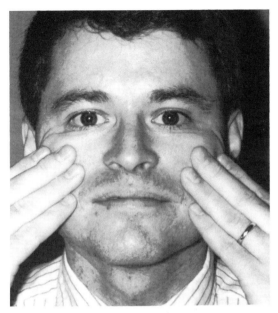

FIGURE 24–9. Cottle's sign.

lage is absent, composite grafts.[24] Sheen introduced the concept of spreader grafts to be placed between the upper lateral cartilage and septum to widen the valve.[65] Johnson and associates have incorporated that into structural grafting, utilizing tip grafting and alar restructuring to provide tip support along with lateral crural and upper lateral stability, thereby improving the airway[37–39] (Fig. 24–10). The treatment of nasal valve airway collapse is a difficult one that depends on an individualized plan based on the deformity.

Vestibular stenosis occurs to a small degree following an endonasal approach as a result of contraction of the incisions high in the vestibule.[1, 65] It also occurs as a result of lower septal incisions that traverse the floor of the nose. Vestibular stenosis severe enough to cause airway compromise is a result of inappropriate resection of vestibular skin and mucosa or traumatic surgical technique leading to vestibular synechiae and stenosis (Fig. 24–11).

Nasal obstruction can be the result of the prolapse of the bony nasal vault.[21] Inappropriate or complete dissection of the periosteum from the nasal bones will allow for the nasal bones to telescope following lateral osteotomy. Excessively low lateral osteoto-

mies can also compromise the airway by repositioning the inferior turbinates medially. Partial turbinectomy is helpful to relieve the symptoms of nasal obstruction secondary to bony vault collapse, but good planning and avoidance are the best measures.[5]

OLFACTORY DISTURBANCES

Anosmia can be present up to 10 per cent of the time and is typically transient, usually lasting 3 to 18 months.[10] It is of value to ask preoperatively about any disturbance in olfaction and to do preoperative testing, if indicated, as baseline documentation. Permanent anosmia is exceedingly rare; in preoperative discussion patients should be made aware but reassured that it is most commonly due to crusting and postoperative edema and, therefore, transient in nature.[2]

UNTOWARD AESTHETIC RESULTS

When the outcome of a surgical procedure is such that it warrants further unplanned surgical intervention, it should be considered a complication.[74] In rhinoplasty this may occur in spite of an uneventful perioperative course without any of the aforementioned events. Preoperatively it is imperative that the rhinoplastic surgeon discuss the realities and occasional unpredictability of the surgical outcome. Tardy and colleagues note that between 10 and 20 per cent of cases will have some irregularity, even minor, that will require revision.[73]

Errors in planning usually result from failure to diagnose. Failure to recognize inadequate tip projection, overprojection, or a low radix prior to rhinoplasty causes an unsatisfactory result.[61] Most errors during the execution of the procedure are either errors of omission, commission, or asymmetry. One can critically evaluate each anatomic area of the postoperative nose with all possible configurations of over-resection, under-resection and asymmetric resection; the net result could be every mishap possible from pollybeak to saddle nose deformity. Correction of every sequelae or aesthetic complication is beyond the scope of this chapter and is best addressed in a revision rhinoplasty text.

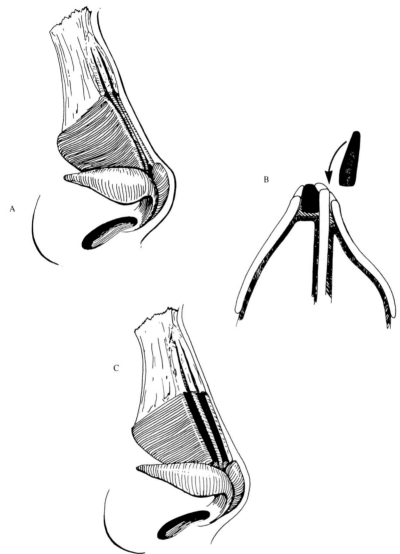

FIGURE 24–10. Bilateral spreader grafts. *A,* Narrowing of the middle third of the nose is due to collapse of the upper lateral cartilages. *B,* Spreader grafts are placed into position between the upper lateral cartilage and the nasal septum. *C,* Bilateral spreader grafts are in position. (From Johnson CM, Toriumi DM: Open Structure Rhinoplasty. Philadelphia, WB Saunders, 1990, p 205.)

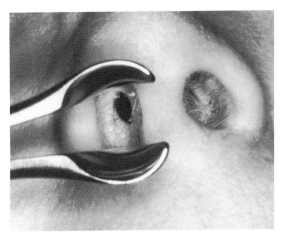

FIGURE 24–11. Moderately severe vestibular stenosis secondary to misplaced nasal floor incisions, bridging to incisions at osteotomy sites.

BLEPHAROPLASTY

Fortunately the incidence of complications following cosmetic blepharoplasty is low. Complications vary from the easily treatable milia to the most dreaded complication of blindness. The prevention of all complications is not possible, but it is important for the surgeon to be well-versed in various etiologies and treatments of these undesired and unexpected results. This process starts at the first consultation with the patient seeking blepharoplasty. A detailed history should be obtained, including the patient's reasons for wanting surgery and their understanding of the procedure. A detailed ophthalmologic history should include any ocular or oculoplastic procedures, ophthalmologic disease, especially dry eye syndrome, blepharitis, glaucoma, corneal abrasions, epiphora, and visual disturbances. Questions regarding the patient's general medical health are important, especially regarding diseases that may affect the eyes, such as diabetes, hypertension, thyroid disease, atopic disease, and dermatologic disorders. The surgeon who inadvertently operates on a patient with uncontrolled thyroid ophthalmic disease will quickly learn that primary management is medical therapy and not surgery (Fig. 24–12).

Physical examination of the eye and orbital adnexa should include visual acuity, confrontation visual field studies, extraocular muscle motility assessment, lacrimal function, tonometry, and evaluation of periorbital morphology. Some surgeons refer all their preoperative blepharoplasty patients to an ophthalmologist for a complete ocular examination. It is essential that an ophthalmologic examination be performed prior to blepharoplasty. The results should be recorded in the patient's file. DeMere and associates surveyed approximately 3000 surgeons regarding eye complications following blepharoplasty.[90] They found that only 15 per cent of the plastic surgeons recorded the results of an ophthalmologic examination.

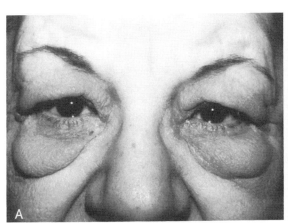
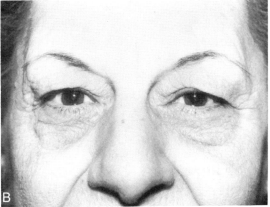

FIGURE 24–12. Ophthalmic thyroid disease. *A*, Patient with hypothyroid. *B*, Improvement with medical management only.

Another compelling reason to perform a preoperative ocular examination is to detect the patient who has an undiagnosed ocular problem. In a study by Moser and coworkers, preoperative ophthalmologic screening turned up four patients with previously undiagnosed unilateral blindness.[127]

For purposes of discussion, complications will be divided into four categories: general complications, dermatologic complications, and specific complications related to the lower eyelids and upper eyelids.

General Complications

CONTOUR DEFECTS

Undercorrection or unequal removal of eyelid skin, fat, or muscle may result in surface irregularities. Preoperative assessment of the fat pads should be performed in an upright position so that the correct amount of fat is removed from the respective compartments. Planned upper lid skin excision is also determined at the same step preoperatively. It is rare for a patient to have perfectly symmetric eyelids preoperatively, and this fact should be specifically pointed out to the patient. Existing asymmetries must be considered in preoperative planning in order to perform the proper procedure. Blepharoplasties done "by the book" are sure to be included in the next book on complications.

DRY EYE SYNDROME

A detailed preoperative ocular history and examination are crucial in attempting to identify the patient who postoperatively may develop dry eye syndrome. A variety of tests (Schirmer's test, tear film break-up time, quantitative tear lysozyme level, and corneal staining with rose bengal solution) are available for evaluating tear production and composition. Unfortunately, none of these tests are 100 per cent accurate and are not readily available to all persons who perform aesthetic blepharoplasty. A study by Rees and La-Trenta found that the periorbital morphology is a more reliable method of identifying a patient at risk for developing dry eye syndrome postblepharoplasty.[136] McKinney and Zukowski compared the Schirmer test and tear film break-up time test as predictors of possible postblepharoplasty dry eye syndrome and found that neither test was extremely accurate in predicting which patients would develop dry eye complications.[123] A positive history of dry eye symptoms and abnormalities of periorbital morphology appear to be the most reliable indicators for identifying a patient at risk of developing postblepharoplasty dry eye syndrome. A patient in this category should undergo further testing prior to elective blepharoplasty. There is a diminution of tear production with increasing age. This should be considered in counseling an older patient who is seeking blepharoplasty. A female patient taking estrogen supplements also may experience decreased tear production and an increase in tear viscosity.[118] Transient postoperative dry eye syndrome is treated with wetting agents or ophthalmologic ointment. Persistent dry eye syndrome may require prolonged use of wetting agents, ointment, or slow-release methylcellulose inserts in the lower cul-de-sac.

INFECTION

Due to the excellent vascularity of the eyelids, postoperative infection following blepharoplasty is extremely rare. Orbital cellulitis has been reported in at least two cases and, in both cases, the patients developed blindness secondary to the infections.[92, 126] Rees and associates reported a case of orbital abscess following blepharoplasty.[135] Allen reported a patient developing orbital cellulitis secondary to dacryocystitis following blepharoplasty.[83] This particular patient had problems with lacrimal drainage to dacryostenosis prior to blepharoplasty. This reinforces the importance of conducting a thorough preoperative history and physical examination. Blepharitis may occur following blepharoplasty, but the incidence is so low that the occurrence may not be related to surgery and only coincidental.[132, 133]

If infection does occur, prompt treatment is necessary. Chronic blepharitis may respond to topical ophthalmologic antibacterial drops. More severe infections such as orbital cellulitis, abscess or dacryocystitis will require surgical drainage and appropriate intravenous antibiotic coverage.

ALLERGIC REACTIONS

To avoid the possibility of topical allergic reactions, patients are asked not to wear any cosmetics for the first 10 postoperative days. The use of antibiotic ointments on the eyelid incisions will help decrease crusting and speed re-epithelialization of the incision line. Only ophthalmologic ointment should be used. Many patients may exhibit a reaction to neomycin, and for this reason many surgeons prefer to use other ophthalmologic ointments such as erythromycin opthalmic ointment. Bacitracin also can be a skin sensitizer, but the incidence is much less than that of neomycin.[109]

EPIPHORA

Transient postoperative epiphora is common and usually resolves within the first several days. Epiphora is caused by increased production of tears due to irritation or dysfunction of the lacrimal drainage system. Postoperative edema may position the punctum away from the globe and interfere with drainage. Lagophthalmos and corneal irritation may produce a reflective increase in tear production.

Persistent epiphora may be the result of punctal or canalicular injury. This usually results from extending the lower eyelid incision too far medially. Direct injury to the canaliculus at the time of surgery should be repaired during the blepharoplasty procedure if recognized. Stenosis of the lacrimal drainage system may require dilation and, on rare occasions, dacryocystorhinostomy. Postoperative ectropion may position the punctum away from the globe. Mild cases of punctal eversion may respond to a posterior wall punctoplasty. More severe eversions associated with ectropion may be corrected with horizontal eyelid tightening procedures. In extreme cases a skin graft may be required

to correct ectropion brought about by over-resection of lower eyelid tissue.[134]

HEMATOMA

Diffuse ecchymosis following surgery is not uncommon. It may be more noticeable in a light-skinned individual, and it usually resolves without complications in 3 to 4 weeks. More severe ecchymosis may occur in the patient who has a coagulopathy or a patient who has been taking drugs that may inhibit platelet aggregation (e.g., aspirin and ibuprofen) (Table 24–1). Patients on these medications should be instructed to discontinue their use 2 weeks prior to operation. Postoperative nausea and vomiting as well as increased physical activity may result in increased vascular pressure, which could lead to more severe ecchymosis. Detailed postoperative instructions outlining the restrictions in physical activity should be given to the patient prior to operation.

Small, discrete hematomas recognized immediately postoperatively should be evacuated through the blepharoplasty incisions. If the hematomas are unrecognized owing to postoperative ecchymosis and edema, they should be allowed to liquefy and then be aspirated or evacuated through small stab incisions in 7 to 10 days (Fig. 24–13). If left untreated, these areas will be replaced with fibrous tissue and can be annoying to both the surgeon and the patient. Massage and small amounts of intralesional triamcinolone may be used to soften these areas.

A subscleral hematoma is another type of

TABLE 24–1. Drugs Inhibiting Platelet Aggregation

Aspirin
Aspirin, buffered
Aspirin, micronized
Nonsteroidal anti-inflammatory agents— prescription drugs
Alcohol
Tobacco

These are categories of drugs that may cause increased bruising with surgical procedures. These drugs are not to be taken for at least 2 weeks prior to operation and not until so instructed following operation.

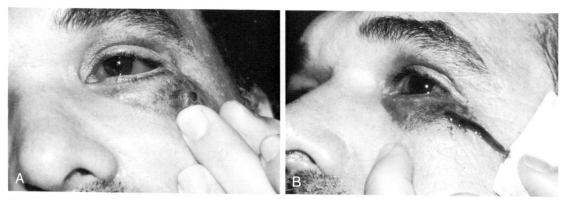

FIGURE 24–13. *A*, Postoperative blepharoplasty patient with liquefied small hematoma. *B*, Evacuation with stab incision.

localized hemorrhage. A patient is frequently distressed at the appearance of this bright-red eye. This hematoma will resolve spontaneously over 3 to 4 weeks, and reassurance is the only treatment necessary. Some surgeons feel that warm compresses to the affected eye may expedite resolution of the hematoma.

The most feared and dreaded complication of hemorrhage following blepharoplasty is retrobulbar hematoma, since it has been associated with visual disturbances.[90, 91, 95, 99–101, 105, 106, 110, 112, 114, 143] Fortunately, the incidence is low. Rees saw four retrobulbar hematomas in 15,000 blepharoplasties.[51] All four patients responded to conservative therapy without any permanent visual disturbances. A direct cause-and-effect relationship between retrobulbar hematoma and blindness has not been established.[90, 91, 95, 99–101, 105, 106, 108, 112, 114, 130, 137, 141]

The salient clinical symptoms are pain, proptosis, mydriasis, and chemosis (Fig. 24–14). Pain is the primary symptom. A patient complaining of severe ocular pain postoperatively should be examined carefully. It is inadvisable to place compressive dressings over the eyes postoperatively because they may increase intraorbital pressure and they prevent easy postoperative examinations. Lightweight iced compresses may be used. As a retrobulbar hematoma progresses, the eye becomes extremely firm and tense to palpation. As proptosis increases it may protrude the globe between the eyelids. Visual acuity testing may or may not reveal abnormalities. Tonometry should be performed and often

will reveal pressures of greater than 80 mm.[117] Normal intraocular pressure is 15 mm Hg.[128]

Retrobulbar hematomas occur only when the orbital septum has been violated in some fashion. The most common cause is puncture of blood vessels from deep injections of local anesthetic through the septum into the fat pads.[132] Blind injection of fat pads should be avoided, and it is recommended that injection be performed under direct vision after opening the orbital septum. Inadequate coagulation of blood vessels in the stump of the orbital fat pads is another possible mechanism. A third possibility is bleeding from the vascular orbicularis muscle extending through the previously opened orbital septum into the retro-orbital space.[99, 116, 117, 138]

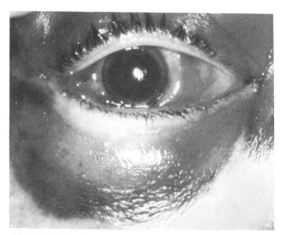

FIGURE 24–14. Retrobulbar hematoma following transconjunctival blepharoplasty resolves without sequelae.

Excessive traction on orbital fat during removal can cause avulsion of deeper orbital vessels. This etiology is supported by Koorneef's work which found delicate soft tissue interconnections in the posterior orbit.[111] Traction of the anterior orbital fat could be transmitted to the posterior fat, which results in avulsion of the small vessels in this region.

Retrobulbar hemorrhage results in increased intraorbital pressure, which causes an increase in the intraocular pressure. Increased intraocular pressure may produce ischemia of the central retinal artery.[95, 99, 104] Increased intraorbital pressure may also compromise blood flow to branches of the postciliary artery, which may result in optic nerve head ischemia and partial visual loss. This could progress to the point of central retinal artery occlusion, which would then lead to complete blindness. However, it has been shown experimentally that the central retinal artery must be occluded for 105 minutes before permanent visual changes are effected.[100, 112]

Once the diagnosis of retrobulbar hematoma has been made, therapy should be instituted as soon as possible. If the retrobulbar hemorrhage is diagnosed during operation, Rees recommends widely opening the septum with a judicious exploration of the fat in an attempt to locate the bleeding vessel. It is not uncommon for the bleeding vessel to be identified; however, widely opening the septum helps in decompressing the orbital contents. Terminating the procedure is not always necessary.[132] Conservative therapy for postoperative retrobulbar hematomas involves observation, compresses, and ophthalmologic consultation. Hematomas that fail to respond to conservative measures should be treated by opening the incision lines and administering a 20 per cent mannitol solution (2 mg/kg), Diamox (500 mg IV stat then 250 mg IV every 6 hours for 24 hours), and Solu-Medrol (Table 24–2).[108] If these measures fail to provide improvement, then lateral canthotomy should be performed. A temporary tarsorrhaphy stitch may be placed to protect the cornea if the eye is extremely proptotic. Paracentesis of the anterior chamber is an extremely contro-

TABLE 24–2. Protocol for Suspected Raised Intraocular Pressure

1. Immediate ophthalmologic consultation for fundoscopy and tonometry

Steps 2 through 4 should be instituted without waiting for the ophthalmologic consultation

2. Diamox (500 mg IV stat; 250 mg IV every 6 hours for 24 hours)
3. Solu-Medrol (1 gm IV stat)
4. Mannitol 20% solution; 2 gm/kg of body weight; 24 hour IV; no more than 12.5 gm in 3–4 minutes

If there is no improvement, proceed to step 5

5. Lateral canthotomy

Make sure that the medications are present in the operating room at all times

versial treatment and should be performed only as a last resort by an experienced ophthalmologist.

BLINDNESS AND VISUAL DISTURBANCES

The importance of obtaining and recording visual acuity examinations preoperatively cannot be overemphasized. Previously undiagnosed visual disturbances and even blindness have been discovered with this preoperative evaluation. The incidence of blindness following blepharoplasty was estimated to be 0.04 per cent in a study performed by DeMere and colleagues in the 1970s.[89, 90]

A single mechanism resulting in blindness following blepharoplasty has not been illustrated. Multiple etiologies have been suggested, and the most common denominator without underlying ocular or central nervous system disease is increased intraocular and intraorbital pressure. Blindness is frequently attributed to retrobulbar hemorrhage. However, experimental studies using animal models have failed to produce permanent blindness.[84, 86, 91, 92, 95, 99, 104, 113]

Idiopathic optic nerve atrophy and retrobulbar neuritis have been suggested as possible causes for postblepharoplasty visual disturbances or blindness.[126] Theoretically, current from a unipolar cautery may cause direct injury of the optic nerve or induce vasospasm of the central retinal or posterior ciliary artery.[87, 127] Orbital cellulitis has been a reported cause of blindness following blepharoplasty, and this is discussed in the section on infection.[126]

Glaucoma may be precipitated by blepharoplasty.[97] The incidence of acute closed-angle glaucoma is 0.09 per cent.[103] There is a female predominance. A careful preoperative history inquiring about visual field defects, blurred vision, halos around lights, ocular pain, and headaches should be obtained. A patient with postoperative acute closed-angle glaucoma may complain of ocular pain, nausea, vomiting, and headaches. Physical findings may include mydriasis, corneal edema, and decreased visual acuity. If glaucoma is suspected in the postoperative period, immediate ophthalmologic consultation should be sought.

Extraocular motility disturbances have been reported following blepharoplasty. These are usually caused by injury to the superior or inferior oblique muscles.[82, 98, 102, 129, 142] Injury of all the oblique and vertical recti extraocular muscles has been reported; however, the inferior rectus and oblique muscles seem to be particularly susceptible during lower lid blepharoplasty.[82] Transient paresis of the extraocular muscles may be the result of hemorrhage, edema, or myotoxicity of the local anesthetic agents.

Complete transection of the inferior rectus has also been reported.[118] If this is recognized at the time of injury, reanastomosis of the severed muscle ends should be performed intraoperatively. Since most extraocular motility problems are transient in nature, conservative therapy is advised. Extraocular motility impairment lasting greater than 6 months may require strabismus surgery to free scarred fibrotic muscles or relocate the muscle attachments.[118]

CORNEAL ABRASION

Corneal injuries usually occur during surgery. For this reason many blepharoplasty surgeons use protective corneal shields, whereas others feel that shields actually may contribute to corneal abrasions. If used, a thin, opaque, sterile corneal shield coated with a bland ophthalmologic ointment such as Lacrilube should be employed. These shields offer the advantage of protecting the patient's eyes from injury, desiccation, and exposure to the intense surgical lights. Before each use the concave surface of the shield should be carefully inspected for surface defects and an ophthalmologic ointment applied to prevent possible iatrogenic corneal abrasions. The thickness of the corneal shield must be taken into consideration when performing any type of lower lid tightening procedure to avoid undercorrection. It is important to avoid the use of abrasive sponges when working around the eye. Desiccation also may be a problem during blepharoplasty surgery if lubricated eye shields are not used. Use of ophthalmologic ointment alone prior to starting the operation may decrease the possibility of drying; however, the eye should be assessed frequently throughout the operation and more ointment applied if needed. A temporary Frost traction suture to protect the eye during lower lid blepharoplasty is a technique used by one of us.

At the completion of the procedure, the eye should be irrigated with balanced salt solution and, if a small amount of lagophthalmos exists, an ointment such as erythromycin or Polysporin ophthalmic ointment should be placed within the inferior cul-de-sac as well as on the eyelid incisions. Pain and a foreign body sensation following operation should make one suspect a corneal abrasion. Diagnosis is made by fluorescein staining and slit lamp examination. If a corneal abrasion is identified, a nonsteroidal antibacterial ophthalmologic ointment should be used and the eye closed and patched for 24 to 48 hours. Ophthalmologic consultation should be obtained if the patient fails to improve after these measures.

SCARRING

Formation of hypertrophic scars in blepharoplasty incisions is extremely rare. True keloids following blepharoplasty have never been reported. Webbing may occur in the upper lid medial canthal region, especially when the incision line is carried across the concavity onto the nasal skin. If this webbing occurs, conservative therapy is advised. Watchful waiting (chronotherapy) and massage should be tried first. The use of steroid tape, Cordran tape, or intralesional injections with dilute triamcinolone acetate (10 mg/ml) may be used for 4 to 6 weeks postoperatively. Rarely Z-plasty or some other type of scar revision technique may be needed to correct the problem if conservative therapy fails.

MILIA

Milia are inclusion cysts that form because of rapid epithelialization of suture tracts. Epithelial desquamation accumulates within the lined suture tracts and presents as a small white nodule. Early suture removal 42 to 72 hours postoperatively will prevent milia formation. If additional support is needed in the lateral aspect of the incisions after early suture removal, small subcutaneous absorbable sutures should be used, and the skin edges may be held in apposition with small Steri-strips. If milia do appear, they are easily treated by unroofing the lesion with a large-gauge needle or a No. 11 blade. Larger inclusion cysts may require excision and reapproximation of skin edges. Complete epithelial-lined tunnels may require unroofing with one blade of a fine scissors inserted the length of the tunnel.[88]

Dermatologic Complications

ECCHYMOSIS

As mentioned in the section on hemorrhage, some degree of periorbital ecchymosis is to be expected following blepharoplasty, and a patient should be advised of this during the preoperative counseling. Normal postoperative ecchymosis usually resolves within 7 to 14 days and may be camouflaged with cosmetics after the sutures have been removed. Women who use cosmetics are advised to use a water-based makeup two shades darker than used normally. Persistent ecchymosis should be treated by reassuring the patient and watchful waiting.

HYPERPIGMENTATION

Hyperpigmentation may be the result of prolonged ecchymosis. Hemosiderin remaining from the degradation of hemoglobin may be deposited in the skin, and this can result in hyperpigmentation. Increased production of melanin may occur following surgery, and this can also result in hyperpigmentation. It is important to inform a patient who has hyperpigmentation preoperatively that the operation will not eliminate the darker color but may, in fact, exacerbate it. Bleaching agents such as Soloquin Forte or Melanex may provide some relief for hyperpigmentation that results from increased melanin production. A periorbital chemical peel or dermabrasion can be used for persistent hyperpigmentation that fails to respond to bleaching agents. Strict avoidance of sunlight and the use of sunblock must be included in the preoperative instructions since sun exposure also can contribute to hyperpigmentation.

TELANGIECTASIA

A patient with pre-existing telangiectasias of the face may experience an increase in the number or size of telangiectasias postoperatively. It is important to make the patient cognizant of any preoperative telangiectasias of the eyelids. Telangiectasias rarely resolve without treatment. Photocoagulation using a yellow wavelength laser (557-585 nm) is an effective treatment for facial telangiectasias. Argon or KTP lasers may be used also. If lasers are not available, then electrocauterization is another option.

LOSS OF EYELASHES

Spontaneous loss of eyelashes with recovery has been reported.[132] More commonly, eyelashes are lost due to lack of meticulous surgical technique. Permanent loss of eyelashes may be caused by heat injury to the eyelash follicles from the use of electrocautery.

EDEMA AND CHEMOSIS

Routinely, postoperative edema is confined to the lower eyelids and the tarsal portion of the upper eyelids. Conservative measures, such as elevation of the patient's head and cold compresses used in the postoperative period, may diminish the amount of postoperative edema and hasten its resolution. McCord advocates the use of steroids by pretreating with steroids the day before surgery and continuing for 3 days postoperatively.[122]

Excessive or prolonged edema lasting longer than 7 to 10 days is thought to be the result of disrupted or impaired lymphatic drainage. This may occur as the result of excessive dissection of the skin muscle flap, both inferiorly and laterally. Overzealous use of electrocautery also may contribute to this problem. Although bothersome, edema usually responds using conservative measures. Chemosis or conjunctival edema can accompany subcutaneous edema. It usually results from extensive dissection or overuse of electrocautery. This conjunctival type of edema may last 6 to 8 weeks. It can be an annoying problem, especially if the patient experiences prolapse of the conjunctiva. Treatment includes a light pressure patch at night, head elevation, diuretics, steroid ophthalmologic solution, and hypertonic saline eye drops, e.g., Murol 128.

WOUND SEPARATION

Meticulous approximation of skin edges of the incision lines will help prevent wound separation. The very thin, delicate skin of the eyelids has a tendency to contract and roll inward, so it is essential for the surgeon to use meticulous surgical techniques and evert the skin edges when suturing. The lateral aspects of blepharoplasty incisions may separate after early suture removal. The possibility of this occurring in the lower lid incision may be decreased by using a very fine absorbable suture in the subcutaneous tissues. If separation does occur, it is treated by resuturing or application of Steri-strips.

ENOPHTHALMOS

Proper preoperative assessment of the patient's periorbital area may help prevent postoperative enophthalmos. A patient with prominent bony orbital rims and deep-set eyes will have a sunken or hollow-eyed appearance postoperatively, especially if excess fat resection has been performed. In such a patient it is important to be extremely conservative in resection of periorbital fat. Once the orbital septum has been opened, only the small amount of fat that protrudes through the septum without aggressive traction should be resected. If the surgeon feels that too much fat has been resected, the fat may be returned and the orbital septum sutured. Free fat grafting has been used to correct this problem, but the long-term results have been less than satisfactory.[96, 107, 119, 120] If a prominent bony orbital rim is contributing to the patient's hollow-eyed appearance, the rim may be reduced using a surgical drill.

Upper Eyelid Complications

LAGOPHTHALMOS

Incomplete eye closure immediately following blepharoplasty is not unusual. The orbicularis muscle may not function adequately to achieve complete eye closure because of edema, surgical trauma, and local anesthetic. The palpebral fissure with eyes closed following blepharoplasty should not be more than 3 mm.[132] Lagophthalmos usually resolves within the first week postoperatively but may continue for months. The patient's main complaint is a "dry eye" and, in severe cases, an exposure keratitis can develop if protective measures are not instituted. Treatment is directed at protecting the eye from desiccation. A mild antibiotic ophthalmologic ointment should be used at night, and wetting agents should be used in the day until complete eye closure is obtained. Temporary lagophthalmos can persist for months, but most often it resolves within the first 2 to 3 weeks. It is not unusual to have 2 to 3 mm of lagophthalmos at the end

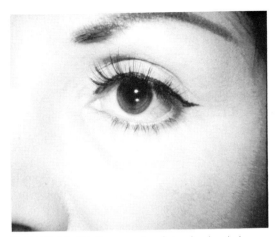

FIGURE 24–15. Preoperative lateral scleral show.

of a procedure owing to muscle hypotonia. This hypotonia is due to edema and the effects of local anesthesia.

The most common cause of permanent lagophthalmos is overzealous resection of upper eyelid skin. For this reason, we stress the importance for beginning blepharoplasty surgeons to refrigerate the upper eyelid skin for 1 week in case over-resection of upper eyelids requires subsequent grafting. A postauricular full-thickness skin graft is another option if grafting is necessary. Other possible causes of lagophthalmos include inadvertent suturing of the orbital septum with the skin closure sutures. This can be corrected by excision of the scar between the skin and the septum.[117]

PTOSIS

Upper eyelid edema may cause what appears to be several millimeters of ptosis postoperatively. This is transient and usually resolves spontaneously. Asymmetric supertarsal fixation can cause a pseudoptosis that usually resolves with time. A permanent postoperative ptosis may be the result of an unrecognized preoperative ptotic condition. This type of ptosis may appear worse postoperatively as a result of skin excision and fat sculpting. A ptosis that persists 4 to 6 months postoperatively usually is due to some derangement of the levator aponeurosis. Injury of the levator at the level of the tarsus occurs more commonly during re-

moval of the medial fat pad. In the elderly patient, routine dissection can unmask a pre-existing dehiscence of the levator.[84] True levator injury causing ptosis necessitates repair. Multiple techniques for ptosis repair are described in the literature. For a minimal amount of ptosis, conjunctival approaches may be used.[131] More severe degrees of ptosis will require some type of external levator resection or repair of the dehiscence.[84, 115]

Lower Eyelid Complications

LATERAL SCLERAL SHOW/ECTROPION

Correct preoperative evaluation will identify many patients with a slight amount of lateral scleral show. Ten per cent of a normal population were found to have superficial scleral show when evaluated with their heads in the primary position of gaze (Fig. 24–15).[121] A certain degree of lateral scleral show is common in the immediate postoperative period. This is caused by edema and orbicularis oculi hypotonia. If it persists it is classified as a mild degree of ectropion and is considered a complication. A persistent ectropion can be classified as cicatricial, paralytic, or mechanical. Postoperative paralytic ectropions can occur as the result of a paretic or paralyzed orbicularis muscle. The majority of postoperative ectropions are mechanical or cicatricial. Causes include scar contracture of the orbicularis muscle, scar formation between the lower lid and bony orbit, scar contracture of the orbital septum, or excess skin or orbicularis muscle (Fig. 24–16).[124, 134, 139]

A more common cause of postoperative ectropion is over-resection of skin after the removal of large amounts of fat. It is essential that the surgeon be conservative in excision of lower eyelid tissue. After fat excision the skin must be properly contoured to the new concave muscle surface. To determine properly the correct amount of skin to be excised, a surgeon may employ various maneuvers, such as having the patient open the mouth, applying light downward traction on the cheek, or sitting the patient in an upright position to ascertain the proper amount of skin and muscle excision.

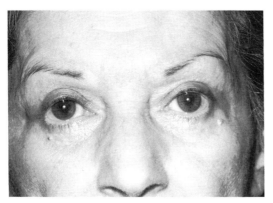

FIGURE 24–16. Postoperative blepharoplasty with ectropion, lateral canthal webbing, and shortening of the palpebral fissure.

flap and lysis of the adhesions. The patient with an established ectropion due to over-resection of lower eyelid tissue should be treated by full-thickness skin grafts. First choice of a donor site for the graft is the upper eyelid if sufficient tissue exists. Other possible donor sites include the postauricular region and supraclavicular area. An ectropion secondary to lower eyelid laxity should be corrected by using some type of lower eyelid tightening procedure. A variety of lower lid tightening procedures have been described, including wedge resection, dermal flap, lateral canthal tendon plication, and tarsal strip.[85, 87, 94, 134, 140]

The best treatment for postoperative ectropion is prevention. Careful preoperative evaluation should note any existing scleral show or lower lid laxity. If these conditions exist preoperatively, they should be discussed with the patient and adjunctive surgical techniques should be performed along with the blepharoplasty to correct them. Treatment for a mild degree of lateral scleral show consists of massage and placement of a lateral tape sling at night (Fig. 24–17). A piece of quarter-inch paper tape or Steri-strip is placed on the skin of the lateral third of the lower eyelid. Tape is gently pulled in a superior and lateral direction and secured to the skin of the lateral canthal region. Wetting agents or mild ophthalmologic ointments should be used if corneal desiccation proves to be a problem.

Most mild degrees of scleral show will respond to conservative measures and watchful waiting, but the surgeon must be prepared to deal with the patient's dissatisfaction until this occurs. If the mild ectropion persists over 6 weeks, intralesional injections of triamcinolone acetate may be helpful if the underlying mechanism is secondary to adverse scarring. If the patient fails to respond to conservative treatment in 6 months postoperatively and is left with a persistent ectropion, then surgical intervention is indicated. Ectropion caused by adherence of the orbital septum to the orbicularis oculi muscle is treated by re-elevation of the skin muscle

SKIN SLOUGH

Skin slough following lower eyelid blepharoplasty is extremely rare due to the excellent vascularity of the area. Hematoma formation is the most common cause. Theoretically, a skin-flap-only blepharoplasty as opposed to a skin-muscle lower eyelid blepharoplasty should be more susceptible to skin slough following wide dissection and hematoma formation. If an area of slough does develop in the lower eyelid, it should be treated conservatively with antibiotic ointment. Re-epithelization occurs more rapidly under an eschar kept soft with an antibiotic ointment. Conservative therapy is indicated, and aggressive debridement of the eschar should not be performed. An area of full-thickness skin loss allowed to heal by secondary intention may result in a cicatricial ectropion, and this is best treated with grafts or local skin flaps.

FACE LIFT

Preventive Measures

Avoidance of complications during or following rhytidectomy begins with the preoperative consultation. It is essential to perform an anatomic analysis of the patient's face, including skin, muscle, and bony structures. Any pre-existing asymmetries in the patient's

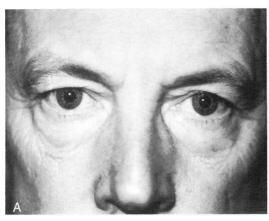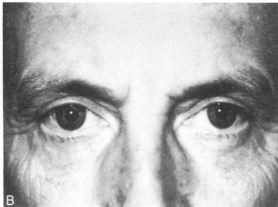

FIGURE 24–17. *A*, Preoperative blepharoplasty patient. *B*, Postoperative photo with some early scleral show. Reassurance, massage, and taping of the lower lid will result in resolution.

face should be pointed out to the patient at this time. The patient's motivation for seeking operation and expectations for the operation are extremely important. It is essential for the surgeon to make sure that the patient understands the difference between redundant skin and fine-line rhytids, the latter of which, of course, the face lift does not eliminate. This procedure should be portrayed as an operation for improvement by correction of excess skin and muscle. Any patient seeking perfection or having unrealistic expectations of the effects of this operation should be dissuaded from it.

Patients should be prepared adequately for the temporary disfigurement and bruising that accompany an uneventful postsurgical course so that it is not interpreted as a complication.

In the preoperative assessment, it is important to attempt to individualize the procedure for the patient. Attention to details of hairline and hairstyle and previous operations may alter incision placement. Accurate diagnosis of the factors contributing to an obtuse cervicomental angle will affect the decision of whether to use chin augmentation, liposuction, platysma/SMAS alterations, or a combination of these modalities.[158, 165, 176, 192–195] Preoperatively obtaining an accurate history, including hypertension, bleeding diathesis, or aspirin ingestion, goes a long way toward avoidance of a hematoma. The complications that will leave us, the surgeons, the least satisfied are those that could have been prevented.

Finally it is important that we place our role in proper perspective. In rhytidectomy, unlike other aesthetic procedures, striving for perfection requires that the experienced surgeon calculate the risk-benefit ratio of all facets of the procedure. Major interventions, such as more extensive undermining of the skin, extensive dissection in the subplatysmal plane, as well as subperiosteal dissection, may result in only minor improvements in the overall net cosmetic result.[164] The increased risks of nerve injury, hematoma, skin slough, infection, and hair loss need to be factored against the patient's individualized needs and potential for improvement (Table 24–3).[177, 192] "Less is more," when used appropriately, is an adage that will result in more satisfaction and create less dissatisfaction.

HEMATOMA

Hematoma is the most common complication following face lift. The reported incidences of hematoma is between 1 per cent and 16%, but more recent studies show the incidence to be around 3 per cent.[147, 169–171] Expanding hematomas occur most commonly within the first 24 hours postoperatively but may occur as much as 2 weeks later.[180, 188] Hematomas requiring postoperative drainage range from 1 per cent to 8 per cent, with men having a greater preponder-

TABLE 24–3. Complications in Rhytidectomy

	No. of Cases	Hematoma		Skin Loss		Hair Loss		Motor Nerve Loss		Infection	
		No.	(%)	No.	(%)	No.	(%)	No.	(%)	No.	(%)
Conway (1970)	300	21	(6.6)	1	(0.3)			2	(0.7)	2	(0.6)
McDowell (1972)	105	3	(3)	1	(1)	0		2	(1.9)		
Barker (1977)	163	6	(4)								
Leist et al (1977)	324	19	(6)	7	(2)	10	(3)	4	(1.2)		
Stark (1977)	500	30	(6)	1	(0.2)			20	(4)	4	(0.8)
Straith et al (1977)	500	13	(3)								
Baker, Gordon, et al (1977)	1500	234	(16)	17	(1.1)	0		8	(0.5)	15	(1)
Pitanguy, Ceravolo (1981)	3202	156	(9.5)								
Klein, Allen (1981)	561	22	(4)	13	(2)						
Thompson, Ashley (1978)	922	44	(5)	3	(0.3)			6	(0.7)	17	(2)
Matsunaga (1980)	427		(4.9)		(0.5)		(0.2)		(0.2)		(0.9)
Kamer et al (1984)	512	4	(0.78)	9	(1.75)						
McCollough et al (1989)	1188		(2.384)		(0.17)	0			(0.084)		

ance, presumably because of the thickness and excellent vascularity of the hair-bearing skin.[145, 163] Etiologic factors include platelet dysfunction and other coagulopathies, hypertension, and postoperative nausea and vomiting.[149, 151, 180, 188] Most hematomas resolve without the sequelae of skin necrosis, but other sequelae have been reported. Cardiac asystole secondary to presumed hematoma compression of the carotid sinus, as well as motor nerve injury secondary to hematoma, has occurred.[183]

Expanding hematomas are characterized by the sudden onset of pain, swelling, and ecchymosis and are usually unilateral. Buccal ecchymosis can be an associated finding.[180] Surgical management of an expanding hematoma begins at bedside with inspection of the wound and removal of the sutures. This relieves pain, which helps lower systemic blood pressure: pressure on the flap is decreased and vascular integrity is restored. Adjunctive analgesics are important in the management of hypertension associated with the pain of an expanding hematoma.[144, 150] The remainder of the evacuation of the hematoma can take place in an operating room with local anesthesia without epinephrine. Generally, only preauricular and postauricular incision sites need be infiltrated with local anesthetic to accomplish the evacuation. If an active bleeding site is found, it is cauterized. Usually there is no active bleeding; a drain is placed and a pressure dressing applied. Other surgeons advocate a more conservative approach with subcutaneous suctioning of the hematoma without opening the entire incision.[179] Most hematomas, if recognized early, should heal without the sequelae of a skin slough. The postoperative course is slightly prolonged and ecchymosis is more than usual, but the result should not be compromised. We feel strongly about utilization of drainage during face lift procedures and light pressure dressings. Some observers feel that delaying closure of rhytidectomy until all dissection and ancillary procedures are performed decreases the incidence of hematoma.[184]

Small, localized hematomas (less than 25 cc) are more common than expanding hematomas and do not represent a surgical emergency. A small, superficial hematoma can be aspirated with a 14-gauge needle transcutaneously as soon as suspected. Liquefaction begins with the seventh day, but waiting for complete liquefaction of these small hematomas risks thinning of the skin and also creates a potential nidus for infection. Later to appear and more difficult to detect, the smaller, deeper hematoma sometimes can be felt with intraoral bimanual palpation. If these go undetected they will organize and become firm within 2 weeks. The lump is distressing to the patient and may cause a distortion of the overlying skin during animation. Intralesional injections of triamcinolone acetonide in concentrations of 5 to 10 mg/ml may be helpful. With the more aggressive superficial musculo-aponeurotic system (SMAS) elevation techniques, violation of the parotid tissue may occur. Bamberg and Krugman report on a parotid sialocele presenting as a soft, fluctuant mass 2 weeks postoperatively that was treated with aspiration and pressure.[148]

Aspirin and aspirin-containing preparations, nonsteroidal anti-inflammatory drugs, and vitamin E products all can inhibit platelet functions. An appropriate history of coagulopathy is obtained, and patients are provided with a list of these products and instructed to avoid their ingestion for 2 weeks prior to surgery. If there is uncertainty with regard to ingestion, a bleeding time is obtained prior to proceeding.

McCollough and group and Webster and group each have demonstrated that the short flap rhytidectomy has a much lower incidence of hematoma.[176, 189] One must weigh the risk-benefit ratio of the longer flap against the patient's desires and surgeon's need for improvement.

INFECTION

The incidence of infection, which varies from 1 to 3 per cent, is rare due to the excellent vascularity of the face and neck.[155, 169] It is most commonly associated with hematoma because of the excellent culture medium the hematoma site provides. Infection is characterized by pain, swelling, localized erythema, and fever. *Staphylococcus aureus* has been implicated in the majority of these infections. Therapy consists of cultures and broad-spectrum antibiotics with antistaphylococcal coverage. Cellulitis of the earlobe and subsequent chondritis of the ear can be seen (Fig. 24–18). Chondritis of the ear must be managed more aggressively with intrave-

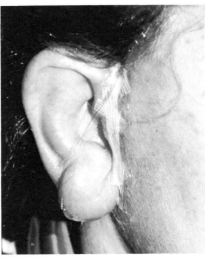

FIGURE 24–18. Cellulitis and early chondritis following rhytidectomy.

nous antibiotics and possible surgical debridement.

NERVE INJURIES

Hypesthesia of the elevated flap in the periauricular area is routine and an expected outcome of face lift. Usually it is transient and resolves within 6 to 12 weeks. The most commonly injured nerve in a face lift is the greater auricular nerve.[146, 171] This occurs if the dissection plane is too deep and one enters the cervical fascia over the sternocleidomastoid muscle. This injury will prolong the numbness and rarely may leave one with permanent numbness of the ear and periauricular area. Fortunately this area has excellent cross-innervation and compensation occurs. Greater auricular nerve injury can be minimized if dissection is performed under direct visualization rather than bluntly. If severance of the nerve is encountered, the nerve should be microanastomosed to maximize the recovery and avoid the sequelae of neuromata.[174] Entrapment with plication sutures may lead to cervical pain lasting several months.[157]

The incidence of motor nerve injury is reported to be from 0 to 3.3 per cent.[156, 169, 170] The facial nerve with its branches is the nerve discussed, although there has been reported injury to the spinal accessory nerve with trapezius dysfunction. Baker and Conley looked at a combined series of motor nerve injuries in which 6551 postrhytidectomy patients were evaluated and facial nerve injury was found in 0.7 per cent.[146] Eighty per cent experienced resolution in 6 months, which left the incidence for permanent injury in this group at 0.1 per cent.

Causes of facial nerve injury following rhytidectomy include but are not limited to the following:

1. Electrocautery injury (especially the frontal branch over the zygoma)
2. Neuropraxia injury during vigorous blunt dissection
3. Compression of the nerve by sutures during SMAS plication
4. Liposuction injuries, aggressive approach inadvertently crossing planes
5. Partial or complete transection during aggressive SMAS elevation (beyond the parotid gland)
6. Distorted anatomy from previous lifting or orthognathic procedures
7. Infection

Preoperatively, it is important to recognize and alert the patient to any pre-existing facial asymmetries. Some patients will have congenital weakness of the marginal mandibular nerve or a hypertrophic frontalis function that goes unnoticed by the patient because it is part of the facial expression.

The most commonly injured branches are the frontal and the marginal mandibular. The frontal branch is most commonly injured as it traverses the zygoma and courses in the SMAS.[146] Avoidance by remaining in the subcutaneous plane during flap undermining and by remaining inferior to the zygoma during SMAS elevation are the keys to preservation. The marginal mandibular branch is most vulnerable as it courses 1 to 2 cm inferior to the midbody of the mandible. Here the patient with a thin platysma may be more vulnerable to injury either from scissor dissection or application of the suction cannula. SMAS elevation below the mandible should be blunt under direct vision. Patients who have had previous operations, such as sagittal split osteotomies, mandibular fracture repair, or submandibular resection and also previous lifting procedures, may have a nerve altered in location. These patients may have an increased predisposition to marginal mandibular injury.[146] SMAS elevation should not be performed in revision face lifts unless it is certain that there was no SMAS treatment in the previous lifting procedure. Since the parotid gland protects the proximal portion of the facial nerve, it is the distal nerve branches that are affected. Recovery is usually spontaneous without surgical intervention.[144]

Patients will require frequent follow-up and reassurance. The weakness will usually resolve within a month but occasionally will require a year for full recovery. Permanent injury is more common with frontal nerve injury. Treatment after 18 months of frontal branch paresis is lysis or crush of the contralateral branch to restore symmetry. In the interim, use of botulinum toxin may achieve symmetry temporarily and relieve patient anxiety.[154]

Injury to the cervical branch of the facial nerve may occur during procedures directed at treating platysmal cording. Occasional depressor angularis function can be affected by platysma dissection causing a pseudomarginal mandibular weakness.[160] Resolution is usually complete without intervention.

SKIN NECROSIS

Skin slough is the most dreaded complication following a rhytidectomy. Its most severe form commonly is a sequelae of an unrecognized hematoma. Its more common form is often noted as a small area of superficial epidermolysis in the postauricular area (Fig. 24–19). The incidence of skin slough is unclear but is between 1 to 6 per cent and is secondary in rhytidectomy complication to hematoma.[162, 176] Etiologic factors that are a result of technique involve excessive tension, thinning, undermining, or pressure on flaps. In those instances, when a larger than discussed amount of skin is excised during tailoring of the postauricular flaps, it may be prudent to allow healing to take place by secondary intention followed by scar revision.[187] Closure under tension may create a

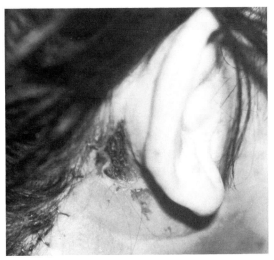

FIGURE 24–19. Postauricular slough in a smoker following long-flap rhytidectomy.

larger segment of necrosis. A history of previous face and neck scars (e.g., submaxillary gland excision) may play a role in the vascularity of the flap.

Smoking has a negative impact on the microcirculation of the skin. Stimulation of the sympathetic ganglia by nicotine results in cutaneous vasoconstriction.[159, 182, 185] Nicotine also increases blood viscosity and platelet adhesiveness. Rees and coworkers retrospectively reviewed 1186 face lifts and demonstrated a 12-fold increase in risk of slough in the smoker.[181] Riefkohl and associates had similar findings (fivefold incidence) but demonstrated that in those smokers with a slough there was little correlation between smoking and nonreversible vascular occlusive changes.[182] Therefore, Riefkohl recommended cessation of smoking 1 day before and 5 days after the lift procedure to clear the vasoconstrictive effects of nicotine. Webster and associates reviewed 407 lifts using the technique of conservative undermining and found no sloughs among smokers, implying that reducing the extent of undermining for smokers would result in less sloughs.[191] Our standard practice is to avoid performing rhytidectomy unless the patient ceases smoking 2 weeks preoperatively and 1 week postoperatively. The majority of the patients are able to do this because they are highly motivated.

An impending slough will initially appear at 24 hours as a mottled discoloration that goes on to demarcate within 48 to 72 hours. Postauricular sloughs tend not to be full thickness and usually heal without scarring, but there may be pigmentary sequelae. The large, full-thickness sloughs that involve pre- and postauricular skin require tremendous reassurance. Antibiotic ointment is used to moisturize the area and promote healing. Despite the large, gaping nature of these wounds and patient insistence to intervene, conservative management, allowing secondary intention healing, will result in a satisfactory outcome. Rarely is surgical intervention, other than minor scar revision, indicated.[169, 188] Since the entire healing process may require several months, it is important that the patient receive the surgeon and staff's utmost in attention and reassurance.

UNFAVORABLE SCARS

To maximize the camouflage of scars, the surgeon must individualize incisions for different gender, hairline characteristics, and previous operations. During the preoperative consultation, patients demonstrate great anxiety about the visibility of scars, and it is important for the surgeon to explain incision placement accurately.[190]

Scars in the postauricular and perilobular area can be unsightly if they migrate into the neck as a result of tension. Maximal tension should be high by the root of the helix and

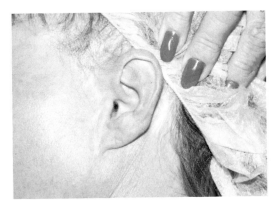

FIGURE 24–20. Postrhytidectomy patient with unsatisfactory scars and "trophy handle" or "pixie" ear.

posteriorly as the incision turns into the hairline, so that the pre- and postauricular skin forms a sling around the ear without tension (Fig. 24–20). Placement of the incision should not be planned in the postauricular sulcus, where it can migrate, but rather 0.5 to 1.0 cm into the backside of the ear, where fixation to cartilage makes migration of scars less likely. Likewise, attention to tailoring the posterior hairline incision to mimic the gentle sloping of a natural hairline will prevent stepoff deformities.[161, 166, 172]

Controversies exist over the results of a pretragal versus a post-tragal incision. Our preference is to use the gentle pretragal crease that exists in most patients who have lost elasticity of their facial skin. The pretragal incision, although potentially being more visible, does not distort or thicken the tragus. The winging of the tragus that can occur in post-tragal incisions represents a stigmata of face lift.[161, 166]

Rarely face lift scars will hypertrophy. Kamer reports a 3.1 per cent incidence.[169] In our practice it is more common in noncaucasians and very fair-skinned, light-haired individuals. Hypertrophied scars in the postauricular site are more common than in the preauricular area. A common site is where the postauricular incision turns back into the postauricular hairline. The usual treatment

consists of massage initially with Cordran taping. If resolution does not occur, intralesional triamcinolone acetonide, 20 mg/ml, may help. Occasionally, scars may require excision or a small Z-plasty postauricularly.

HAIR DEFORMITIES

The incidence of alopecia varies in the literature from 0.2 per cent to 2.8 per cent.[155, 178] The location is usually in the temporal area, following incisions that extend into the temporal hair, rather than along the perimeter of sideburn and temporal hair. Tension on closure and excessive thinning of the flaps with injury to the hair bulbs contributes to alopecia. Hair loss is usually transient and will take 3 to 6 months to regrow spontaneously. It is unclear whether minoxidil (Rogaine) may be of some therapeutic benefit. If hair growth is not complete and an area of alopecia remains, scar excision and closure or punch grafting could be considered at 1 year (Fig. 24–21).

Hair deformities secondary to surgery are more common in men than women. These deformities do not always institute a complication but represent a normal unavoidable sequelae of operation. It is important that patients be cognizant preoperatively of the changes that will occur with their hair.

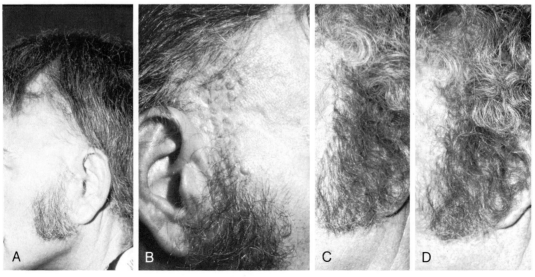

FIGURE 24–21. *A*, Temporal alopecia secondary to face lift. *B*, Early result in punch grafting. *C*, Punch grafting at six months. *D*, Punch grafting with hair styling.

Women need to be made aware that the sideburn tuft of hair will be slightly elevated, but incision planning must be such that it is not eliminated.[166, 173] Removal of the sideburn and temporal tuft gives the face a wider appearance in the AP view. Men will experience narrowing of the width of the sideburn in the preauricular area. Men must be warned that they may have to shave the postauricular area. The hair of the skin in the perilobular area can be minimized by thinning the flap and cutting the hair bulbs, and also through electrolysis.[163]

EDEMA

Edema within the first several weeks following a rhytidectomy is not a complication, and the patient should be educated to expect it. Edema persistent beyond 3 weeks may be localized or generalized. When it is localized, treatment may consist of massage. Dilute concentrations (3 mg/ml) of triamcinolone acetonide may be beneficial but must be used judiciously and sparingly to avoid atrophy. The majority of the edema will resolve in time and merely requires reassurance.

Zaworski reports a case of massive edema at 48 hours postoperatively.[196] The mechanism is believed to be a nonspecific histamine release reaction triggered by the local tissue injury.

PIGMENTARY CHANGES

Patients with a predisposition to telangiectasia and who are fair skinned should be forewarned that they may develop further telangiectasias and may require cutaneous yellow wavelength laser ablation. Although it is rare, this same population can develop a persistent erythema over the lateral neck area that is permanent and amenable only to cosmetics.

Hyperpigmentation can be seen as a sequelae in patients who have extensive postoperative ecchymosis. Localized ecchymosis routinely seen after face lift recedes in 1 to 2 weeks. Patients who develop extensive, diffuse ecchymosis may require 2 to 3 months for it to resolve and may acquire residual changes of hyperpigmentation. Patients with darker complexions are more likely to develop hyperpigmentation and should be forewarned. The discoloration may be related to hemosiderin pigment staining of the skin and eventually should resorb. In those patients with superficial hyperpigmentation, 4 per cent hydroquinones are of some benefit. In persistent cases, trichloroacetic or phenol peeling may be used for blending.

PAIN

Most patients experience minimal pain following rhytidectomy and rarely require analgesics. All patients with significant unilateral pain in the immediate postoperative period should be evaluated for a hematoma. Occasionally, upon removal of the dressing, on inspection one will discover a malpositioned ear that was folded, causing ischemic pain. Pain that persists for the first few weeks may be related to platysmal overtightening. This is described as a "tight band from ear to ear." It will loosen with time and reassurance is all that is necessary. As sensation returns, patients may experience needle jab–like pain in the periauricular area. Again, reassurance that this is part of a routine postoperative course, and analgesics, will resolve this. Neuromata of the greater auricular nerve, which has been shown to cause pain, can be palpated as masses in the lateral neck.[174] Their presentation can be many years after the procedure; the treatment of choice is excision.

MINOR CONTOUR DEFORMITIES

Earlobe deformities are a result of excessive tension placed on the closure during tailoring of the face lift flaps. Most commonly the deformity manifests as a downward pull toward the neck on the earlobe so that it mimics a "trophy handle." Tension of the closure should be at the most superior aspect of the pre- and postauricular skin so that this skin forms a sling about the ear without any tension at the lobe or in the pre- and postauricular areas.

Tragal deformities are usually a result of

previous post-tragal incisions. The skin about the tragus must be thin and without tension, otherwise the tragus may appear thick and lateralized. We prefer pretragal incisions to avoid these potential tragal distortions unless the patient has had a previous post-tragal incision.

Submental deformities are usually related to uneven fat removal (Fig. 24–22) and an inadequate treatment of platysmal banding.[168] Submental deformities encountered with liposuction are covered elsewhere in this chapter. Treatment of a prominence of the platysma muscle may involve horizontal sectioning of the muscle or suturing the muscle midline followed by a SMAS lift. Accurate clinical diagnosis preoperatively, followed by a surgical plan, will help avoid the complication of persistent platysmal banding.[165]

Another submental deformity that is a result of sculpting is the increased noticeability of a ptotic submaxillary gland. Cervical fat, which may have previously camouflaged the submandibular gland ptosis, is removed in conjunction with a superior elevation of the SMAS.

Persistent nasolabial folds are a source of patient dissatisfaction postrhytidectomy. Extended SMAS dissection provides some improvement.[164] Submalar hollowness from buccal fat resorption also contributes to patient dissatisfaction with this facial subunit. Binder has described a technique of submalar augmentation that adds to this complex.[152, 153]

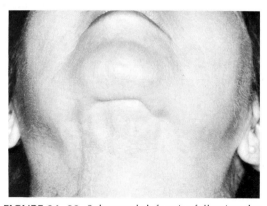

FIGURE 24–22. Submental deformity following rhytidectomy with nonsuction lipectomy and uneven fat removal.

Patients often complain of temporal swelling or bumps, which represent the pivot points of rotation of the preauricular flaps. This swelling also can exist postauricularly at the posterior limits of the hairline incision. The temporal areas can be quite distressing to the patient because, in the AP view, their face appears widened and swollen. Reassurance is usually all that is necessary. Occasionally dilute injection of Kenalog, 3 mg/ml, may improve the area and rarely excision may be necessary.

SUCTION LIPECTOMY

Although the technique is not new, suction lipectomy has gained wide acceptance only in the past decade. Cervical or facial liposuction may be done as an isolated operation but more often it is performed in conjunction with other facial procedures, especially rhytidectomy or chin augmentation. When discussing the complications associated with suction lipectomy, it is important to distinguish between combined procedures and liposuction alone. As with other surgical procedures, the individual surgeon's technique and experience in performing this procedure undoubtedly affect the complication rate. A survey by Pitman and Teimourian[204] revealed a lower overall complication rate for surgeons who performed 50 or more liposuction procedures a year.

INFECTION

The incidence of postoperative infection following facial or cervical liposuction is extremely low. In a series of 49 patients undergoing suction lipectomy of the neck only, there were no reported cases of infection.[199] The excellent vascularity of the face and cervical regions seems to provide some protection against infection. Although the infection rate is low, it is important that suction lipectomy be done in a sterile fashion. Cannulas must be thoroughly cleaned after each procedure. Commercial solutions are available to help dissolve any entrapped fat within the lumen of the cannulas. Disposable cannulas are also available from certain manufacturers. Disposable sterile tubing should be used to connect the suction machine and the suction cannula. All suction machines should have some type of filter to prevent contamination by aerosolized bacteria and viruses. It is important that this filter be checked on a routine basis and cleaned or replaced when necessary.

The use of prophylactic antibiotics is controversial. If the surgeon chooses to use them, the selection should be of one that provides adequate coverage for *Staphylococcus aureus* and other skin flora.

Unrecognized seromas or hematomas may serve as a nidus for infection, and therefore patients should be followed closely within the immediate postoperative period. If an infection does occur, the area may require drainage either by aspiration or through the incision used to introduce the cannula. Cultures of any drainage should be performed to ensure that the correct antibiotic is administered. Other adjunctive measures such as elevating the head of the patient's bed and applying warm compresses to the affected area should be instituted.

SEROMA-HEMATOMA

Small seromas of the facial or cervical areas usually will respond to aspiration and application of a pressure dressing. Reaccumulation and persistence of a seroma may indicate infection. If liposuction of the cheeks has been performed and a persistent fluid accumulation occurs over the parotid region, the fluid should be analyzed for salivary amylase to rule out the possibility of a salivary fistula. This is unlikely to occur if the surgeon has performed the suction procedure in the proper plane. Hematoma formation following cervical suction lipectomy varies from 1 to 2 per cent.[204, 205] Intuitively, it seems more likely for a hematoma to occur in the patient in whom the skin is widely undermined with the cannula, than to the patient in whom an array of tunnels are made with the cannula, leaving intervening partitions or septa of connective and adipose tissue.

A small hematoma may be aspirated transcutaneously using a syringe and a large-bore needle. A larger hematoma may be treated with the suction cannula and reapplication of a tighter pressure dressing. Placement of a closed-suction drainage system may be indicated in certain cases. A massive cervical hematoma may compromise a patient's airway and require an emergency tracheotomy.[204]

SKIN DISCOLORATION

Hyperpigmentation of the skin may occur in the area having undergone liposuction. Deposition and persistence of hemosiderin in the dermal layer is the most common cause. This type of discoloration will usually resolve within 3 to 6 months, but in some patients it may persist much longer. Trauma to the skin may induce hyperactivity of the melanocytes, resulting in increased production and deposition of melanin. This type of discoloration may be treated with some type of bleaching agent, such as Melanex or Eldoquin Forte.

SKIN SLOUGH

Necrosis of skin in the area of facial or cervical liposuction usually occurs because of some technical error in performing the procedure or in the postoperative care. Overaggressive suctioning of adipose tissue may damage the subdermal plexus of the skin. This is especially true if the operator turns the suction port outward toward the undersurface of the skin and vigorously suctions at this level. As mentioned in the discussion on hematomas, wide undermining of the skin flap with the suction cannula may also compromise the blood flow to the overlying skin. If the connective tissue septa are left intact by creating an array of individual tunnels, then the possibility of vascular compromise is less likely. Overzealous application of a cervical pressure dressing may compromise blood flow and lead to necrosis. Untreated seromas or hematomas may also cause tissue damage and subsequent necrosis. If a large, bulky pressure dressing is necessary, it is recommended that it be removed at 24 hours or that the surgeon consider replacing it with a lighter dressing in conjunction with the use of a closed-suction drainage system.

Aesthetic Complications

SKIN EXCESS

Traditionally it has been taught that patients with redundant skin and submental collection of adipose tissue were not suitable candidates for suction lipectomy because removal of the fat would excerbate the appearance of the redundant cervical skin. More recent studies have shown that older patients and those with decreased skin tone may still benefit from cervical suction lipectomy as long as it is understood that the procedure will not remove excess skin but will result in some retraction and redraping of the cervical skin.[205] Goddio reviewed skin retraction following suction lipectomy by treatment site in 458 patients.[202] In 81 cases of cervical suction lipectomy, no patient developed or had increased skin laxity as a result of the procedure. In fact, postoperative skin laxity decreased in 27.2 per cent of the patients.

Isolated facial liposuction has decreased in popularity as surgeons have begun to look critically at their long-term success rate. Facial skin does not exhibit the same amount of retraction following suction lipectomy as the cervical skin does and therefore suctioning the cheek and nasolabial fold regions should probably be reserved for a very young patient without any evidence of skin laxity.[197]

DERMAL SCARRING

Dermal scarring or dimpling is usually due to overaggressive removal of adipose tissue, which allows the dermis to scar to the platysma or facial musculature. Certain patients have facial or cervical scars as a result of cystic acne or other skin conditions. These irregularities should be pointed out and discussed preoperatively so that the patient does not mistakenly attribute them to the operation. It is also important for the patient

to realize that these imperfections will not be corrected by suction lipectomy, and they may even be more noticeable.[205]

Scarring of the skin to the underlying musculature may respond to massage or other noninvasive techniques. Dilute triamcinolone injections may also be helpful, but these should be used judiciously. Severe scarring may require lysis of the scar tissue and placement of a facial or dermal graft between the skin and musculature.

CONTOUR DEFECTS

Postoperative depressions may occur following suction lipectomy of the facial or cervical regions. Failure to feather the edges of the areas to be liposuctioned may result in a discrete ridge between the treated and untreated area. The transition area can be feathered either by using a smaller cannula at the edge or by performing fewer tunnels with the cannula. Unequal removal of subcutaneous adipose tissue also may create contour deformities. The amount of fat removed from the facial and cervical regions is usually not great, but the surgeon should use some means to quantify the amount removed from each side of the face or neck. The average fat volume removed by facial and cervical liposuction is 18 ml and 31 ml, respectively.[204] Postoperative depressions or asymmetries may be improved by injections of autogenous fat grafts, but long-term results are variable.[206, 207]

Underlying anatomic structures may present as contour defects following cervical suction lipectomy. Prominent platysmal bands and ptotic submandibular glands both may be unmasked by the removal of cervical fat. Platysmal banding may be corrected by a variety of cervical procedures performed either through a submental incision or along with rhytidectomy. Ptosis of the submandibular gland may be corrected by tightening and plication of the platysma via a rhytidectomy. In an extreme case, resection of the ptotic submandibular gland may be performed.[201]

Neurologic Complications

HYPESTHESIA

Numbness of part or all of the skin over the area treated with suction lipectomy is to be expected. The patient should be informed of this prior to undergoing the procedure. Transient postoperative hypesthesia should be viewed as an undesired sequelae of the procedure.[198] Skin numbness still present 1 year postoperatively may be viewed as a complication. Courtiss and Donelan evaluated skin sensation after suction lipectomy.[200] A patient's skin sensation was tested pre- and postsuction lipectomy. All patients experienced some numbness in the treated area, but the majority had normal sensation by 6 to 8 months postoperatively. It is interesting that many patients tested preoperatively were found to have areas of decreased skin sensation that they had not previously recognized, leading to the conclusion that some of the numbness in postsuction lipectomy patients may have been present initially and had nothing to do with the operation.

MARGINAL NERVE INJURY

Facial nerve injury during an elective facial plastic procedure is always a dreaded complication. Fortunately, the incidence of marginal nerve injury associated with cervical or facial liposuction is extremely low. Paresis of the marginal branch with return to normal function has been reported.[205] Permanent paralysis of the marginal branch undoubtedly has occurred as a result of this procedure; however, it has not been documented in the literature to our knowledge. Based on an anatomic study to define the course of the marginal mandibular nerve, it is recommended that dissection superficial to the platysma be limited to a point 2 cm lateral to the lower lip.[203] The marginal mandibular nerve takes a more superficial pathway as it courses medial to this point and is therefore more susceptible to injury.

FOREHEAD LIFT

True complications from the treatment of the aging forehead are few and infrequent.

The relatively abundant blood supply of the scalp offsets any threat of infection from the hairbearing tissues. The relatively thick and inelastic skin of the forehead, when applied tightly against the cranium, does not provide the same potential space to allow a hematoma to occur. The horizontal rhytids of the forehead, the hairline, and the hair itself provide an excellent backdrop for the necessary incisions in this area (Fig. 24–23). Depending on the forehead procedure, certain alterations in sensation and hairline occur, and these should be represented to the patient as tradeoffs for the benefits of eliminating forehead rhytids, glabellar infrowning, and brow ptosis.[211, 216, 222–224, 228] Proper patient selection and planning prevail, and the minor complaints related to brow position, hairline, and sensory disturbances in the acute postoperative period subside. Surgical management of the aging forehead is gratifying to both the surgeon and patient.

HEMATOMA

Hematoma is much less common than with lower rhytidectomy, presumably because of the relatively avascular plane of the subgaleal lift.[209, 213, 217, 227] The tight, inelastic skin envelope applied against the cranium does not allow for a significant potential space. True expanding hematomas are rare.[218] Their hallmark is excruciating pain resistant to any analgesic therapy, including supraorbital block. Swelling may be minimal relative to pain. Treatment consists of removing the scalp sutures at the bedside, which restores vascularity of the flap and also relieves the pain that may be causing hypertension. Appropriate drainage and cautery of bleeding sites is then performed in the operating room. More commonly, patients will present with small hematomas in the temporal area that are amenable to daily aspiration with a 14-gauge needle until resolved. Preventive and etiologic factors for hematoma in the forehead are similar to those of rhytidectomy and are discussed in that section.

INFECTION

Infection is exceedingly rare, due to the abundant vascular supply of the scalp. Most

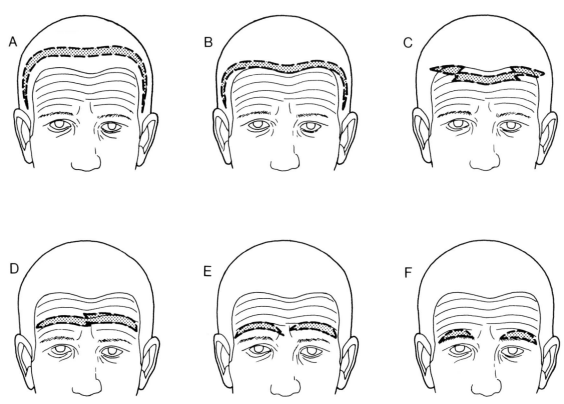

FIGURE 24–23. Incisions for treatment of the aging brow. *A,* Coronal; *B,* pretrichial lift; *C,* high midforehead lift; *D,* midforehead lift; *E,* midforehead brow lift; *F,* direct brow lift.

observers report a near-zero infection rate in hundreds of cases. Connell reports two infections in 500 patients (0.4 per cent).[213] The organism involved was *Staphylococcus aureus*. Treatment consisted of culture, drainage, and appropriate antibiotics. As a prophylaxis against infection, patients' hair is washed with Hibiclens preoperatively, and patients routinely receive a 3-day prophylactic course of cephalosporin.

SKIN NECROSIS

Sloughs of skin are an exceedingly rare complication following forehead rhytidectomy when performed in the subgaleal plane.[213, 215, 217] Vinas and associates report a case of an undetected hematoma that caused an extensive slough of the scalp with concomitant alopecia.[229] They reported a smaller slough related to a scalp infection. Small areas of superficial slough in the suture line are more common with the high midforehead

lift performed in the subcutaneous plane.[216] Excessive thinning of this large flap and injury to the subdermal plexus are the probable mechanisms of injury. The plane of dissection should be immediately above the frontalis and supraorbital neurovascular bundle to ensure the thickest, most substantial flap possible.

NERVE INJURIES

Transient sensory disturbances of the forehead skin and scalp are normal sequelae to forehead lifting. Patients' complaints regarding paresthesias are directly related to the degree of paresthesia experienced as a result of incision placement and plane dissection. The coronal incision with dissection in the subgaleal plane preserves the supraorbital neurovascular bundle from the notch to the midscalp and, hence, results in the least amount of paresthesia. Patients will experience transient paresthesia as a result of corrugator dissection and sacrifice of the subtrochlear branches. Prolonged and excessive paresthesia with this procedure indicates either neuropraxia from traumatic undermining or direct injury from either sharp dissection or cautery. If this occurs at the notch, the patient may experience paresthesia for up to 1 year. Some permanent alterations in sensation may remain. As the flap dissection proceeds toward the orbital rim, it is best continued with blunt dissection to avoid this mishap. The pretrichial lift with dissection in the subgaleal plane severs the supraorbital neurovascular bundle at the hairline, thereby leaving the patient with considerable numbness from the hairline to the midscalp. It is always interesting that some patients hardly complain about the numbness whereas for others it becomes an obsession. The midforehead lift[216] and the midforehead brow lift, discussed by Cook and associates[214] and others,[223, 224] are performed with dissection in the subcutaneous plane, leaving the supraorbital neurovascular bundle intact and minimizing postoperative paresthesia. Injury to the nerve may occur in excising or incising strips of the frontalis muscle. Care must be taken to note the position of the supraorbital nerves and avoid severing them.

Perhaps worse than the paresthesia is the itching that follows the paresthesia; this may last 2 to 3 months. Patients must be warned about the paresthesia and itching preoperatively and also the possibility of permanent numbness. Patients are reminded postoperatively to avoid scratching because it will contribute to thinning of the hair and may excoriate the scalp.[213, 217, 218] Hydroxyzine (Atarax), 10 to 20 mg at bedtime, provides symptomatic relief. Patients may require much reassurance that paresthesias and itching will resolve.

Pain, which is sometimes a complaint in the early postoperative period, is described as a band across the forehead. This sensation usually spontaneously resolves in 6 to 8 weeks. If the pain is unilateral and has a trigger point, a neuralgia of the supraorbital nerve might be present and may be amenable to local blocks and Tegretol.

The incidence of motor nerve injury to the temporal branch of the facial nerve, as reported by Connell, is 0.4 per cent (500 cases) with no permanent paralysis noted.[213] The mechanism of injury is neuropraxia, direct injury during elevation of the flap, or the result of excisions made in the frontalis lateral to the supraorbital neurovascular bundle. Kaye reports that incisions lateral to the supraorbital rim will not injure the nerve if they are made not lower than 3 cm superior to the orbital rim.[217] One must remember that the nerve travels from a point 0.5 cm below the tragus of the ear and intersects 1.5 cm superior to the lateral end of the eyebrow.[219, 221] It is in this temporal area lateral to the eyebrow that nerve injury can occur. Liebman and Webster defined its depth at the lateral brow area as covering the SMAS immediately above the temporalis fascia[219] (Fig. 24–24). It behooves the surgeon to dissect directly off the temporalis fascia to preserve the frontal branch of the facial nerve within the flap.

If permanent injury (more than 18 months) were to occur, lysis or crush of the opposite side should be considered. Botulinum toxin could be considered as an interim step in obtaining temporary contralateral paresis.[212]

HAIR ABNORMALITIES

Hairline alterations are generally not complications but compromises of the procedure.[208–210] Preoperatively the patients must be educated that post-trichial incisions will elevate the hairline. The sensory disturbances and potentially visible scar must be presented and weighed against the patient's desire not to elevate the frontal hairline. Hairline incisions can be camouflaged by slightly beveling incisions to allow hair growth through scar, and also by meticulous techniques.[213]

Some patients will experience thinning of the hair in the anterior flap, which generally is transient. Close questioning of patients may uncover the fact that they are scratching the head, thereby contributing to the hair loss. Cessation of the scratching is usually accompanied by return of hair growth.[217]

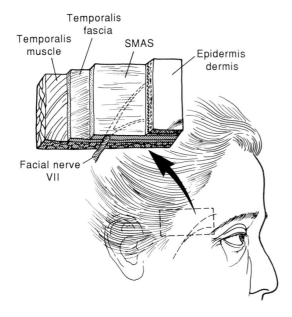

FIGURE 24–24. The danger area for the temporal branch of nerve VII as it courses in the thin superficial musculoaponeurotic system (SMAS) immediately lateral to the temporalis fascia.

Hair loss may occur transiently, especially in those patients with a history of alopecia areata, but watchful waiting for 3 to 6 months should see complete restoration of hair growth (Fig. 24–25). Permanent hair loss is more likely to be seen when skin necrosis and infection are factors.[229] Following full scar maturation, re-excision of scar or punch grafting techniques could be employed. Occasionally areas of traction alopecia will develop around the pilot suture because of tension.[217, 227] We prefer to remove pilot sutures following closure of the incision.

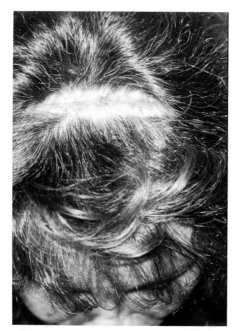

FIGURE 24–25. Telogen effluvium at the midline portion of coronal incision.

UNFAVORABLE SCARS

The superiority of midforehead incisions over direct brow incisions has been demonstrated by several investigators.[214, 216, 223–225] The surgeon must demonstrate good patient selection, and the patients must be warned that occasionally these scars do not heal favorably and may need dermabrasion. The patient with sebaceous skin and minimal forehead rhytids generally does not do well and should be discouraged from a midforehead excision.

Pretrichial incisions can look "surgical" if they are made linearly in the hairline so that the fine hairs and irregularities of the hairline are lost. Some surgeons recommend a W-plasty type of closure at the hairline to maintain the irregularity.[220]

Occasionally coronal incisions will spread, revealing a patch of alopecia in the lateral temporal portion of the incisions (Fig. 24–26). Assuming that the patients have no abnormalities of skin elasticity, the surgeon may re-excise these areas when the scar has reached full maturation.

LAGOPHTHALMOS

Prudence must be used when performing a forehead lift in an unhappy postblepharoplasty patient with persistent brow ptosis. Often when the diagnosis of brow ptosis is missed, the skin excision during blepharoplasty will be excessive to compensate. Subsequent forehead lifts may be performed conservatively or not at all, depending on the patient's ability to achieve lid closure following brow elevation. Likewise, the surgeon's predetermined excision of eyelid skin for blepharoplasty is reduced by the forehead lift, so that the forehead lift should be performed first.[213, 226] We prefer, in the ideal setting, to perform the upper lid procedure months after the forehead lift.

UNTOWARD RESULTS

As with any aesthetic procedure, the errors in judgment are either in the planning or execution stage. During the execution of the procedure the surgeon may be too aggressive or too conservative, or too asymmetric in the skin excision. Unfortunately, this equates directly into a change in facial expression. Aggressive skin excision results in a startled look. Differentially, more excision laterally than medially, when not indicated, may create an "angered" brow. Preoperative thought and planning in conjunction with adherence to the "less is more" philosophy will result in greater patient satisfaction.

DERMABRASION

Patient selection and proper preoperative consultation can help avoid many of the complications associated with dermabrasion. Blacks, orientals and Mediterranean patients with olive-colored skin should be alerted that there may be pigmentary changes.[242, 243] A slight pigmentary change may be an acceptable exchange for smooth skin in someone who uses cosmetics. Patients with active infections of the face should not have dermabrasion until they are treated. Patients with keloids or hypertrophic scars will probably experience limited improvement or may even worsen. All patients should be questioned regarding a previous history of perioral herpetic infections and receive appropriate prophylaxis.

Noncompliant patients and those with unrealistic expectations should be avoided. It is essential that, through good patient-physician rapport, the degree of improvement is accurately communicated so that patient satisfaction can be achieved. A noncompliant patient who does not follow postoperative skin care and sun avoidance instructions is more likely to have a complication with scarring and changes in pigmentation.

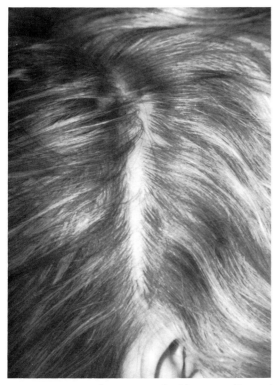

FIGURE 24–26. Alopecia postrhytidectomy. Coronal incision with spreading of scars.

PIGMENTARY ALTERATIONS

Hyperpigmentation to some extent can be seen in all noncaucasian dermabrasions, and the overall incidence is about 20 per cent. Oriental skin, in our experience, is the most problematic. Hypopigmentation usually results from melanocytic injury and is more commonly seen with deeper dermabrasions.[241] Treatment of hypopigmentation in selective dermabrasions consists of dermabrading the entire face for blending purposes.

Hyperpigmentation should be treated at its earliest sign—as the erythema becomes slightly tan in color, which is described to the patient as "tea staining" of the skin. Hydroquinones, tretinoin, and triamcinolone acetonide should be instituted.[235] Fluorescent lighting tends to camouflage early detection, so patients are best evaluated in natural daylight. Sun avoidance for 6 months should be regimentally adhered to with the use of protective clothing and sunscreens. Patients should be pretreated with tretinoin for 2 weeks and resume it 1 week postdermabrasion to minimize hyperpigmentation.[236]

SCARRING

Healing with occlusive dressing is within 7 days.[238] Delayed healing is the first sign of impending scar. Deep dermabrasions into and beyond the reticular dermis can cause scarring. Although the dermabrasion may not violate the reticular dermis, thermal injury from repeated use of the skin refrigerant may. Careful consideration of choice of skin refrigerants is warranted; several have been demonstrated to cause excessive scarring.[230, 232-234] Hypertrophic scarring is most commonly seen over bony prominences such as the malar areas, as well as the angle and body of the mandible (Fig. 24–27).

Topical hydrocortisone creams can be used as initial treatment for suspicious areas of delayed healing and hypertrophic scars. Cordran taping of scars at night is also beneficial. Those scars that not respond may require intralesional steroids such as triamcinolone

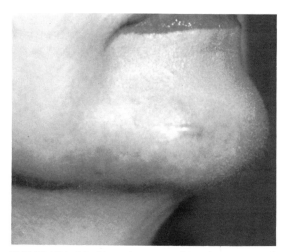

FIGURE 24–27. Mental scar resulting from perioral dermabrasion.

acetonide (10 to 30 mg/ml) injected at 4-week intervals.[239]

Dermabrasion of active acne cysts can result in scarring, so severe cases of cystic acne should be treated medically first. Postoperative infections such as herpetic eruptions can cause scarring.

Although somewhat controversial, delayed healing and subsequent scarring have been noted by some surgeons in those patients recently using Acutane (isotretinoin) for acne.[237, 240] It is unclear as to what is a satisfactory period of time to wait following Acutane therapy because some observers have had uneventful healing. At present we recommend a 12-month delay following the cessation of Acutane therapy.

INFECTIONS

Although infrequent, dermabrasion can result in postoperative infection of the skin. The most commonly offending bacterial organism is *Staphylococcus aureus*. Bacterial infection is usually accompanied by fever and is seen 48 to 72 hours following dermabrasion. Increased swelling and a honey crusting of the skin can be evidenced. Antistaphylococcal antibiotics are to be instituted immediately to avoid scarring.

All patients with a history of herpes simplex should receive pretreatment with acyclovir. If an outbreak should occur in a patient without a previous history, the outbreak can be controlled by instituting oral acyclovir (200 mg five times a day) in conjunction with topical acyclovir ointment during the postoperative epithelialization phase.

Occasionally a candidal infection can manifest by diffuse facial swelling and delayed healing. The exudate can be cultured for a predominance of yeast. Treatment consists of topical ketoconazole treatment.

THERMAL INJURY

Thermal injury to the skin and subsequent scarring can be the result of inappropriate selection of topical refrigerants[232–234] or repeated spraying of a dermabraded area. Care should be taken to protect the previously dermabraded area with gauze while spraying the next area to be dermabraded.[231] Skin necrosis with subsequent scarring can be a result of excessive or inappropriate use of topical skin refrigerant. Freon 12 and Freon 11 products should be avoided. Dichlorotetrafluoroethane (Frigiderm) and ethyl chloride–dichlorotetrafluoroethane mixture (FluroEthyl) are time tested and proven safe.[233]

MILIA

Milia are the most common event occuring after dermabrasion, seen in over half the patients at 3 to 4 weeks. These small whiteheads represent epithelial inclusion cysts that sometimes can cause anxiety; patients may wonder if they are experiencing an outbreak of acne. The incidence of milia can be reduced with pre- and post-treatment with tretinoin.[236, 239] The milia are usually self-limiting, and facial washing in conjunction with tretinoin usually is all that is necessary. Occasionally persistent milia can be incised with an 18-gauge needle.

ERYTHEMA

Patients should be prepared for a 4- to 12-week course of erythema postoperatively. Patients should be instructed in covering this with cosmetics. Cosmetic foundations with green toner help camouflage the redness. Unusually severe erythema that persists beyond 8 weeks should be treated with topical steroid creams, such as 2 per cent hydrocortisone.

SUPERFICIAL DERMATITIS

This is an allergic dermatitis whose etiology is unclear. This pruritic rash, similar to a diaper rash, will spread beyond the confines of the dermabraded area. Topical steroid creams and hypoallergenic soaps are helpful during this process. Encouraging the patient to use hypoallergenic skin care products postoperatively may reduce the incidence of occurrence.

POOR PATIENT SELECTION

The novice dermabrader may undertreat a patient, who then may require subsequent dermabrasion 1 year later. However, it is not uncommon with dermabrasion that a patient expects more than the procedure can provide. A thorough understanding of all preoperative and postoperative instructions is imperative. It is essential for the surgeon to communicate clearly how the patient will appear postoperatively and the length of time for resolution. The limitations of the procedure, more so than in other cosmetic procedures, must be stressed, for often a patient expects more than can be achieved.

CHEMICAL PEEL

To ensure safety and an efficacious outcome with chemical exfoliation, patient selection and education, as well as appropriate selection of peel solutions, is paramount. In general, patients with fair complexions and dry skin have a more uniform absorption of the peel solution and less problem with pigmentary changes. In addition to not being able to camouflage with makeup, men also have thicker and more sebaceous skin that does not allow for adequate absorption of the peel solution. Dark-skinned patients and those with much superficial pigmentation may make poor candidates for a phenol peel because of visible dermarcation; however, the choice of trichloroacetic (TCA) peel may have some benefit.[247] Patients must be properly prepared for their change in appearance during the postoperative period and also for the length of the resolution phase. Patient expectations must be realistic, and the goals be made clear. This is particularly important as it relates to choosing a peel solution. The patient expecting complete rhytid removal will be unhappy following a TCA peel; likewise, a patient who does not wear makeup may be unhappy with certain skin aberrations following a phenol peel. Even with adequate selection of patients and type of peel solutions, complications will occur, and the surgeon must be prepared to treat them.

PHENOL TOXICITY

Unlike TCA peels, which have no known systemic side effects, phenol has significant cardiac, renal, hepatic, and neural toxicity when not used judiciously.[244, 250, 251] Another, much less common, complication from phenol is laryngeal edema.[248] The majority of the phenol is slowly excreted unchanged by the kidney; some is metabolized by the liver. Signs of toxicity include cardiac arrhythmias, syncope, fatigue, depressed respiratory status, coma, and death.[250] All patients undergoing full face phenol peels should have cardiac monitoring and adequate hydration. They should be screened for previous history of cardiac and renal disease.

The occurrence of cardiac arrhythmias is directly related to the amount and rate of application of the peel solution. Life-threatening cardiac arrhythmias are more likely to occur if the peel solution is applied to over half the face in a 30-minute period. It has been demonstrated that cardiac arrhythmias will not occur if the same area is done in twice the time.[253] It is recommended that the face be approached segmentally (cheeks, forehead, perioral, periorbital) and that a 15-minute recovery time be allowed between

segments; the entire facial phenol peel then will take 1.5 hours.

In the event of an arrhythmia, the procedure should be terminated and a bolus of intravenous lidocaine given. Most arrhythmias will resolve quickly; with return of normal sinus rhythm for continuous 15-minute intervals, the peel application may be resumed at a slower rate of application.

SCARRING

Overall scarring from TCA or phenol peel is uncommon[244, 245, 247, 250] provided established formulas and guidelines are adhered to. The areas most often involved are the perioral area and along the mandible. Baker phenol solution causes a deeper injury that extends into the midreticular dermis and can cause hypertrophic scarring more commonly than does TCA (50 per cent), which extends only into the upper reticular dermis. Scarring is influenced by factors that affect the depth of penetrations, such as differences in skin preparation, occlusive taping, recent history of dermabrasion or peel, and differences in application techniques.[244, 245] Patients are instructed to avoid a constrictive headband, such as a shower cap, which may lead to scarring.[252] The patients are warned against using any chemicals in the hair for 2 weeks prior to the procedure, as the reaction may affect the depth of peel penetration and result in hairline scarring.

Early signs of scar formation are manifested by delayed healing and persistent erythema. These areas should be treated with topical nonfluorinated steroid creams as soon as there is suspicion. When a scar forms, initial measures consist of massage compression and a trial of taping with a steroid-impregnated tape such as Cordran. If this treatment is unsuccessful, intralesional steroid injection of triamcinolone acetonide (Kenalog), 10 to 30 mg/ml, may be used judiciously. Most scarring resolves satisfactorily with these measures and rarely requires scar revision.

We prefer a 6-month interval following rhytidectomy and blepharoplasty before peeling over these areas, to avoid the potential for scarring and possible ectropion. However, perioral and periorbital peeling can be performed at the same time as rhytidectomy.[244]

PIGMENTARY CHANGES

Hypopigmentation is a common occurrence following phenol peel, and the patients should be educated in this regard. A demarcation line between peeled and nonpeeled areas almost always occurs; this represents a difference in pigmentation as well as texture.

When one performs a regional peel, these lines can be diminished by feathering the solution with a dry applicator 0.5 cm beyond the nasolabial fold or orbital rim. When performing a full-face peel, it is also wise to feather 0.5 cm beyond the mandibular margin to allow for a more subtle transition from face to neck.[252]

Blotchy hyperpigmentation postoperatively can be due to inappropriate exposure to the sun, concomitant use of oral contraceptives, pregnancy, or uneven application or absorption of the peel solution. All patients are encouraged to avoid sun exposure for 3 to 6 months; a daily moisturizer with sunscreen is recommended. Early hyperpigmentation can best be detected with frequent postoperative observation in natural light and should be treated when there is early suspicion. A formula popularized by Kligman and Willis that consists of hydroquinone 7.0 per cent, retinoic acid cream 0.05 per cent, and triamcinolone cream 0.1 per cent in equal parts should be instituted as a bleaching agent.[249] The patient is to use the preparation for 8 to 12 weeks. If there is a concern about the formation of telangiectasia, the triamcinolone may be omitted. Spotty pigmentation that is not responsive to these measures may respond to a repeat peel of the affected area in 6 months.

Persistent erythema is considered a complication if it extends beyond 3 months. The patients should be reassured that it will eventually resolve. Topical hydrocortisone creams may be used to accelerate the resolution and improve the pruritus that sometimes accompanies it.

INFECTION

Fortunately, infection is an uncommon occurrence following chemical peeling in the otherwise healthy patient. Chemical peeling should be postponed in those individuals who have active bacterial or viral infections of the skin. The most common bacterial and viral organisms are *Staphylococcus* and herpes simplex, respectively. Patients should be screened for previous history of herpetic infections of their lips or mouth, because peel in this area can cause the virus to resurface. The preferred regimen of prophylaxis is acyclovir (200 mg five times a day orally), starting 48 hours prior to the procedure and continued for 7 days postpeel.

Topical acyclovir ointment is also used during the re-epithelialization phase. It has been rare in our experience to have herpetic eruptions using prophylaxis. Herpetic outbreaks that develop in those patients without antecedent history cause intense pain and superficial ulceration of the skin on about the fourth or fifth day postpeel. Cultures and acyclovir therapy should be instituted immediately. If pain is not a significant complaint and it is unclear as to whether the lesions are herpetic, then adequate antistaphylococcal antibiotic coverage should also be provided until definite culture results are obtained. Most of these infections are quite amenable to therapy; however, untreated infection can progress to life-threatening problems such as toxic shock syndrome.[246] Untreated infections postpeel can result in scarring; however, this is rarely a problem with prompt, appropriate therapy (Fig. 24–28).

Occasionally an allergic contact dermatitis may be mistaken for an infection. Dermatitis distinguishes itself by its late appearance (at 7 to 10 days postoperatively) and associated intense pruritus. Treatment consists of a detailed history to ascertain and eliminate the offending agent. Topical hydrocortisone creams can be useful for symptoms.

ABERRATIONS IN SKIN CHARACTERISTICS

Patients should be forewarned that there may be certain changes in skin characteristics

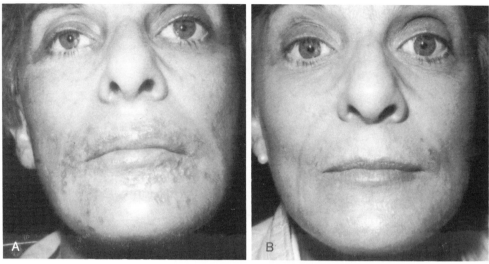

FIGURE 24–28. *A,* Herpetic outbreak following Baker chemical peel. *B,* Resolution without scarring: note the obvious line of demarcation, which improved with dermabrasion for blending.

that are beyond technical control. Existing nevi may become darker, and pore enlargement may be an unwanted side effect of chemical peeling. Telangiectasia may be more apparent or actually increase in number and require laser intervention.

Milia are less common than with dermabrasion and usually resolve with routine face cleansings. Occasionally when the milia are numerous and persistent, they may require unroofing with an 18-gauge needle. As with dermabrasion, a 2-week pretreatment with tretinoin, resuming when epithelialization occurs, markedly decreases the incidence of milia.

OTOPLASTY

A variety of procedures exist to correct congenitally prominent ears. The surgeon's choice of a particular technique depends upon careful preoperative evaluation and diagnosis of the anomalies that are causing the ear to protrude. No single technique is suitable for every patient, and each technique has its own advantages and disadvantages. The two main types of procedures used in otoplasty are cartilage incision techniques and the horizontal mattress suture method.[259, 265]

Early Complications

PAIN

Pain may be a sign of hematoma, infection, or excessive pressure. Unrelenting postoperative pain, especially if unilateral, should alert the surgeon of a possible complication, and inspection of the ear must be performed. An excessively tight dressing or a dislodged dressing may fold the ear or apply undue pressure, both of which may result in devitalization of the tissue. Increasing pain not relieved by narcotics also may be a sign of hematoma or chondritis.

HEMATOMA

The incidence of postoperative hematoma ranges from 0.08 per cent to 3.0 per cent.[256, 261, 264] Possible causes include rebound vasodilation following anesthesia with vasoconstrictors, inadequate hemostasis, or improper application of postoperative dressings. Unilateral pain is one of the cardinal signs. A patient suspected of having a hematoma should have the dressings removed and the ears examined. If a hematoma is identified, the patient should be returned to the operating room for evacuation under sterile conditions. Any identified bleeding points should be cauterized. A small closed-suction drainage system or a rubber band drain should be used and the dressing reapplied. Since a hematoma formation may serve as a nidus for infection, the patient should be placed on broad-spectrum antibiotics.

INFECTION

Skin and soft tissue infection following otoplasty should be treated vigorously in an attempt to prevent chondritis. Chondritis following operation is a dreaded complication, and for that reason many surgeons give the patient prophylactic antibiotics.[254, 260] Irrigation of the wound with an antibiotic solution prior to closure and application of an antibiotic ointment to the incision lines postoperatively may help prevent a postoperative infection.

If the diagnosis of infection is made, aggressive treatment should be undertaken. Treatment includes culture and sensitivity determination of any drainage material, evacuation of a hematoma if one is present, intravenous antibiotics, and warm compresses to the affected ear.

Chondritis, a feared but fortunately rare complication following otoplasty, occurs in fewer than 1 per cent of the cases.[256, 261, 264] Pain, swelling, and erythema are signs of chondritis. Possible etiologies include hematoma;[267] the use of braided suture, especially silk in the horizontal mattress suture technique;[276] or primary wound infection. Treatment includes hospitalization and administration of appropriate intravenous antibiotics after culture and sensitivity testing of any drainage. Incision and drainage should be performed when indicated, and any necrotic cartilage should be debrided. Persistent perichondritis may necessitate the placement of an auricular catheter to irrigate the wound with antibiotic solution. Resolution of pain may be used as an indication of the effectiveness of treatment. Even following successful treatment of chondritis, large portions of auricular cartilage may be missing through necrosis or debridement, and the ultimate postoperative result will be unsatisfactory.[268]

ALLERGIC REACTION

Skin reactions, characterized by pruritus, pain, and erythema, may indicate a local reaction to antibiotic ointment, dressing material, or skin sutures. Treatment consists of identifying and removing the causative agent.

SKIN NECROSIS

Skin loss following otoplasty is fortunately rare due to the excellent vascularity of the area. Excessive pressure caused by bolsters, overtightened or malpositioned dressings, hematoma, or infection may result in skin loss (Fig. 24–29). Small, superficial areas of skin necrosis should be treated with systemic antibiotics and an antibiotic ointment such as Bactroban.[267] Aggressive debridement of any eschar should not be performed unless there is evidence of overt infection.

Late Complications

HYPERTROPHIC SCARS/KELOIDS

In a study by Baker and Converse, the incidence of hypertrophic scars was 0.7 per

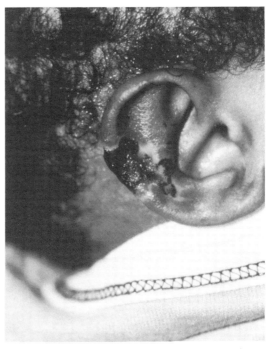

FIGURE 24–29. Skin necrosis following otoplasty. Bolsters were used with an excessively tight mastoid dressing.

cent; however, the incidence of keloid formation in black patients in the same study was 11 per cent.[256] Since the majority of otoplasty techniques are performed using postauricular incisions, if an unacceptable scar does occur it usually is well concealed. Procedures that make use of anterior auricular incisions should be avoided in patients with skin types V and VI (darkly pigmented). To avoid excessive tension of the postauricular incision, conservative skin excision should be performed. Closure of the postauricular incision may be difficult, especially if a conchal bowl setback procedure has been performed. To facilitate the closure, the excision may be outlined so that upon closure the suture line lies just above the postauricular crease. A patient with a preoperative history of hypertrophic scar or keloid formation should be counseled carefully prior to undergoing surgery.

If keloid formation does occur, gentle massage and intralesional injection of triamcinolone acetonide may be helpful. Persistent large postauricular keloids may require excision and reapproximation of the skin edges along with triamcinolone injections. Furnas reported two cases that required radiation therapy in conjunction with surgical excision and triamcinolone injections.[259] Radiation therapy for postauricular keloids should not be considered as routine treatment because the side effects, i.e. chondritis, may be more deleterious than the keloid being treated.[267]

RECURRENCE OF DEFORMITY

A unilateral recurrence of the auricular deformity occurs in approximately 6 per cent of otoplasties.[271] The choice of surgical technique may play a role, depending on the preoperative abnormalities; however, most relapses are due to the surgeon and not the technique. Adults may have thicker and more noncompliant auricular cartilage that requires the use of a technique to break the spring of cartilage as well as repositioning with suturing.[257, 263, 273] Children with more pliable cartilage may respond quite well with use of the Mustardé[265, 266] or the Furnas'[259] technique. When using the Mustardé tech-

nique, the auricular deformity may recur if the horizontal mattress sutures are improperly placed or an insufficient number of sutures are used. The suture must pass from posterior to anterior through the auricular cartilage but without penetrating the skin of the anterior auricle.

Patient noncompliance is another cause for recurrence of the deformity. A patient is asked to wear a terrycloth headband continuously for the first week following removal of the dressing. For the next 6 weeks postoperatively the patient should wear the headband at night to provide support and to prevent inadvertent trauma and folding of the ear during sleep. No contact or racket sports should be played for the first 6 weeks postoperatively to reduce the possibility of accidental trauma.

Postoperative hematomas or infections can compromise the procedure seriously and lead to a recurrence or worsening of the presurgical deformity. Immediate correction of a recurrent deformity is not indicated until adequate healing and scar formation has occurred.

ACUTE AURICULOCEPHALIC ANGLE

Formation of an acute auriculocephalic angle will result in an ear that appears to be excessively set back in relation to the skull. A study by Spira calculated that the average distance between the helical rim and the mastoid was 1.8 to 2.0 cm.[272] It was also noted that in the "normal" ear the helix is in a position lateral to the antihelix. Excessive resection of conchal cartilage may result in this deformity. Overtightening of the Mustardé sutures in the middle one third of the auricle and excessive postauricular skin excision can contribute to this deformity, which is sometimes called the "reverse telephone ear." If recognized at the time of surgery, Mustardé sutures can be removed or readjusted. Excessive conchal cartilage removal may require augmentation with an autogenous or homologous graft to increase the auriculocephalic angle. Excess skin excision can be corrected by grafting.

TELEPHONE DEFORMITY

This deformity results when the upper and lower poles of the auricle protrude from the head, and the middle third of the auricular deformity has been overcorrected. This type of deformity is more likely to occur in patients with large ears and with wide scaphas. The deformity may occur for any of the following reasons: improper placement of the horizontal mattress sutures in the superior third; inadequate excision of cartilage or skin from the upper and lower auricular pole; overzealous excision of contralateral cartilage from the middle one third.

The surgeon should reassess continually the position of the ear before any of the critical sutures are tightened. Insufficient removal of postauricular skin is addressed by carefully planning the preoperative incision. Since the deformity consists of protrusion in the superior and inferior poles of the ear, it is often necessary to excise more skin in these areas. The same holds true for conchal cartilage excision. Hatch describes a technique to decrease the angle between the root of the helix and the scalp that involves suturing the root of the helix to the temporal fascia.[262] Persistent protrusion of the earlobe may be corrected using simple skin excision[275] or placement of a horizontal mattress suture between the cauda and the conchal cartilage.[255] The spring of the cauda may be weakened by an incision, but complete excision should not be performed because control of the cauda with a suture would not then be possible.[258]

DISTORTIONS OF THE EXTERNAL AUDITORY CANAL

Improper placement of conchal mastoid sutures, as used in the Furnas conchal bowl setback technique, may cause narrowing of the external auditory canal, especially if the conchal bowl is large.[259, 274] The surgeon should check the external auditory canal for narrowing before the conchal mastoid sutures are secured. Excision of a portion of the medial cartilage also has been proposed.[270]

SUTURE COMPLICATIONS

Tenting of the postauricular skin over the sutures used in the Mustardé technique may occur years after the initial surgery. In thin-skinned individuals, dyed sutures may be visible. The suture need not be removed unless it becomes infected or begins to extrude. This usually will not compromise the result of surgery if adequate scarring has occurred to hold the auricle in proper position. The best suture material to use during otoplasty is a matter of personal preference. Rigg reviewed his use of buried sutures in otoplasty and reported an 8 per cent incidence of granulation formation using Mersilene to reconstruct the antihelical fold.[269] Braided, nonabsorbable sutures resist untying and stretching better than monofilament, nonabsorbable sutures, but the former also have a greater tendency to be a nidus for infection.

SENSORY DEFICITS

Postauricular numbness and hypesthesia are common following otoplasty. Normal sensation usually returns within weeks or months. Permanent postauricular numbness may occur following excision of the postauricular muscle during a conchal set-back technique. Elliott also noted that relatively few patients complained of this symptom postoperatively.[258]

References

Rhinoplasty

1. Adamson JE: Constriction of the internal nasal valve in rhinoplasty: Treatment and prevention. Ann Plast Surg 18(2):114, 1987.
2. Adamson PA: Open rhinoplasty. Otolaryngol Clin North Am 20(4):837, 1987.
3. Adamson P, Smith O, Cole P: The effect of cosmetic rhinoplasty on nasal patency. Laryngoscope 100(4):357, 1990.
4. Anderson R, Sprinkle PM, et al: Complication of septorhinoplasty. Benign or malignant? Arch Otolaryngol 109(7):489, 1983.
5. Beekhuis GJ: Nasal obstruction after rhinoplasty: Etiology and techniques for correction. Laryngoscope 86(4):540, 1976.
6. Beekhuis GJ: Saddle nose deformity: Etiology, prevention and treatment. Laryngoscope 84(1):2, 1974.

7. Bridger GP: Split rib graft for alar collapse. Arch Otolaryngol 107:110, 1981.
8. Burgess LP, Everyton DM, et al: Complications of the external (combination) rhinoplasty approach. Arch Otolaryngol 112(10):1064, 1986.
9. Casaubon J-N, Dion MA, Larbrisseau A: Septic cavernous sinus thrombosis after rhinoplasty. Plast Reconstr Surg 59(1):119, 1977.
10. Champion R: Anosmia associated with corrective rhinoplasty. Br J Plast Surg 19(2):182, 1966.
11. Cheney ML, Blair PA: Blindness as a complication of rhinoplasty. Arch Otolaryngol 113(7):768, 1987.
12. Churukian MM, Zemplenyi J, et al: Postrhinoplasty epistaxis. Role of Vitamin E? Arch Otolaryngol 114(7):748, 1988.
13. Cies WA, Baylis HI: Epiphora following rhinoplasty and Caldwell-Luc procedures. Ophthalmic Surg 7(1):77, 1976.
14. Coursey DL: Staphylococcus endocarditis following septorhinoplasty. Arch Otolaryngol 99:454, 1974.
15. Courtiss EH, Goldwyn R: The effects of nasal surgery on air flow. Plast Reconstr Surg 72:9, 1983.
16. Dicken CH: Argon laser treatment of the red nose. J Dermatol Surg Oncol 16(1):33, 1990.
17. Eschelman LT, Schleuning AJ, Brummett R: Prophylactic antibiotics in otolaryngologic surgery: A double-blind study. Trans Am Acad Ophthalmol 75:387, 1971.
18. Fabricant ND: Cavernous sinus thrombosis following submucous resection. Arch Otolaryngol 17:635, 1933.
19. Fairbanks DN: Closure of nasal septal perforations. Arch Otolaryngol 106:509, 1980.
20. Flowers RS, Anderson R: Injury to the lacrimal apparatus during rhinoplasty. Plast Reconstr Surg 42:577, 1968.
21. Ford CN, Battaglia DG, Gentry LR: Preservation of periosteal attachment in lateral osteotomy. Ann Plast Surg 13(2):107, 1984.
22. Goldwyn RM, Shore S: The effects of submucous resection and rhinoplasty on the sense of smell. Plast Reconstr Surg 41:427, 1968.
23. Goldwyn RM: Unexpected bleeding after elective nasal surgery. Ann Plast Surg 2(3):201, 1979.
24. Goode RL: Surgery of the incompetent nasal valve. Laryngoscope 95(5):546, 1985.
25. Goode RL: Resection of obstructing inferior turbinates (letter). Plast Reconstr Surg 86(6):1236, 1990.
26. Goodman WS, Strelzow VV: The surgical closure of nasoseptal perforations. Laryngoscope 92:121, 1982.
27. Griffies WS, Kennedy K, et al: Steroids in rhinoplasty. Laryngoscope 99:1161, 1989.
28. Grocutt M, Fatah ME: Recurrent multiple epidermoid inclusion cysts following rhinoplasty—an unusual complication. J Laryngol Otol 103(12):1214, 1989.
29. Guyuron B, Licota L: Arteriovenous malformation following rhinoplasty. Plast Reconstr Surg 77(3):474, 1986.
30. Hallock GG, Trier WC: Cerebrospinal fluid rhinorrhea following rhinoplasty. Plast Reconstr Surg 77(1):109, 1983.
31. Harley EH, Erdman JP: Dorsal nasal cyst formation. A rare complication of cosmetic rhinoplasty. Arch Otolaryngol 116(1):105, 1990.
32. Herzon FS: Bacteremia and local infections with nasal packing. Arch Otolaryngol 94:317, 1971.
33. Hoffman DF, Cook TA, Quatela VC, et al: Steroids and rhinoplasty: A double blind study. In Stucker FJ (ed): Plastic and Reconstructive Surgery of the Head and Neck: Proceedings of the Fifth International Symposium. Philadelphia, BC Decker, 1991, p 7.
34. Holt GR, Garner ET, McLarey D: Postoperative sequelae and complications of rhinoplasty. Otolaryngol Clin North Am 20(4):853, 1987.
35. Jacobson JA, Kasworm EM: Toxic shock syndrome after nasal surgery. Arch Otolaryngol 112(3):329, 1986.
36. Johnson CM Jr, Anderson J: The deviated nose—its correction. Laryngoscope 87:1680, 1977.
37. Johnson CM Jr, Quatela VC: Nasal tip grafting via the open approach. Facial Plast Surg 4(4):301, 1987.
38. Johnson CM Jr, Quatela VC, Toriumi DM: Open structure rhinoplasty: The basic technique. In Johnson CM, Toriumi DM (eds): Open Structure Rhinoplasty. Philadelphia, WB Saunders, 1990.
39. Johnson CM Jr, Quatela VC, Toriumi DM, Biggerstaff R: The tip graft. In Johnson CM, Toriumi DM (eds): Open Structure Rhinoplasty. Philadelphia, WB Saunders, 1990.
40. Kamer FM: Pseudomonas after nasal and facial surgery (letter). Plast Reconstr Surg 71(2):285, 1983.
41. Kamer FM, Binder WJ: Pseudomonas infection of the nose. Arch Otolaryngol 106(8):505, 1980.
42. Kamer FM, Churukian MM: High septal hemitransfixion for the correction of caudal septal deformities. Laryngoscope 94:391, 1984.
43. Kamer FM, Churukian MM, Hansen L: The nasal fossa: A complication of rhinoplasty. Laryngoscope 96(3):303, 1986.
44. Klabunde HE, Falces E: Incidence of complications in cosmetic rhinoplasties. Plast Reconstr Surg 34:192, 1964.
45. Kridel RWH, Appling WD, Wright WK: Septal perforation closure utilizing the external septorhinoplasty approach. Arch Otolaryngol Head Neck Surg 112:168, 1986.
46. Lacy GM, Conway H: Recovery after meningitis with convulsions after rhinoplasty. Cause for Pause. Plast Reconstr Surg 36:254, 1965.
47. Lavine DM, Lehman JA, Jackson T: Is the lacrimal apparatus injured following cosmetic rhinoplasty? Arch Otolaryngol 105:719, 1979.
48. Lawson W, Kessler S, Biller HF: Unusual and fatal complications of rhinoplasty. Arch Otolaryngol 109(3):164, 1983.
49. Levin ML, Argamaso RV, Friedman S: Localized cerebritis following and esthetic rhinoplasty. Plast Reconstr Surg 64(5):720, 1979.
50. Mabry RL: Visual loss after intranasal corticosteroid injection. Arch Otolaryngol 107:484, 1981.
51. Marshall DR, Slattery PG: Intracranial complications of rhinoplasty. Br J Plast Surg 36(3):342, 1983.
52. McKinney P, Cook JQ: A critical evaluation of 200 rhinoplasties. Ann Plast Surg 7(5):357, 1981.
53. Meyer M, Moss ALH, Cullen KW: Infraorbital nerve palsy after rhinoplasty. J Craniomaxillofac Surg 18:173, 1990.
54. Miller T: Immediate postoperative complications of septoplasties and septorhinoplasties. Trans Pacific Coast Otoophthalmol Soc 57:201, 1976.
55. Noe JM, Finley J, Rosen S, Arndt KA: Postrhinoplasty "red nose:" Differential diagnosis and treatment by laser. Plast Reconstr Surg 65(5):661, 1981.

56. Osborne JE, Blair RL, Christmas HE, McKenzie H: Actinomycosis of the nasopharynx: A complication of nasal surgery. J Laryngol Otol 102:639, 1988.

57. Osguthorpe JD, Calcaterra TC: Nasolacrimal obstruction after maxillary sinus and rhinoplastic surgery. Arch Otolaryngol 105(5):264, 1979.

58. Parkes ML, Borowiecki B, Binder W: Functional sequelae of rhinoplasty. Ann Plast Surg 4(2):116, 1980.

59. Parkes ML, Griffiths CO Jr: Atrial-venous aneurysm after rhinoplastic surgery. Arch Otolaryngol 86:91, 1967.

60. Parkes ML, Kanodia R: Avulsion of the upper lateral cartilage: Etiology, diagnosis, surgical anatomy and management. Laryngoscope 91(5):758, 1981.

61. Quatela VC, Cook TA: Difficult decisions: Problems in nasal tip projection. Operative Techniques Otolaryngol Head Neck Surg 1(3):204, 1990.

62. Romo T III, Foster CA, Korovin GS, Sach ME: Repair of nasal septal perforation utilizing the midface degloving technique. Arch Otolaryngol 114:739, 1988.

63. Rosenvold LK: Intracranial suppuration secondary to disease of the nasal septum. Arch Otolaryngol 40:1, 1944.

64. Sessions RB: Membrane approximation by continuous mattress sutures following septoplasty. Laryngoscope 94:702, 1984.

65. Sheen JH: Special problems. In Sheen JH, Sheen AP (eds): Aesthetic Rhinoplasty. St. Louis, CV Mosby, 1987, p 807.

66. Silk KL, Ali MB, et al: Absence of bacteremia during nasal septoplasty. Arch Otolaryngol 117(1):54, 1991.

67. Slavin SA, Goldwyn RM: The cocaine user: The potential problem patient for rhinoplasty. Plast Reconstr Surg 86(3):436, 1990.

68. Slavin SA, Rees TD, Guy CL, Goldwyn RM: An investigation of bacteremia during rhinoplasty. Plast Reconstr Surg 71(2):196, 1983.

69. Slavitt DR, Quatela VC, Wang TO: Aesthetic refinement in significant nasal augmentation. In Stucker FJ (ed): Plastic and Reconstructive Surgery of the Head and Neck: Proceedings of the Fifth International Symposium. Philadelphia, BC Decker, 1991, p 41.

70. Song IC, Bromberg BE: Carotid-cavernous sinus fistula occuring after a rhinoplasty. Plast Reconstr Surg 55(1):92, 1975.

71. Stucker FJ: Prevention of post-rhinoplasty edema. Laryngoscope 84(4):536, 1974.

72. Sykes JM, Toriumi D, Kerth JD: A devitalized tooth as a complication of septorhinoplasty. Arch Otolaryngol 112(7):765, 1987.

73. Tardy ME Jr, Cheng EY, Jernstrom V: Misadventures in nasal tip surgery; Analysis and Repair. Otolaryngol Clin North Am 20(4):797, 1987.

74. Tardy ME Jr, Kron TK, Younger R, Key M: The cartilaginous pollybeak: Etiology, prevention, and treatment. Facial Plast Surg 6(2):113, 1989.

75. Teichgraeber JF, Riley WB, Parks DH: Nasal surgery complications. Plast Reconstr Surg 85(4):527, 1990.

76. Thomas GG, Toohill RJ, Lehman RH: Nasal actinomycosis following heterograft; A case report. Arch Otolaryngol 100(5):377, 1974.

77. Thomas JR, Griner N: The relationship of lateral osteotomies in rhinoplasty to the lacrimal drainage system. Otolaryngol Head Neck Surg 94(3):362, 1986.

78. Thomas JR, Tardy ME Jr: Complications of rhinoplasty. ENT J 65:19, 1986.

79. Thompson AC: Nasal tip numbness following rhinoplasty. Clin Otolaryngol 12(2):143, 1987.

80. Toback J, Fayerman JW: Toxic shock syndrom following septorhinoplasty. Implications for the head and neck surgeon. Arch Otolaryngol 109(9):627, 1983.

81. Wagner R, Toback JM: Toxic shock syndrome following septoplasty using plastic septal splints. Laryngoscope 96(6):609, 1986.

Blepharoplasty

82. Alfonso E, Levada AJ, Flynn JT: Inferior rectus paresis after secondary blepharoplasty. Br J Ophthalmol 68:535, 11984.

83. Allen MV, Cohen IK, Grimson B, et al: Orbital cellulitis secondary to dacryocystitis following blepharoplasty. Plast Reconstr Surg 73:126, 1984.

84. Anderson RL, Dixon RS: Aponeurosis ptosis surgery. Arch Ophthalmol 97:1127, 1979.

85. Anderson RL, Gordy DD: The tarsal strip procedure. Arch Ophthalmol 97:2192, 1979.

86. Callahan NA: Prevention of blindness after blepharoplasty. Ophthalmology 90:1048, 1983.

87. Carroway JH, Mello CG: The prevention of lower lid ectropion following blepharoplasty. Plast Reconstr Surg 85:6, 1990.

88. Converse JN: Treatment of epithelialized suture tracts of eyelids by marsupialization. Plast Reconstr Surg 48:47, 1966.

89. DeMere M: Blindness and eyelid surgery. Aesthet Plast Surg 53:634, 1974.

90. DeMere M, Wood T, Austin W: Eye complications with blepharoplasty or other eyelid surgery. Plast Reconstr Surg 53:634, 1974.

91. Rees TB, Newell FW: "Discussions by Lemoine, A. N. Jr." 52:12, 1973.

92. Donohue HC: Cellulitis followed by total blindness. Am J Ophthalmol 29:1574, 1946.

93. Edgerton MT, Hansen FC: Matching facial color with split thickness skin grafts from adjacent areas. Plast Reconstr Surg 21:455, 1960.

94. Edgerton MT, Wolfort FG: The dermal flap canthal lift for lower eyelid support. Plast Reconstr Surg 43:42, 1969.

95. Fry JH: Reversible visual loss after proptosis from retrobulbar hemorrhage. Reproduction of syndrome in Cynomolgus monkey. Plast Reconstr Surg 44:480, 1969.

96. Golcman B, Friedhofer H, Anger M, Golcman R: Surgical indications for sunken eyelids. Aesthet Plast Surg 5:123, 1981.

97. Green MF, Kadri SWM: Acute closed angle glaucoma; A complication of blepharoplasty. Br J Plast Surg 27:25, 1974.

98. Harley RD, Nelson LB, Glannagan JC, Callahan JH: Ocular motility disturbances following cosmetic blepharoplasty. Arch Ophthalmol 104:542, 1986.

99. Hartley JH, Lester JC, Schatten WE: Acute retrobulbar hemorrhage during elective blepharoplasty. Plast Reconstr Surg 52:8, 1973.

100. Hartman E, Morax PV, Vergez A: Severe visual

complications in blepharoplasty. Ann Ocul 195:142, 1962.

101. Hayreh SS, Kolder HE, Weingeist TA: Central retinal artery occlusion and retinal tolerance time. Ophthalmology 87:75, 1980.

102. Hayworth RS, Lisman RD, Muchnick RS, et al: Diplopia following blepharoplasty. Ann Ophthalmol 16:4484, 1984.

103. Hollows FC, Graham AP: Intraocular pressure, glaucoma and glaucoma suspects in a defined population. Br J Ophthalmol 50:570, 1966.

104. Huang TT, Horowitz B, Lewis ST: Retrobulbar hemorrhage. Plast Reconstr Surg 59:39, 1977.

105. Hueston JT, Heinze JB: A second case of relief of blindness following blepharoplasty. Case Report. Plast Reconstr Surg 59:430, 1977.

106. Hueston JT, Heinze JB: Successful early relief of blindness occurring after blepharoplasty. Plast Reconstr Surg 53:588, 1972.

107. Iverson RE, et al: Correction of enophthalmos in the enophthalmic orbit. Plast Reconstr Surg 51:545, 1973.

108. Jackson IT: Letters to the editor. Plast Surg Outlook 2(5), 1988.

109. Katz BE, Fisher AA: Bacitracin: A unique topical antibiotic sensitizer. J Am Acad Dermatol 17:1016, 1987.

110. Klatsky SA, Manson PN: Blepharoplasty—Management of complications and patient dissatisfaction. In Goldwyn RM (ed): The Unfavorable Result in Plastic Surgery: Avoidance and Treatment. Boston, Little, Brown, 1984.

111. Koorneef L: The architecture of musculo-fibrosis apparatus in the human orbit. Acta Morphol Neerl Skand 15:35, 1971.

112. Kraushar MF, Seelenfreund MH, Frelich DB: Closure of the central artery following retrobulbar injection. Trans Am Acad Ophthalmol Otolaryngol 78:65, 1974.

113. Kroll AJ: Experimental central retinal artery occlusion. Arch Ophthalmol 79:453, 1968.

114. Lemoline AN Jr, Rees TD, Newell FW: Discussion of acute retrobulbar hemorrhage during elective blepharoplasty. Plast Reconstr Surg 52:12, 1973.

115. Levine MR: Traumatic ptosis. Adv Ophthalmol Plast Surg 1:195–204, 1982.

116. Levine MR, Baynton J, Tenzel RR, et al: Complications of blepharoplasty. Ophthalmic Surg 6:53, 1975.

117. Levine MR: Prevention and management of complications of blepharoplasty. Facial Plast Surg 1:311, 1984.

118. Lisman RD, Hyde K, Smith B: Complications of blepharoplasty. Clin Plast Surg 15:309, 1988.

119. Loeb R: Corrections of subpalpebral depression with small free grafts. In Transactions of the Seventh International Congress of Plastic and Reconstructive Surgeons. Sao Paulo, Cartgraft, 1981.

120. Loeb R: Fat pad sliding and fat grafting for leveling lid depressions. Clin Plast Surg 8:757, 1981.

121. Mackinnon SE, Fielding JC, Delton AL, Fisher DM: The incidence and degree of scleral show in the normal population. Plast Reconstr Surg 80:20, 1987.

122. McCord CD: Complications of orbital surgery. Otolaryngol Clin North Am 21(1):184, 1988.

123. McKinney P, Zukowski ML: The value of tear film breakup and Schirmer's test in preoperative blepharoplasty evaluation. Plast Reconstr Surg 84:572, 1989.

124. Millay DJ, Larrabee WF: Ptosis and blepharoplasty surgery. Arch Otolaryngol 115:198, 1989.

125. Mitchell JP, Lumb JN: A Handbook of Surgical Diathermy. Bristol, England, John Wright & Sons, 1966, pp 56–57.

126. Morgan SC: Orbital cellulitis and blindness following blepharoplasty. Plast Reconstr Surg 64:823, 1979.

127. Moser MH, Dipirro E, McCoy FJ: Sudden blindness following blepharoplasty. Plast Reconstr Surg 51:364, 1973.

128. Moses RA: Adler's Physiology of the Eye. 7th ed. St. Louis, CV Mosby, 1981.

129. Neely KA, Ernest TJ, Mottier M: Combined superior oblique paresis and Brown syndrome after blepharoplasty. Am J Ophthalmol 109(3):347, 1990.

130. Puterman AM: Temporary blindness after cosmetic blepharoplasty. Am J Ophthalmol 80:1081, 1975.

131. Putterman AM, Urist MJ: Mueller's muscle conjunctival resection, a method for treatment of blepharoptosis. Arch Ophthalmol 92:614, 1975.

132. Rees TD: Blepharoplasty; postoperative considerations and complications. In Aesthetic Plastic Surgery. Philadelphia, WB Saunders, 1980.

133. Rees TD: Complications following blepharoplasty. In Symposium on Plastic Surgery in the Orbital Region. St. Louis, CV Mosby, 1976.

134. Rees TD: Correction of ectropion resulting from blepharoplasty. Plast Reconstr Surg 50:1, 1972.

135. Rees TD, Craig SM, Fisher Y: Orbital abscess following blepharoplasty. Plast Reconstr Surg 73:126, 1984.

136. Rees TD, LaTrenta GS: The role of the Schirmer's test and orbital morphology in predicting dry-eye syndrome after blepharoplasty. Plast Reconstr Surg 82:619, 1988.

137. Stasior OG: Blindness associated with cosmetic blepharoplasty. Clin Plast Surg 8:793, 1981.

138. Suttcliff I, et al: Bleeding in cosmetic blepharoplasty: An anatomic approach. Ophthal Plast Reconstr Surg 1:107, 1985.

139. Tenzel R: Cosmetic blepharoplasty. In Soll DB (ed): Management of Complications in Ophthalmic Plastic Surgery. Birmingham, AL, Aesculapius Publishing Co, 1976, Chap 8.

140. Tenzel RR, Buffam FV, Miller GR: The use of the "lateral canthal sling" in ectropion repair. Can J Ophthalmol 2:199, 1977.

141. Waller R: Is blindness a realistic complication in blepharoplasty procedures? Trans Am Acad Ophthalmol Otolaryngol 85:730, 1978.

142. Wesley RE, Pollard ZF, McCord CD Jr: Superior oblique paresis after blepharoplasty. Plast Reconstr Surg 66:283, 1980.

143. Wust K: Therapy of threatening optic atrophy due to retrobulbar hematoma. Klin Monatsbl Augenheilkd 114:140, 1949.

Face Lift

144. Baker DC: Complications of cervicofacial rhytidectomy. Clin Plast Surg 10(3):543, 1983.

145. Baker DC, Aston SJ, Guy CL, Rees TD: The male rhytidectomy. Plast Reconstr Surg 60(4):514, 1977.

146. Baker DC, Conley J: Avoiding facial nerve injuries

in rhytidectomy. Plast Reconstr Surg 64(6):781, 1979.

147. Baker TJ, Gordon HL, Mosienko P: Rhytidectomy: A statistical analysis. Plast Reconstr Surg 59(1):24, 1977.

148. Bamberg SF, Krugman ME: Parotid salivary fistula following rhytidectomy. Ann Plast Surg 24(1):61, 1990.

149. Barker DE: Prevention of bleeding following a rhytidectomy. Plast Reconstr Surg 54(6):651, 1974.

150. Beekhuis GJ: How I do it—plastic surgery: Face-lift—postoperative hematoma; Prevention and management. Laryngoscope 90:164, 1980.

151. Berner RE, Morain WD, Noe JM: Postoperative hypertension as an etiological factor in hematoma after rhytidectomy. Plast Reconstr Surg 57(3):314, 1976.

152. Binder WJ: Submalar augmentation. An alternative to face-lift surgery. Arch Otolaryngol 115(7):797, 1989.

153. Binder WJ: Submalar augmentation: A procedure to enhance rhytidectomy. Ann Plast Surg 24(3):200, 1990.

154. Clark RP, Berris CE: Botulinum toxin: A treatment for facial asymmetry caused by facial nerve paralysis. Plast Reconstr Surg 84(2):353, 1989.

155. Cohen SR, Webster RC: Primary rhytidectomy—Complications of the procedure and anesthetic. Laryngoscope 93:654, 1983.

156. Conway H: The surgical facelift—Rhytidectomy. Plast Reconstr Surg 45:124, 1970.

157. Dedo DD: Preliminary report on complications of the extended cervicofacial rhytidectomy. Laryngoscope 93:272, 1983.

158. Deutsch HL: Resection of platysma bands in face-lift surgery. J Dermatol Surg Oncol 6(12):1003, 1980.

159. Dillman DB: Cigarette smoking in face lift patients. Plast Reconstr Surg 75(3):445, 1985.

160. Ellenbogen R: Pseudo-paralysis of the mandibular branch of the facial nerve after platysmal face-lift operation. Plast Reconstr Surg 63:364, 1979.

161. Franco T: Face-lift stigmas. Ann Plast Surg 15(5):379, 1985.

162. Fredricks S, Faires R: Postauricular skin slough in cervical facial rhytidectomy. Ann Plast Surg 16(3):195, 1986.

163. Gonzalez-Ulloa M: Rhytidectomy in men: A new approach. Arch Otolaryngol 96:325, 1972.

164. Hamra ST: The deep-plane rhytidectomy. Plast Reconstr Surg 86(1):53, 1990.

165. Hugo NE: Rhytidectomy with radical lipectomy and platysmal flaps. Plast Reconstr Surg 65(2):199, 1980.

166. Johnson CM Jr, Adamson PA, Anderson JR: The face-lift incision. Arch Otolaryngol 110:371, 1984.

167. Kamer FM: Sequential rhytidectomy and the two stage concept. Otolaryngol Clin North Am 13(2):305, 1980.

168. Kamer FM, Binder WJ: Avoiding depressions in submental lipectomy. Laryngoscope 90(8):1396, 1980.

169. Kamer FM, Damiani J, Churukian M: Five hundred twelve rhytidectomies: A retrospective study. Arch Otolaryngol 110:512, 1984.

170. Klein DR, Allen R: A comparison of complications between in-hospital patients and outpatients for aesthetic surgical procedures: A ten-year study. Plast Reconstr Surg 67:17, 1981.

171. Kridel RWH, Aguilar EA III, Wright WK: Complications of rhytidectomy. Ear Nose Throat J 64:44/584, 1985.

172. Leist FD, Masson JK, Erich JB: A review of 324 rhytidectomies, emphasizing complications and patient dissatisfaction. Plast Reconstr Surg 59(4):525, 1977.

173. Lewis CM: Preservation of the female sideburn. Aesthetic Plast Surg 8(2):91, 1984.

174. Manstein CH, Manstein G: Bilateral neuromata of the great auricular nerves 8 years following face lift. Plast Reconstr Surg 76(6):937, 1985.

175. Matsunaga RS: Rhytidectomy employing a two-layered closure: Improved results with hidden scars. Otolaryngol Head Neck Surg 89:496, 1981.

176. McCollough EG, Perkins SW, Langsdon PR: SAS-MAS suspension rhytidectomy. Rationale and long-term experience. Arch Otolaryngol 115(2):228, 1989.

177. McDowell AJ: Effective practical steps to avoid complications in face-lifting. Plast Reconstr Surg 50(6):563, 1972.

178. Parkes ML, Kamer FM, Bassilios MI: Treatment of alopecia in temporal region following rhytidectomy procedures. Laryngoscope 87(6):1011, 1977.

179. Pitanguy I, Ceravolo MP: Hematoma postrhytidectomy: How we treat it. Plast Reconstr Surg 67:526, 1981.

180. Rees TD, Lee YC, Coburn RJ: Expanding hematoma after rhytidectomy. Plast Reconstr Surg 51:149, 1973.

181. Rees TD, Liverett DM, Guy CL: The effect of cigarette smoking on skin-flap survival in the face lift patient. Plast Reconstr Surg 73(6):911, 1984.

182. Riefkohl R, Wolfe JA, Cox EB, McCarty KS Jr: Association between cutaneous occlusive vascular disease, cigarette smoking and skin slough after rhytidectomy. Plast Reconstr Surg 77(4):592, 1986.

183. Rose EH, Laub DR, Avakoff J: Cardiac asystole secondary to carotid sinus compression in the face-lift operation. Plast Reconstr Surg 59(2):252, 1977.

184. Schnur PL, Burkhardt BR, Tofield JJ: The second-look technique in face lifts—does it work? Plast Reconstr Surg 65(3):298, 1980.

185. Solmer R: Cigarette smoking and skin flap survival in the face lift patient. Plast Reconstr Surg 75(2):282, 1985.

186. Stark RB: A rhytidectomy series. Plast Reconstr Surg 59:373, 1977.

187. Straith RE, Raghava R, Hipps CJ: The study of hematomas in 500 consecutive face lifts. Plast Reconstr Surg 59(5):694, 1977.

188. Thompson DP, Ashley FL: Face-lift complications. Plast Reconstr Surg 61(1):40, 1978.

189. Webster RC, Davidson TM, White MF, et al: Conservative face lift surgery. Arch Otolaryngol 102:657, 1976.

190. Webster RC, Fanous N, Smith RC: Male and female face-lift incisions. Arch Otolaryngol 108:299, 1982.

191. Webster RC, Kazda G, Hamdan US, et al: Cigarette smoking and face lift: Conservative versus wide undermining. Plast Reconstr Surg 77(4):596, 1986.

192. Webster RC, Smith RC, Smith KF: Face Lift, Part I: Extent of undermining of skin flaps. Head Neck Surg Jul/Aug:525, 1983.

193. Webster RC, Smith RC, Smith KF: Face Lift, Part III: Plication of the superficial musculoaponeurotic system. Head Neck Surg Nov/Dec:696, 1983.

194. Webster RC, Smith RC, Smith KF: Face Lift, Part IV: Use of superficial musculoaponeurotic system

suspending sutures. Head Neck Surg Jan/Feb:780, 1984.

195. Webster RC, Smith RC, Smith KF: Face Lift, Part V: Suspending sutures for plastysma cording. Head Neck Surg Mar/Apr:870, 1984.
196. Zaworski RE, Noriega CJ: Massive postoperative facial edema in a rhytidectomy. Plast Reconstr Surg 62(4):622, 1978.

Suction Lipectomy

197. Courtiss EH: Suction lipectomy: A restrospective analysis of 100 patients. Plast Reconstr Surg 73:780, 1986.
198. Courtiss EH: Suction lipectomy: Complications and results by survey (discussion). Plast Reconstr Surg 76:70, 1985.
199. Courtiss EH: Suction lipectomy of the neck. Plast Reconstr Surg 76:882, 1985.
200. Courtiss EH, Donelan MB: Skin sensation after suction lipectomy: A prospective study of 50 consecutive patients. Plast Reconstr Surg 81:550, 1988.
201. de Pina DP, Quinta WC: Aesthetic resection of the submandibular salivary gland. Plast Reconstr Surg 88:779, 1991.
202. Goddio AS: Skin retraction following suction lipectomy by treatment site: A study of 500 procedures in 458 selected subjects. Plast Reconstr Surg 87:66, 1991.
203. Liebman EP, Webster RC, Gaul JR, Griffin T: The marginal mandibular nerve in rhytidectomy and liposuction surgery. Arch Otol Head Neck Surg 114:179, 1988.
204. Pitman GH, Teimourian B: Suction lipectomy: Complications and results by survey. Plast Reconstr Surg 76:65, 1985.
205. Teimourian B: Complications associated with suction lipectomy. Clin Plast Surg 16:385, 1989.
206. Teimourian B: Repair of soft-tissue contour deficit by means of semiliquid fat graft. Plast Reconstr Surg 78:123, 1986.
207. Yues-Gerard: The fat cell "graft:" A new technique to fill depressions. Plast Reconstr Surg 78:122, 1986.

Forehead Lift

208. Adamson PA, Johnson CM Jr, Anderson JR, Dupin CL: The forehead lift. A review. Arch Otolaryngol 111(5):325, 1985.
209. Beeson WH, McCollough EG: Complications of the forehead lift. Ear Nose Throat J 64:575/27, 1985.
210. Brennan HG: The frontal lift. Arch Otolaryngol 104:26, 1978.
211. Castanares S: Forehead wrinkles, glabellar frown and ptosis of the eyebrows. Plast Reconstr Surg 34(4):406, 1964.
212. Clark RP, Berris CE: Botulinum toxin: A treatment for facial asymmetry caused by facial nerve paralysis. Plast Reconstr Surg 84(2):353, 1989.
213. Connel BF, Lambros VS, Neurohr GH: The forehead lift: Techniques to avoid complications and produce optimal results. Aesthetic Plast Surg 13:217, 1989.
214. Cook TA, Brownrigg PH, Wang TD, Quatela VC: The versatile midforehead browlift. Arch Otolaryngol 115(2):163, 1989.
215. Ellenbogen R: Transcoronal eyebrow lift with con-

comitant upper blepharoplasty. Plast Reconstr Surg 71(4):1983.
216. Johnson CM Jr, Waldman R: Midforehead lift. Arch Otolaryngol 109:155, 1983.
217. Kaye BL: The forehead lift. Plast Reconstr Surg 60(2):161, 1977.
218. Kaye BL: The forehead lift: Problems and complications. In Goldwyn RM (ed): The Unfavorable Result in Plastic Surgery. Boston, Little Brown, 1984, p 611.
219. Liebman EP, Webster RC, Berger AS, DellaVecchia M: The frontalis nerve in the temporal brow lift. Arch Otolaryngol 108:232, 1982.
220. Mayer T: Personal communication, Jan 1992.
221. Pitanguy I: Indications for and treatment of frontal and glabellar wrinkles in an analysis of 3,404 consecutive cases of rhytidectomy. Plast Reconstr Surg 69:167, 1981.
222. Quatela VC, Larrabee WF: Forehead and brows revisited. Arch Otolaryngol 114(11):1236, 1988.
223. Rafaty FM, Brennan G: Current concepts of browpexy. Arch Otolaryngol 109:152, 1983.
224. Rafaty FM, Goode RL, Abramson NR: The browlift operation in a man. Arch Otolaryngol 104:69, 1978.
225. Rafaty FM, Goode RL, Fee WE Jr: The brow-lift operation. Arch Otolaryngol 101:467, 1975.
226. Reifkohl R: The forehead brow lift. Ann Plast Surg 8:55, 1982.
227. Reifkohl R, Kosanin R, Georgiade GS: Complications of the forehead-brow lift. Aesthetic Plast Surg 7(3):135, 1983.
228. Toledo GA, Tate JL: Coronal approach for rejuventation of the eyes and forehead. Arch Otolaryngol 112(7):738, 1986.
229. Vinas JC, Caviglia C, Cortinas JL: Forehead rhytidoplasty and brow lifting. Plast Reconstr Surg 57(4):445, 1976.

Dermabrasion

230. Alt TH: Technical aids for dermabrasion. J Dermatol Surg Oncol 13:638, 1987.
231. Dzubow LM: Survey of refrigerant and surgical techniques used for facial dermabrasion. J Am Acad Dermatol 12:287, 1985.
232. Hanke CW, O'Brien JJ: A histologic evaluation of the effects of skin refrigerant in an animal model. J Dermatol Surg Oncol 13:664, 1987.
233. Hanke CW, O'Brien JJ, Solow EB: Laboratory evaluation of skin refrigerants used in dermabrasion. J Dermatol Surg Oncol 11:45, 1985.
234. Hanke CW, Roenigk HH, Pinske JB: Complications of dermabrasion resulting from excessively cold skin refrigeration. J Dermatol Surg Oncol 11:896, 1985.
235. Kligman A, Willis I: A new formula for depigmenting human skin. Arch Dermatol 111:40, 1975.
236. Mandy SH: Tretinoin in the pre- and postoperative management of dermabrasion. J Am Acad Dermatol 15:878, 1986.
237. Moy R, Zitelli J, Uitto J: Effect of 13 cis-retinoic on dermal wound healing. J Invest Dermatol 88:508, 1987.
238. Pinski JB: Dressings for dermabrasion: Occlusive dressings and wound healing. Cutis 37:471, 1986.
239. Roenigk HH Jr: Dermabrasion: State of the art. J Dermatol Surg Oncol 11(3):306, 1985.

240. Rubenstein R, Roenigk HH Jr: Atypical keloids after dermabrasion of patients taking isotretinoin. J Am Acad Dermatol 15:280, 1986.

241. Stegman SJ: A study of dermabrasion and chemical peels in an animal model. J Dermatol Surg Oncol 6:490, 1980.

242. Yarborough JM: Dermabrasion by wire brush. J Dermatol Surg Oncol 13:610, 1987.

243. Yarborough JM Jr, Beeson WH: Dermabrasion. In Beeson WH, McCollough EG: Aesthetic Surgery of the Aging Face. St. Louis, CV Mosby, 1986, p 142.

Chemical Peel

244. Baker TJ: Chemical face peeling and rhytidectomy: A combined approach for facial rejuvenation. Plast Reconstr Surg 29:199, 1962.

245. Beeson WH, McCollough EG: Chemical face peeling without taping. J Dermatol Surg Oncol 11:985, 1985.

246. Dmytryshyn JR, Gribble MJ, Kassen BO: Chemical face peel complicated by toxic shock syndrome. Arch Otolaryngol 109(3):179, 1983.

247. Goldman PM, Freed MI: Aesthetic problems in chemical peeling. J Dermatol Surg Oncol 15(9):1020, 1989.

248. Klein DR, Little JH: Laryngeal edema as a complication of chemical peel. Plast Reconstr Surg 71:419, 1983.

249. Kligman AM, Willis I: A new formula for depigmenting human skin. Arch Dermatol 111:40, 1975.

250. Koopman CF: Phenol toxicity during face peels. Otolaryngol Head Neck Surg 90:383, 1982.

251. Litton C: Chemical face lifting. Plast Reconstr Surg 29:371, 1962.

252. McCollough EG, Beeson WH: Chemical peel. In Beeson WH, McCollough EG: Aesthetic Surgery of the Aging Face. St. Louis, CV Mosby, 1986, p 182.

253. Truppman ES, Ellenby JD: Major electrocardiographic changes during chemical face peeling. Plast Reconstr Surg 63:45, 1979.

Otoplasty

254. Adamson PA: Complications of otoplasty. Ear Nose Throat J 64:16, 1985.

255. Adamson PA: Complications of otoplasty. Ear Nose Throat J 64:23, 1985.

256. Baker DC, Converse JM: Otoplasty: A twenty year retrospective. Aesthetic Plast Surg 2:36, 1979.

257. Converse JM, Wood-Smith D: Technical details in the surgical correction of the lop ear deformity. Plast Reconstr Surg 31:118, 1963.

258. Elliott RA Jr: Complications in the treatment of prominent ears. Clin Plast Surg 5:479, 1978.

259. Furnas DW: Correction of prominent ears by conchal mastoid sutures. Plast Reconstr Surg 24:189, 1968.

260. Furnas DW: Complications of surgery of the external ear. Plast Surg 17:306, 1990.

261. Goode RL, Profitt SD: Complications of otoplasty. Arch Otolaryngol 91:352, 1970.

262. Hatch MD: Common problems of otoplasty. J Int Coll Surg 30:171, 1958.

263. Luckett WJ: A new operation for prominent ears based on the anatomy of the deformity. Surg Gynecol Obstet 10:635, 1910.

264. Manigula AJ, Witten BR: Otoplasty—an electric technique. Laryngoscope 87:1359, 1977.

265. Mustardé JC: The correction of prominent ears using simple mattress sutures. Br J Plast Surg 16:170, 1963.

266. Mustardé JC: The treatment of prominent ears by buried mattress sutures: A 10 year survey. Plast Reconstr Surg 39:382, 1967.

267. Rees TD, Wood-Smith D: Complications and untoward results. In Rees TD, Wood-Smith D (eds): Cosmetic Facial Surgery. Philadelphia, WB Saunders, 1973, p 556.

268. Reynaud JP, Gary-Bobo A, Maten J, et al: Chondritis post-operatories de l'oreille externe: Two cases from a Series of 200 Patients (387 Otoplasties). Ann Chir Plast Esthet 31:170, 1986.

269. Rigg BM: Suture materials in otoplasty. Plast Reconstr Surg 63:409, 1979.

270. Small A: Prevention of meatal stenosis in conchal set back otoplasty. Laryngoscope 85:1782, 1985.

271. Spira M: Reduction otoplasty, In Goldwyn RM (ed): The Unfavorable Results in Plastic Surgery; Avoidance and Treatment. Boston, Little, Brown, 1984, p 307.

272. Spira M, McCrea R, Gerow FJ, et al: Correction of the principal deformities causing protruding ears. Plast Reconstr Surg 44:150, 1969.

273. Stenstrom SJ: A "natural" technique for correction of congenitally prominent ears. Plast Reconstr Surg 32:509, 1963.

274. Webster R: Conchal set back operation for protruding ears. Arch Otolaryngol 92:572, 1970.

275. Wood-Smith D, Converse JM: The lop ear deformity. Surg Clin North Am 51:417, 1971.

276. Zohar Y: Otoplasty (letter). Arch Otolaryngol 96:187, 1972.

CHAPTER 25

Facial Reanimation Surgery

MONTE S. KEEN, MD
SCOTT L. KAY, MD

A man finds room in a few square inches of his face for the traits of all his ancestors; for the expression of all his history, and his wants.

R. W. Emerson[1]

The facial nerve innervates the muscles of expression and therefore, controls the ability to communicate emotion. To suddenly lose the use of the mimetic muscles strips the patient of vital functions, protection of the eye, and maintenance of oral competence, and also causes a disfiguring asymmetry of the face. As physicians we sometimes underestimate the damage an injury of this kind has on the patient's psyche. Nevertheless, we have the ability to significantly improve and sometimes restore facial mobility; however it must be clear to the patient that the face will never be normal again.

Many innovative and ingenious surgical procedures have been developed to restore movement to the paralyzed face. Traditionally, facial reanimation surgery is divided into four distinct categories: (1) physiologic neural restoration, (2) dynamic muscle flap procedures, (3) static procedures, and (4) eye protective procedures. Providing a previously paralyzed face with mimetic capability and aesthetic quality surely is an art. However, knowing when to operate and deciding which operation is appropriate for a particular clinical situation separates the surgeon from the technician. Certainly, the management of an immediate facial palsy after blunt trauma differs drastically from that of the patient presenting with a facial paralysis 5 years after an acoustic neuroma resection. The surgeon has to gather prognostic data, such as the condition of the proximal segment of the nerve, the site of injury, fibrotic changes occurring in the distal segment of the nerve, the presence of intact myoneural junctions capable of restoring muscular function, and so on. The physician also should have an understanding of the individual patient's expectations and desires. Will the patient survive long enough for nerve regeneration to take place? Does the patient require immediate improvement of facial mobility at the expense of physiologic function? To perform the operation that will best serve the patient, we need to answer these questions and have reanimation techniques at our fingertips.

Once the presence and function of the proximal portion of the facial nerve are established, the timing of the procedure is the major issue. Physiologic restoration of mimetic function implies voluntary and emotional movement of the individual muscles of the face in a coordinated pattern. The only way to accomplish this goal is to restore neural communication from the facial nucleus. This can be done by primary neural repair, cable grafting, or, if the proximal portion of the facial nerve is absent, faciofacial cross-face graft. Neural repair should be performed as soon as discontinuity of the facial nerve is discovered. When discontinuity is uncertain, repair can be delayed, in the hope of spontaneous recovery, up to 1 year. After 1 year, May has reported little success with primary neurorrhaphy.[2]

Beyond this point, neural or muscle flap procedures, which transfer nerve or innervated muscle from another region to the paralyzed mimetic muscles, are indicated. The more common examples are hypoglossal–facial nerve crossover, neuromuscular pedicles based on the ansa hypoglossi, and transposition of the temporalis and masseter muscles. Generally, results of hypoglossal-facial crossover are best if performed within 2 years of the initial injury. Nevertheless, Conley has reported successful cases 7 years postinjury.[3] If the facial musculature has undergone extensive fibrosis or atrophy or if a disfiguring deficiency due to trauma exists, then temporalis and masseter transpositions are more appropriate. This technique offers the advantages of voluntary control, immediate results, facial symmetry, and separation of eyelid closure from mouth movement.

The "static" operations, such as face lift, brow lift, fascial suspension, and canthopexy, can be used any time in the course of facial paralysis, but it is essential not to compromise function for cosmesis—for example, raising the brow to the point where lagophthalmos is accentuated.

This brings us to the last, but most important, category of procedures, namely those that serve to protect the eye. Even with a temporary paralysis, the cornea can sustain irreparable injury owing to exposure. When the so-called BAD syndrome is evident, an operation to protect the eye is warranted. "B" represents the *lack* of a *B*ell phenomenon, which constitutes a protective reflex of rolling the globe superiorly, keeping the cornea covered by a paralytic upper lid. "A" is for *A*nesthesia of the cornea, occurring when patients suffer a concurrent fifth cranial nerve palsy. Finally, "D" stands for *D*ryness caused by diminished lacrimation. The procedures employed to prevent the progression of the BAD syndrome to eventual blindness include tarsorrhaphy, lid-loading techniques, canthopexy, and lid shortening. Since most of these procedures are reversible and relatively minor, we recommend taking patients to the operating room early after the onset of a complete facial paralysis.

The purpose of this chapter is to familiarize the reader with the type of complications one might expect to encounter in facial reanimation surgery, how to treat them, and how to avoid them.

PHYSIOLOGIC NEURAL PROCEDURES

Nerve Repair

It is axiomatic that microsurgical repair of the facial nerve be carried out in an atraumatic manner. The use of the operating microscope at a magnification of 10 to 16 × has facilitated this procedure. The strategy is for repair by coapting the nerve with a minimal number of nonreactive sutures. The anastomosis should be tension free, and the nerve should be handled gingerly with atraumatic microsurgical instruments. Before performing the anastomosis, we remove the epineurium and maintain a cuff of perineurium of approximately 5 mm. Careful preparation of the proximal and distal ends of the nerve with a sharp blade are crucial to a successful outcome. Nevertheless, the type of repair, fascicular (perineural) or end-to-end (epineural), is still a point of controversy. Based on work done by Mellesi, the epineurium has been shown to be the collagen-producing layer responsible for potential disruption of an anastomosis by fibrosis.[4] Ingrowth of scar tissue within the anastomotic site that prevents or misdirects axonal growth is probably the most common reason for failure. In addition, reapproximation of corresponding fascicular ends could restore spatial orientation of the facial nerve and limit the development of synkinesis. However, as pointed out by Conley and May, there has never been any demonstrative difference between the two procedures when compared clinically.[5, 6] This is because the neural fibers spiral down the nerve and are spatially aligned. When a segment of nerve is trimmed for anastomosis, invariably the fibers will be out of phase and the resultant anastomosis will yield some synkinesis. Certainly the repair that can be performed the fastest, with the least amount of trauma and tension, will limit scar formation and provide the best results.

Any complication that arises in the normal course of surgery will have devastating effects on the regeneration of the nerve and, hence, the restoration of facial mobility. The technique must be aseptic, and extra attention should be given to hemostasis since infection and hematoma formation will ruin the operation. We recommend careful placement and removal of drainage systems. Before closure, the wound is copiously irrigated with an antibiotic solution and parenteral antibiotics covering skin flora are given in the perioperative period. The bed upon which the anastomosis lies also requires consideration, especially in radical parotidectomy in which the neural repair could rest upon bone. Swinging a small muscle flap into the region will buffer the nerve from trauma with mastication and head turning. A cautious surgeon may even choose to keep the patient on a liquid diet some time after the procedure to limit the amount of mastication and movement in this area. With respect to the tissue bed, remaining or recurring tumor not only adversely affects the result, but also bears a grave prognosis. Postoperative radiation, however, has not been

shown to affect the neural repair if performed several weeks after the surgery; thus, withholding this treatment should not be a consideration.[7]

Even with the best microsurgical technique, some synkinesis results. This is due to the fact that the nerve fibers regrow in aberrant pathways. In mild cases, a slight uncontrollable twitching of the eye may occur when the patient is smiling.

In more severe cases, mass movement of the entire cheek or facial spasm may occur when the patient attempts to smile or close the eyes (Figs. 25–1 and 25–2). If the synkinesis is mild and tolerable, it is best left alone. Patients can learn to hide minimal deformities. Surgical intervention consists of selective neurolysis and should be reserved for only the most severe cases, i.e., when the synkinesis becomes a hemifacial spasm, and only after more conservative measures such as biofeedback and physical therapy have failed. In some cases a faciofacial crossover can be performed at the time of neurol-

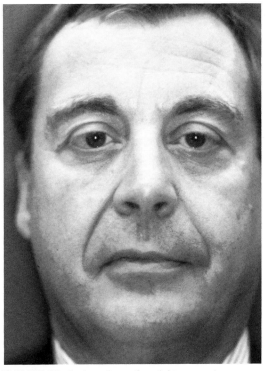

FIGURE 25–1. A patient after right acoustic neurectomy, with facial paralysis demonstrating hypertonicity at rest.

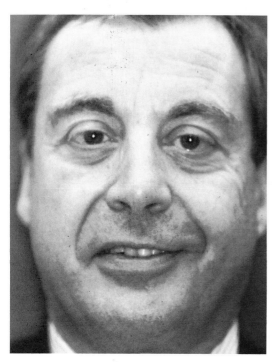

FIGURE 25–2. The patient shown in Figure 25–1 attempting to smile. Note synkinesis and facial spasm on the affected side, due to aberrant nerve growth.

ysis to provide dual innervation, especially to the eye. Botulinum toxin in low doses may also prove to be a promising tool to correct this problem.[8]

During the course of facial nerve rehabilitation, it may be necessary to use a cable graft. Surely a repair that appears to be under tension would fare much better with a cable graft despite the fact that an additional anastomosis is required. The cervical plexus, the greater auricular nerve in particular, serves as a suitable donor for grafting. If several branches of this nerve can be harvested as well, these can be plugged into several distal stumps, which is preferable to multiple cable grafts. Rarely more than 10 cm of greater auricular nerve is obtainable. In that case, the sural nerve provides ample length, with several branches. When a radical neck dissection is performed in conjunction with a cancer operation such as a parotidectomy, the surgeon has a choice between using the sural nerve and going to the opposite side of the neck for the greater auricular nerve. One disturbing complication that occurs 6 months

to 2 years after the procedure at the donor site is the formation of neuromas. Since the sensory nerve is affected, not only are these neuromas cause for alarm regarding recurrent tumor, but they can be extremely painful. After being assured of the diagnosis with a biopsy, an injection of lidocaine or Marcaine mixed with a steroid solution provides some relief. Excision is the definitive treatment; however, it is important to bury the newly transected end in nearby muscle to avoid recurrence.

Faciofacial Grafting

When the proximal stump of the facial nerve is unavailable, as may be the case in acoustic neuroma resection, the surgeon can call upon the contralateral facial nerve to provide physiologic excitation of the mimetic muscles. Several variations of faciofacial cross-grafting techniques have been described and advocated by Scaramella,[9] Anderl,[10] and Fisch.[11] Theoretically this procedure would allow emotional and involuntary control of the paralyzed side. If several crossgrafts are employed, separation of eyelid closure from the rest of facial movement is possible. Needless to say, our results with this technique have not been as favorable. This procedure requires the use of multiple operations, with more incisions to the face, greater operating time, and longer cable grafts with tunnels that may traverse over bony prominences, i.e., the nasal bones. Finding the distal aspect of the peripheral branches on both sides can be extremely difficult. Probably the greatest deterrent is causing dysfunction to the normal facial nerve, especially in the frontal and mandibular branches, which typically do not receive communicating twigs from the other branches. Some paralysis of the normal side invariably occurs, and for this reason we do not advocate this approach. Clearly this procedure should not be attempted by an inexperienced surgeon.

Hypoglossal Crossover

When the proximal stump is lost or primary repair has failed, transferring the ipsi-

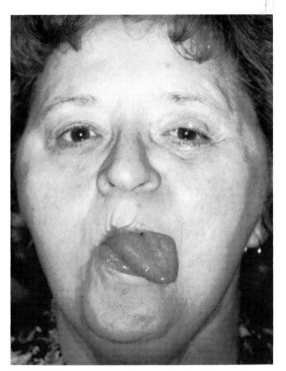

FIGURE 25–3. Patient with paralysis of the right side of the tongue following hypoglossal–facial nerve crossover.

lowing mechanism and visualization of a functional larynx are imperative before proceeding. Patients who have cranial neuropathies on the basis of progressive diseases such as diabetes, multiple sclerosis, or von Recklinghausen disease should be advised against hypoglossal crossover.

Although the percentage of patients with remaining dysphagia or dysarthria is low, incapacitating tongue dysfunction could prompt the surgeon to explore corrective measures (Fig. 25–3). A midline Z-plasty of the tongue that interdigitates innervated intrinsic muscle with deinnervated lingual musculature has produced favorable results in our hands (Fig. 25–4). Most likely myoneurotization occurs; thus, with time, there is not only passive movement of the deinnervated side but also resumption of tongue muscle tone. Patients need to be reminded of, and motivated to engage in, a period of training in order to regain tongue mobility

lateral hypoglossal nerve to the distal portion of the facial nerve can provide adequate efferent stimulation. A majority of patients will experience restoration of facial tone, although few procedures result in division of mimetic movement. When consulting with patients, remember the "rule of 25." Twenty-five per cent will be dissatisfied with the reanimation. Approximately 50 per cent achieve reasonable facial movement, and the last 25 per cent have synkinesis or hyperactivity due to excessive innervation. Conley reported a 15 per cent incidence of this last group of patients, who complain of spasm and random motion of the affected side.[6] Another commonly encountered complication, occurring in roughly 25 per cent of those with a hypoglossal crossover, is persistent speech or swallowing deficits from loss of tongue innervation. This procedure is absolutely contraindicated in patients possessing other cranial neuropathies, especially ninth and tenth nerve palsies, who are at risk for aspiration. Thus, examination of the swal-

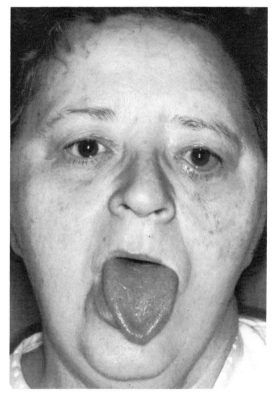

FIGURE 25–4. The patient shown in Figure 25–3 6 months after an intramuscular Z-plasty. Note the improvement in tongue function.

and facial movement as well. A degree of plasticity is required as new nerves are now innervating these muscles. In the operating room, the surgeon can attempt to spare the descendens hypoglossus if enough length of the proximal portion of the nerve exists. This may provide alternative pathways for reinnervation to the tongue. May has suggested an interesting method of sparing tongue function—by partially dividing the hypoglossal nerve and cable grafting in the form of a "jump graft" to the distal segment of the facial nerve.[12] An alternative is to use the spinal accessory nerve as a source of efferent innervation. However, since motor control of the trapezius is not as fine as that of the tongue, one would expect less gratifying results. In addition, the paralysis of the trapezius is usually more disabling.

Good results can be encouraged before proceeding with the hypoglossal transfer by following several simple guidelines. Perform the operation as soon as possible. Excellent results can be obtained by operating up to 2 years after the onset of paralysis. May reports successful reanimations.[13] Although beyond this point, one has to bear in mind the condition of the distal nerve and musculature being reinnervated. By making biopsies of the distal stump, the surgeon can guarantee the existence of Bungner bands over which growing axons advance. Certainly fibrotic changes in the distal nerve stump have to be ruled out. Likewise the facial musculature can be examined histologically to avoid reinnervating atrophic or fibrotic muscles.

Cervical Neuromuscular Pedicles

The technique of harvesting neuromuscular pedicles based on the ansa cervicalis nerve and swinging them up to attach to facial musculature has been well described by Tucker.[14] After allowing myoneurotization to occur, he has reported a 77 per cent success rate. Because of limited experience with this technique, we cannot comment on the complications. However, the reader should be aware of this procedure and is referred to Dr. Tucker's article for further explanation.

DYNAMIC MUSCLE FLAPS

Muscle transpositions of the temporalis and masseter muscles, complete with their neural innervation, can be utilized in long-standing facial paralysis (greater than 2 years), in facial trauma with a loss of mimetic muscle and facial fullness, or in congenital absence of the facial nerve and corresponding musculature. As mentioned, atrophic and fibrotic facial muscle no longer lends itself to successful reinnervation, and therefore muscle transposition is essential for reanimation. Within 3 weeks of the operation the patient senses facial movement. Since the muscles of mastication are innervated by the trigeminal nerve, voluntary control can be masterfully incorporated into emotional facial expression by the highly motivated patient. In this manner, he or she can maintain facial symmetry. However, it is most important to guide the patient's expectations to realistic levels preoperatively in order avoid disparagement and distraction from the physical therapy task ahead.

Knowledge of the anatomy, especially the neurovascular bundles of the temporalis and masseter muscles, is of supreme importance to avoid complications. Since these are viable muscle flaps, the circulation and innervation can be disrupted while raising and transferring the flap. The blood supply to the temporalis muscle is the deep temporal vessels, which are branches of the first division of the internal maxillary artery. The artery and vein course obliquely along the undersurface of the temporalis muscle in an anterior and superior direction. The nerve originates from the motor division of the mandibular branch (V_3) of the trigeminal nerve. It enters the muscle at the midsection of the zygoma and then branches out superiorly, following the direction of the muscle fibers. When elevating this flap, detach the muscle along with periosteum from the temporal bone. Continue the dissection down to the level of the zygoma. When preparing slips of muscle for insertion, incise the superficial temporalis fascia to a greater extent than the muscular component and keep the incision in the direction of the muscle fibers to avoid transecting the nerve. A scalpel is preferred over electrocautery during this step. Likewise, to avoid damaging the nerve to the masseter muscle, Baker and Conley recommend placing the incision in the center of the muscle and extending the length of the incision only approximately a third of the distance from the inferior margin.[15]

More common than injuries to the neurovascular supply is a dehiscence of one or more of the fascial slips from either the muscle or its approximation to the nasolabial skin (Fig. 25–5). This complication is manifested by drooping of the corner of the mouth postoperatively. The diagnosis is confirmed when the examiner places the hands over the muscle and notes muscle contraction and an absence of mouth motion when the patient is requested to clench the teeth. At this point, we recommend exploration and resuturing with nonabsorbable 4–0 clear nylon, utilizing an interrupted vertical mattress suture technique (Fig. 25–6). Preoperatively, obtain consent for a fascia lata graft in case the temporalis fascia is macerated or atrophic. This complication can be avoided by delicate handling of the fascia, making

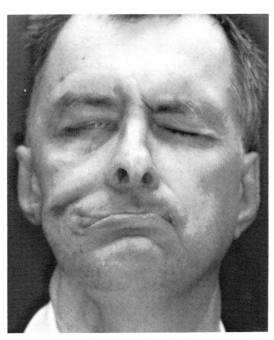

FIGURE 25–6. The same patient in Figure 25–5 after reinsertion of the fascia to the corner of the lip and nasolabial fold.

sure not to detach it from the muscle. If it is necessary to elevate the fascia off the muscle to obtain more length, the fascia should be reinforced by suturing it to the muscle. Rubin advises the creation of a fascial button to sandwich the muscle and provide greater strength to the reinforcing sutures.[16] Distally, the fascial slips could be sutured to both the nasolabial fold and farther on to the vermilion border. This provides "double" protection against dehiscence. Postoperatively, the tension on the fascial-skin sutures can be reduced by Steri-stripping the nasolabial skin in a superior direction and applying a supportive dressing with Elastoplast tape. Maintain the patient on a liquid diet for the first postoperative week to prevent mastication and movement of the transposed muscles.

At first, the inexperienced operator is overly concerned with achieving enough length to plug into the nasolabial skin and corner of the mouth. Remember, it is almost impossible to overcorrect too much. Overcorrect to the point where the gingiva is visible with the mouth retracted superiorly. Inevitably, the position of the mouth drops. If this

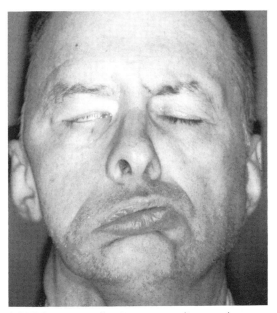

FIGURE 25–5. Following temporalis muscle transposition, this patient demonstrates a sudden dehiscence of the temporalis fascia at the insertion of the oral commissure and nasolabial fold.

occurs, re-exploration and trimming of fascia are employed to reposition the mouth. Several techniques are available if length is in fact a problem. As mentioned, folding the temporalis fascia along its superior connection affords the operator more length at the increased risk of dehiscence. Baker and Conley instruct the inexperienced operator to extend the temporal incision superiorly to include 1 to 2 cm of pericranium.[15] Or, if need be, the fascia lata should be harvested for grafting. Keep in mind that joining fascia lata graft to temporalis fascia presents the fascial slip with another area of weakness. Gortex strips also can be substituted for fascia lata grafts, but we prefer autogenous material. Lastly, one can remove the zygomatic arch for greater length; however, this is discouraged because the mandibular nerve is vulnerable during this maneuver and the fulcrum action of the arch is eliminated.

Although a drain is no substitute for complete hemostasis, the cut edges of the muscle flap and scalp wound edges can bleed profusely. Active suction drains for a minimum of 3 days are recommended. Hematomas of the donor site should be drained, since the subgaleal area communicates with the facial cutaneous flap and the hematoma could collect in the nasolabial region. We have observed collections such as these almost 2 weeks postoperatively (Fig. 25–7). Devastating complications from dissecting hematoma can ensue, such as alopecia and skin flap necrosis. Thus treat hematoma aggressively and be certain to avoid or ligate significant vessels, e.g., the superficial temporal artery. If a hematoma develops, operative drainage is imperative.

Every attempt to avoid infection should be made, since the outcome, as in hematoma formation, could be catastrophic. Perioperative antistaphylococcal antibiotics, as well as anti-infective agents against oral flora, play a role to decrease the incidence of infection. May copiously washes the hair with povidone-iodine (Betadine).[13] Abscess formation on postoperative days 6 to 10 may be difficult to diagnose initially, since the swelling from the temporalis swung over the zygoma hides any minor collection. If patients begin to

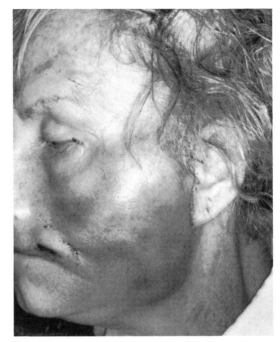

FIGURE 25–7. A patient with a developing hematoma 5 days after a temporalis muscle transposition.

complain of increased pain, fever, or redness without obvious masses or edema, obtain a CT scan immediately. Do not hesitate to incise and drain as soon as the diagnosis is confirmed.

One of the primary goals of reanimation surgery is to restore the patient's appearance. Immediately after the operation, the face will again assume an asymmetric look, only instead of drooping the face will appear contracted and contorted. Over time, gravity will pull the face into a more symmetric position. The patients require repeated reassurance of this fact. The patient may complain of bulging over the malar eminence, which is highlighted by severe depression over the temporalis muscle donor site (Fig. 25–8). Augmentation of this area with allografts such as fat or artificial material such as Silastic is particularly critical in men or short-haired women. It is easiest to accomplish this augmentation during the initial procedure; however, it can be performed at a later date. Some surgeons routinely resect a portion of the zygomatic arch in order to lay the muscle flatter against the cheek, although, for the

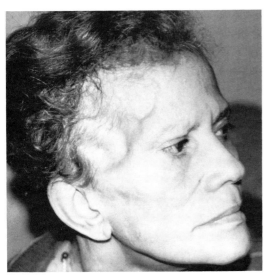

FIGURE 25–8. Many years after a temporalis muscle transposition, this patient displays a large defect over the temporal region.

reasons already mentioned, it is not recommended.

Basic principles that apply to aesthetic surgery apply in reanimation surgery as well. Thus try to keep most of the scars hidden behind the hairline. Use anatomic divisions of facial regions to camouflage incisions. If possible, make the incision for the fascial slips along the vermilion border. Muscle flaps that are sutured to the lip in the area of the corner of the mouth produce a natural crease at the nasolabial fold. The surgeon can test this intraoperatively. Because of fibrosis and loss of the natural crease, it may be necessary to re-create the fold, which is best done by anchoring the flap 5 mm anterior to the desired fold. Rubin advocates preoperative evaluation of the smile on the normal side to determine the vectors of force acting on the lips and carefully positioning the fascial slips along the lip to match those vectors.[16]

Controversy exists over the use of the masseter transposition flap. When performed in conjunction with a total parotidectomy, the masseter flap is easily elevated and swung into position. It does not create a bulging deformity like the temporalis transposition, and it is utilized to counteract the pulling effect of the normal side. The major drawback, however, is gapping of the infe-rior portion of the corner of the mouth, causing drooling and diminished oral competence. The overall vector of force of the masseter muscle is in a horizontal direction, in contrast to a superior vertical force produced by the temporalis.

STATIC PROCEDURES

Included in this category of static procedures are fascial slings, face lift, brow lift, and canthopexy. These procedures play an important role in reanimation surgery; however, the expected complications are not different from standard aesthetic surgery and are covered elsewhere in this book. Thus, we will refer the reader to other chapters covering these topics, except to reiterate and forewarn the aggressive surgeon not to sacrifice function for cosmesis.

EYELID PROCEDURES

Tarsorrhaphy

The technique of routinely suturing the eyelids together to protect the cornea, namely tarsorrhaphy, has fallen into disfavor among facial reanimation surgeons for a variety of reasons. Any compromise of visual fields by tarsorrhaphy is unnecessary and is strongly discouraged. Adhesions of the lid margins can form, further limiting vision and the ability to reverse the procedure. Irregularities of the lid margins develop, producing trichiasis and constant irritation to the cornea, with weeping and possible ulceration. Lastly, the objectionable aesthetic results cannot be underestimated by the physician, as the patient already has a heavy psychologic burden to bear with the facial paralysis. If tarsorrhaphy is absolutely necessary, employ a technique that spares the lateral commissure, to avoid further complications.

Lid-Loading Techniques

By introducing a force to push the upper eyelid down, in the form of a weight, spring action, and even magnetic attraction, surgeons have been able to provide corneal protection. The placement of a gold weight in the upper eyelid is a simple, elegant, and reversible method of restoring function to the paralyzed eyelid. Choosing the correct amount of weight preoperatively is critical to achieving adequate closure postoperatively. In the office, the surgeon should tape weights of various sizes to the patient's eyelid to determine the appropriate weight. Sizing ought to be performed with the patient sitting up. The weight often is not sufficient to maintain eyelid closure when the patient is recumbent. Although the gold weight establishes eyelid closure when voluntarily closing the eyes, it does not restore the blink function, and some workers report poor results during sleep unless the patients are instructed to use more than one or two pillows.[17] Since gravity acts on the weighted eyelid for closure, elevation of the head ensures a greater force on the lid. We achieve successful eyelid closure (80 per cent or greater) without complications in 83 per cent of our patients, while May reports a success rate of 91 per cent.[18]

Although not technically demanding, complications arise owing to technical errors. Most of the surgical misadventures can be avoided by adequate knowledge of the regional anatomy and meticulous hemostasis and vasoconstriction. It is essential to operate in a bloodless field. Thus, we inject with 1 per cent lidocaine with 1:50,000 epinephrine solution, followed by a 10-minute delay before proceeding to the skin incision. The weight should be placed in a pocket deep to the orbicularis oculi muscle, superficial to the levator superioris muscle, and on the posterior aspect of the tarsal plate. Injury to the septum orbitale will cause a bothersome herniation of orbital fat that will make the operation more difficult but will not alter function or the cosmetic results. Closure of a defect in the septum orbitale could transform a preseptal hematoma into a postseptal hematoma, compressing the orbital contents, and for this reason it is not recommended. Transection of the levator aponeurosis can result from making an incision too deep,

leaving the patient with a severely ptotic eyelid. If it is felt to be significant, repair can be performed with several simple 7–0 nylon sutures. The weight should be secured to the tarsal plate inferiorly and the levator aponeurosis superiorly. Migration of the weight results if it is not sutured properly. To avoid gapping of the lids medially, the medial edge of the weight should lie slightly medial to the pupil, approximately two thirds the distance from the lateral canthus. The closing stitch should incorporate the orbicularis oculi muscle along with skin to provide a myocutaneous closure to prevent extrusion of the weight.

Aseptic technique and irrigation of the wound area with sterile saline are a must when one is implanting a foreign body. We employ perioperative antistaphylococcal antibiotics, one dose intravenously prior to the skin incision and oral antibiotics 3 days postoperatively. A wound infection will lead to the extrusion of the weight (Fig. 25–9). Routinely, patients are instructed to apply bacitracin ophthalmic ointment over the incision two to three times daily. We advise against using Neosporin-containing ointments as lid weights have been extruded after the patient developed an allergic reaction to this compound (Fig. 25–10). Once the wound be-

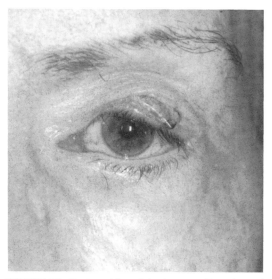

FIGURE 25–9. A gold weight is extruding through the skin due to a superficial infection and inadequate closure by suturing skin only.

comes infected, local care can be attempted; however, typically the only way to manage this problem is to remove the implant. If extrusion occurs in the absence of infection, the weight can be removed and placed in a deeper pocket. However, in the face of infection complete removal of the weight with a temporary tarsorrhaphy stitch is the safest approach. Likewise, any hematoma formation should be evacuated immediately to avoid secondary infection. Prevention of hematomas can begin preoperatively, by stressing the importance of avoiding aspirin, nonsteroidal anti-inflammatory medications, and other drugs that have an adverse effect on coagulation.

Persistent lagophthalmos is a common, under-reported complication of the procedure. Often, incomplete closure results from placing the weight too far superiorly, so that it is partially resting upon the globe or not employing a sufficient amount of weight. Before repositioning or replacing the weight, the surgeon should be certain that the lower lid is not responsible for incomplete closure. A developing paralytic ectropion causing malposition of the lower lid would lead to inadequate approximation of the lids. The management of this problem is discussed in the next section.

Persistent lagophthalmos after gold weight insertion can be attributed to insufficient amount of weight, position of the implant,

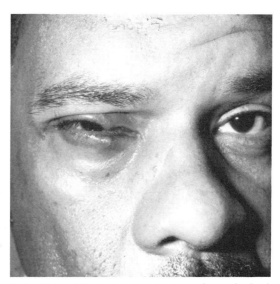

FIGURE 25–11. Eminent extrusion of a palpebral spring in the upper eyelid.

and occasionally a recessed or retracted upper lid, a circumstance in which gold weights will be of no use. These clinical situations call for the insertion of the palpebral spring, a cosmetically acceptable procedure providing a constant degree of inferior force to the upper eyelid, thus capable of restoring the blink mechanism. This procedure is fraught with complications in inexperienced hands. May, who probably has the largest series of patients with palpebral springs, has published a thorough description of the technique.[18] One of the major complications directly associated with the spring is extrusion of the tips of the spring through the eyelid skin (Fig. 25–11). Migration of the spring poses another problem. To avoid this, May recommends applying a dacron glove to cover the tips and providing an area for the ingrowth of surrounding fibrotic connective tissue, thus protecting and fixating the spring. Strong, nonabsorbable sutures are required to fix the fulcrum of the spring to the periosteum of the supraorbital rim. If ptosis or incomplete closure results, the palpebral spring can be readjusted in a second local procedure. Once the surgeon has mastered the technique, the complication rate is only slightly greater than that of the gold weight insertion. May reports a success rate

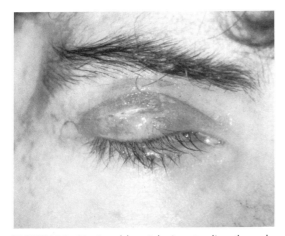

FIGURE 25–10. A gold weight is extruding through the skin owing to an antibiotic ointment neomycin allergy.

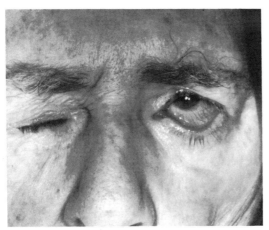

FIGURE 25–12. An older patient with facial nerve paralysis and poor tissue turgor is developing a paralytic ectropion of the lower eyelid.

of 87 per cent, which improved from 33 per cent after he modified the procedure in 1983.

Other methods of lid-loading, such as eyelid magnets, exist; however, they do not offer the advantage of the simplicity and cosmesis of the previously discussed techniques.

Lower Eyelid Procedures

When eyelid paralysis extends beyond 3 to 6 months, especially in the elderly with poor lid tone, ectropion develops, causing exposure keratitis and blepharitis (Fig. 25–12). Left unaddressed, persistent lagophthalmos will result even in the presence of adequate lid-loading (Fig. 25–13). Several techniques have emerged to correct this problem: lateral canthopexy, lid-shortening procedures, and inferior "lid-loading." Numerous bothersome complications can arise, often requiring further surgery for correction.

Tightening the lower eyelid with a canthopexy or lid-shortening procedure early in the course of eyelid paralysis may be futile. As the paralysis progresses, the orbicularis oculi muscle continues to undergo atrophy, allowing the lower lid to relax, droop, and evert. An eyelid procedure performed early will not alter this progression, and thus ectropion will recur. We advise observing the ectropion and treating the patient medically with lubricants, artificial tears, and taping until the amount of exposed sclera below the limbus has stabilized. Once the position of the eyelid is stable, the surgeon can better estimate the amount of suspension necessary to correct the abnormality. An abrupt reappearance of ectropion following a canthopexy can only mean dehiscence of the suspension sutures.

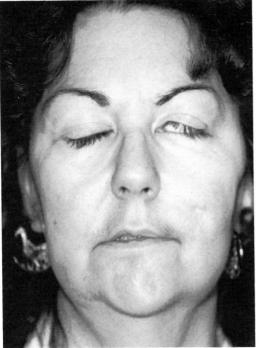

FIGURE 25–13. Four months after temporalis muscle transposition and gold weight insertion, this patient developed lagophthalmos and an ectropion from progression of the paralysis.

The lateral canthal ligament should be suspended to the periosteum of the orbital rim above the lateral orbital tubercle with a non-absorbable or slowly dissolving suture. A healthy bite of both tarsal plate and periosteum is mandatory, and a mattress suture is recommended. Needless to say, reoperation is in order if this stitch should loosen.

Occasionally patients will complain of excessive tearing immediately following a lower eyelid procedure. The lacrimal apparatus is usually away from the operative field and safe from surgical injury. However, the inferior eyelid mechanically pumps tears across the globe to the punctum and canaliculi of the lacrimal sac. By tightening the lower eyelid, this pumping mechanism should improve. Temporary edema after eyelid manipulation could disturb this action, resulting in a transient epiphora lasting from 3 to 4 weeks. Persistent epiphora requires diagnostic intervention with lacrimal probes or radiographic dye studies to rule out lacrimal duct obstruction. Examine the punctum to confirm its proper position abutting the globe. Intraoperatively, an abnormally positioned punctum secondary to lid laxity can be corrected by resecting a small wedge or diamond from the conjunctiva just below the opening. This serves to rotate the punctum toward the globe, allowing tears to drain more easily. The punctum also can be widened by introducing one blade of the Westcott scissors into the aperture, directed inferiorly, and snipping approximately 3 to 4 mm of conjunctiva. Gapping of the punctum will be noted if success is to be obtained.

Blepharitis can occur after surgical correction of ectropion. Mild degrees of infection can be treated with baby shampoo and water scrubs in a ratio of 1:2 shampoo to water. These scrubs should be applied to the lashes three times daily, with bacitracin ophthalmic ointment placed on the eyelids at night. Eye drops and systemic antistaphylococcal antibiotics should be reserved for refractory cases.

SUMMARY

A variety of techniques abound in the surgical literature to reanimate the paralyzed face. The surgeon can play an exceedingly important role in helping the stricken patient regain function and self-esteem. The procedures that comprise this armamentarium are exacting and unforgiving. Thus even a minute complication could have devastating effects on the end results. In this chapter, we have identified the commonly occurring complications associated with each procedure. It is our hope to warn the surgeon of common pitfalls and errors so that he or she may avoid them. Early recognition of these complications may fend off the ruin of arduous work and patient expense. Once it is recognized, understanding the mechanism of a complication can lead to a simple correction. Accomplishing the goal of facial reanimation, we feel, is a worthwhile endeavor, both gratifying and much appreciated by the afflicted patient.

References

1. Emerson RW: Behavior. The Conduct of Life. 1860.
2. May M: Facial reanimation after skull base trauma. Am J Otol Suppl Nov:62–67, 1985.
3. Conley J: The treatment of longstanding facial paralysis: A new concept. Trans Am Acad Ophthalmol Otolaryngol 78:386–392, 1974.
4. Millesi H: Nerve suture and grafting to restore the extratemporal facial nerve. Clin Plast Surg 6(3):333–341, 1979.
5. May M: Trauma to the facial nerve. In May M (ed): The Facial Nerve. New York, Thieme Inc, 1986, pp 421–440.
6. Conley J: Perspectives in facial reanimation. In May M (ed): The Facial Nerve. New York, Thieme Inc, 1986, pp 615–663.
7. McGuirt WF, Welling DB, McCabe BF: Facial nerve function following irradiated cable grafts. Laryngoscope 99(1):27–34, 1989.
8. May M, Croxson GR, Klein SR: Bell's palsy: Management of sequelae using EMG rehabilitation, botulinum toxin, and surgery. Am J Otol 10(3):220–229, 1989.
9. Scaramella LF: Preliminary report on facial nerve anastomosis. Read before the Second International Symposium on Facial Nerve Surgery, Osaka, Japan, 1970.
10. Anderl H: Reconstruction of the face through cross-facial nerve transplantation in facial paralysis. In Converse JM (ed): Reconstructive Plastic Surgery. 2nd ed. Philadelphia, WB Saunders, 1977.
11. Fisch U: Facial nerve grafting. Otolaryngol Clin North Am 7:517–24, 1974.
12. May M: Facial paralysis: Surgical restoration—total approach. Instructional course at the American Academy of Otolaryngology–Head and Neck Surgery Annual Meeting, San Diego, CA, Sept 10, 1990.

13. May M: Surgical rehabilitation of facial nerve palsy: Total approach. In May M (ed): The Facial Nerve. New York, Thieme Inc, 1986, pp 695–777.

14. Tucker HM: Restoration of selective facial nerve function by the nerve-muscle pedicle technique. Clin Plast Surg 6(3):293–300, 1979.

15. Baker DC, Conley J: Regional muscle transposition for the rehabilitation of the paralyzed face. Clin Plast Surg 6(3):317–331, 1979.

16. Rubin LR: Temporalis and masseter muscle transposition. In May M (ed): The Facial Nerve. New York, Thieme Inc, 1986, pp 665–677.

17. Levine RE: Eyelid reanimation surgery. In May M (ed): The Facial Nerve. New York, Thieme Inc, 1986, pp 681–894.

18. May M: Gold weight and wire spring implants as alternatives to tarsorrhaphy. Arch Otol Head Neck Surg 113:656–660, 1987.

Tissue Transfer in Head and Neck Reconstruction: Skin Grafts, Skin Flaps, and Myocutaneous Flaps

DANIEL B. KURILOFF, MD

SHAN R. BAKER, MD

Reconstruction of the head and neck area following trauma, congenital defects, or tumor extirpation continues to evolve and challenge our surgical skills. In the last quarter century, we have seen great advances in tissue transfer techniques, from regional pedicled myocutaneous flaps to the more complex microsurgical composite free grafts. Primary reconstruction of massive defects following cancer ablation with nonirradiated, well-vascularized tissue, best suited for the restoration of form and function, is now routine in most centers. The use of tissue expansion, pharmacologic manipulations, microvascular surgery, and viability monitoring has further enhanced these procedures.

Our attempts to restore the essential cosmetic and functional attributes of the preoperative or pretraumatic state have become more sophisticated, necessitating reconstructive efforts which are more complex, often time-consuming, and technically challenging. As the number and type of tissue transfers continue to grow, more objective means of classifying and assessing the anatomic and functional deficit, along with objective measures of postoperative cosmetic and functional outcome, must be established.[1] The success or failure of tissue transfer can no longer be determined strictly by the survival of the flap or graft, and our concept of reconstructive complications must now include failure to achieve the desired functional and aesthetic result.

No single flap will serve all reconstructive needs, and even technically well-performed tissue transfers will sometimes fail. Therefore, the contemporary head and neck surgeon must have a working knowledge of an assortment of reconstructive options in order to make eclectic decisions regarding the best reconstruction for a particular problem. In some situations, multiple flaps will be required to achieve primary reconstruction or to salvage an initial failed attempt. At other times, one must exercise restraint in planning a complex reconstruction when a simpler method is equally effective. The impaired detection of early tumor recurrence beneath large bulky flaps is a compromise that must carefully be considered for every reconstruction. For many advanced head and neck neoplasms, surgical salvage for recurrent tumor is not a viable option, and well-vascularized tissue transfer following primary resection serves to protect against potential complications of adjuvant radiotherapy and chemotherapy (e.g., osteoradionecrosis, meningitis, carotid artery blowout). Although it is not cost-effective, these patients can be effectively monitored for recurrent disease by serial imaging (computed tomography or magnetic resonance imaging).

In addition to the general risk of complications associated with anesthesia, advanced age, systemic disease, trauma, malnutrition, infection, and irradiation, every surgical procedure has its own attendant threat of complications. These complications can occur at the donor or recipient site and result in immediate or delayed sequelae, some of only minor consequence and others causing severe cosmetic and functional disability, or even death. Some complications are not preventable and can be unpredictable. However, with careful preoperative planning, attention to meticulous operative technique, and vigilant postoperative care, many of these complications can be avoided or ameliorated.

Crucial to the prevention of complications is a thorough understanding of patient-related factors that have an impact on flap or graft viability, indications and limitations of each type of flap or graft selected for a particular defect, technical and anatomic problems, flap design, donor site morbidity, and postoperative surveillance and care. This chapter will focus on the conditions and preconditions leading to complications of tissue transfer, their management, and prevention.

PATIENT SELECTION

Patient-related factors that might influence flap or graft survival should be considered in preoperative planning. The presence of systemic disease, including collagen vascular disorders, peripheral vascular disease (e.g., Raynaud phenomenon), sickle cell disease, and polycythemia, could have adverse effects on flap circulation. Polycythemia can be associated with cigarette smoking and have deleterious effects on flap survival.[2] Clinical and experimental studies have shown decreased flap blood flow, hypercoagulation, and decreased wound healing in cigarette smokers, which can persist for weeks despite cessation of nicotine use.[3-5] Cigarette smoking, therefore, should be strongly discouraged for at least one week prior to surgery and must be forbidden in the early postoperative period. In noncompliant individuals, a preoperative urine nicotine level can be obtained with the understanding that a positive result might force cancellation of surgery. For elective procedures, this threat could serve as an incentive to stop smoking.

Blood coagulopathies must be routinely screened for and corrected prior to any surgical procedure. Hematoma formation can cause excessive pressure, wound dehiscence, and flap necrosis. It is important to question patients regarding their intake of aspirin or other nonsteroidal anti-inflammatory drugs, which may increase the risk of intraoperative and postoperative bleeding. If possible these medications should be discontinued for at least 2 weeks prior to surgery.

Advanced age, although not a contraindication for tissue transfer, is often associated with hypertension, hypercholesterolemia, and arteriosclerosis, which contribute to thickening of the walls of small arteries and overall compromised flap and recipient bed perfusion. In addition, the aging patient with head and neck cancer often has complex problems that affect function and self-image after treatment.[6] These problems must be addressed by the total health care team.

Preoperative metabolic disorders associated with liver disease, diabetes mellitus, and malnutrition represent significant contributory factors leading to complications.[7] Uncomplicated diabetes mellitus generally does not adversely affect tissue transfer. However, advanced or long-standing diabetes is a known cause of microangiopathy and severe segmental arteriosclerosis in larger vessels. Ohtsuka and colleagues described subintimal proliferation and elastolysis of the internal elastic lamina causing increased vessel fragility in diabetic patients.[8] Flap necrosis, especially involving the more distal regions, is not uncommon. Flap elevation and handling must be performed with minimal trauma in this patient population (Fig. 26–1). Malnutrition associated with hypoproteinemia, and severe anemia may lead to excessive flap edema, infection, and poor healing. Hypo-

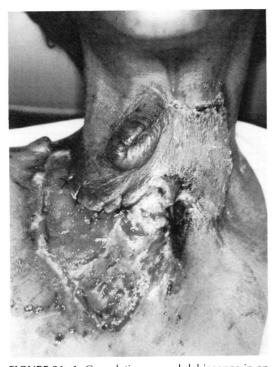

FIGURE 26–1. Granulating wound dehiscence in an insulin-dependent diabetic after second-stage closure of a laryngotracheal trough for laryngotracheal stenosis. The patient's postoperative course was complicated by numerous wound infections that prolonged reconstruction.

thyroidism occurs in a significant number of head and neck cancer patients, especially when neck irradiation is combined with total laryngectomy and ipsilateral thyroidectomy, and may lead to impaired wound healing and fistulization.[9] Every attempt should be made to normalize nitrogen balance and to restore the patient to a euthyroid state prior to operation. Patients with a compromised immune system and those receiving immunosuppressive therapy will often encounter problems with wound healing and increased complications when flap surgery is performed. In patients with normal cardiac output and cerebral blood flow, the hematocrit can be maintained at 30 per cent or below, since optimal blood viscosity, flow, and oxygen delivery occur at this level.[10, 11]

Previous irradiation to the recipient bed or to the flap or graft itself can be deleterious. It is well known that cancericidal doses of radiotherapy produce vascular and fibrotic changes in normal tissue that could interfere with healing.[12] Radiation injury to large and medium-sized arteries consists of transmural fibrosis, elastic degeneration, severe atheromatous plaque formation, and calcific atherosclerosis. Scanning electron microscopy reveals an overall increase in arterial wall thickness, especially in the tunica media. Fibrin deposits, microthrombi, and dehiscence of intercellular bonds are appreciably greater in irradiated vessels compared with nonirradiated controls.[13–15] Induction chemotherapy, in combination with conventional surgery and postoperative radiotherapy, also has been shown to increase wound complications, including flap necrosis.[16]

All tissue beds exposed to upper aerodigestive tract secretions are contaminated by a broad spectrum of microorganisms, the most important groups represented by the gram-positive aerobic cocci (streptococcus) and the anaerobes, fusobacterium, bacteroides, and peptostreptococcus species. Infection can be minimized by the use of perioperative antibiotic prophylaxis.[17, 18] Infection accompanied by a salivary fistula can lead to partial or complete flap necrosis, especially in an already compromised flap. Early wound exploration, debridement, and drainage in the operating room at the first sign of impending postoperative infection or fistulization can salvage some flaps. Every attempt should be made to divert saliva from the vascular pedicle, which must not be exposed in order to prevent desiccation and thrombosis. Circumferential dressings must never be used, to avoid vascular pedicle compression. Infected and heavily irradiated wounds may retard or prevent neovascularization of the transferred tissue and cause delayed healing or flap failure. For this reason, only nonirradiated flaps that carry their own blood supply should be used for infected or irradiated wounds. If possible, prior to tissue transfer, infected wounds should be aggressively debrided until clean, healthy granulation tissue develops. Extensive osteomyelitic bone that does not respond to conservative local treatment or hyperbaric oxygen therapy must be resected and replaced with well-vascularized bone or soft tissue.[19] Systemic antibiotics play a limited role in this setting.

Preoperative planning must include careful consultation with the patient and family. A multidisciplinary approach to the pre- and postoperative care of the head and neck cancer patient is essential for success.[20] The surgeon, as well as other members of the treatment team, should be involved in preoperative counseling, outlining the various aspects of the resection as well as reconstructive options. Expectations for restoration of form and function must be realistically conveyed to the patient. The patient must understand that the benefits and risks of the reconstruction are far outweighed by the morbidity of no reconstruction, or any functional and cosmetic deficit related to the flap or graft donor site. Surgical scars and distortion of normal anatomy (e.g., breast malposition for chest flaps) should be discussed. A plan for total postoperative rehabilitation should be outlined at this time. The risk of infection, flap failure, and the need for additional procedures should also be addressed.

RECONSTRUCTIVE STRATEGY

Complications in reconstructive surgery result from errors in flap selection, errors in flap design, and technical errors related to flap elevation and inset that ultimately impair flap perfusion. A well-planned surgical strategy, with consideration given to all possible intraoperative complications, is of paramount importance for a successful tissue transfer. Despite careful planning, unexpected events can occur that dictate the need for modifications of the original flap selection or design. For example, the defect may be larger than expected or require composite tissue, necessitating the use of an alternate pedicled flap, multiple combined flaps, or a free flap. Overskeletonization of the vascular pedicle may cause irreversible vascular spasm or injury, requiring use of another flap. Anatomic variations in the vascular pedicle may limit the arc of rotation or require tailoring of flap design to include additional blood supply.

FLAP SELECTION

The choice of one particular flap in preference to another should not be limited by the experience of the surgeon, but rather determined by the specific advantages or disadvantages inherent in each reconstructive option. A thorough understanding of the regional anatomy and blood supply to each flap is essential for treatment planning. Characteristics including bulk, color match, innervation, hair growth, and length of the vascular pedicle should be considered. The amount of tissue available for safe transfer, and wound closure without excessive tension, must be known for each flap. The simplest flap that will satisfy the requirements of the reconstruction is the best flap to use. For example, partial glossectomy or floor of mouth resections may be more amenable to simple skin-grafting techniques, which prevent tethering and allow maximal tongue mobility.[21, 22] In contrast, following total glossectomy, a bulky, myocutaneous flap may be advantageous for speech and deglutition. In this setting, attempts should be made to preserve muscle innervation so that denervation atrophy can be minimized. This can best be achieved with free muscle transfer (e.g., free latissimus dorsi and primary neurorrhaphy between the hypoglossal and thoracodorsal nerves). A free latissimus dorsi myocutaneous transfer, unlike a pedicled flap, is less subject to the downward pull of gravity and is more likely to maintain a tissue mound resembling the tongue. In this manner, deglutition and speech are improved, and pooling of saliva and aspiration are minimized.

Flap hair growth may be advantageous for reconstruction of cheek or upper lip defects in men. However, the transfer of hair-bearing skin to a normally nonhair-bearing area of the face or neck can be psychologically devastating to the patient, who must shave or use epilating creams to avoid embarrassment (Fig. 26–2). Hair growth in a reconstructed

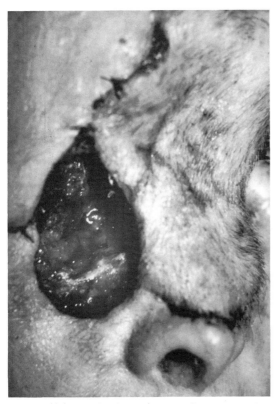

FIGURE 26–2. Orbital exenteration for an extensive erosive basal cell carcinoma of the midface. After a free flap failed, a scalping flap was used to cover exposed anterior cranial fossa dura. Adequate soft tissue coverage was achieved but, unavoidably, hair-bearing skin was transferred. The flap required repeated epilation.

pharyngoesophageal segment can be a limiting factor in the selection of flap donor sites.[23-25] Despite postoperative radiotherapy, hair-bearing skin may have more prolific hair growth than at the original donor site as a result of a stimulation process associated with graft revascularization.[26] Ectopic hair growth may exacerbate problems of deglutition related to loss of sensation, lack of lubrication, and poor elasticity of adynamic flaps (Fig. 26–3).[27] When radiotherapy is not a part of the original treatment plan, its use for epilation is not advisable since it may be needed to treat subsequent tumor recurrence. Postoperative CO_2 laser epilation can be effective in discouraging hair growth; however, precautions must be taken to prevent circumferential cicatrix and stenosis.[28] The de-epithelialization of myocutaneous flaps, and other flaps where a skin bridge must be buried, has also been effectively achieved using the CO_2 laser.[28, 29] Occasionally, intractable dysphagia due to flap hair growth will require excision and replacement with a new nonhair-bearing flap or graft. Prevention of hair growth is best achieved by the initial use of nonhair-bearing skin in the reconstruction. However, this may not be possible in the hirsute man. Deep de-epithelialization of myocutaneous flaps results in unpredictable epilation, and dermal fibrosis often causes undesirable contraction of the flap.[30] Split-thickness or dermal skin grafting of a muscle flap is probably a better alternative.

In some situations, the type of reconstruction might influence certain aspects of the resection. For example, one might be more inclined to excise the sternocleidomastoid muscle when performing a functional neck dissection in order to help accommodate the muscular pedicle of a myocutaneous flap without creating excessive bulkiness and difficulties with skin closure.

DONOR SITE MORBIDITY

Donor site morbidity is an important consideration in flap selection. Shoulder dys-

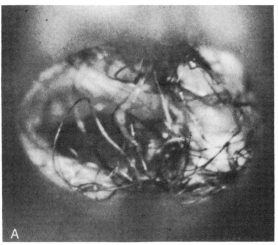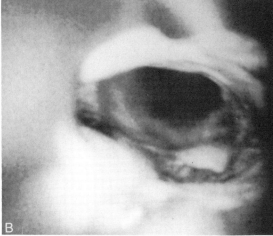

FIGURE 26–3. *A,* Exuberant hair growth on a deltopectoral flap 2 years after pharyngoesophageal reconstruction. Esophageal trichobezoar caused persistent regurgitation, emesis, and weight loss. Endoscopic view demonstrates coarse black hair in the hypopharynx. *B,* Repeated endoscopic hair removal with forceps and the CO_2 laser was required for relief of symptoms. Endoscopic view of the hypopharynx following epilation. (From Kuriloff DB, Finn DG, Kimmelman CP: Pharyngoesophageal hair growth: The role of laser epilation. Otolaryngol Head Neck Surg 98:342, 1988, with permission.)

function following radical neck dissection may be exacerbated by functional loss of the pectoralis major or latissimus dorsi muscles.[31] In this situation, a trapezius myocutaneous flap or a free flap can be used with little additional shoulder morbidity.[32, 33] Closure of the donor site under tension and excessive motion during healing of the shoulder and back can lead to wound dehiscence and wide, hypertrophic scars. Breast distortion may be an unacceptable complication when a chest flap is used for reconstruction. This is especially true in women, for whom the donor site closure should fall into the inframammary fold. Tattoos transferred with the flap may be more conspicuous and unsightly for the patient (Fig. 26–4).

TECHNICAL CONSIDERATIONS

Skin Incisions

The design of the operation should begin with careful placement of cervical incisions to permit adequate exposure while respecting the superior and inferior blood supply to the skin.[34–36] Since no one incision will always fulfill these criteria, it is essential to be familiar with several different utility incisions (e.g., Conley modified Schobinger, apron flap, arena half-H, and so on). When skin perfusion is already compromised by previous operation and radiation injury, careful planning of these incisions is essential to reduce the risk of skin necrosis, fistulization, and exposure of the carotid artery. Trifurcate junctions, known to be at increased risk of necrosis, should be placed away from the carotid artery or eliminated by using single transverse or vertical midline incisions.[37, 38] When designing neck incisions, position and volumetric changes of the underlying soft tissue also should be taken into account. Cosmesis should be maximized by placing incisions in relaxed skin tension lines. A scar placed within or parallel to a skin crease will be thinner and will possess greater tensile strength.[39] Severely damaged skin may need to be resected and replaced with cervical skin flaps outside the irradiated field.[40] For resections involving heavily irradiated tissues and entry into the upper aerodigestive tract, the formation of a temporary orostome or pharyngostome should be considered in the over-

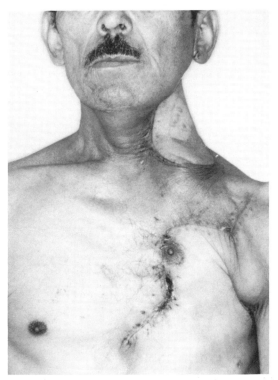

FIGURE 26–4. Full-thickness defect of the anterolateral neck following extirpation of recurrent squamous cell carcinoma with skin involvement, reconstructed with an ipsilateral pectoralis major myocutaneous flap. A large skin island required undesirable transfer of a tattoo and marked distortion of the breast.

all reconstructive plan.[41] A fluid-tight closure, by preventing undermining of cervical skin flaps and infection adjacent to the vascular pedicle, will decrease the potential for vascular thrombosis.

Flap Design, Elevation, and Inset

Flap design requires a three-dimensional perspective. The flap skin paddle may need to be folded or rotated to accommodate the defect. The position of the vascular pedicle relative to its origin must continually be assessed to avoid twisting, kinking, or stretching, all of which could compromise perfusion. If the flap is passed beneath a skin bridge or through a muscular tunnel, an adequate space must be created to prevent pressure on the pedicle and to allow for slight

swelling of the flap and adjacent soft tissues. Tight closure of cervical flaps over the muscle pedicle of a myocutaneous flap will also compromise perfusion; therefore, a split-thickness skin graft should be used instead to cover the exposed muscle.

The flap should be designed slightly larger than the defect to allow for tissue shrinkage and adjustments during wound closure. To protect the musculocutaneous perforating vessels, the skin incision should be beveled in an outward direction and the skin island stabilized with several tacking sutures to the underlying muscle to prevent shearing. Furthermore, gentle handling of the skin island with traction sutures or skin hooks, especially when tunneling under cervical skin to reach the neck, will prevent injury to these vessels.

Excessive skin shrinkage causes constriction of the subdermal plexus, impeding blood flow in the microcirculation.[42] An excessively thick flap that is forced to accommodate a small defect will also be compressed at the periphery, causing ischemia. These conditions may explain partial flap failure with superficial epidermolysis, despite viability of the underlying muscle. Redundant flap skin can easily be tailored to fit the defect. However, overly aggressive excision of tissue at the donor site can result in excessive wound tension. Occasionally, despite aggressive undermining, retention sutures or a skin graft must be used.

Some workers have advocated flap development prior to tumor extirpation based on an estimate of the defect size.[43] Although this approach has the advantage of allowing assessment of flap perfusion for several hours prior to inset, a larger-than-needed flap generally must be harvested to prevent errors in judgment. The potential for increased donor site morbidity, especially for larger flaps, cannot be ignored. In the case of the lateral island and lower trapezius myocutaneous flaps, the transverse cervical vessels must be preserved during neck dissection. If inferior neck disease is present, a commitment to use this flap prior to neck dissection would encourage a less oncologically complete operation. For these reasons, we do not advocate flap design and elevation prior to completion of the tumor extirpation. Once the defect is created, the appropriate flap design is formulated based on exact measurements.

FLAP PERFUSION

With the advent of axial pattern skin flaps, myocutaneous flaps, and free flaps, the use of surgical delay to increase survival is seldom necessary. Every attempt should be made to perform a primary single-stage reconstruction at the outset. This can usually be achieved in over 90 per cent of the cases, is more cost-effective, and reduces the need for multiple procedures and prolonged hospitalization.[44] However, delaying even myocutaneous flaps may be useful to extend the random cutaneous circulation nourished by the subdermal plexus, allowing a greater flap area for tissue transfer.[45] When the risk of flap failure is high or additional surgery is anticipated for new or recurrent disease, incisions should be planned to allow delay of one flap at the time of primary reconstruction. For example, when raising a pectoralis major myocutaneous flap, the deltopectoral flap can easily be delayed without sacrificing cosmesis (Fig. 26–5).

Experimental and clinical soft tissue expansion techniques have been applied to myocutaneous flaps with mean increases in length of 32 per cent and in width of 51 per cent.[46, 47] The use of controlled tissue expansion over several weeks can increase flap vascularity and allow single flap coverage of larger defects than was previously possible. While useful for elective reconstructive surgery, this technique is not suitable for the urgent treatment of head and neck cancer.

DELAYED FLAP FAILURE

Delayed failure of myocutaneous flaps beyond 7 to 10 days following operation occurs more frequently in oral cavity or pharyngoesophageal reconstruction, especially when

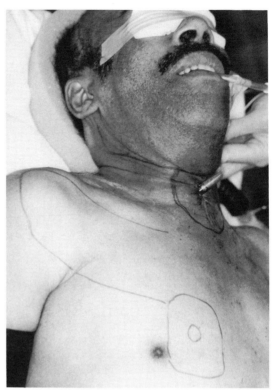

FIGURE 26–5. Initial flap design for immediate reconstruction of anterior neck soft tissue following laryngectomy, manubrial resection, and mediastinal dissection for squamous cell carcinoma of the larynx with subglottic extension. A pectoralis major myocutaneous flap is used for reconstructing the stoma and for great-vessel protection. The deltopectoral flap is delayed for potential later use in this heavily irradiated patient at risk for wound breakdown and fistulization.

bulky flaps are tubed. When the mandible is intact or a mandibular reconstruction plate is used, compression of a bulky myocutaneous flap may lead to delayed skin loss or total flap necrosis. Overskeletonization of the vascular pedicle without leaving a wide muscle strip may contribute to vascular spasm or vessel injury. Cho and colleagues reported a series of 39 pectoralis major myocutaneous flaps in which 50 per cent of the delayed failures were due to narrow-based flaps.[48] Local factors, including salivary fistula, infection, and local pressure, are also thought to play a major role in delayed flap loss. Any suggestion of vascular compromise in tubed flaps supports the use of a controlled fistula, which also serves as a window for postoperative monitoring.

Although gravity has a salubrious effect on the flap in terms of venous and lymphatic drainage, larger, bulky flaps are subjected to a downward pull. This places suture lines under tension and promotes wound separation, which can be counteracted with suspension sutures and attention to patient positioning in the early postoperative period.

Vascular spasm can be minimized by preventing overskeletonization of the vascular pedicle, desiccation and heating from electrocautery, or excessive cooling. The patient's core temperature and room temperature must be maintained at normal levels throughout the procedure. When vascular spasm is suspected, the flap and pedicle should be irrigated with warm physiologic saline. Adequate intravascular fluid volume must be strictly maintained throughout the procedure and in the postoperative period to prevent hypotension and peripheral vasoconstriction. After all precipitating factors have been eliminated, irreversible vascular spasm may necessitate the use of an alternate flap.

Flap perfusion should be assessed at regular intervals during elevation and insetting. Poor capillary refill and dermal bleeding demand careful scrutiny of the "lie" and tension of the vascular pedicle, pressure under cervical flaps, and the possibility of vascular spasm. Tension may also be relieved by flexing the neck and head toward the origin of the flap's vascular pedicle, which on occasion can be maintained with heavy silk sutures from the chin to the shoulder.[43]

POSTOPERATIVE CARE

Extrinsic neck pressure in the postoperative period can also cause compression of the vascular pedicle, compromising flap viability. A tensile force of only 1 ounce will cause venous obstruction and flap necrosis within 4 hours. As little as 2 pounds per square inch of extrinsic pressure to the skin paddle will lead to epidermolysis and dermatolysis.[49] With all pedicled flaps to the neck, tracheotomy tapes, gown ties, and mist collar straps must be avoided to prevent strangulation of

the vascular pedicle. Tracheotomy tubes must be sutured to the skin to avoid this complication. Circumferential dressings should never be used, and the patient must not lie on the flap. The education of the nursing staff and house staff regarding these points cannot be overemphasized.

The excellent vascularity of axial-pattern flaps increases the possibility of hematoma formation. Therefore, excellent hemostasis and the use of large-bore suction drains are important. Strategic drain placement will help eliminate dead space and prevent injury to neurovascular structures. Postoperative surveillance of drain function should be emphasized. Deep hematomas beneath the flap pedicle may go unnoticed and compromise perfusion. Early identification of the problem can be maximized by noting any swelling, discoloration, excessive bloody drainage, or a falling hematocrit level. Once detected, hematomas must be immediately evacuated in the operating room, and attempts made to identify any active bleeding sites. When bleeding is diffuse, suction drains are also essential to avoid reaccumulation of blood. Occult coagulopathies must be investigated and rapidly corrected.

Hypothermia and hypovolemia are most likely to occur during transport from the operating room to the recovery room. Heating blankets and central venous pressure monitoring are crucial. Peripheral vasoconstriction greatly enhances the possibility of vascular compromise and thrombosis.

FLAP MONITORING

Careful postoperative monitoring of flap viability is important, since early detection of ischemia may allow pharmacologic, mechanical, or surgical intervention for flap salvage. Although subjective and often inaccurate, clinical methods for assessing flap perfusion, such as skin color, turgor, capillary refill, temperature, and dermal bleeding, are widely used. The salient manifestations of arterial insufficiency include a cold, pale flap with poor capillary refill and diminished tissue turgor, with minimal or no dermal bleeding following needle puncture. Venous obstruction generally occurs more gradually, heralded by a sudden increase in swelling of the flap and a change in color to a pink-red hue. Progressive thrombosis leads to further edema, development of diffuse skin petechiae, vesicles, and progressive bluish discoloration of the skin. Needle puncture causes brisk dark bleeding.

Continuous clinical monitoring is not practical, and, therefore, various objective methods for flap viability monitoring have evolved, some with direct clinical utility and others relegated to investigational use.[50–58] Each method monitors a different parameter of flap viability: blood flow, temperature, oxygenation, tissue metabolism (see Table 27–3). Objective monitoring techniques are not designed to replace clinical judgment, but rather serve to facilitate early detection of problems. To date, there is no consensus regarding the best monitoring parameter to use, and no single method has been universally successful in predicting flap viability or the timing for salvage attempts. The majority of methods are limited by expense, bulkiness, need for elaborate instrumentation, lack of prolonged continuous on-line monitoring capabilities, and lack of implantability. Poor correlations between measures of flap ischemia and ultimate survival further limit their usefulness.

At present, we rely on clinical judgment, supplemented by information from a needle stick and a portable ultrasound Doppler for assessing both vascular pedicle and direct cutaneous blood flow. This system, although not entirely reliable, serves as a simple, inexpensive, and readily available bedside tool for use by house staff and nurses.

FLAP SALVAGE

Early detection of hypoperfusion and identification and correction of specific etiologic factors will permit salvage of ischemic flaps. Hypotension, hypoxia, hypothermia, and peripheral vasoconstriction will jeopardize flap viability and must be rapidly corrected. A search for a possible deep hematoma, tension, kinking, compression, or torsion of the vascular pedicle is mandatory. Release of a tight suture line or patient repositioning occasionally will improve the situation. Although most axial pattern flaps will tolerate several hours of ischemia, total flap salvage is often not possible by the time arterial insufficiency is detected. On occasion, skin necrosis alone occurs with preservation of underlying viable muscle. Early debridement and skin grafting of the remaining muscle prior to skin necrosis may prevent secondary infection and potential loss of the entire flap.

Various animal studies have demonstrated that tissue necrosis can be minimized and flap survival enhanced by the use of free radical scavengers (deferoxamine, allopurinol, and superoxide dismutase), vasodilators (nitroglycerin), and steroids (methylprednisolone).[59–63] Hypothermia and hyperbaric oxygenation have also proved to be effective techniques for reducing ischemic flap necrosis.[64, 65] However, the efficacy of these methods as adjuvant therapy for ischemic flaps in clinical practice needs further evaluation before they can be recommended.

Flap ischemia due to venous insufficiency generally takes longer to develop. Successful flap salvage might be achieved with medicinal leeches. Flap salvage using leeches has an estimated success of 60 to 70 per cent.[66] Barnett and associates described the "chemical leech" technique, which involves bloodletting from the compromised flap using subcutaneous heparin injections.[67] Continuous bleeding from the wound edge is titrated by dosage adjustment. The use of systemic heparinization in venous insufficiency remains controversial because of the risk of hemorrhagic complications but has been effective in selected cases.

When mechanical and pharmacologic attempts fail, the flap is allowed to demarcate, nonviable tissue is debrided, and the wound is resurfaced with another flap or skin graft. As small areas of peripheral necrosis generally heal by secondary intention, they rarely cause problems. Wound separation in the anterior floor of the mouth should be debrided and advanced early to prevent a salivary fistula. Heavily infected wounds should be managed with topical agents and systemic antibiotics until a clean, granulating bed is achieved. When flap necrosis occurs over the great vessels, immediate debridement and coverage with another well-vascularized flap is the only preventive measure against vessel rupture and exsanguination.

SPECIFIC GRAFTS AND FLAPS

Skin Grafts

Other than healing by secondary intention and primary closure, the skin graft represents the simplest of all soft tissue reconstructions. Color match, texture, and contour are never as good as adjacent normal skin, and the patient must be counseled regarding these limitations prior to operation. In addition, split-thickness skin grafts are prone to contraction and generally leave an unsightly scar at the donor site. On occasion, however, skin grafts may be the most expedient method of closure and provide cosmetic results that are comparable to the use of local or regional skin flaps. Skin grafts may be combined with local pedicled flaps to provide inner lining for mucosal defects. The advantages of skin grafting include ease of application, cost-effectiveness, and single-stage reconstruction that does not require additional local incisions or scars. Skin grafts for oral cavity reconstruction are advantageous in that they are thin and tend to cause less tethering of the tongue than regional pedicled flaps.[21, 22]

Full-thickness skin grafts better approximate normal recipient skin in color, texture, hair growth, and failure to contract than split-thickness skin grafts. Since the donor site must usually be closed primarily, only small areas can be resurfaced at one time. Because they are thicker, full-thickness skin grafts require meticulous defatting and a well-vascularized recipient bed to insure complete "take." The postauricular, upper eyelid, nasolabial, pretragal, and supraclavicular areas are excellent inconspicuous head and neck donor sites. The nasal tip is probably the most common recipient site for full-thickness skin grafts because of good tissue match and the failure of most local flaps to reach this area in a single stage.

Split-thickness skin grafts can be divided into thin, medium, or thick, depending on their widths, which range from 0.008 to 0.025 inch. The advantages of split-thickness skin grafts include ease of harvest and application, availability of donor sites for coverage of large defects (including the ability to mesh for even greater coverage), and a better likelihood of thin grafts to "take" on poorly vascularized beds (e.g., perichondrium, and periosteum). Disadvantages of split-thickness skin grafts include poor color and texture match (adnexal structures are not usually transferred), the need to use a dermatome, the need for bulky dressings (bolsters), and a painful donor site that must heal by secondary intention, resulting in poor cosmesis. In general, donor site healing is more rapid and less noticeable when thin (Thiersch) grafts are taken. Commonly used donor sites include the lower abdomen or upper thigh areas that are usually concealed by bathing suits or other clothing.

Dermal grafts have been used for carotid artery protection and resurfacing of oral cavity defects.[68] The technique for harvesting a dermal graft is simple and results in less donor site morbidity in terms of pain and cosmesis. The dermal graft "takes" better than a split-thickness skin graft of equivalent thickness and is less prone to contraction. It eventually re-epithelializes to normal-appearing oral mucosa without histologic evidence of dermal elements.[69] Recently, the perichondrial cutaneous graft was introduced for nasal tip reconstruction. In a rabbit model, the perichondrial cutaneous graft was found to undergo more rapid revascularization and to have a better survival rate than full-thickness skin grafts.[70] In addition, the perichondrial cutaneous grafts were less prone to contraction. Perichondrial cutaneous grafts may become a useful alternative to full-thickness skin grafts for small defects.

The healing of skin grafts involves two important phases. Within the first 24 hours, plasmatic imbibition takes place and involves diffusion of nutrients from the recipient bed to the graft. At about 48 hours, inosculation and ingrowth of blood vessels from the recipient bed begin, and stabilize the graft. The conditions that favor a graft "take" include (1) a noninfected, well-vascularized recipient bed; (2) rapid diffusion of metabolic waste and nutrients between tissues; (3) rapid revascularization from the recipient site; and (4) adequate immobilization of the graft to prevent disruption of the delicate neovascularization network.[71]

The success or failure of a skin graft or "take" depends to some degree on the quality of the recipient bed and the thickness of the graft. Skin grafts transferred to poorly vascularized recipient beds (i.e., exposed bone, cartilage, nerves and tendons without their associated periosteum, perichondrium, epineurium, or paratenon) compromise survival. The most important causes for skin graft failure include hematomas or seromas beneath the flap and excessive tension (both of which pull the graft away from the recipient bed), lack of immobilization, and infection.[72] Small skin grafts are usually immobilized with nonadherent pressure dressings, usually in the form of tie-over bolsters, for one week. A less cumbersome technique involves a multilayered Telfa dressing secured circumferentially with skin staples.[73] The use of this type of bolster creates an airtight seal, allowing placement of adjacent suction drains. Split-thickness skin grafts applied to the neck and chest may not be amenable to immobilization with bulky pressure dressings, which may cause excessive friction and actually impair graft "take." In this situation, the graft is meshed or "pie-crusted" to allow escape of blood and serum, and tacked in place with multiple absorbable sutures. Soiling from secretions and desiccation are prevented with xeroform gauze. Skin grafts used in the oral cavity can be immobilized with a stent made of dental compound.[74] This prevents putrefaction of gauze bolsters in the mouth. Group A beta-hemolytic streptococcus, coagulase-positive *Staphylococcus*, and *Pseudomonas* infections are commonly cultured from infected skin grafts, and may cause necrosis. To increase the chances of skin graft survival in the presence of infection and poor vascularity, delayed skin grafting after improvement in the recipient bed should be considered.[75]

Donor site complications are rarely encountered following skin graft harvest. Ex-

cessive bleeding usually can be controlled with either topical thrombin spray or a dilute solution of epinephrine. Gauze sponges are applied to the wound, which is wrapped with an Ace bandage until the end of the procedure. Once hemostasis is obtained, a transparent membrane dressing (e.g., Op-Site) is applied, followed by an Ace wrap. This nonadherent dressing is more comfortable and prevents the need to soak off blood-petrified gauze sponges. In addition, the transparent membrane allows wound inspection for early signs of infection.

Although skin grafts tend to decrease wound contraction, the graft itself is prone to some degree of contraction during healing, which may continue for up to 6 months.[71] This is especially problematic for resurfacing circumferential defects in the pharynx, esophagus, or trachea. Excessive mobility of the recipient site, infection, and fluid collection during healing may contribute to this problem. Contraction is generally less severe for full-thickness and thick split-thickness grafts and for those skin grafts placed on bone or cartilage, than for thin grafts. Prolonged stenting, massage, and the judicious use of steroid injections may be beneficial. Skin graft contraction can be minimized in the oral cavity by the use of oversized split-thickness skin grafts or dermal grafts and stenting with a large bolster for 10 to 14 days.[7]

Hyperpigmentation occasionally can be a problem after skin grafting; it is more prevalent in dark-skinned individuals and with thin split-thickness skin grafts.[72] Sun exposure following skin grafting must be avoided for several months and sunscreen ointments used liberally. The judicious use of dermabrasion can be useful for unsightly areas of hyperpigmentation. A small test area should be treated initially.

Composite Grafts

Composite grafts, consisting of cartilage and skin or cartilage and mucosa, are usually harvested from various areas of the auricle and nasal septum. The antihelical fold, fossa triangularis, cavum concha, and tragus are commonly used donor sites. These grafts are ideal for reconstructing small defects (less than 2 cm) of the nasal ala, nasal valve, and columella and provide skeletal support for turn-in, nasolabial, and midline forehead flaps.[76] The survival of composite auricular grafts larger than 1 cm is often precarious.[77, 78] Cigarette smoking is especially deleterious to the "take" of these grafts and should be prohibited in the perioperative period. The senior author has found that early cooling of composite grafts with iced saline compresses for the first 72 hours after harvest decreases metabolic requirements of the tissue and may improve survival.

Local and Regional Skin Flaps

Defects of the face and neck that cannot be closed primarily without significant compromise of form and function can be reconstructed with a skin graft. However, local skin flaps (e.g., rotation, transposition, advancement) are preferred because they provide optimal color and texture match with adjacent skin and contract less severely. Unlike skin grafts, local flaps bring their own blood supply to the defect and "take" is usually not an issue.

As with most flaps, complications generally result from technical errors or poor judgment in design. Poor hemostasis causing a hematoma, and wound closure under excessive tension, are errors in technique that can be prevented. A flap that is too small for the defect, extends beyond its blood supply, or is excessively bulky is destined to give a poor result. Tumor recurrence is unacceptable when it results from compromise of oncologic margins to make the defect accommodate a preconceived flap. Considerable planning is required to design a flap that will restore form and function without sacrificing distortion, asymmetry, and dysfunction of normal anatomic structures.

Various local transposition, rotation, and advancement flaps are quite useful for reconstructing head and neck defects and are usually based on a random cutaneous blood supply from the subdermal plexus. The design and elevation of these flaps must respect this vascular architecture. When raising flaps near the temporal and submandibular areas of the face, the subcutaneous plane of elevation must be deep enough to avoid injury to the subdermal plexus yet superficial enough to prevent injury to the peripheral branches of the facial nerve. Heavily scarred or previously operated sites are especially prone to vascular compromise, and flap elevation or excessive undermining should be avoided in these areas. Because the lymphatic drainage to cutaneous flaps is impaired by the nature of the flap design, it is not uncommon for local flaps to have persistent edema over several months. Longstanding lymphedema and tissue thickening may require one or more debulking procedures to achieve a more aesthetically pleasing result.

The general systemic and local conditions that jeopardize the viability of regional flaps also apply to local skin flaps. However, because of their random blood supply, local flaps are more fragile and are easily traumatized by the effects of crushing forceps, tension, pressure, and torsion. Because of the excellent blood supply to the skin of the head and neck area, local skin flaps seldom fail as a result of infection. However, diabetes mellitus and other immunocompromised conditions will increase the potential for infection, and for these patients antibiotic prophylaxis should be considered.

When designing local skin flaps, one must consider camouflage of incisions, tension across suture lines, and preservation of anatomic units. Excessive pedicle or suture line tension must be avoided to prevent flap necrosis. Experimentally, flaps closed with wound tensions exceeding 250 g predictably undergo necrosis.[79] Although tensile strength is often increased with high wound closing tension, this is often achieved at the expense of a wider scar.[80] Wide undermining is often necessary to prevent these complications. The direction and relative amount of tension produced after the flap is transposed or rotated must be considered in the initial design. Excessive force vectors around the lower eyelid, oral commissure, or naris may lead to ectropion with epiphora, lip deformity with oral incompetence, and nasal deformity with airway obstruction, respectively. Flap modifications are often necessary to reduce tension at either the recipient or donor sites. This may require the use of Z-plasties and subsequent scar revision.

The use of a local anesthetic without epinephrine will prevent potentially harmful vasoconstriction when flap perfusion is marginal. Electrocautery near the base of the pedicle should be avoided, since excessive heat may damage feeding vessels or cause vasospasm. Small bolsters are sometimes used with transposition flaps to help recreate a natural fold or sulcus, such as the nasolabial fold or nasoalar groove. When flap edema becomes significant, excessive pressure from these bolsters can compromise flap circulation and may occur in a delayed fashion (Fig. 26–6). Therefore, when bolsters are used, all local flaps should be carefully monitored for at least 24 hours, to allow early intervention prior to the onset of irreversible ischemia.

Local flaps for facial reconstruction are often subject to revision surgery for recontouring. Overzealous defatting of these flaps can compromise perfusion and result in necrosis. Merging of unequal adjacent wound margins often results in cones of Limberg or "dog ears."[49] Some of these raised areas will settle with time. Others will require a wedge excision or Burow triangle. Care must be taken in tailoring the Burow triangle so that the flap's pedicle is not violated or narrowed.

When a local flap exhibits obvious signs of ischemia, attempts must be made to improve perfusion. Release of several sutures may decrease flap tension. When a hematoma is encountered, the wound must be explored, hemostasis obtained, and drainage established. If these maneuvers fail, the flap occasionally may be salvaged by returning it to the donor site, in essence effecting a "delay" for subsequent reconstruction.

A detailed discussion of all the local flaps used in head and neck reconstruction is beyond the scope of this chapter. We will focus on several of the more commonly used local flaps and their various complications.

Rhombic Transposition Flaps. The rhombic transposition flaps (e.g., Limberg, Dufourmental, and Webster 30°) are especially

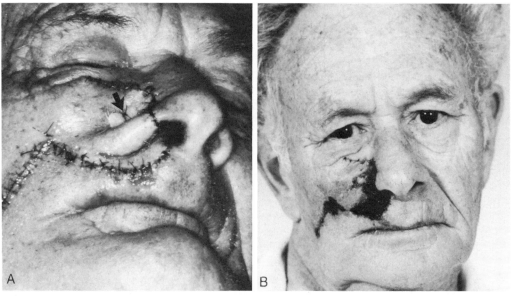

FIGURE 26–6. *A*, Reconstruction of lateral nose, alar rim, and nasal sill with a superiorly based transposition flap following surgical extirpation of a basal cell carcinoma using the Mohs technique. A bolster *(arrow)* was used to re-create the nasoalar groove. *B*, Vascular compromise and subsequent distal necrosis of the flap due to excessive compression by the bolster.

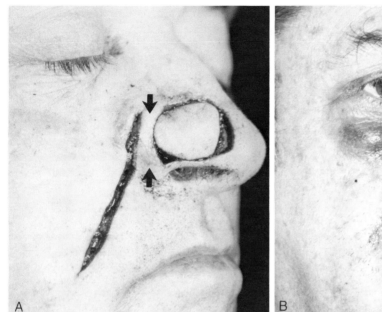
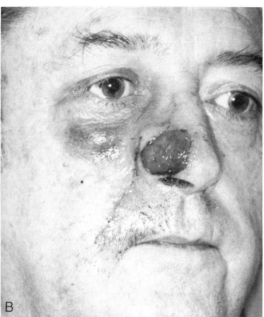

FIGURE 26–7. *A,* A superiorly based nasolabial flap is tunneled beneath skin bridge *(arrows)* to reconstruct a defect of the nasal ala following surgical extirpation of a basal cell carcinoma. *B,* Forty-eight hours later, the flap shows signs of venous congestion from vascular pedicle compression beneath the skin bridge.

useful in facial reconstruction. This type of flap is often preferred among transposition flaps because of its precise geometric design and method of transposition, combining both a lateral shift and rotation, which aids in closure of the donor site.[81] The size of the flap is limited only by the laxity and amount of skin available at the donor site. In a series of 30 facial reconstructions, it was found that the cheek, temple, and nose were the most useful anatomic areas for the application of the rhombic flap.[82] The acute angles created by the flap design may be subject to ischemia, and the geometric scar is difficult to camouflage. When excessive tension is required to close the donor site, a depression along this line of closure may occur. Although this depression usually fills out in time, closure over a bony prominence may create an unsightly deformity.[82]

Nasolabial Flap. The nasolabial flap is a well-vascularized flap ideally suited for nasal reconstruction. Advantages include its immediate proximity to the defect, excellent texture and color match, and inconspicuous donor site scar. The superiorly based flap may be folded on itself for alar reconstruction

or bilateral flaps used for columellar reconstruction.[83] It also can be partially de-epithelialized and tunneled subcutaneously, obviating the need to divide the pedicle at a later stage.[84] The island flap, however, may be more subject to venous congestion and persistent lymphedema (Fig. 26–7). Effacement of the nasoalar groove is another disadvantage of this flap that may require subsequent revision. Large nasolabial flaps may cause distortion and asymmetry of the oral commissure, requiring resection of skin in the opposite nasolabial fold to restore symmetry.[85] In men, it may be necessary to use a higher nasolabial flap than usual to avoid the inclusion of hair-bearing skin.

Midline Forehead Flap. The midline forehead flap is an axial-pattern myocutaneous flap primarily based on the paired supratrochlear vessels. Historically, it is one of the oldest-described flaps for nasal reconstruction and has undergone numerous modifications. In older patients, a flap measuring approximately 3.5 cm in width can be harvested with primary closure of the donor site. In younger patients, donor site closure is more difficult and may require a narrower pedicle or wide undermining and vertical relaxing incisions in the frontalis muscle fascia. A flap length of 6 to 8 cm will generally ιeach the nasal tip and allow folding on itself for alar reconstruction. Modifications of the flap (e.g., oblique and hairline extensions) will allow increases in length.[86] Elevation of this flap must be done bluntly in the area of the supratrochlear vessels to avoid injury. Although the flap can survive on only one vessel, every attempt should be made to preserve both. The distal end of the flap may be safely thinned primarily, preserving the subdermal plexus, to better match the thickness of the nasal skin. The median forehead flap remains attached to the recipient site for 3 weeks and is then detached. The perfusion of the flap in the recipient site should be tested by temporary pedicle occlusion just prior to division.[87] Only the portion of the flap between the eyebrows need be returned to restore normal eyebrow glabellar dimensions.

Further extensions of this flap when needed and improvement in blood supply may be obtained by the use of tissue expansion.[88] The disadvantages of this technique include possible forehead skin necrosis dur-

ing expansion, skin depigmentation, deformity during expansion, increased number of operative procedures, and delay in final reconstruction (Fig. 26–8). Rapid, intraoperative tissue expansion also has been used with the forehead flap.[89] Up to a 20 per cent increase in width can be obtained by this method, providing more tissue than the unexpanded flap without the usual 5- to 6-week delay involved in conventional tissue expansion. In addition, donor site closure can be performed under less tension, improving the forehead scar. The transfer of hair-bearing skin to the nose when the flap is extended past the frontal hair-line is a potential complication of this flap. The midline scar may spread laterally if the wound is closed under excessive tension. Although dermabrasion may be useful in selected patients, problems with depigmentation and unpredictable results often make direct scar revision a better alternative.

Cervical Flaps. One of the oldest reconstructive methods in head and neck surgery, skin flaps were described as early as 1842[90] and have been used for intraoral reconstruction as well as external cervical resurfacing. The McGregor forehead flap, nape of neck

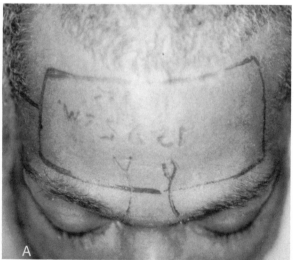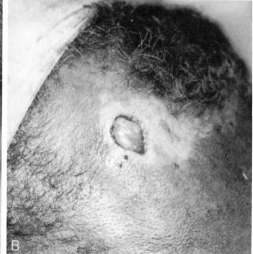

FIGURE 26–8. *A*, A rectangular tissue expander is placed subcutaneously in preparation for later use of an expanded midline forehead flap to reconstruct a large nasal defect. *B*, Full-thickness necrosis of forehead skin and exposure of the Silastic tissue expander one week following insertion, necessitating early removal of the expander. Note the surrounding area of skin depigmentation. The patient was a heavy cigarette smoker and was smoking during the early postoperative period, despite numerous admonitions to abstain.

flap, lateral cervical flap, and thoracoacromial flap have all been replaced by more reliable myocutaneous flaps. Although cervical flaps provide excellent color match, their location within the usual portals of irradiation and their occasional need for surgical delay make them less attractive for contemporary head and neck reconstruction.[91] Cervical rotation flaps remain useful for resurfacing the anterior neck. The forehead flap leaves an unacceptable cosmetic deformity and has been replaced by other flaps for intraoral reconstruction.

Since their blood supply is tenuous, based on random anastomoses within the subdermal plexus, these flaps will not tolerate tension, torsion, compression, or kinking at their base. Skin necrosis, therefore, represents the major complication of these flaps. Major losses occur in 5 to 10 per cent of cases and partial losses in up to 20 per cent.[92] Division of cutaneous nerves will cause areas of anesthesia, and extensive undermining or tunneling beneath facial skin may cause facial nerve injury.

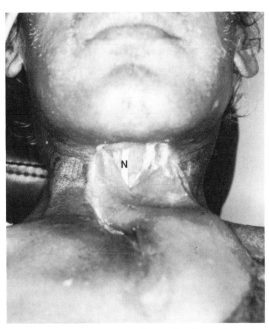

FIGURE 26–9. Necrosis of the distal portion of a deltopectoral flap used to repair a pharyngocutaneous fistula after total laryngectomy. N, nasogastric tube.

Deltopectoral Flap

The medially based deltopectoral flap (DPF) was originally described by Bakamjian in 1965 for pharyngoesophageal reconstruction.[93] The DPF is based on the first three or four perforating branches of the internal mammary artery. It provides thin, relatively hairless skin that is readily accessible without the need for surgical delay, unless the distal cutaneous skin extends beyond the mid-deltoid region of the shoulder. Its disadvantages include the need to skin graft a portion of the donor site, with its attendant scarring and upper chest wall deformity, and a high rate of necrosis (Fig. 26–9).[94] When used in the presence of a tracheostoma to resurface the anterior neck or repair a pharyngocutaneous fistula, the DPF may cause partial airway obstruction and require the prolonged use of a laryngectomy tube or later stomal revision (Fig. 26–10).

When elevating this flap, it is important to include the fasciae overlying the pectoralis major and deltoid muscles to prevent injury to the overlying vasculature. The base of the flap is initially kept wide enough to include at least four internal mammary artery perforators. The intercostal spaces at the sternal junction should be marked and careful scissor dissection performed as this area is approached. Occasionally, sacrifice of the fourth intercostal perforator with a back cut at the base of the flap is necessary to allow rotation of the DPF into the defect without excessive tension. Sacrifice of more than one of the four intercostal vessels could result in flap necrosis. When used without delay, the distal portion of the DPF is not extended beyond the mid-deltoid region of the shoulder.

In combined series, pharyngoesophageal reconstruction utilizing the tubed DPF had an 83 per cent success rate of achieving swallowing.[95] However, this result was achieved with a 56 per cent incidence of postoperative complications, including flap necrosis, fistula formation, and stenosis. An average of 3.8 procedures per patient, a hospital stay of 8 to 16 weeks, and an average

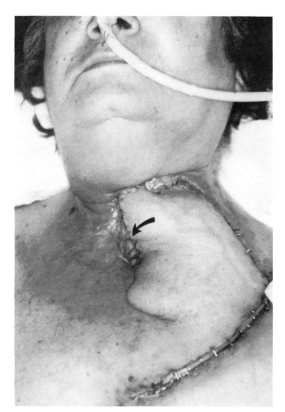

FIGURE 26–10. A deltopectoral flap (DPF) is used to salvage a necrotic wound resulting from failure of a bulky, tubed pectoralis major myocutaneous flap. The bulkiness of the DPF caused partial obstruction of the stoma *(arrow)*, requiring permanent use of a laryngectomy tube.

time of 10 weeks to initial swallowing were also required.[95] The need for multiple stages and prolonged hospitalization has made the use of the Wookey and the DPF for circumferential pharyngoesophageal defects less desirable. The tubed pectoralis major myocutaneous flap, gastric transposition, and free jejunal grafts have supplanted these earlier techniques.

Despite the widespread use of the pectoralis major myocutaneous flap, the DPF still has a useful role in head and neck reconstruction. It can be elevated rapidly, causes no shoulder disability, and does not distort breast position in women. It can be inset without violation of the neck when a neck dissection is not performed. It is thin and supple, allowing contouring for complex defects, and lies outside of most radiation therapy portals. It has distinct advantages for

resurfacing limited anterior mandibular defects, posterior and lateral pharyngeal defects, and complex resections involving the palate. It is particularly useful for resurfacing cervicofacial skin, where bulk is not needed and would obscure oncologic follow-up examinations.[96]

MYOCUTANEOUS FLAPS

Pectoralis Major Myocutaneous Flap

The pectoralis major myocutaneous flap (PMMF), originally described by Ariyan[97] and Baek and associates,[98] is presently the most widely used myocutaneous flap for head and neck reconstruction following cancer extirpation. The PMMF has an excellent and constant blood supply from the pectoral branch of the thoracoacromial artery. A minor contribution comes from the lateral thoracic artery.

The major advantages of the PMMF include its ease and speed of elevation with the patient supine, direct visualization of the vascular pedicle, proximity to most head and neck defects, preservation of shoulder function, and low donor site morbidity. The PMMF allows immediate single-stage reconstruction of most defects with primary closure of the donor site. Although transfer of the 4th or 5th rib as a compound osteomyocutaneous flap is possible, a high incidence of bone necrosis and poor functional results have been reported.[99]

Disadvantages of the PMMF include excessive bulkiness in women, transfer of hair-bearing skin in men, breast malpositioning and chest wall deformity, and exacerbation of shoulder dysfunction following radical neck dissection.[100] The muscle mass of the PMMF pedicle, while useful following radical neck dissection to eliminate the contour defect, may prevent early detection of tumor recurrence. The bulkiness of the PMMF also can be a complicating factor when the skin paddle is tubed for pharyngoesophageal reconstruction in obese patients. Despite the use of thin, parasternal random skin as described by Sharzer and associates,[101] the PMMF can be difficult to tube. Compression of this bulky flap and excessive suture line tension result in fistulization (Fig. 26–11). A 25 per cent to 30 per cent incidence of stenosis at the mucocutaneous anastomotic site has been reported for pharyngoesophageal reconstruction using the tubed PMMF.[102–104] However, proper flap design, ensuring ample lumen and tension-free closure, has been reported to yield a lower incidence of this complication.[105] Lam[106] reported anastomotic stricture in fewer than 6 per cent of tubed PMMFs when an interdigitating mucocutaneous suture line was created.[106] Fabian described the use of a partially tubed PMMF sutured directly to the prevertebral fascia, which reduced the incidence of stenosis to 6 per cent.[106a]

Problems with stenosis are further exacerbated in men when intraluminal hair growth occurs despite postoperative radiotherapy. This factor alone may cause significant dysphagia, regurgitation, and patient distress. A

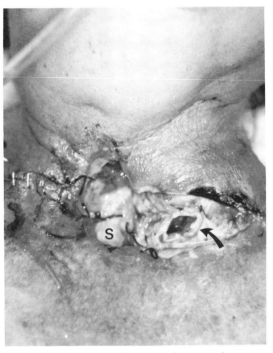

FIGURE 26–11. A bulky, tubed pectoralis major myocutaneous flap was used in a female patient for reconstruction following total laryngopharyngectomy. Early flap necrosis and a pharyngocutaneous fistula (arrow) necessitated staged reconstruction with cervical turn-in and deltopectoral flaps. *S*, stoma.

skin-grafted pectoralis major muscle or the use of muscle alone also allows epithelialization from adjacent mucosa and has been used with variable success to circumvent both of these problems.[107–109] Smith and Collins encountered problems with stenosis despite the use of skin-lined myogenous flaps for pharyngoesophageal reconstruction.[110] Skin-grafted muscle or muscle alone is prone to wound contraction. Therefore, its use probably should be limited to small oral cavity and oropharyngeal defects.

Flap necrosis, suture line separation, and orocutaneous fistulae are the most common complications reported for the PMMF. Total falp necrosis occurs in 3 to 7 per cent of PMMFs.[111] Shah and co-workers[111a] found a 29 per cent incidence of partial necrosis among 214 PMMFs. The majority of these were characterized by distal partial thickness flap loss (regions where cutaneous blood supply may be random). The majority of defects owing to necrosis healed by secondary intention. Significant risk factors for necrosis included age greater than 70 years, female gender, obesity, hypoalbuminemia <4g/dl, oral cavity sites, glossectomy, concurrent systemic disease, and preoperative radiotherapy.[112, 113]

Congenital absence of the pectoralis major muscle, as in Poland syndrome, should be assessed preoperatively and rarely will require selection of an alternate flap. Previous mastectomy, involving removal of the pectoralis muscle, or disruption of myocutaneous perforating vessels would prevent use of an ipsilateral PMMF. Further cosmetic deformity and excessive skin tension at the donor site closure also would discourage use of this flap following mastectomy. Injury to the thoracodorsal vessels following axillary dissection could jeopardize the viability of the PMMF. Preoperative arteriography or selection of an alternate flap might be necessary.

When raising the skin paddle of the PMMF, the incision should be beveled away from the underlying muscle to incorporate as many myocutaneous perforators as possible. The placement of temporary tacking sutures from the skin to the muscle fascia helps protect these vessels from shearing forces during flap elevation. Care should be taken to create incisions that will allow surgical delay of a deltopectoral flap and preservation of its blood supply. Undermining of the chest skin in the area of the DPF to accommodate passage of the PMMF should be done deep to the fascia of the pectoralis major muscle. The medial limit of dissection should be several centimeters lateral to the costosternal junction, to preserve the perforating branches of the internal mammary artery. Inferior and medial extensions of random skin beyond the muscle edge are reliable for several centimeters. Skin extensions over the rectus abdominis muscle should include rectus fascia to protect the integrity of the distal cutaneous blood supply. In women, the skin paddle should be designed at the medial aspect of the inframammary fold to maintain normal breast contour and conceal the scar. The design of the flap should be larger than the measured defect to accommodate skin shrinkage and to prevent suture line tension, especially when tubed for pharyngoesophageal reconstruction. Suspension sutures for both the skin paddle and muscle pedicle will help counteract the downward pull of gravity and tension across the suture line. This is especially important when the skin paddle is draped over a mandibular reconstruction plate. Excessive pressure from a fixed, firm prosthesis will result in flap necrosis and early fistulization (Fig. 26–12). When the sternocleidomastoid muscle is present, excessive bulkiness in the neck may prevent cervical skin closure without excessive tension and pressure on the vascular pedicle. In this instance, the cervical skin should be sutured to the edges of the muscle and a split-thickness skin graft applied.

Primary closure of the donor site is almost always possible when a single flap is used. Suction drains are used routinely to prevent hematomas or seromas. Inadvertent entry into the pleural space during PMMF elevation or rib harvest is rarely encountered.[96] Shoulder disability has not been significant with the PMMF unless radical neck dissection or an ipsilateral latissimus dorsi myocutaneous flap has also been raised. When intact, the latissimus dorsi muscle continues to provide adduction of the arm, and medial rotation is maintained by preservation of the clavicular fibers of the pectoralis major muscle.[99]

Trapezius Myocutaneous Flap

The trapezius myocutaneous flap (TMF) encompasses three separate flaps, deter-

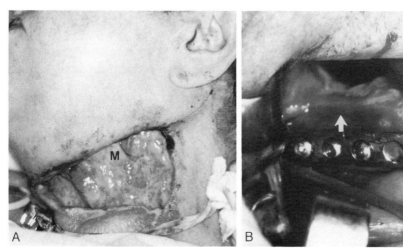

FIGURE 26–12. *A,* Composite resection for an advanced squamous cell carcinoma of the tongue and floor of the mouth, reconstructed with a pectoralis major myocutaneous flap (PMMF) and a mandibular reconstruction plate. Compression of the vascular pedicle against the reconstruction plate led to total necrosis of the skin paddle and an orocutaneous fistula. The muscle of the PMMF *(M)* remained viable proximal to the plate and served to protect the carotid artery. *B,* Complete exposure of the reconstruction plate and mandible *(arrow).*

mined by their blood supply and donor site location. These include the superior trapezius, the lateral island trapezius, and the lower trapezius flaps.

The superior trapezius flap, a modification of the Mutter shoulder skin flap, was first conceived by Conley in 1972[114] and subsequently popularized by Ariyan,[115] McGraw and group,[116] and Panje.[117] The excellent blood supply from the occipital artery and paraspinous muscular perforators, location in a nonirradiated field, and proximity to the lower face and lateral and anterior neck make this one of the most versatile and reliable myocutaneous flaps for head and neck reconstruction. The superior trapezius flap is limited by its wide, bulky base, which limits the arc of rotation beyond 110°, and potential trapezius muscle paralysis with resulting shoulder disability. A slight increase in the arc of rotation may be achieved by extending a random portion of skin, elevated deep to the deltoid fascia, for up to 10 cm beyond the trapezius muscle.[118] Ideally, this flap should be used following radical neck dissection when the spinal accessory nerve has already been sacrificed. The TMF, unlike an ipsilateral PMMF, would not cause additional shoulder disability. When at least four paraspinous perforators are included in the flap design, sacrifice of the occipital artery during an ipsilateral neck dissection does not compromise the superiorly based TMF. Netterville and associates reported no major tissue losses in 28 patients using the superiorly based TMF, making this variation of the trapezius flap the most reliable.[119] Primary skin closure is not usually possible for donor site defects wider than 6 to 8 cm, and a split-thickness skin graft is necessary. Delayed or incomplete skin graft "take" can be a problem, due to difficulties immobilizing the skin graft in the presence of shoulder motion. Delayed skin grafting on a bed of granulation tissue helps lessen the cosmetic deformity. Healing by secondary intention is occasionally necessary and usually results in a poor scar.

The lateral island TMF was first described by Demergasso and Piazza in Argentina[120] and by Panje in the United States.[117] This flap, as well as the lower island trapezius flap, receives its primary blood supply from the transverse cervical artery (TCA). The skin island can be designed beyond the acromial insertion of the trapezius muscle to provide thin, supple skin for difficult reconstructions of the oral cavity and pharynx. However, variations in the vascular anatomy of the lateral island TMF may be a limiting factor in its use. When the TCA branches off the dorsal scapular artery in a lateral position, the arc of rotation of this flap may be limited.[119] Intentional preservation of the TCA during neck dissection may not be oncologically safe when inferior neck disease is present. Furthermore, Goodwin and Rosenberg found that in approximately one third of their dissections, the transverse cervical vein drained directly into the external jugular vein.[121] Therefore, prior neck dissection, even with preservation of the TCA, may severely jeopardize venous drainage to this flap. Prior to the design of the lateral island TMF, the integrity and entry point of the transverse cervical vessels must be carefully assessed. Neck exploration and intraoperative use of a Doppler probe must be performed routinely. A dominant dorsal scapular artery or stenotic TCA following neck dissection may necessitate inclusion of the former vessel in the flap design.

When the spinal accessory nerve enters the trapezius muscle medial to the transverse cervical vessels, occasionally it may be preserved. Although one or more of the several distally located spinal accessory nerve branches are often divided when isolating the transverse cervical artery, the proximal branches to the trapezius can be preserved with maintenance of muscle function.[122] However, when reconstructing large defects, it is often impossible to preserve innervation to the trapezius muscle.[32] Again, either a split-thickness skin graft or healing by secondary intention is required for donor site defects of greater than 6 to 8 cm.

The lower island TMF was first described by Baek and colleagues and is based on the descending branch of the TCA.[123] This flap, primarily for reconstruction of upper face and scalp defects, was developed as an alternative to split-thickness skin grafts, scalp flaps, and deltopectoral flaps. The advantages of the lower island TMF include a long pedicle length, a thin, hairless skin paddle, and an inconspicuous donor site scar on the back. Krespi and colleagues modified the original design of the lower island TMF to incorporate the dorsal scapular artery and rhomboid muscles.[124] This modification increases tissue bulk when needed, allows harvest of a skin paddle distal to the scapular angle, spares upper trapezius muscle function, increases pedicle length, and improves vascularity. In addition, up to 18 cm of medial scapular bone can be harvested as a compound flap for mandibular reconstruction. Although additional shoulder morbidity with scapular winging was encountered in the early postoperative period, this improved with intensive physical therapy.

The disadvantages of the lower island TMF include the need for cumbersome lateral decubitus positioning or repositioning during flap elevation, potential shoulder disability, and problems related to excessive donor site closing tension. Of all the myocutaneous flaps, the trapezius flap has the greatest potential for donor site morbidity, plagued by persistent seromas, late wound dehiscence,

and wide, hypertrophic scars. Donor site problems are more frequently encountered with the rhombotrapezius flap, especially when large amounts of skin and muscle are transferred (Fig. 26–13). The variable anatomy of the TCA and its absence following neck dissection can be a significant problem. Cummings and colleagues experienced a high incidence of flap necrosis; 21 per cent and 35 per cent, respectively, for major and minor flap losses.[43] They attributed this to previous surgery and radiation therapy, atherosclerosis, and compromised venous outflow related to postoperative patient positioning. Urkin and associates reported one total flap failure and three partial failures among 35 lower island TMFs.[125] All flap losses, with the exception of one partial loss, occurred when previous ipsilateral neck dissection had been performed. Therefore, if the lower island TMF must be used following ipsilateral neck dissection, preservation of the dorsal scapular blood supply should be considered.

To circumvent potential trapezius muscle paralysis and shoulder dysfunction, Panje introduced the trapezius musculocutaneous "paddle" flap.[122] Extension of random skin beyond the muscle border (up to 20 cm in

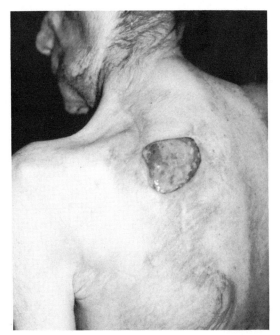

FIGURE 26–13. Seroma formation and wound dehiscence following harvest of a large rhombotrapezius musculocutaneous flap and skin closure under excessive tension. (Courtesy of Yosef P. Krespi, MD.)

length) is possible when supported by a 4 × 4-cm square of trapezius muscle overlying the transverse cervical artery. Preservation of the TCA and spinal accessory nerve when fashioning the superior trapezius flap limits the muscle's arc of rotation but allows the extended skin paddle to rotate into the defect. The trapezius muscle carrier (handle) subsequently can be returned to its original position following training of the distal cutaneous portion of the flap, further reducing shoulder disability.

With the advent of tissue expansion, microvascular free tissue transfer, and an assortment of more easily raised flaps, the trapezius flap based on the TCA is generally not the flap of choice for most head and neck reconstructions. Krespi and colleagues[126] and Baker[127] found free flaps to be superior to pedicled myocutaneous flaps for reconstruction of the upper face and orbit when a microvascular surgical team is available.

Latissimus Dorsi Myocutaneous Flap

The latissimus dorsi myocutaneous flap (LDMF) is one of the most versatile and widely used flaps in reconstructive surgery. Although it was first described by Iginio Tansini in 1896, it was not until 1978 that Quillen and associates described its utility in head and neck reconstruction.[128, 129] The sacrifice of this muscle causes little functional morbidity, due to compensation by numerous other muscles, such as the pectoralis major, teres minor, deltoid, and subscapularis. Shoulder disability, however, may be significant when this flap is combined with ipsilateral radical neck dissection or previous or concurrent PMMF harvest.[130] In this situation, the contralateral side should be chosen as a donor site.

The LDMF receives its main blood supply from the thoracodorsal artery, a terminal branch of the subscapular artery arising from the axillary artery. This vessel supplies the upper two thirds of the muscle, the lower one third being supplied segmentally by the 9th through 11th intercostal arteries. The neurovascular pedicle enters the undersur-

face of the muscle approximately 8 to 10 cm below the axillary vessels. The thoracodorsal artery usually splits 8 to 9 cm from the hilum, forming a medial and lateral division at right angles to each other. The lateral branch parallels the muscle border 1 to 4 cm medial to the edge. The medial division parallels the upper muscle border 3.5 cm inferior to the edge. The motor nerve to this muscle, the thoracodorsal nerve, divides 1 to 2 cm more proximally and parallels the arterial branches. This consistent neurovascular anatomy generally allows splitting of the muscle into two independent myocutaneous flaps, each with its own innervation and blood supply.[131] This flap can be used reliably as a pedicled or free myocutaneous or muscle only flap.

The advantages of the LDMF include a large, hairless, cutaneous skin island outside the usual irradiated fields, a long arc of rotation with the ability to reach virtually any site in the head and neck, a consistent neurovascular pedicle, the ability to maintain motor innervation to minimize muscle atrophy for tongue reconstruction and carotid artery protection, and low donor site morbidity and functional loss (especially in women) compared with the PMMF. Disadvantages include cumbersome lateral patient positioning during flap elevation, location of the donor site out of the operative field, poor color match with facial skin, excessive flap bulk, and difficult axillary dissection in obese patients. The bulkiness of this flap may be partially circumvented by developing a smaller muscle segment and extending the thin cutaneous portion of the flap beyond the muscle boundary. This skin has a reliable, random blood supply based on the musculocutaneous perforators nourishing the subdermal plexus for a distance of up to 10 cm.[132] Alternatively, a muscle flap may be harvested without its overlying skin and a split-thickness skin graft applied for lining. When a previous or concurrent neck dissection has not been performed, excessive muscle bulk often will prevent closure of cervical skin flaps. When this problem arises, primary or delayed split-thickness skin grafting may be needed for muscle coverage.

Donor site defects of up to 10 cm usually can be closed primarily. The back skin should be pinched prior to flap elevation to determine its laxity and the prospect for primary closure. As with the lower island TMF, excessive donor site closing tension may cause skin necrosis and wound breakdown. Although retention sutures may be useful to relieve skin tension, further impairment of local skin perfusion may occur, resulting in necrosis and wound dehiscence (Fig. 26–14). Because of the constant tension and mobility of the back skin with respiration and shoulder motion, these wounds are difficult to manage and may result in delayed healing and hypertrophic scarring. Larger defects require coverage with a split-thickness skin graft but cause an unsightly contour defect and poor color match.

A high incidence of seroma formation at the donor site has been reported with this flap. This may be due to excessive mobility of the shoulder girdle and scapula in the early postoperative period. A short period of shoulder immobilization, and prolonged suction drainage beyond one week may be of benefit. However, seroma formation may be a recalcitrant problem despite prolonged suction drainage. Persistent or recurrent seromas often will form a bursa-like cavity, which may require abrasion of the opposing surfaces or excision to allow the chest wall skin to adhere to the underlying musculature. Lumbar herniation and late hematoma formation are rarely reported complications of the LDMF.[133] Compression of the brachial plexus between the clavicle and the cervical vertebrae is believed to cause a temporary neurapraxia associated with excessive arm abduction during the axillary dissection. Injury to the long thoracic nerve and scapular winging are rarely seen.

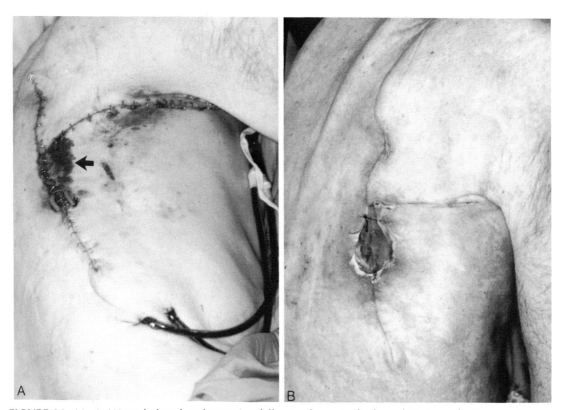

FIGURE 26–14. *A*, Wound closed under tension following harvest of a large latissimus dorsi myocutaneous flap (LDMF) for floor of mouth reconstruction. Demarcation of an ischemic area of back skin developed 48 hours after surgery *(arrow)*. *B*, Seroma formation and skin necrosis left a large skin defect that required debridement and closure with a local rhombic flap.

Most of the complications related to flap necrosis are caused by technical errors that result in compression, torsion, stretching, or spasm of the vascular pedicle. The LDMF is usually transferred to the neck through a tunnel between the pectoralis major and minor muscles, and then brought out subcutaneously over the clavicle. This space must amply accommodate the vascular pedicle without compression, taking into account any subsequent tissue edema (Fig. 26–15). Division of the humoral attachment of the latissimus muscle must be done with the neurovascular pedicle in direct view to avoid inadvertent injury or transection. Division of the tendinous insertion of the pectoralis minor muscle decreases compression of the pedicle between the two chest muscles. The central clavicular portion of the pectoralis major muscle must also be detached to allow flap transfer over the clavicle. Dissection in this area must be done carefully to avoid injury to the thoracoacromial vessels, in the event that a PMMF would be necessary in the future. The long vascular pedicle of the LDMF must be carefully guided through the muscular and subcutaneous tunnels without torsion. Placing long guide sutures often helps this maneuver. Division of the circumflex scapular vessels to increase pedicle length must be done with caution because kinking or compromised venous drainage may result.

When the integrity of the vascular pedicle is in doubt, such as following previous mastectomy with axillary dissection, a preliminary upper incision is recommended for exploration of the vascular pedicle. Use of a Doppler probe is often helpful in identifying the location of the vascular pedicle and to assure an adequate density of musculocutaneous perforators to the proposed skin paddle. Careful handling of the myocutaneous flap and placement of tacking sutures from the skin island to the muscle will prevent shearing of the musculocutaneous perforating vessels and skin necrosis. Other reported factors causing flap necrosis have included a distally placed skin paddle beyond the primary thoracodorsal blood supply, hematoma beneath the pedicle, and flap compression in the oral cavity (Fig. 26–16).[134, 135]

Ligation of the serratus anterior branch of the thoracodorsal artery too close to the main trunk can cause irreversible vasospasm and thrombosis. Total flap loss occurs in 5 per cent to 10 per cent of cases. Partial flap losses have occurred in up to 20 per cent but are usually minor in nature, consisting of suture line necrosis or epidermolysis.[136] Although the reported incidence of major flap loss is higher than for the PMMF, this is likely due to the relative inexperience with this flap among most head and neck surgeons.

Sternocleidomastoid Myocutaneous Flap

The sternocleidomastoid myocutaneous flap (SCMMF) was first described for use in

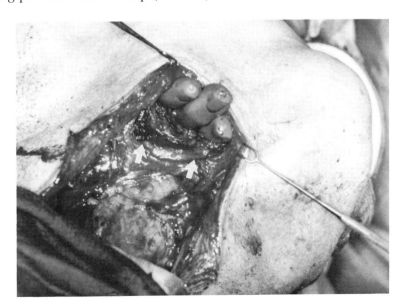

FIGURE 26–15. A tunnel between the pectoralis major and minor muscles was created large enough to accommodate the vascular pedicle of the LDMF. The clavicular origin of the pectoralis muscle (arrows) is divided laterally, allowing preservation of the thoracoacromial vessels.

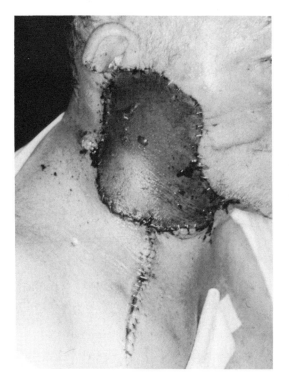

FIGURE 26–16. Venous thrombosis of an LDMF used for reconstruction following a lateral temporal bone resection for squamous cell carcinoma. The flap is ecchymotic with vesicle formation, oozing dark red blood from the staple line. Vascular pedicle compression or kinking was the likely cause for this complication. (Courtesy of Gregory T. Wolf, MD.)

head and neck reconstruction by Owens in 1955.[137] Since that time, the utility of the SCMMF has been expanded by many workers.[138, 139] It provides a thin, compound flap consisting of sternocleidomastoid and platysma muscles with relatively hairless overlying skin. The close proximity of the SCMMF to the oral cavity, oropharynx, and pharynx facilitates superiorly or inferiorly based transpositions and donor site closure with cervical advancement flaps. A portion of the clavicle may be transposed with the SCM muscle for mandibular reconstruction.[140] The SCMMF has been most useful for oral cavity and oropharyngeal defects not exceeding 6 cm in diameter, for closure of pharyngocutaneous fistulas, and for protection of the great vessels.[141, 142] The SCMMF is not a true axial pattern flap since it has a tripartite blood supply, superiorly from the occipital and postauricular arteries, inferiorly from branches of the thyrocervical trunk, and in its midportion from a branch of the superior thyroid artery.[143, 144]

Reported total or partial flap necrosis ranges from 20 per cent to 66 per cent.[48, 142, 143] The high incidence of skin slough may be diminished by including the platysma muscle along the length of the SCM muscle.[145] The reluctance to use this flap following cancer extirpation stems from concerns regarding the oncologic safety of selective neck dissections that preserve the sternocleidomastoid muscle. In addition, the flap cannot be used reliably after previous neck dissection or radiation therapy that interferes with its blood supply. Muscle atrophy, the small size of the skin paddle, the high incidence of complications, and the availability of other more reliable myocutaneous flaps have limited the usefulness of the SCMMF in head and neck reconstruction.

Platysma Myocutaneous Flap

The platysma myocutaneous flap (PMF) provides a thin, pliable skin island for resurfacing small intraoral or facial defects. Its proximity to the reconstructive site and its 180° arc of rotation are advantageous.[146] Primary closure of the donor site is usually possible with little morbidity. When based superiorly, the flap's primary blood supply

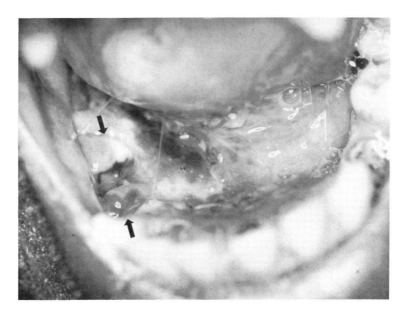

FIGURE 26–17. Partial necrosis of a platysma myocutaneous flap used to reconstruct a small anterior floor of mouth squamous cell carcinoma. An orocutaneous fistula (*arrows*) eventually closed without surgical intervention.

is derived from branches of the facial artery. Additional blood supply comes from the occipital and superior thyroid arteries. The use of the PMF is less desirable following neck dissection and major ablative procedures, in which the integrity of these vessels is at risk, and flap viability may be tenuous (Fig. 26–17). The PMF also should be avoided following radiotherapy to the neck, since radiation-induced endarteritis and fibrosis may further jeopardize flap viability. In elderly patients, or following long-standing facial paralysis, the platysma muscle may be atrophic, and the required soft tissue bulk and vascular support to the skin may be inadequate.[147] Overthinning of the cervical skin during harvest of the PMF may lead to necrosis and exposure of the carotid artery. In men, flap hair growth further limits the usefulness of this flap. Skin grafting is often a better option for reconstructing small oral cavity defects.

References

1. Schusterman MA: The proof of the pudding is in the eating, or the functional evaluation of surgical reconstruction (editorial). Head Neck 11:203–204, 1989.
2. Kaufman T, Eichenlaub EH, Levin M, et al: Tobacco smoking: Impairment of experimental flap survival. Ann Plast Surg 13:468–472, 1984.
3. Lawrence WT, Murphy RC, Robson MC, Heggers JP: The detrimental effect of cigarette smoking on flap survival: An experimental study in the rat. Br J Plast Surg 37:216–219, 1984.
4. Rao VK, Morrison WA, O'Brien BM: Effect of nicotine on blood flow and patency of experimental microvascular anastomosis. Ann Plast Surg 11:206–209, 1983.
5. Engelberg H, Futterman M: Cigarette smoking and thrombotic coagulation of human blood. Further in vitro studies. Arch Environ Health 14:266–270, 1967.
6. Endicott JN, Cantrell RW, Kelly JH, et al: Head and neck surgery and cancer in aging patients. Otolaryngol Head Neck Surg 100:290–291, 1989.
7. Schechter GL: Complications of flaps and grafts in the oral cavity and pharynx. Laryngoscope 93:306–309, 1983.
8. Ohtsuka H, Kamiishi H, Shioya N: Successful free flap transfers in two diabetics. Plast Reconstr Surg 61:715–718, 1978.
9. Palmer BV, Gaggar N, Shaw HJ: Thyroid function after radiotherapy and laryngectomy for carcinoma of the larynx. Head Neck Surg 4:13–15, 1981.
10. Hansen EB, Gellett S, Kirkegard L, et al: Tissue oxygen tension in random pattern skin flaps during normovolemic hemodilution. J Surg Res 47:24–29, 1989.
11. Earl AS, Fratianne RB, Nunez FD: The relationship of hematocrit levels to skin flap survival in the dog. Plast Reconstr Surg 54:341–344, 1974.
12. Marchetta FC, Sako KS, Maxwell W: Complications after radical head and neck surgery performed through previously irradiated tissues. Am J Surg 114:835–838, 1967.
13. Guelinckx PJ, Boeckx WD, Fossion E, Gruwez JA: Scanning electron microscopy of irradiated recipient blood vessels in head and neck free flaps. Plast Reconstr Surg 74:217–226, 1984.
14. Murros KE, Toole JF: The effect of radiation on carotid arteries. Arch Neurol 46:449–455, 1989.
15. Butler MJ, Lane RHS, Webster JH: Irradiation injury to large arteries. Br J Surg 67:341–343, 1980.
16. Corey JP, Calderelli DD, Hutchinson JC, et al: Surgical complications in patients with head and neck cancer receiving chemotherapy. Arch Otolaryngol Head Neck Surg 112:437–439, 1986.

17. Johnson JT, Yu VL: Antibiotic use during major head and neck surgery. Ann Surg 207:108–111, 1988.

18. Johnson JT, Yu VL: Role of aerobic gram-negative rods, anaerobes, and fungi in wound infection after head and neck surgery: Implications for antibiotic prophylaxis. Head Neck 11:27–29, 1989.

19. Dolezal RF, Baker SR, Krause CJ: Treatment of the patient with extensive osteoradionecrosis of the mandible. Arch Otolaryngol 108:179–183, 1982.

20. Goepfert H: The "multidisciplinary approach" (editorial). Head Neck 11:109–110, 1989.

21. Schramm VL, Myers EN: Skin grafts in oral cavity reconstruction. Arch Otolaryngol 106:528–532, 1980.

22. Schramm VL, Johnson JT, Myers EN: Skin grafts and flaps in oral cavity reconstruction. Arch Otolaryngol 109:175–177, 1983.

23. Montgomery WW: Reconstruction of the cervical esophagus. Arch Otolaryngol Head Neck Surg 77:55–66, 1963.

24. McLean GK, Laufer I: Hairy esophagus: A complication of pharyngoesophageal reconstructive surgery in two cases. Am J Roentgenol 132:269–270, 1979.

25. Maisel RH, Liston SL, Adams GL: Complications of pectoralis myocutaneous flaps. Laryngoscope 93:928–930, 1983.

26. Conley JJ: Skin flap and skin graft complications. In Conley JJ (ed): Complications of Head and Neck Surgery. Philadelphia, WB Saunders, 1979, p 457.

27. Kuriloff DB, Finn DG, Kimmelman CP: Pharyngoesophageal hair growth: The role of laser epilation. Otolaryngol Head Neck Surg 98:342–345, 1988.

28. Hallock GG: Extended applications of the carbon dioxide laser for skin deepithelialization. Plast Reconstr Surg 83:721, 1989.

29. Krespi YP, Weiss MH, Bhatia P: Laser de-epithelialization of muscle-based flaps. Laryngoscope 100:661–662, 1990.

30. Eliachar I, Kraus DH, Bergfeld WF, Tucker HM: Prevention of hair growth in myocutaneous flap reconstruction. Arch Otolaryngol Head Neck Surg 116:923–927, 1990.

31. Har-El G, Krespi YP, Har-El R: Physical rehabilitation after myocutaneous flaps. Head Neck 12:218–224, 1990.

32. Demergasso F, Piazza MV: Trapezius myocutaneous flap in reconstructive surgery for head and neck cancer. Am J Surg 138:533–536, 1979.

33. Krespi YP, Baek SM, Surek CL: Flap reconstruction of the upper face: Free flaps vs. lower trapezius myocutaneous flap. Laryngoscope 93:485–488, 1983.

34. Arena S: Incisions. Laryngoscope 85:823–828, 1975.

35. Rabson JA, Hurwitz DJ, Futrell J: The cutaneous blood supply of the neck: Relevance to incision planning and surgical reconstruction. Br J Plast Surg 38:208–219, 1985.

36. Appiani E, Delfino M: Plastic incisions for facial and neck tumors. Ann Plast Surg 13:335–352, 1984.

37. Becker GD: Extended single transverse neck incision for composite resections: An update of technique and results. Laryngoscope 94:605–607, 1984.

38. Dissanayaka L: A modified single flap for neck dissection in oral cancer. Head Neck 12:75–76, 1990.

39. Bernstein L: Incisions and excisions in elective facial surgery. Arch Otolaryngol 97:238–243, 1973.

40. Schuller DE: Cervical skin flaps in head and neck reconstruction. Am J Otolaryngol 2:62–68, 1981.

41. De Souza FM, Fredrickson JM: Planned pharyngostome. Laryngoscope 85:848–852, 1975.

42. Panje WR, Schuller DE, Shagets FW: Musculocutaneous flap reconstruction of the head and neck. In Panje WR, Schuller DE, Shagets FW (eds): Physiological and Practical Considerations in Musculocutaneous Flap Reconstruction. New York, Raven Press, 1989, pp 6–9.

43. Cummings CW, Eisele DW, Coltrera MD: Lower trapezius myocutaneous island flap. Arch Otolaryngol Head Neck Surg 115:1181–1185, 1989.

44. Conley JJ: Skin flap and skin graft complications. In Conley JJ (ed): Complications of Head and Neck Surgery. Philadelphia, WB Saunders, 1979, p 450.

45. Haughey B, Panje WR: Extension of the musculocutaneous flap by surgical delay. Arch Otolaryngol 111:234–240, 1985.

46. Forte V, Middleton WG, Briant TD: Expansion of myocutaneous flaps. Arch Otolaryngol 111:371–374, 1985.

47. Thornton JW, Marks MW, Izenberg PH, Argenta LC: Expanded myocutaneous flaps: Their clinical use. Clin Plast Surg 14:529–534, 1987.

48. Cho HT, Mignogna F, Garay K, Blitzer A: Delayed failure of myocutaneous flaps in head and neck reconstruction. Laryngoscope 93:17–19, 1983.

49. Tenta LT, Keyes GR: Biogeometry: The logic in the process of selection, insetting, design, construction, and transfer of flaps. Clin Plast Surg 12:423–452, 1985.

50. Barron JN, Laing JE, Colbert JG, Veall N: Observations on the circulation of tubed skin pedicles using the local clearance of radioactive sodium. Br J Plast Surg 5:171, 1952.

51. Silverman DG, LaRossa DD, Barlow CH, et al: Quantification of tissue delivery and prediction of flap viability with the fiberoptic dermofluorometer. Plast Reconstr Surg 66:545–553, 1980.

52. Weisman RA, Silverman DG: Fiberoptic fluorometer for skin flap assessment. Otolaryngol Head Neck Surg 91:377–379, 1983.

53. Glogovac SV, Bitz MD, Whiteside LA: Hydrogen washout technique in monitoring vascular status after replantation surgery. J Hand Surg 7:601–605, 1982.

54. Batchelor A, Kay S, Evans D: A simple and effective method of monitoring free muscle transfers: A preliminary report. Br J Plast Surg 35:343–344, 1982.

55. Fischer JC, Parker PM, Shaw WW, Colen SR: Dynamic computed tomography determining the patency of buried free flaps. Microsurg 7:190–192, 1986.

56. Harrison DH, Girling M, Mott G: Methods of assessing the viability of free flap transfer during the postoperative period. Clin Plast Surg 10:21–36, 1983.

57. Sloan GM, Sasaki GH: Noninvasive monitoring of tissue viability. Clin Plast Surg 12:185–195, 1985.

58. Jones NF: Postoperative monitoring of microsurgical free tissue transfers for head and neck reconstruction. Microsurgery 9:159–164, 1988.

59. Pokorny AT, Bright DA, Cummings CW: The effects of allopurinol and superoxide dismutase in a

rat model of skin flap necrosis. Arch Otolaryngol Head Neck Surg 115:207–212, 1989.

60. Sagi A, Ferder M, Levens D, Strauch B: Improved survival of island flaps after prolonged ischemia by perfusion with superoxide dismutase. Plast Reconstr Surg 77:639–642, 1986.

61. Pokorny AT, Bright DA, Cummings CW: The effects of allopurinol and superoxide dismutase in a rat model of skin flap necrosis. Arch Otolaryngol Head Neck Surg 115:207–212, 1989.

62. Waters LM, Pearl RM, Macaulay RM: A comparative analysis of the ability of five classes of pharmacologic agents to augment skin flap survival in various models and species: An attempt to standardize skin flap research. Ann Plast Surg 23:117–122, 1989.

63. Esclamado RM, Larrabee WF, Zel GE: Efficacy of steroids and hyperbaric oxygen on survival of dorsal skin flaps in rats. Otolaryngol Head Neck Surg 102:41–44, 1990.

64. Zamboni WA, Roth AC, Russell RC, et al: The effect of acute hyperbaric oxygen therapy on axial pattern skin flap survival when administered during and after total ischemia. J Reconstr Microsurg 5:343–347, 1989.

65. Nylander G, Lewis D, Nordstrom H, Larsson J: Reduction of postischemic edema with hyperbaric oxygen. Plast Reconstr Surg 76:596–603, 1985.

66. Kraemer BA, Korber KE, Aquino TI, Engleman A: Use of leeches in plastic and reconstructive surgery: A review. J Reconstr Microsurg 4:381–386, 1988.

67. Barnett GR, Taylor GI, Mutimer KL: The "chemical leech": Intra-replant subcutaneous heparin as an alternative to venous anastomosis. Report of three cases. Br J Plast Surg 42:556–558, 1989.

68. Reed GF: The use of dermal grafts in otolaryngology. Ann Otol Rhinol Laryngol 74:769–784, 1965.

69. Smiler D, Radack K, Bilovsky P, Montemarano P: Dermal graft: A versatile technique for oral surgery. Oral Surg 43:342–350, 1977.

70. Portuese W, Stucker F, Grafton W, et al: Perichondrial cutaneous graft. Arch Otolaryngol Head Neck Surg 115:705–709, 1989.

71. Swanson NA: Advanced techniques: Local skin grafts. In Swanson NA: Atlas of Cutaneous Surgery. Boston, Little, Brown, 1989, pp 128–149.

72. Converse JM, McCarthy JG, Brauer RO, Ballantyne DL: Transplantation of skin: Grafts and flaps. In Converse JM, McCarthy JG (eds): Reconstructive Plastic Surgery. Vol 1. 2nd ed. Philadelphia, WB Saunders, 1977, pp 152–240.

73. Hoffman HT, La Rouere M: A simple bolster technique for skin grafting. Laryngoscope 99:558–559, 1989.

74. Teichgraeber J, Larson DL, Castaneda O, Martin JW: Skin grafts in intraoral reconstruction: A new stenting method. Arch Otolaryngol 110:463–467, 1984.

75. Bumsted M, Panje R, Ceilley Rl: Delayed skin grafting in facial reconstruction. Arch Otolaryngol 109:178–184, 1983.

76. Baker SR, Swanson NA: Management of nasal cutaneous malignant neoplasms. Arch Otolaryngol 109:473–479, 1983.

77. Maves MD, Yessenow RS: The use of composite auricular grafts in nasal reconstruction. J Dermatol Surg Oncol 14:994–999, 1988.

78. Brown JB, Cannon B: Composite free graft of skin and cartilage from ear. Surg Gynecol Obstet 82:253–255, 1946.

79. Larrabee WF, Holloway GA, Sutton D: Wound tension and blood flow in skin flaps. Ann Otol Rhinol Laryngol 93:112–115, 1984.

80. Burgess LP, Morin GV, Rand M, et al: Wound healing: Relationship of wound closing tension to scar width in rats. Arch Otolaryngol Head Neck Surg 116:798–802, 1990.

81. Gunter JP, Carder HM, Fee WE: Rhomboid flap. Arch Otolaryngol 103:206–211, 1977.

82. Becker FF: Rhomboid flap in facial reconstruction: New concept of tension lines. Arch Otolaryngol 105:569–573, 1979.

83. Baker SR: Options for reconstruction in head and neck surgery. In Cummings CW, Fredrickson JM, Krause CJ, et al (eds): Otolaryngology–Head and Neck Surgery Update. St. Louis, CV Mosby, 1989, pp 192–248.

84. Toomey JM, Spector GJ: The buried nasolabial flap. Laryngoscope 89:847–848, 1979.

85. Baker SR, Swanson NA: Regional and distant skin flaps in nasal reconstruction. Facial Plast Surg 2:33–44, 1984.

86. Baker SR, Swanson NA: Oblique forehead flap for total reconstruction of the nasal tip and columella. Arch Otolaryngol 111:425–429, 1985.

87. Thomas JR, Griner N, Cook TA: The precise midline forehead flap as a musculocutaneous flap. Arch Otolaryngol Head Neck Surg 114:79–84, 1988.

88. Adamson JE: Nasal reconstruction with the expanded forehead flap. Plast Reconstr Surg 81:12–20, 1988.

89. Hoffman HT, Baker SR: Nasal reconstruction with the rapidly expanded forehead flap. Laryngoscope 99:1096–1098, 1989.

90. Mutter TD: Cases of deformity from burns, relieved by Aboration. Am J Med Sci 4:66–70, 1842.

91. Schuller DE: Cervical skin flaps in head and neck reconstruction. Am J Otolaryngol 2:62–68, 1981.

92. Conley JJ, Patow C: Cervical flaps. In Conley JJ, Patow C (eds): Flaps in Head and Neck Surgery. New York, Thieme Inc, 1989, p 156.

93. Bakamjian VY: A two-stage method for pharyngoesophageal reconstruction with a primary pectoral skin flap. Plast Reconstr Surg 36:173–184, 1965.

94. Krizek TJ, Robson MC: Potential pitfalls in the use of the deltopectoral flap. Plast Reconstr Surg 50:326–331, 1972.

95. Surkin MI, Lawson W, Biller HF: Analysis of the methods of pharyngoesophageal reconstruction. Head Neck Surg 6:953–970, 1984.

96. Price JC, Davis K: The deltopectoral flap vs the pectoralis major myocutaneous flap: Which one? Arch Otolaryngol 110:35–40, 1984.

97. Ariyan S: Further experiences with the pectoralis major myocutaneous flap for the repair of defects from excision of head and neck cancers. Plast Reconstr Surg 64:605–612, 1979.

98. Baek SM, Biller HF, Krespi YP, Lawson W: The pectoralis major myocutaneous island flap for reconstruction of the head and neck. Head Neck Surg 1:293–300, 1979.

99. Biller HF, Baek SM, Lawson W, et al: Pectoralis major myocutaneous island flap in head and neck surgery: Analysis of complications in 42 cases. Arch Otolaryngol 107:23–26, 1981.

100. Schuller DE: Limitations of the pectoralis major

myocutaneous flap in head and neck cancer reconstruction. Arch Otolaryngol 106:709–714, 1980.

101. Sharzer LA, Kalisman M, Silver CE, Strauch B: The parasternal paddle: A modification of the pectoralis major myocutaneous flap. Plast Reconstr Surg 67:753–762, 1981.

102. Schuller DE: Pectoralis myocutaneous flap in head and neck cancer reconstruction. Arch Otolaryngol 109:185–189, 1983.

103. Cusumano RJ, Silver CE, Brauer RJ, Strauch B: Pectoralis myocutaneous flap for replacement of cervical esophagus. Head Neck 11:450–456, 1989.

104. Schuller DE: Reconstructive options for pharyngeal and/or cervical esophageal defects. Arch Otolaryngol 111:193–197, 1985.

105. Silver CE, Cusumano RJ, Fell SC, Strauch B: Replacement of the upper esophagus: Results with myocutaneous flap and with gastric transposition. Laryngoscope 99:819–821, 1989.

106. Lam KH, Ho CM, Lau WF, et al: Immediate reconstruction of pharyngoesophageal defects: Preference or reference. Arch Otolaryngol Head Neck Surg 115:608–612, 1989.

106a. Fabian RL: Pectoralis major myocutaneous flap reconstruction of the laryngopharynx and cervical esophagus. Laryngoscope 98:1227–1231, 1988.

107. Murakami Y, Saito S, Ikari T, et al: Esophageal reconstruction with a skin-grafted pectoralis major muscle flap. Arch Otolaryngol 108:719–722, 1982.

108. Robertson MS, Robinson JM: Immediate pharyngoesophageal reconstruction: Use of a quilted skin-grafted pectoralis major muscle flap. Arch Otolaryngol 110:386–387, 1984.

109. Robertson MS, Robinson JM: Pharyngoesophageal reconstruction: Is a skin-lined pharynx necessary? Arch Otolaryngol 111:375–376, 1985.

110. Smith PG, Collins SL: Repair of head and neck defects with thin and double-lined pectoralis flaps. Arch Otolaryngol 110:468–473, 1984.

111. Baek SM, Lawson W, Biller HF: An analysis of 133 pectoralis major myocutaneous flaps. Plast Reconstr Surg 69:460–467, 1982.

111a. Shah J, Haribhakti V, Loree TR, Sutaria P: Complications of the pectoralis myocutaneous flap in head and neck reconstruction. Am J Surg 160:352–355, 1990.

112. Ossoff RH, Wurster CF, Berktold RE, et al: Complications after pectoralis major myocutaneous flap reconstruction of head and neck defects. Arch Otolaryngol 109:812–814, 1983.

113. Mehrhof AI, Rosenstock A, Neifeld JP, et al: The pectoralis major myocutaneous flap in head and neck reconstruction: Analysis of complications. Am J Surg 146:478–482, 1983.

114. Conley J: Use of composite flaps containing bone for major repairs in the head and neck. Plast Reconstr Surg 49:522–526, 1972.

115. Ariyan S: One-stage repair of a cervical esophagostome with two myocutaneous flaps from the neck and shoulder. Plast Reconstr Surg 63:426–429, 1979.

116. McGraw JB, Magee WP, Kalwaic H: Uses of the trapezius and sternomastoid myocutaneous flaps in head and neck reconstruction. Plast Reconstr Surg 63:49–59, 1979.

117. Panje WR: Myocutaneous trapezius flap. Head Neck Surg 2:206–212, 1980.

118. Panje WR, Schuller DE, Shagets FW: Musculocutaneous flap reconstruction of the head and neck. In Panje WR, Schuller DE, Shagets FW (eds): Trapezius Musculocutaneous Flap. New York, Raven Press, 1989, pp 25–44.

119. Netterville JL, Panje WR, Maves MD: The trapezius myocutaneous flap: Dependability and limitations. Arch Otolaryngol Head Neck Surg 113:271–281, 1987.

120. Demergasso F, Piazza MV: Trapezius myocutaneous flap in reconstructive surgery for head and neck cancer: An original technique. Am J Surg 138:533–536, 1979.

121. Goodwin WJ, Rosenberg GJ: Venous drainage of the lateral trapezius musculocutaneous island flap. Arch Otolaryngol Head Neck Surg 108:411–413, 1982.

122. Panje WR: A new method for total nasal reconstruction: The trapezius myocutaneous island 'paddle' flap. Arch Otolaryngol 108:156–161, 1982.

123. Baek S, Biller HF, Krespi YP, et al: Lower trapezius myocutaneous flap. Ann Plast Surg 5:108–114, 1980.

124. Krespi YP, Oppenheimer RW, Flanzer JM: The rhombotrapezius myocutaneous and osteocutaneous flaps. Arch Otolaryngol Head Neck Surg 114:734–738, 1988.

125. Urkin ML, Naidu RK, Lawson W, Biller HF: The lower trapezius island musculocutaneous flap revisited. Arch Otolaryngol Head Neck Surg 117:502–511, 1991.

126. Krespi YP, Baek SM, Surek CL: Flap reconstruction of the upper face: Free flaps vs. lower trapezius myocutaneous flap. Laryngoscope 93:485–488, 1983.

127. Baker SR: Closure of large orbital-maxillary defects with free latissimus dorsi myocutaneous flaps. Head Neck Surg 6:828–835, 1984.

128. Lassen M, Krag C, Nielsen IM: The latissimus dorsi flap: An overview. Scand J Plast Surg 19:41–51, 1985.

129. Quillen CG, Shearin JC, Georgiade NG: Use of the latissimus dorsi myocutaneous island flap for reconstruction in the head and neck area. Plast Reconstr Surg 62:113–117, 1978.

130. Russell RC, Pribaz J, Zook EG, et al: Functional evaluation of the latissimus dorsi donor site. Plast Reconstr Surg 78:336–344, 1986.

131. Tobin GR, Schusterman M, Peterson GH, et al: The intramuscular neurovascular anatomy of the latissimus dorsi muscle: The basis for splitting the flap. Plast Reconstr Surg 67:637–641, 1981.

132. Hayashi A, Maruyama Y: The reduced latissimus dorsi musculocutaneous flap. Plast Reconstr Surg 84:290–295, 1989.

133. Lineaweaver WC, Buncke GM, Buncke HJ: Hematoma in a latissimus dorsi donor site 21 months after surgery. Ann Plast Surg 21:143–144, 1988.

134. Barton FE, Spicer TE, Byrd HS: Head and neck reconstruction with the latissimus dorsi myocutaneous flap: Anatomic observations and report of 60 cases. Plast Reconstr Surg 71:199–204, 1983.

135. Chowdhury CR, McLean NR, Harrop-Griffiths K, Breach NM: The repair of defects in the head and neck region with the latissimus dorsi myocutaneous flap. J Laryngol Otol 102:1127–1132, 1988.

136. Maves MD, Panje WR, Shagets FW: Extended latissimus dorsi myocutaneous flap reconstruction of major head and neck defects. Otolaryngol Head Neck Surg 92:551–558, 1984.

137. Owens N: Compound neck pedicle designed for repair of massive facial defects. Plast Reconstr Surg 15:369–389, 1955.

138. Conley J, Gullane PJ: The sternocleidomastoid muscle flap. Head Neck Surg 2:308–311, 1980.

139. Gupta AK, Bhasin D, Shah R: Closure of post laryngectomy pharyngocutaneous fistula with sternocleidomastoid muscle flap. Ann Acad Med 12:407–410, 1983.

140. Barnes DR, Ossoff RH, Pecaro B, Sisson GA: Immediate reconstruction of mandibular defects with a composite sternocleidomastoid musculoclavicular graft. Arch Otolaryngol 107:711–714, 1981.

141. Sasaki CT: The sternocleidomastoid myocutaneous flap. Arch Otolaryngol 106:74–76, 1980.

142. Rubin JS: Sternocleidomastoid myoplasty for the repair of chronic cervical esophageal fistulae. Laryngoscope 96:834–836, 1986.

143. Jabaley ME, Heckler FR, Wallace WH, Knott LH: Sternocleidomastoid regional flaps: A new look at an old concept. Br J Plast Surg 32:106–113, 1979.

144. Ariyan S: One-stage reconstruction for defects of the mouth using a sternomastoid myocutaneous flap. Plast Reconstr Surg 63:618–625, 1979.

145. Charles GA, Hamaker RC, Singer MI: Sternocleidomastoid myocutaneous flap. Laryngoscope 97:970–974, 1987.

146. Futrell JW, Johns ME, Edgerton MT, et al: Platysma myocutaneous flap for intraoral reconstruction. Am J Surg 136:504–507, 1978.

147. Persky MS, Kaufman D, Cohen NL: Platysma myocutaneous flap for intraoral defects. Arch Otolaryngol 109:463–467, 1983.

Free Tissue Transfer in Head and Neck Reconstruction

DANIEL B. KURILOFF, MD
SHAN R. BAKER, MD

Microvascular free tissue transfer has become an increasingly popular technique in head and neck reconstruction.[1] Free tissue transfer offers greater versatility in selecting the best possible tissue replacement for complex defects following trauma or tumor extirpation.[2-6] Continuing investigation in regional anatomy and flap physiology over the past decade has led to an explosion in the variety of free tissue transfers available for head and neck reconstruction (Table 27–1). In the past, extensive tumor resections following radiotherapy, chemotherapy, or both, often involving loss of external skin, subcutaneous fat, mucosa, muscle, and bone, would have necessitated staged reconstructions employing local or regional pedicled flaps. However, these defects can now be reconstructed primarily in one stage using microvascular free grafts with a predictable high rate of success. Free tissue transfers based on large-caliber vessels can provide well-vascularized, nonirradiated skin, mucosa, bone, and composite tissue, including neurofaciocutaneous, musculocutaneous, osteocutaneous, and osteomusculocutaneous units, and have now become routine, with overall success rates approaching 95 per cent.[7-9] In addition, microvascular free flaps allow for soft tissue augmentation of the head and neck with restoration of normal contour and symmetry, without the problem of subsequent resorption or atrophy associated with nonrevascularized free grafts.[10] Superior functional and cosmetic single-stage reconstructions can now be achieved, with low complication rates and minimal donor site morbidity.

Although free tissue transfer allows increased freedom and economy of tissue in reconstruction relative to pedicled flaps, not every defect in the head and neck is optimally reconstructed with free flaps. These procedures are labor-intensive and must be individualized for each patient. More traditional reconstructive techniques, using pedicled, regional, or local flaps, may be a better option in selected patients. Perhaps more so than in

TABLE 27–1. Microvascular Free Flaps and Grafts

Cutaneous and Fasciocutaneous Flaps	Muscle and Musculocutaneous Flaps
Scalp and forehead	Latissimus dorsi
Deltopectoral	Serratus anterior
Lateral thoracic	Rectus femoris
Scapular, parascapular	Rectus abdominis
Deltoid	Pectoralis major
Forearm	Pectoralis minor
Medial arm	Tensor fascia lata
Lateral arm	Gracilis
Lateral thigh	**Osteomusculocutaneous Flaps**
Groin	Tensor fascia lata
Osteocutaneous Flaps	Deep circumflex iliac
Groin skin and iliac crest	Internal mammillary intercostal muscle
Chest skin and anterior rib	**Osteomuscular Flaps**
Dorsal foot skin and metatarsal bone	Tensor fascia lata
Lower leg skin and fibular bone	Serratus anterior
Back skin and scapular bone	Internal mammillary intercostal muscle
Forearm skin and radius bone	Iliac crest internal oblique muscle
Bone Grafts	**Other Grafts**
Rib	Omentum
Fibula	Jejunum
Iliac crest	Nerve (neurofasciocutaneous)
Radius	Toe transfer

(Modified from Baker SR: Microvascular free flaps in soft-tissue augmentation of the head and neck. Arch Otolaryngol Head Neck Surg 112:733, 1986. Copyright 1986, American Medical Association.)

any other surgical endeavor, patient selection, preoperative planning, and attention to the preparatory aspects of the procedure are crucial for achieving a successful outcome.

HISTORICAL BACKGROUND

Jacobson and Suarez are generally credited with the development of modern microvascular surgery.[11] They validated the technical feasibility of small vessel suture repair by using an operative microscope which they had seen used by otologic surgeons at the Mary Fletcher Hospital. Ultimately, this application led to the development of a Carl Zeiss double binocular microscope system. Other refinements in microvascular instrumentation pioneered in their laboratory included new microsutures, needles, and various small vessel approximating clamps. The first successful replantation of a severed arm was performed in 1962, by Malt and McKhann on a boy injured in a train accident.[12] Using 6.0 polyester suture for vascular anas-

tomoses, microvascular salvage ultimately resulted in a functional limb.

The first clinical application of free tissue transfer dates back to 1957. Following extirpation of a recurrent esophageal carcinoma, Seidenberg and colleagues performed a single-stage reconstruction of the cervical esophagus using a free segment of revascularized jejunum.[13] A nonsuture tantalum ring technique was used for the venous anastomosis, and a "continuous over-and-over" 7–0 silk suture technique for the arterial anastomosis. Despite this early report, free tissue transfer for head and neck reconstruction was rapidly overshadowed by the introduction of regional axial pattern skin flaps, such as the McGregor forehead flap (1963) and the Bakamjian deltopectoral flap (1965). The later introduction of well-vascularized myocutaneous flaps, based on the work by McGraw and coworkers,[14] Ariyan,[15] and Baek and colleagues[16] (pectoralis major, latissimus, trapezius) constituted a major advance in head and neck reconstruction.

Microsurgical tissue transplantation was reintroduced in 1972 with several clinical reports of free, vascularized, fasciocutaneous flap transfers.[17-19] McLean and Buncke, in the same year, reconstructed a large scalp defect using free revascularized omentum.[20] Fujino and Saito[21] and Panje and colleagues[22] introduced revascularized skin flaps for reconstruction of pharyngoesophageal and intraoral defects, respectively.

The introduction of the revascularized composite osteocutaneous groin flap by Taylor and colleagues[23] (1979), later modified by Urken and colleagues[24] (1989), and the scapular osteocutaneous free flap by Dos Santos[25] (1984), Swartz and colleagues[26] (1986), and Baker and Sullivan[27] (1988) contributed a new dimension to primary mandibular reconstruction. Lukash and associates (1987) reported the first use of osseointegrated implants in revascularized bone for dental rehabilitation.[28] Using implant-assisted or implant-borne dentures, Urken and associates (1989) recently described their encouraging experience with intraoperative placement of osseointegrated implants at the time of free tissue transfer.[29] In addition to obviating a second surgical procedure, primary implant placement offers a potentially more rapid attainment of total oromandibular reconstruction.

The recent use of neurofasciocutaneous free flaps has added yet another level of sophistication to head and neck reconstruction.[30, 31] Although still being assessed, revascularized sensate flaps may soon play a major role in improving deglutition, oral competence, aspiration, and speech following extirpation of head and neck cancer.

quelae of partial or complete vascular compromise. Although the success or failure of the reconstructive effort rests almost entirely on the technical proficiency of the microvascular surgeon, complications are occasionally unavoidable, with sequelae ranging from minor wound problems to anastomotic failure and total graft necrosis. Following complex and time-consuming reconstructive efforts, total flap loss can be catastrophic, causing considerable morbidity, prolonged hospitalization, severe functional and cosmetic deformity, and the need for additional surgical procedures. In the worst situation, death may occur due to flap failure, carotid artery rupture, or sepsis.

In addition, free tissue transfer for head and neck reconstruction is fraught with complicating factors not encountered by microvascular surgeons in other disciplines. The excessive mobility of the head and neck region, the cramped working area, the complicated orientation of the recipient vessels, problems associated with previous treatment (surgery, irradiation, and chemotherapy), and the complex three-dimensional nature of the defects to be reconstructed are among the many challenges posed by this advanced technique.

This chapter focuses on the conditions and preconditions leading to complications in free tissue transfer, their management, and their prevention. Patient selection, selection of appropriate donor tissues, technical and hemodynamic factors related to both microvascular anastomoses and flap inset, postoperative monitoring for early detection of thrombosis, anastomotic revision, and flap salvage, will be discussed in detail.

COMPLICATIONS

Microvascular surgery, because of the small dimensions of the structures involved and its technical difficulty, demands an extremely small margin of error. The survival of free tissue transfer depends on adequate tissue perfusion, which is dictated by the patency of arterial and venous microvascular anastomoses. Ultimately, most complications in microvascular surgery result from the se-

PATIENT SELECTION

Age

Microvascular tissue transfer has been successfully performed in patients ranging in age from 18 months to over 70 years.[32, 33] Free tissue transfer in the pediatric age group is often technically more difficult to perform

due to smaller recipient and donor vessels. However, with meticulous preoperative planning and technique, complications should be no greater than in the adult population. Advanced age alone is usually not a deterrent to microvascular surgery.[32] However, aging is often associated with diabetes mellitus, hypercholesterolemia, and arteriosclerosis, which may result in thickening of the walls of small arteries and overall increased vessel fragility and friability. Ohtsuka and colleagues described subintimal proliferation and elastolysis of the internal elastic lamina, causing increased vessel fragility in diabetic patients undergoing free tissue transfer.[34, 35] Despite this problem, free tissue transfers have been successfully performed in diabetic patients by use of meticulous microvascular technique. Experimentally, Van Gelder and Klopper found that the combination of vessel trauma associated with microvascular anastomoses and induced hypercholesterolemia in rabbits led to an accelerated formation of atherosclerosis.[36] The increased vessel fragility associated with atherosclerotic lesions, probably caused by abnormal collagen, tends to expose more connective tissue to the blood stream, thus increasing the risk of thrombosis. Brittle, calcified, atherosclerotic lesions may lead to heightened difficulties at the time of vessel anastomoses, resulting in technical failures.

Systemic Factors

Some systemic illnesses have a negative influence on the results of free tissue transfer. Patients with blood coagulopathies, collagen vascular disorders, sickle cell disease, and polycythemia in general are not candidates for microvascular surgery. Clinical and experimental studies have shown decreased flap blood flow, hypercoagulation, and decreased wound healing in cigarette smokers.[37–40] Cigarette smoking, therefore, should be strongly discouraged for at least one week prior to surgery and forbidden in the postoperative period. Obesity may influence successful surgery, particularly when it relates to the transfer of direct cutaneous flaps from the groin or chest areas. The increased adipose tissue makes dissection of the vascular pedicle difficult and interferes with proper placement and tailoring of the flap following transfer to the head and neck. This is particularly true when the oral cavity is the recipient site for the flap. Although the flap may be defatted at the time of transfer, extensive defatting increases the risk of injury to the vascular pedicle. In the case of the groin flap, subcutaneous fat overhangs the vascular pedicle, thereby making the vascular anastomoses problematic. Extreme obesity may necessitate the use of enteric grafts. However, fatty deposits in the mesentery of the jejunum can also make dissection of the vascular pedicle difficult.

Radiation Effects

Previous irradiation to the recipient bed or donor site can contribute to problems related to graft inset and vascular anastomoses. It is well known that cancericidal doses of radiotherapy produce vascular and fibrotic changes in normal tissue, which may interfere with healing.[41] Radiation injuries to large arteries (axillary, iliac, carotid) have been reported and consist of transmural fibrosis, elastic degeneration, severe atheromatous plaque formation, and calcific atherosclerosis.[42, 43] Compound flaps transferred by microvascular anastomoses are nourished by vascular pedicles that consist of small muscular arteries and venae comitantes. These vessels may be as small as 0.8 to 2.0 mm in diameter. Such small vessels are moderately radiosensitive and are susceptible to thrombosis following microvascular anastomoses.

Early effects of irradiation on small vessels include degeneration, swelling, and necrosis of the endothelium. The swollen endothelial cells narrow the lumen, and when necrosis occurs, loss of the endothelium allows the blood to come in contact with the subendothelial connective tissue, thus promoting thrombosis. In addition, radiation damage to small vessels and capillaries causes increased permeability, resulting in increased perivascular fluid, lumen narrowing, and, ultimately, thrombosis.

Late effects of radiation injury to small blood vessels include fibrosis and increased interstitial connective tissue in the tunica media, along with endothelial proliferation and progressive fibrosis. This further thickens the vessel wall and narrows the lumen, eventually causing occlusion. Even in cases of slowly progressive vessel fibrosis, the obstructive nature of these changes may severely compromise the vascular supply to a particular area. These areas may then succumb to necrosis when subjected to an additional injury or increased functional demand.

Numerous animal studies examining the effects of radiation therapy on microvascular anastomoses have yielded conflicting results. Baker and associates[44] and De Wilde and Donders[45] found histologic evidence of vessel injury but no decrease in anastomotic patency rates when radiation was given preoperatively. Histologic changes following irradiation and microvascular anastomosis consisted of increased fibrosis and increased smooth muscle proliferation in response to injury at the anastomotic site (Fig. 27–1). Scanning electron microscopy revealed decreased epithelial regeneration, increased fibrin and platelet deposition, as well as a higher incidence of microthrombi compared with controls. Fried[46] and Cunningham and Shons[47] transferred nonirradiated free flaps to irradiated recipient sites. Again, although histologic evidence of vessel injury was found in the irradiated groups, no deleterious effects on anastomotic patency could be

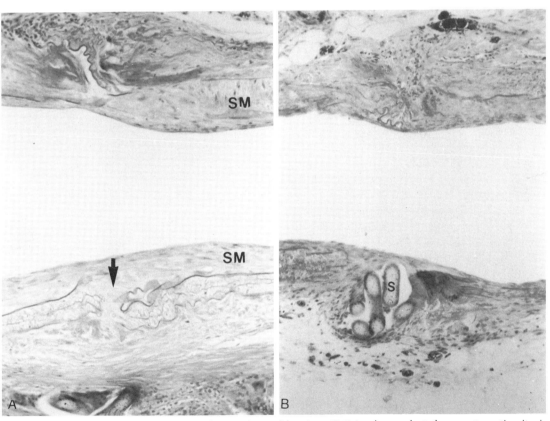

FIGURE 27–1. *A,* Subendothelial smooth muscle proliferation *(SM)* is observed at the anastomotic site in response to preoperative irradiation (1000 rad once a week for 6 weeks). Disruption of the internal elastic membrane is well demonstrated *(arrow).* (Hematoxylin and eosin, ×20.) *B,* Collagen deposits and smooth muscle proliferation are less notable in this control vessel. *S,* Suture. (Hematoxylin and eosin, ×20.) (From Baker SR, Krause CJ, Panje WR: Radiation effects on microvascular anastomosis. Arch Otolaryngol 104:103, 1978, with permission. Copyright 1978, American Medical Association.)

demonstrated. In contrast, Watson found decreased venous patency rates but normal arterial patency rates compared with nonirradiated control femoral vessels.[48] Tan and associates delivered a single dose of 2000 rads to the femoral vessels of rabbits.[49] At 6 and 16 weeks following irradiation, nonirradiated groin flaps were transferred to the irradiated recipient sites. For both groups, flap survival was only 50 per cent. Krag and associates irradiated the carotid artery and jugular vein in rabbits (5000 rads over 5 weeks).[50] Free groin flaps were anastomosed to both irradiated and control vessels. All flaps anastomosed to the normal vessels survived, whereas only 68 per cent of flaps anastomosed to the irradiated neck vessels remained viable.

In a clinical study, Guelinckx and associates examined irradiated recipient vessels in the neck (5000 rads, fractionated to 200 rads/day over 5-day periods) sampled just prior to microvascular anastomoses.[51] Using scanning electron microscopy, they found an overall increase in arterial wall thickness, especially in the tunica media. Fibrin deposits, microthrombi, and dehiscence of intercellular bonds were appreciably greater in the irradiated vessels compared with nonirradiated controls. Irradiated vessels were surrounded by a large amount of periadventitial fibrosis. Despite gentle tissue handling during vessel dissection, intimal pieces became dislodged from several irradiated vessels when their ends were cut. Irregularities in the vessel end complicated anastomoses. Total intimal separation was noted in two heavily irradiated facial arteries while the end was trimmed. These investigators now recommend the use of an inside-to-outside perforating technique for suturing irradiated blood vessels, which helps prevent further dehiscence of the damaged intima or calcific plaque in the media (Fig. 27–2).

Following full-course radiotherapy to the head and neck, varying degrees of adventitial and periadventitial fibrosis make atraumatic recipient vessel dissection more difficult. Encasement of recipient vessels in thick fibrous tissue often requires more aggressive proximal adventitial dissection to allow dilatation

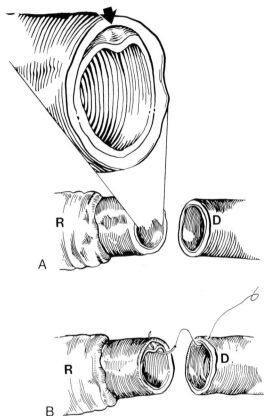

FIGURE 27–2. *A,* Separation of intima from wall of damaged irradiated recipient blood vessel *(arrow). B,* An inside-to-outside perforating technique for suturing an irradiated recipient blood vessel. This method helps prevent further dehiscence of the damaged intima or calcific plaque in the media. *R,* Recipient irradiated vessel; *D,* healthy donor vessel.

and prevention of vessel kinking and torsion. Vessel selection to achieve a good match between recipient and donor vessel diameters can be misleading when examining irradiated vessels. For similar outer diameters, irradiated vessels have lower flow rates than nonirradiated vessels.[52] In our experience at the University of Michigan, in patients previously irradiated with or without induction chemotherapy, the need for more extensive periadventitial dissection, combined with the increased friability of previously irradiated vessels, makes vascular spasm an important complicating factor in performing microvascular anastomoses. In several cases, despite aggressive use of various topical vasodilating agents, vascular spasm could not be broken and alternate recipient vessels had to be used.

There has been relatively little investigation concerning neovascularization of free tissue transfers. Black and associates,[53] Tsur and associates,[54] and Serafin and colleagues[55] demonstrated experimentally that adequate neovascularization from the recipient site to support survival of a free tissue graft normally occurs within 5 to 8 days following transfer. Rothaus and Acland reported complete flap survival when the arterial inflow to a free groin flap failed on the ninth postoperative day.[56] This time-frame, however, may vary depending on the status of the recipient bed and the type of donor tissue. Fisher and Wood described delayed necrosis of a latissimus dorsi free muscle graft 7 months after microvascular transfer.[57] Blunt trauma, resulting in hematoma formation and pedicle occlusion, was the likely etiology in this case. Neovascularization from the recipient bed was not sufficient to support the muscle.

Malnutrition, commonly seen in the head and neck cancer patient, may play an important role in poor healing and subsequent delayed neovascularization of the free tissue graft. The endarteritis and fibrosis induced by radiotherapy has a profound deleterious effect on the microcirculation of the recipient bed, which may prolong the time needed for neovascularization beyond 8 days. Clark and associates studied the radiation effects on neovascularization of normal groin free flaps placed into an irradiated recipient site in rats.[58] They subsequently ligated the vascular pedicle to evaluate early neovascularization of the free flap from the irradiated bed. In rats with irradiated recipient sites, significantly less tissue survived complete occlusion of the vascular pedicle by the second to fourth postoperative day than occurred in nonirradiated controls. This difference in survival was not observed if the vascular pedicles were ligated beyond 5 days following free flap transfer, suggesting adequate neovascularization at that time.

The threshold for primary or secondary ischemia time for each type of free tissue transfer has yet to be elucidated. Free enteric grafts, for example, due to a segmental blood supply, tubular anatomy, and thick serosa, may be less tolerant of prolonged ischemia times and may require longer periods for neovascularization than do fasciocutaneous flaps (Table 27–2).

Although both clinical evidence and experimental evidence demonstrate that irradiation causes significant irreversible damage to recipient blood vessels and to the microvasculature of the recipient bed, these factors alone are not sufficient to cause failure of free tissue transfer. However, in combination with other deleterious technical or physiologic conditions, radiation may indeed be responsible for anastomotic failure or delayed neovascularization, making late graft failure possible. The effects of radiation therapy create technically more difficult anastomoses, requiring extraordinary care in vessel handling, preparation, and suturing.

Dense fibrosis in the neck, either from previous surgery or irradiation, may limit the availability or adequacy of donor vessels and is an important consideration in patient selection and preoperative planning. The status of the superficial and deep venous systems, as well as the external carotid artery and its branches following previous neck dissection, may need to be assessed preoperatively by angiography. Despite the well-known toxic effects of radiocontrast media on blood vessels,[59] experimental data evaluating the use of Renografin-76 in rats showed no increased

TABLE 27–2. Maximal Ischemia Time Compatible with Survival for Various Tissues

Tissue	Maximal Ischemia Time (Hr)
Skin (pig)	21
Nerve (rat)	>8
Digit (human)	6
Muscle (human)	6
Fibroblast (culture)	>4
Gut (dog)	2–4
Endothelium (rabbit)	0.04

(From Panje WR, Schuller DE, Shagets FW: Musculocutaneous flap reconstruction of the head and neck. *In* Panje WR, Schuller DE, Shagets FW (eds): Physiological and Practical Considerations in Musculocutaneous Flap Reconstruction. New York, Raven Press, 1989, p 13.)

rate of anastomotic failure.[60] Using a rabbit model, Sheppard and Dell found that if injection pressures of arteriography were carefully controlled, there was no histologic effect on vascular endothelium.[61] Furthermore, the survival of composite tissue transfer was not affected by arteriography performed 24 hours prior to replantation. Despite these findings, it would be prudent to limit the dose and concentration of the radiocontrast medium to the minimum required for adequate vessel imaging. Operation also should be delayed for 3 to 5 days following angiography to allow some reversal of the potential vascular effects of radiocontrast media.

TECHNICAL CONSIDERATIONS

Surgical precision is perhaps the single most important factor in dictating a successful free tissue transfer. Most surgeons who have no training in microvascular surgery tend to think of the technique as a challenge in anastomosing small blood vessels. In fact, this is only a small part, and at times, the easier part of the whole procedure, which has numerous other detailed facets. The entire process can be divided into seven important stages:

1. Extirpation of disease. The extent of resection must be dictated by the extent of tumor. Oncologic margins must never be compromised to accommodate the reconstruction.
2. Preparation of the recipient vessels in the neck. This may actually begin at the start of the resection by preservation of the external or internal jugular veins or transverse cervical vessels, if oncologically sound.
3. Harvesting the donor tissue graft. This stage may have been initiated prior to completion of the resection and left pedicled until actual transfer.
4. Initial insetting, bone contouring, and preliminary fixation. The free graft is often secured in place with tacking sutures or reconstruction plates to determine proper orientation and placement of the vascular pedicle.

5. Microvascular anastomoses.
6. Reperfusion and assessment.
7. Final flap inset, tailoring, and closure, with attention to drain placement.

Ideally, a two-team approach should be used to prepare the recipient and donor sites. In addition, an assistant with training in microsurgical technique is indispensable for performing the microvascular anastomoses. This approach helps decrease operative time, helps assure good coordination between flap harvesting and inset, and allows the microvascular surgeon to focus on the task at hand with minimal fatigue.

General Factors

It is essential that the patient be kept warm (heating blanket), normotensive, and well-hydrated throughout the procedure. A hematocrit of 30 is adequate for oxygen transport and delivery and is optimal in terms of low viscosity flow.[62] Maintaining these parameters will help prevent peripheral vasoconstriction and vascular spasm. Placement of ipsilateral peripheral venous catheters that enter the subclavian vein may cause retrograde internal jugular vein thrombosis and should be avoided prior to or following free tissue transfer. Warm physiologic saline must be available throughout the procedure for frequent irrigation of the flap and vessels.

Patient Positioning and Instrumentation

The patient is usually positioned on a Mayfield headrest and turned 180° to allow unrestricted access to the neck. When needed, the patient is also positioned over a deflatable beanbag mattress to facilitate precise, secure positioning. All pressure points are padded with foam cushions, the legs are wrapped with Ace bandages to prevent venous stasis, and an axillary roll is placed to protect the brachial plexus when a lateral decubitus position is needed for flap harvest. Eventually, a second set of surgical instruments will be needed to avoid contamination of the donor site. If an antiplatelet agent is to be used (Rheomacrodex), then it should be available in the operating room at the outset.

Well in advance of the vessel anastomoses, a back table must be set up with the microsurgical instruments, warm irrigating solutions, background material, Weck-Cel surgical spears, and microsutures. The microscope should always be checked (light source, objective lens, power zoom, etc.) prior to the procedure, and draped sterilely in advance. A sterile intraoperative Doppler probe should be available to aid in vascular pedicle identification and confirmation of vessel patency following the microvascular anastomoses. A scrub nurse well-versed in microvascular surgery is essential if primary ischemia time is to be minimized. Handling of the expensive, delicate instruments must be done carefully to avoid damage. The reconstruction, in terms of the choice of donor sites, timing of flap harvest, and final insetting, must be thoroughly discussed with both the patient as well as all members of the surgical team prior to operation. In addition, a preconceived alternative reconstructive plan must be ready for implementation in the event of unsuitable recipient vessels or unsalvageable primary graft failure.

Preparation of Recipient Vessels

Which specific recipient vessels are used is usually dictated by the operation performed at the recipient site. The superficial temporal, facial, lingual, superior thyroid, and transverse cervical arteries commonly serve as recipient arteries for free tissue transfer. The superficial temporal, facial, lingual, external and internal jugular, transverse cervical, and cervical cutaneous veins most frequently serve as recipient veins.

The recipient vessels are carefully dissected using gentle vascular technique. Minimal handling of the vessel wall itself may be facilitated by grasping adjacent tissue. Periadventitial fibrous tissue and adventitia are dissected proximally for several millimeters to prevent vessel spasm and kinking and to insure flexibility for good vessel geometry. To maximize the length of the recipient vessels, small branches are ligated with vascular clips or carefully coagulated away from the main vessel with the bipolar electrocautery. The vessels are not divided or clamped until the free graft has been harvested and the microscope and instrument table are ready. Throughout the dissection, warm physiologic saline is used for irrigation, along with topical vasodilators to prevent vascular spasm. The recipient artery must demonstrate brisk pulsatile flow upon release of the vascular clamp prior to anastomosis. Vessel spasm, especially in fragile irradiated vessels, may require more aggressive proximal adventitial dissection. Occasionally, despite warming and use of vasodilators, persistent vasospasm or inadequate flow will necessitate selection of an alternate recipient artery, which may require an interpositional vein graft.

Interpositional Vein Grafting

Vein grafts are needed when the vascular pedicle is short, the contralateral neck must be reached due to recipient vessel unavailability, or vessel geometry is unsatisfactory. Blair and colleagues demonstrated experimentally that although hemodynamic characteristics are altered, volumetric flow can be restored after interpositional vein grafting in small arteries.[63] Excessively long vein grafts, however, may have a tendency toward thrombosis in low-flow states, which should be a consideration in overall planning. Melka and associates studied the fate of microarterial grafts versus microvenous grafts in rabbits.[64] Based on morphologic aspects, patency rates, and histologic features, the arterial grafts gave better long-term results than the venous grafts. Venous grafts were noted by 15 days postoperatively to undergo intimal hyperplasia, with proliferation of smooth muscle cells and elastic fibers. By 3 months the lumen of the vein grafts became narrowed, and smooth muscle proliferation was replaced by subintimal fibrotic changes. Despite these histologic changes, interpositional vein grafts still gave a high patency rate (90 per cent at 2 weeks and 80 per cent at 3 months) after the operation.

Superficial veins are used in preference to

arterial grafts because of their widespread availability and ease of harvest. Vein grafts are commonly harvested from the superficial saphenous system of the thigh, or from the cephalic or basilic system of the arm. The cephalic vein can serve as a recipient vessel when transposed from the upper arm into the neck.[65] Vein harvesting must be performed using meticulous and gentle microvascular technique. Minimal handling of the vessel may be facilitated by grasping adjacent tissue during dissection, instead of the vessel adventitia. Vasospasm is best treated with topical vasodilators. Side branches are clipped, or ligated close enough to the vessel wall to prevent long stumps but without narrowing the lumen. An estimation of vessel diameter is made immediately after exposure, prior to the onset of vascular spasm, assuring a maximum 2:1 discrepancy in vessel diameter at the anastomosis. Diameter mismatches of greater than 2:1 are associated with turbulent flow and a greater risk of anastomotic failure.

Vein grafts are irrigated with heparinized saline to remove gross clot and twist in the vein prior to performing the anastomosis. High-pressure hydrostatic dilatation, however, must be avoided, since this may damage the vessel wall.[66] The direction of flow should be carefully noted by placing a suture on the proximal end (by convention), since valves will prevent reversed flow in a vein graft. Vein grafts are reversed for arterial anastomoses (Fig. 27–3). Valves should be resected when close to the suture line to prevent turbulence and the potential for thrombosis. Potential donor sites for vein graft harvest should be prepped at the start of surgery when the need for vein grafting is anticipated.

Graft Harvest and Preparation

Considerable thought and preoperative planning must go into selection of the appropriate donor site to be used, which will be discussed later in this chapter. Ideally, the donor tissue graft should be harvested prior to, or simultaneously with, preparation of the recipient vessels. This serves to minimize primary ischemia time and hasten overall operative time. Surface landmarks are identified; the size of the skin island to be transferred, either as a monitor or for soft tissue coverage, is measured, overestimating by 2 to 3 cm to allow for shrinkage and facilitate insetting. Flap elevation proceeds at a slower pace as the vascular pedicle is approached. The pedicle dissection is aided by the use of loupes, especially when dealing with smaller vessels 1 to 2 mm in diameter. The vascular pedicle should not be excessively skeletonized to avoid direct vessel injury or precipitate vasospasm. The vascular pedicle is dis-

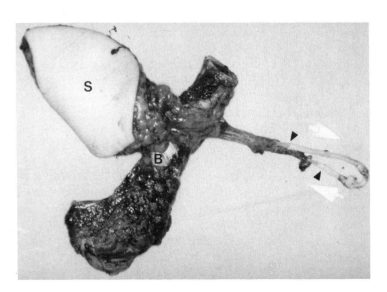

FIGURE 27–3. Osteocutaneous scapular free flap with a single vein graft anastomosed to the vascular pedicle *(arrowheads)*. S, Skin paddle; B, scapular bone. The vein graft will be divided prior to anastomosis to recipient vessels in the contralateral neck. This method avoids confusion with valve orientation and assures proper direction of blood flow *(white arrows)*.

sected as far as possible to its parent vessels to gain maximum length. Large side branches are carefully ligated. Hemoclips and bipolar cautery are often used for smaller side branches and can speed up the dissection. Bleeding vessels from the graft tissue must be carefully ligated or electrocoagulated to prevent subsequent bleeding and the potential for hematoma formation after revascularization.

The conventional monopolar cautery may be used away from the vascular pedicle. However, bipolar cautery is used exclusively for cauterizing vessels near the pedicle or for side branches. We have found that the bipolar cautery is a valuable tool for increasing the speed of dissection along the vascular pedicle. Unlike the monopolar cautery, current passes primarily between the tips of the forceps, avoiding spread of injury to structures more than 1 to 2 mm away.[67, 68] Some of this spread may be due to thermal injury. Caffee and Ward found that vessel side branches could be coagulated using the bipolar device without damaging the parent vessel or adversely affecting an adjacent anastomosis.[69] They stressed the importance of using a device whose output produces a continuous sine wave current to minimize voltage. In addition, the equipment should be designed to sense impedance and automatically shut down at the point of desiccation, thus avoiding sparking, charring, and adherence of tissue to the forceps. Caffee and Ward concluded that this form of bipolar energy was safe for use in microvascular surgery.

The donor tissue is left pedicled until the recipient site and vessels are ready for transfer. At this time the perfusion of the graft is assessed by both inspection (capillary refill, dermal bleeding, color, peristalsis for jejunum) and direct Doppler probe flow signals. The distal end of the pedicle is clamped. The proximal end is divided sharply with tenotomy scissors, preventing a crush injury that would require vessel resection and undesirable shortening of the vascular pedicle. The ends of the donor vessels are gently irrigated with heparinized saline (20 U/ml of saline) to remove gross clots.[70] Clamp time is

recorded to monitor the duration of primary ischemia.

Perfusion of free flaps with various solutions prior to transfer has not been shown to increase safe primary ischemia times and is not recommended. In fact, Gould and associates, using a rabbit model, found that early perfusion, prior to cold storage, had a detrimental effect on flap survival.[71] Chait and associates demonstrated that early perfusion was also detrimental to flap survival following normothermic storage.[72]

The exact "safe" primary ischemia time for various clinical free tissue transfers has not been elucidated. It is thought that more metabolically active tissue is less resistant to the effects of ischemia. Intestinal grafts such as free jejunum will tolerate only 60 to 90 minutes of warm ischemia.[73] Skeletal muscle will tolerate up to 6 hours of warm ischemia and cutaneous flaps, up to 8 hours.[74] May and associates, using the rabbit as an animal model, demonstrated 100 per cent flap survival after 4 hours of normothermic ischemia, 80 per cent flap survival after 8 hours, and total necrosis following 12 hours of normothermic ischemia[75] (see Table 27–2).

Hypothermia may increase tissue viability. This is most useful for limb and digit replantation when ischemia times are often prolonged. Clinically successful digit replantation has been reported following 6 hours of normothermia (20 to 25° C) or 24 hours of hypothermia (0 to 4° C).[76] Ballantyne and coworkers found that rat groin flaps tolerated up to 72 hours of cold ischemia (4° C) with a high survival rate following revascularization.[77] Donski and associates reported a 50 per cent free flap survival following 3 to 5 days of hypothermic storage.[78] Histologically, however, fat, muscle, and microvessels were generally inflamed, fibrotic, or necrotic. Longer periods of ischemia, even with cooling, led to extensive tissue injury, especially in the microvasculature, ultimately resulting in necrosis. In actual clinical practice, with the exception of free jejunum (discussed later), and when excessively long warm ischemia times are unavoidable (more than 4 hours), hypothermia is rarely necessary. Unplanned interruption of surgery following flap harvest, caused by patient instability, would require cold storage for flap survival. Revascularization would then be performed as soon as the patient was stabilized.[79]

Donor Site Closure and Graft Insetting

The donor site is closed immediately after flap harvest. In some situations, wide skin undermining is necessary to prevent excessive wound tension. On occasion, retention sutures are placed. The radial forearm donor site generally requires split-thickness skin grafting, which must be anticipated prior to operation. Abdominal wall closure, as with the rectus abdominis and iliac crest grafts, must be carefully performed to avoid herniation or wound dehiscence and on occasion will require reinforcement with Marlex mesh. Suction drains are carefully placed and a multilayered closure is performed.

The first step after flap transfer is insetting. The soft tissue, with or without bone, is positioned within the defect and temporarily secured with tacking sutures. If bone is transfered, ostectomies are performed for contour and then rigidly fixed to a previously placed mandibular reconstruction plate prior to performing the anastomoses. Securing the graft initially will prevent accidental avulsion following completion of the anastomoses. In addition, this preliminary three-dimensional positioning insures that vascular pedicle geometry will not cause torsion, kinking, compression, or excessive tension across the anastomoses.

VASCULAR PEDICLE GEOMETRY AND ANASTOMOTIC TECHNIQUE

Geometry

When feasible, the free tissue graft is positioned so that the vascular pedicle lies closest to available recipient vessels, both in an attempt to minimize the use of vein grafts and to create the best vascular geometry for blood flow.[80] When suitable recipient vessels are not available in the operated neck or excessive tension would result, interposi-

tional vein grafts may be required to reach recipient vessels from the contralateral side or to reach the transverse cervical vessels low in the ipsilateral neck. If excessively long, the vascular pedicle must be trimmed to prevent kinking. When oncologically sound, we generally prefer to preserve the internal jugular vein for end-to-side anastomosis. The superior thyroid artery, along with several other branches of the external carotid system, can be transposed into the ipsilateral neck, where they generally serve as adequate recipient vessels. The transverse cervical vessels are also useful because they are often less heavily irradiated. In addition, when transposed cephalad, they lie in the axis of neck rotation, making vessel kinking less likely. The recipient artery should demonstrate brisk pulsatile flow.

Attention to vessel geometry is crucial at this juncture. Ideally, both recipient artery and vein should run along the same axis. The so-called "lie" of the vessels must be studied carefully and adjustments made when needed prior to vessel shortening or clamp placement. This is especially true for long vascular pedicles and interpositional vein grafts. The excessive mobility of the head and neck region may cause vessel kinking or twisting with certain head positions. This should also be assessed prior to vessel anastomoses. Following reperfusion, vessel kinking or suboptimal angulation of end-to-side anastomoses occasionally occurs and requires placement of adventitial tacking sutures (Fig. 27–4). Rarely, more than one artery, and commonly more than one vena comitans, are present. When two arteries are present, the more central vessel is chosen.

Selection of an end-to-end versus an end-to-side anastomosis depends on vascular geometry, including the overall size of the vessel diameters, their degree of diameter mismatch, and the availability of recipient vessels. End-to-end anastomoses are preferred when there is little size discrepancy between the recipient and donor vessels. This is usually possible for most arterial anastomoses. Large discrepancies in vessel size cause bunching, exposure of collagen, and increased risk of thrombosis. A vessel size mismatch greater than 2:1 but less than 3:1 requires spatulation or angulation of one ves-

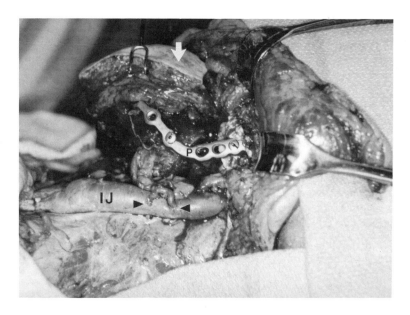

FIGURE 27–4. Osteocutaneous scapular free flap with two venae comitantes anastomosed end-to-side to the internal jugular vein *(IJ)*. Skin paddle *(arrow)* rests on top of the mandibular reconstruction plate *(P)*, immobilizing the scapular bone. The "lie" of the donor veins relative to the IJ is adjusted with tacking sutures to prevent vessel kinking *(arrowheads)*.

sel end. In this situation an end-to-side anastomosis is preferable if vascular geometry permits this. Theoretically, anastomotic angles exceeding 30° may cause excessive turbulence, intimal injury, and subsequent thrombosis. Despite the theoretic increase in turbulence for end-to-side anastomoses, experimental and clinical results show no decrease in patency rates with this method.[81, 82]

Bas and associates compared end-to-end with end-to-side venous anastomoses for similar and size-discrepant vessels in a rat model.[83] Patency rates were higher for the end-to-side technique for size-discrepant veins—85 per cent versus 50 per cent patency rates, respectively. Advantages of end-to-side anastomoses include the "stenting" effect of the venotomy on the smaller vessel acting to counteract spasm, the "washing" effect of high flow in the larger vein discouraging platelet aggregation, preservation of existing vessels, and greater freedom in operative planning.[81, 84] We prefer an end-to-side venous anastomosis to the internal jugular vein whenever possible. When the recipient artery is small and pulsatile flow is poor, end-to-side anastomosis of the donor artery to the external carotid artery, or a large branch, is performed. Anastomoses performed adjacent to bifurcations or large side branches should be avoided but experimentally have not shown a significant risk of thrombosis from increased turbulence.[85]

Anastomotic Technique

The details of performing microvascular anastomoses are beyond the scope of this chapter, and the reader is encouraged to consult other excellent texts devoted to this topic.[86] Several technical points, however, should be stressed, as they relate to preparation, atraumatic vessel handling, suturing technique, and prevention of clot formation.

Careful preparation of the operative site is essential. This includes proper microscope placement to avoid awkward hand and arm positions during suturing, building up the undersurface of the background material to raise the approximating clamp slightly out of the wound, and packing off surrounding tissue that tends to obscure a wide field of vision. Minimal vessel handling is important throughout. Appropriate microvascular approximating clamps should be used to avoid excessive transmural pressures (more than 30 g/mm²) and crush injury. Vessel dilatation should be gentle, especially with fragile, irradiated vessels in which the intima has a tendency to fracture away from the media. Atheromatous plaque is not removed since this would injure the intima and lead to thrombosis. If pedicle length is not critical, these areas can be resected.

Suturing Methods

We generally prefer the interrupted suture technique, especially when the vessels are not well matched. For vessels larger than 2.5 mm in diameter, a continuous suture technique can save operative time. However, when vessel mismatch is significant and lumen size is small, the continuous suture technique may result in excessive narrowing of the anastomoses. We prefer a continuous suture technique for end-to-side anastomoses to the internal jugular vein. The risk of lumen narrowing here is minimal. Experimentally, patency rates for the two techniques are identical.[87] Telescoping end-in-end or sleeve anastomoses have been described by Siemionow and others for small arteries.[88] Since only two sutures are tied at 180° apart from each other, operative time may be reduced. Healing was rapid and long-term patency rates equal to traditional end-to-end techniques.[89] We have no experience with this method, which does cause initial narrowing at the anastomotic site (18 per cent to 25 per cent) and the potential for early failure. The increase in speed is advantageous only when multiple arterial anastomoses are required, as in limb replantation.

Generally, the deepest of the vessel anastomoses is performed first, and all clamps are left in place until completion of both anastomoses. Microvascular clamps are released in such a way that lower pressure flow occurs first—e.g., donor vein clamp first, then recipient vein, then donor artery, then recipient artery. This avoids tissue engorgement and may demonstrate large vessel leaks early. Venous leaks are generally less common than arterial leaks and often stop after a minute or two. Often anastomotic leakage requires one additional suture that may be carefully placed without reclamping the recipient vessels. Placing a through-stitch, although diminished with the vessel lumen fully distended, must be avoided. Occasionally, continued leak from the anastomosis

will necessitate reclamping of vessels to facilitate additional suturing. For arterial anastomotic revision, reclamping of the artery only is necessary. When revising a venous anastomosis, however, both recipient artery and vein should be clamped to prevent donor vein engorgement and potential endothelial injury.

Fahmy and Moneim, using a rat femoral artery model, found that the "safe limit" for blood stasis in a repaired artery of 0.8 mm was 90 minutes.[90] In their study, only 10 minutes was allowed for blood flow across the anastomosis prior to vessel reclamping for the specified intervals. Pottie and associates found that proximal reclamping of vessels 15 minutes following completion of microvascular anastomoses, for periods of up to 4 hours, had no adverse affect on short- or long-term anastomotic patency despite prolonged blood stasis.[91] They postulated that technically well-performed anastomoses that remain patent after 15 minutes of blood flow can be regarded and treated as normal vessels. Static blood across the anastomosis of pedicle vessels should not affect their patency up to the time when the no-reflow phenomenon sets in.

Thrombogenesis

In the absence of a hypercoagulable state, the primary factors involved in microvascular thrombosis are stasis and vessel injury with subsequent platelet aggregation (white clot). Collagen fibers are routinely exposed following transection of the vessel wall, manipulation, and clamping. Morecraft and associates showed that extensive endothelial loss occurs spanning the lumen from clamp site to clamp site, especially at the suture region, as early as 1 hour after microvascular anastomoses.[92]

Complete endothelial regeneration across a microvascular anastomosis occurs within 7 to 14 days (Fig. 27–5).[93, 94] Until endothelialization is complete, collagen exposure within the vessel lumen, which is richly distributed in the media and adventitia of the vessel wall, serves as a potent stimulator of platelet aggregation and mediator release. In addi-

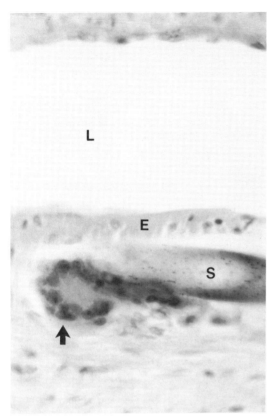

FIGURE 27–5. Complete regeneration of the endothelium *(E)* across a microvascular anastomosis takes up to 2 weeks. A subendothelial multinucleated foreign body giant cell *(arrow)* is seen adjacent to a suture *(S)*. L, Lumen. (Hematoxylin and eosin, × 40.) (From Baker SR, Krause CJ, Panje WR: Radiation effects on microvascular anastomosis. Arch Otolaryngol 104:103, 1978, with permission. Copyright 1978, American Medical Association.)

tion, adventitial strands resulting from inadequate dissection at vessel ends may become incorporated into the vessel lumen following completion of anastomoses. Thrombus formation is initiated by platelet aggregation, membrane deformation with granule release, fibrinogen binding, and activation of thrombin. Fibrinogen, adenosine diphosphate (ADP), serotonin, and thromboxane A_2 are released and perpetuate platelet aggregation. Arachidonic acid derivatives are converted by cyclo-oxygenase to prostaglandin endoperoxides, which ultimately form thromboxane A_2 and prostacycline. Prostacycline, primarily produced by the vessel wall, has powerful antiaggregation effects that serve

to prevent the progression to thrombus formation.

When vascular injury is slight, the normal equilibrium between thromboxane and prostacycline is shifted toward the former. This allows the formation of a reparative platelet plug to arrest hemorrhage but does not allow progression of an occluding thrombus. When vascular injury is severe, extensive exposure of platelets to vessel wall collagen initiates thromboxane synthesis and the simultaneous activation of the vascular coagulation cascade that may overwhelm the antiaggregation effect of prostacycline. The resulting widespread platelet aggregation, vasoconstriction, fibrin formation, and thrombus propagation lead to irreversible vessel occlusion.[95]

Therefore, it should be the goal of every microvascular surgeon to perform technically perfect anastomoses. This requires the absolute minimum of endothelial trauma and collagen exposure. In summary, this can be achieved by handling vessels gently, use of high-quality low-pressure microvascular clamps, and assuring proper vessel geometry to avoid sluggish or excessively turbulent blood flow.

Vasospasm

Vasospasm may play an important role in thrombus formation by decreasing flow rates across anastomoses and increasing concentrations of platelet-aggregating factors. Severe vasospasm may cause intimal injury or separation. Therefore, vasospasm must be prevented throughout all microvascular procedures, including flap or graft harvest. Vasospasm is thought to be caused by several factors, including excessive intraoperative manipulation of the cut vessels, tension across the anastomosis, exposure of the extraluminal vessel surface to fresh blood, desiccation of the vessel, excessive heating in the field of cauterization, or exposure to cold. Each one of these issues must be addressed by the microvascular surgeon. Vessel manipulation must be gentle without handling of the vessel ends, the surgical field should be kept free of fresh blood, warm physiologic saline should be used continuously to avoid vessel desiccation and cooling, and the patient's core temperature and room temperature must be maintained at normal levels.

Irrigating Solutions

There has been conflicting evidence concerning the experimental effects of different irrigating solutions on the endothelium of small vessels.[96] Mazer and colleagues, in an exhaustive study, found normal saline to be less irritating to vascular endothelium than Ringer solution.[97] This is in contrast to Acland's group, who found the reverse to be true.[98] Various topical spasmolytic agents, including Chlorpromazine HCl (Thorazine), 2 per cent to 20 per cent plain lidocaine (Xylocaine), reserpine, 0.3 per cent papaverine, and magnesium sulfate, have been evaluated experimentally. Acland suggested that magnesium sulfate solution reduced both vasospasm and platelet adhesion.[99] He demonstrated increased patency rates of microvascular anastomoses compared with controls, by irrigating the anastomosed vessels with isotonic magnesium sulfate for 20 minutes following anastomosis. Hoe and group, using a rat femoral artery model, found that topical 0.3 per cent papaverine and 20 per cent lidocaine were more effective spasmolytics than lower concentrations of lidocaine or normal saline.[100] Geter and associates, in an epinephrine-induced vasospasm model in the rat tail, demonstrated that 20 per cent lidocaine and chlorpromazine (25 mg/ml) (a calmodulin inhibitor) were the most effective topical spasmolytic agents compared with bupivacaine (Marcaine), nifedipine (calcium channel blocker), Carbacyclin (a prostacycline analog), Forskolin (adenylate cyclase stimulator), and phentolamine (Regitine) (an alpha-receptor blocker). Chlorpromazine was found to have a greater potential to relieve vasospasm and improve anastomotic patency rates than 20 per cent lidocaine. We have had success using 2 per cent lidocaine, which is less likely to cause toxicity problems than higher concentrations.

Anticoagulation

The use of systemic prophylactic anticoagulation and antiplatelet agents remains controversial and has not proved to increase microvascular patency rates for technically well-performed anastomoses between normal vessels. Davies surveyed anticoagulation practices in clinical microvascular surgery in over 100 centers throughout the world.[102] He found no standardized practice with routine use of 21 different agents, not taking into account any differences in dosage or duration. A comparison between those centers routinely using no anticoagulation at any stage in the operation and those centers practicing anticoagulation revealed no statistical difference in anastomotic patency rates. However, when anastomoses of diseased vessels (irradiated recipient vessels, atherosclerotic or diabetic vessels) are unavoidable, and when excessive vessel injury has occurred, use of these agents may be beneficial.[103]

At present, three classes of agents are frequently used. Heparin accelerates the action of antithrombin. We empirically use subcutaneous heparin in its minidose form (5000 USP unit doses) preoperatively. Postoperative use of heparin is not recommended because of the potential increased risk of hemorrhagic complications, including hematoma and vascular compression. Anti-prostaglandin agents such as aspirin may be beneficial for prophylaxis of small vessel thrombosis after microvascular anastomoses. We routinely use 10 grains of aspirin twice daily during the first 2 postoperative weeks.

Low molecular weight dextran (Rheomacrodex), originally introduced as a plasma volume expander in 1944, was later found to have antiplatelet properties useful for prophylaxis of deep vein thrombosis and fatal pulmonary embolism following orthopedic procedures.[104] In addition to a reduction in platelet adhesiveness, dextran has been shown to increase blood flow by decreasing viscosity and to alter the structure of fibrin, making it more easily lysed by plasmin in vitro.[105, 106] No formal study on the efficacy of various doses and dosing schedules for dextran use in microvascular surgery has been published; this remains a fertile area of research. Dextran 40 is probably equally as effective as dextran 70, but in Europe dextran 70 is used for thromboembolic prophylaxis because of its longer duration of action.[107] The maximum reduction in platelet adhesiveness and aggregation following an infusion of dextran occurs 2 to 4 hours after the completion of the infusion.[108] Therefore, the timing of infusion should allow peak antiplatelet activity to occur at the time of vascular clamp release. We routinely administer dextran 40 at 25 to 50 ml/hour prior to reperfusion and continue it for 5 days postoperatively. Judicious use of this drug is important since rare cases of anaphylaxis have been reported (approximately 1 in 40,000 treated patients), and fluid overload resulting in congestive heart failure may occur in elderly patients.[109, 110] An apparent hemodilution that may prompt overtransfusion of blood products occurs.

ANASTOMOTIC FAILURE

The success or failure of free tissue transfer depends on adequate tissue perfusion, which is dictated by the patency of arterial and venous microvascular anastomoses. Approximately 5 to 15 per cent of free tissue transfers are unsuccessful due to anastomotic failure.[8, 111, 112] Despite the use of perioperative antiplatelet agents,[102] failure of a free graft owing to thrombosis usually occurs within the first 24 to 72 hours following reperfusion.[113] Thrombosis unrelated to the anastomotic technique may occur several days later from vascular pedicle tension, kinking, extrinsic compression (due to tissue edema or hematoma), vasospasm, and infection.[57, 80, 114] Hematoma formation underneath a free tissue graft can be avoided by suction drainage and meticulous hemostasis during flap harvest.

Flap ischemia is most critical during the first 8 days following transfer. Experimentally, it has been shown that beyond 8 days free tissue transfers can be perfused by neovascularization from the recipient site. Prior

to that time, the free flap depends completely on its own vascular pedicle for survival.[53] Irradiated, infected, or severely traumatized recipient tissue beds, commonly seen in the head and neck, may delay effective neovascularization beyond this time frame.

It has been shown, both experimentally and clinically, that although revascularized tissue is extremely resistant to infection, the vascular pedicle is not. Local wound infection or salivary fistula near the vascular pedicle of a free flap can rapidly lead to thrombosis. Luk and colleagues have shown experimentally that in the presence of infection the rate of microvascular thrombosis was inordinately high. If the anastomosis was placed near the area of infection but did not traverse it, the failure rate was 19 per cent. However, if the anastomotic site traversed the area of infection, failures as high as 75 per cent were seen. Harii, in his review of 319 free tissue transfers, attributed three total flap failures to local infections.[7] When free tissue transfer must be used for an infected recipient site, the anastomosis ideally should be positioned outside the infected area. We strongly advocate early wound exploration, debridement, and drainage at the first sign of impending postoperative infection or fistulization. Every attempt should be made to divert saliva away from the vascular pedicle, which must not be exposed, in order to prevent desiccation and thrombosis. Traditional methods of fistula management may need to be modified for free tissue transfer. Circumferential dressings must never be used to avoid vascular pedicle compression, and wound drainage or exploration at the bedside is contraindicated.

Partial necrosis of a free tissue transfer is more common than total graft loss and may be unrelated to anastomotic failure. Although partial necrosis may result from compression or kinking of the vascular pedicle, more often it is due to inadequate cutaneous circulation at the periphery of the flap from excessive surgical trauma or extension of the graft beyond the vascular territory of the donor vessels. Partial flap necrosis often results in superficial epidermolysis without loss of underlying muscle or bone. In these situations, healing will usually occur by secondary intention. As with pedicled flaps, excessive free flap compression or tension across the suture line may also result in partial tissue loss (Figs. 27–6 and 27–7).

MONITORING FREE TISSUE TRANSFERS

Clinical Monitoring

Monitoring of free tissue transfer is critical during the first few days following transfer and must be performed by trained personnel on an hourly basis. Early detection of anas-

tomotic failure demands continuous evaluation of fine nuances in perfusion parameters that easily can go unrecognized by even the most experienced microvascular surgeon. It often happens that the least experienced member of the surgical team is left with the important responsibility of flap monitoring. Continuous clinical monitoring is not practical, and further inaccuracies in judgment are compounded by interobserver biases.

Close systemic monitoring is also crucial, especially in the early postoperative period when hypothermia, hypotension, and intense peripheral vasoconstriction are likely and compromise graft perfusion.

Although commonly used, clinical meth-

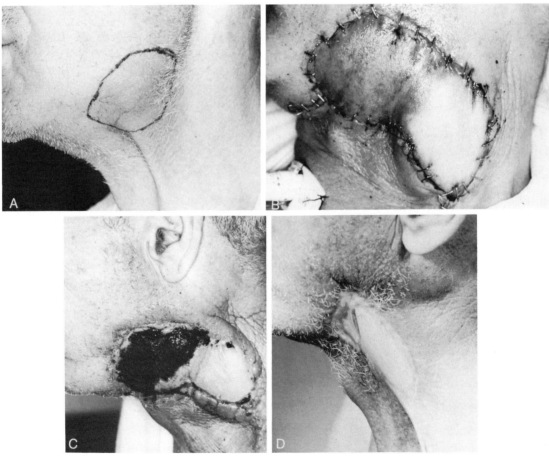

FIGURE 27–6. *A,* Squamous cell carcinoma of the submandibular gland, with invasion of the mandible. *B,* Forty-eight hours after surgery, early venous stasis suggests inadequate cutaneous circulation of the distal portion of the free revascularized osteomusculocutaneous flap. *C,* Full-thickness skin loss of distal flap. *D,* Twelve months after surgery, although partial skin loss resulted from vascular compromise, the underlying subcutaneous tissues and bone graft remained viable, and the wound healed by secondary intention. (From Baker SR: Microvascular surgery. *In* Johns ME (ed): Complications in Otolaryngology–Head and Neck Surgery. Vol 2: Head and Neck. Toronto, BC Decker, 1986, with permission.)

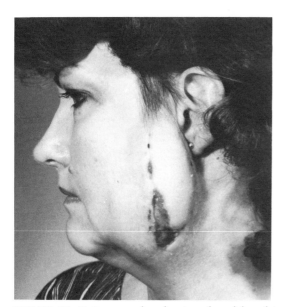

FIGURE 27–7. Four weeks after transfer of free fat dermis graft to left face. Excessive tension along the suture line resulted in partial necrosis of the cutaneous portion of the free flap. (From Baker SR: Microvascular surgery. *In* Johns ME (ed): Complications in Otolaryngology–Head and Neck Surgery. Vol 2: Head and Neck. Toronto, BC Decker, 1986, with permission.)

ods of assessment, such as skin flap color, turgor, capillary refill, temperature, and dermal bleeding, are subjective and often inaccurate. The salient manifestations of arterial insufficiency include a cold, pale flap with poor capillary refill and diminished tissue turgor, with minimal or no dermal bleeding following needle puncture (Fig. 27–8). Venous obstruction generally occurs more gradually, heralded by a sudden increase in swelling of the flap with a change in color to a pink-red tone. Progressive thrombosis leads to further edema, development of diffuse skin petechiae, vesicles, and progressive bluish discoloration of the skin (Fig. 27–9). Needle puncture causes brisk dark bleeding. Assessment of flap color and capillary refill is difficult for deeply pigmented or normally appearing pale skin islands placed introrally. Following pedicle division, capillary refill has been demonstrated even when the flap is detached from its donor site.[116] Thin skin flaps and those placed intraorally have negligible temperature drops (0.9 to 3°C),

especially with isolated venous thrombosis, which usually lags behind actual flap ischemia.[117, 118] Furthermore, flap temperature, influenced by fluctuations in surface, peripheral, and core body temperature, may be misleading. Tissue turgor is difficult to assess, especially when postoperative flap edema confounds the issue. Flaps placed intraorally are often inaccessible to direct observation in the early postoperative period due to swelling, secretions, and deep posterior placement. Although a portion of the transferred flap may be exteriorized for monitoring purposes, this often complicates flap inset and may require subsequent surgical revision owing to poor color match or excessive bulk.[119] Furthermore, the viability of indicator skin may not always reflect the viability of the underlying tissue.

The bone of a composite graft may remain viable despite thrombosis of the microcirculation of the overlying soft tissue (see Fig. 27–6). Bone scintigraphy with technetium-99m–methylene diphosphonate, performed within the first week postoperatively, can be valuable in predicting the survival of revascularized composite bone grafts. Scintigraphy is unreliable if performed beyond one week. Single photon emission computed tomography (SPECT) allows a three-dimensional view of the transferred bone and may be a more reliable indicator of bone viability than conventional planar imaging.[120] The transfer of buried bone without soft tissue can only be monitored using scintigraphy. Buried fat or enteric tissue for head and neck reconstruction precludes early detection of anastomotic failure by conventional methods.

Objective Continuous Monitoring

Over the past decade numerous objective monitoring systems have evolved, some with direct clinical utility and others relegated to investigational use (Table 27–3).[121–129] Each method monitors a different parameter of flap viability: blood flow, temperature, oxygenation, and tissue metabolism. The majority are limited by expense, bulkiness, need for elaborate instrumentation, lack of prolonged continuous on-line monitoring capabilities, and lack of implantability. In addi-

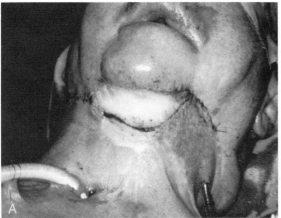
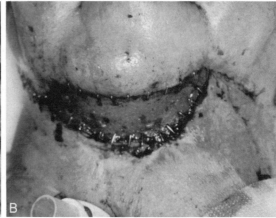
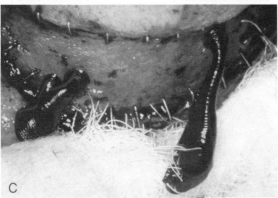

FIGURE 27–8. *A*, Arterial thrombosis of free osteocutaneous scapular flap 12 hours after transfer. Indicator skin is pale, and capillary refill is absent. Reperfusion was successfully established after a kink in the arterial anastomosis was revised. *B*, Progressive congestion of the flap 24 hours following anastomotic revision, indicating venous outflow obstruction. *C*, Attempted flap salvage using systemic heparinization and medicinal leeches was unsuccessful. (Courtesy of Michael J. Sullivan, MD.)

tion, poor correlations between measures of flap ischemia and ultimate survival further limit their usefulness.

Miniature implantable sensors for continuous on-line monitoring, using differential thermometry, continuous wave ultrasound, or laser Doppler, have had limited success. May and Halls implanted thermocouple sensors proximal and distal to arterial anastomoses in free flaps.[130] An almost immediate temperature drop occurred following arterial occlusions, with return to baseline upon reperfusion. Venous obstruction caused a more gradual temperature drop, approaching arterial occlusion by 30 minutes. Venous occlusion temperature changes preceded clinical signs of flap compromise by several hours. A differential temperature between flap and control tissue exceeding 0.3°C, and sustained for 1 hour, was felt to be highly predictive of anastomotic failure. There were several problems with this technique. Sensor malfunction occurred in 11 per cent of 36 monitored flaps.

Reliable differential temperatures could not be obtained prior to an initial equilibration period of 3 to 6 hours following sensor placement in deep tissues, precluding detection of anastomotic failure in the immediate postoperative period. Meticulous positioning of the thermocouples required special training and practice in the laboratory. Roberts and associates implanted miniature thermocouples adjacent to the vascular pedicle of rat island and free flaps.[131] They were unable to reliably predict venous or arterial occlusions because of temperature effects of surrounding soft tissues.

Marks and associates utilized laser Doppler velocimetry to study blood flow in rat skin flaps.[132] They noted some severe limitations of this technique, including positive flow readings in excised, nonviable rat and human skin. Fernando and colleagues investigated a miniature implantable laser Doppler for continuous free flap monitoring.[133] Despite high sensitivity to changes in muscle capillary

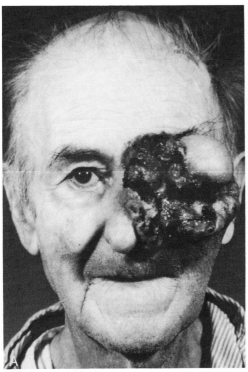
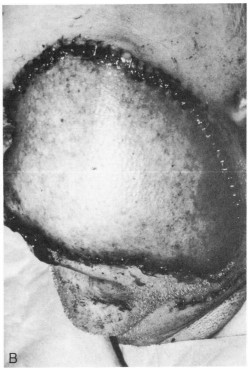
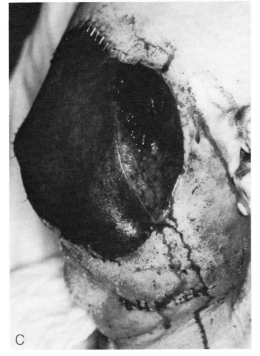

FIGURE 27–9. *A*, Extensive basal cell carcinoma of the midface. *B*, Defect resulting from orbital exenteration and maxillectomy was reconstructed with a free revascularized scapular flap. Flap has developed diffuse petechiae 12 hours postoperatively, suggesting partial thrombosis of the venous anastomosis. *C*, The free flap 24 hours postoperatively is markedly engorged and cyanotic as a result of progressive thrombosis of the venous outflow of the flap. (From Baker SR: Microvascular surgery. *In* Johns ME (ed): Complications in Otolaryngology–Head and Neck Surgery. Vol 2: Head and Neck. Toronto, BC Decker, 1986, with permission.)

TABLE 27–3. Objective Flap Monitoring Techniques

Fluorescein	Differential thermometry
Radioisotope clearance	Interstitial fluid pressure
Hydrogen washout	Photoplethysmography
Tissue pH	Continuous wave Doppler
Transcutaneous oximetry	Laser Doppler flowmetry
Direct tissue oximetry	Pulsed ultrasound velocimetry
Muscle contractility	Electromagnetic flowmetry

blood flow and rapid response times, the optical sensor was extremely susceptible to motion artifact, causing wide reading fluctuations with patient motion. Muscle edema caused a decrease in signal intensity. Furthermore, blood flow from recipient tissue vessels near the sensor gave false readings. Differentiation of venous from arterial thrombosis was not possible with this device. Walkinshaw and colleagues found laser Doppler measurements to be less predictive of flap failure (55 per cent) than clinical assessment (100 per cent) in 23 free tissue transfers.[134]

Sensors that require exact, stable positioning for accuracy are not suitable for monitoring in head and neck reconstruction. Sensor dislodgment would be difficult to prevent owing to neck mobility and variabilities in vascular pedicle geometry. Motion artifact would cause inaccurate and misleading sensor information.

The Ideal Monitoring System

To date, there is no consensus regarding the best monitoring parameter to use, and no single method has been universally successful in predicting flap viability or the timing for salvage attempts. An ideal monitoring system would enable near-instantaneous detection of anastomotic failure by recording subtle changes in blood flow or tissue metabolism compared with a safe intraoperative baseline from the flap or surrounding normal tissues. It would allow continuous on-line monitoring for the first several days following tissue transfer. Specificity and sensitivity would be high, enhanced by a verification system to assure proper sensor function and insure a high correlation between predicted

flap survival (based on unambiguous threshold readings) and actual outcome. The measuring sensor would be relatively noninvasive and biocompatible. The instrumentation would be portable for bedside and ambulatory monitoring, simple to use and interpret by all members of the surgical team, relatively inexpensive (disposable implantable sensors), and allow interface with computer and telemetry systems for data analysis and remote monitoring.

Recent advances have allowed miniaturization of various chemical sensors for in vivo physiologic measurements.[135] Sensors for both tissue and intravascular use are now available for on-line continuous monitoring of PCO_2, PO_2, and pH.

Development of pH Monitoring

Tissue pH determination has proved to be a consistently sensitive and reliable monitor of tissue ischemia. Determination of tissue pH to assess the viability of pedicle flaps was first utilized by Glinz and Clodius.[136] Subcutaneous pH was measured using a glass electrode 60 to 75 minutes following flap elevation. Although subjective clinical parameters, such as degree of cyanosis or paleness, did not permit precise prediction of final flap survival, changes in tissue pH were reproducible and rapidly obtained. Extracellular acidosis, reflected by a pH difference greater than 0.35 unit, predicted necrosis in 83 per cent of 36 flaps. Trauma to local tissues during electrode insertion caused a transient negligible acidosis.

Raskin and associates utilized a continuous pH monitoring system, originally designed for neonatal use, to monitor island flaps in a murine model.[116] Percutaneous glass electrodes were used to monitor both island flaps and normal control tissues for up to 3 hours of pedicle occlusion. An immediate drop in pH was demonstrated for arterial, venous, and combined occlusions. Venous occlusion alone resulted in a less pronounced initial rate of pH decline over the first hour and to a higher final pH value. Upon reperfusion, flap pH rapidly rose to preocclusion values over a 10-minute period. Nine patients undergoing free tissue transfer were monitored over a 24-hour period following completion of anastomoses. A pH differential of 0.21 unit or less predicted survival in six of nine flaps. In the failure group, a pH difference of 0.35 unit occurred within 2 hours following vessel thrombosis and slightly increased over the next 10 hours of monitoring. In one patient, a pH reading of 0.35 unit predicted anastomotic failure 10 hours before obvious clinical parameters of flap failure.

Dickson and Sharpe obtained virtually identical results in a murine model using a different glass pH electrode over a 30-minute monitoring period.[137] Again, pH values following venous occlusion fell more slowly and to a higher final value than arterial occlusions: a possible useful criterion for distinguishing arterial from venous occlusions.

Warner and associates used pH monitoring to compare ischemic responses of flap muscle and subcutaneous tissue.[117] Changes in pH during vessel occlusions were similar, suggesting a parallel utilization of anaerobic metabolism at both tissue levels. Prolonged continuous monitoring (100 hours) was achieved in two patients following free tissue transfers. A progressive decrease in pH during flap transfer and microvascular anastomosis was followed by a rapid rise to near-pretransfer levels.

A consistently decreasing pH value in free tissue transfers appears to be a reliable and almost immediate indicator of failed microvascular patency in an otherwise hemodynamically stable patient.

Development of Po_2 Monitoring

Like pH monitoring, technical advancements in oxygen monitoring have made clinical oximetry a reality.[138] Achauer and colleagues[139, 140] and Matsen and associates[141] demonstrated the utility of continuous transcutaneous Po_2 ($TcPo_2$) for monitoring flaps and limb replantations. They used electrodes incorporating a heating element to cause cutaneous vasodilatation and enhancement of oxygen transport through the skin. The sensors were sensitive to changes in tissue Po_2 and responded rapidly to supplemental oxygen (oxygen challenge test). Serafin and associates found that variabilities in the regional microcirculation of skin flaps necessitated the use of a control sensor for reliable flap monitoring.[142] All flaps with a Po_2 greater than 25 mm Hg survived in their series. Several second-degree burns occurred when ischemic flaps were monitored over a prolonged period. Smith and associates evaluated continuous transcutaneous Po_2 monitoring for 65 replantations and 18 free tissue transfers.[143] Po_2 changes preceded temperature drops or clinical signs of flap ischemia by several hours. The oxygen challenge test provided reliable information about the patency of the arterial anastomoses. Transcutaneous oximetry, despite being noninvasive and allowing continuous monitoring, requires an external skin island. The heated $TcPo_2$ sensor may cause burns in nonsensate flaps over prolonged periods and has questionable reliability in ischemic tissues. Eickhoff and Jacobsen found that $TcPo_2$ was affected by relatively minor changes in systemic and local blood flow through monitored tissues.[144] Raskin and associates compared tissue pH with $TcPo_2$ as indices of perfusion in rabbit epigastric island flaps.[145] Although transcutaneous Po_2 measurement was a more rapid indicator of diminished perfusion than tissue pH, $TcPo_2$ became unreliable in ischemic tissues. Reductions in blood flow of greater than 50 per cent led to numerous false positive $TcPo_2$ predictions of flap necrosis. Raskin and group again attributed these findings to local physiologic changes in the microcirculation of the flaps.

An implantable tPo_2 sensor was investigated by Mahoney and Lista for continuous free tissue transfer monitoring.[146] Experimentally, measured tPo_2 in rabbit epigastric island flaps rapidly declined from a mean pre-clamp value of 34.9 mm Hg to 11.3 mm Hg over 20 minutes. PO_2 values returned to baseline after reperfusion periods of from 17 to 23 minutes for arterial and venous occlusions, respectively. All flap PO_2 values rapidly increased severalfold in response to an inspired oxygen challenge, confirming both sensor function and flap perfusion. The sensor was used clinically over a 3- to 5-day period as a trend monitor, without a control, for 12 free tissue transfers. An absolute tPO_2 of less than 20 mm Hg and lack of response to an inspired oxygen challenge accurately predicted three anastomotic failures.

Tissue oxygen tension responds almost instantaneously to total acute vessel occlusion and may be the earliest indicator of anastomotic failure. Continuous determination of tissue pH also has stood the test of time as a reliable viability monitor. These techniques appear to represent state-of-the-art in free tissue monitoring. Which parameter will provide the most sensitive and reliable monitoring system has yet to be elucidated. The use of a miniature, implantable, combined pH/PO_2 sensor for continuous on-line monitoring of free tissue transfers may offer several advantages over single-parameter monitoring systems and is presently being investigated by Kuriloff and associates.[147]

It is stressed, however, that objective monitoring techniques are not designed to replace clinical judgment, but rather serve to facilitate early detection of problems. At the present time we utilize a 20-MHz handheld portable Doppler probe for assessing patency of the vascular pedicle and cutaneous blood flow when possible. This system is not entirely reliable but serves as a simple, inexpensive, and readily available bedside tool for house staff and nurses. When possible, capillary refill and percutaneous needle sticks, with assessment of the quality of bleeding from the graft, remains the standard.

ANASTOMOTIC REVISION AND FLAP SALVAGE

There is a finite period during which pharmacologic (thrombolytic and anticoagulant therapy)[148–150] or microsurgical revision or both will allow flap salvage.[151] In Harii's experience, if revascularization following warm ischemia occurs within 4 hours, complete recovery without necrosis is possible.[152] After 4 to 8 hours of warm ischemia, despite revascularization, some degree of necrosis is inevitable. Flap survival is rarely achieved beyond 8 to 12 hours of warm ischemia because of the "no-reflow phenomenon."[72] Several factors, including the generation of superoxide free radicals leading to intimal injury, increased capillary permeability, flap edema, hyperviscosity, sludging, and microemboli in the microcirculation, are all thought to play a role in this irreversible process.[153–155]

Various pharmacologic manipulations have been tried in an attempt to increase flap tolerance to primary warm ischemia with varying results. Several free radical scavengers, as well as agents that block the production of oxygen-derived free radicals, experimentally have shown promise for improving survival of ischemic tissue and perhaps prolonging the time of onset for the no-reflow phenomenon. Deferoxamine, a compound derived from the bacterium *Streptomyces pilosus*, is an iron chelator and free radical scavenger that has been used intravenously to prolong ischemic flap survival. Both modes of action appear to play a role in its ability to enhance flap survival.[156, 157] Allopurinol and superoxide dismutase act at two different sites to decrease the presence of free radicals in ischemic tissue. Allopurinol, a xanthine oxidase enzyme inhibitor, used in the past for the treatment of gout, prevents production of the superoxide radical generated in the conversion of hypoxanthine to uric acid. Superoxide dismutase converts superoxide free radicals to hydrogen peroxide. Pokorny and associates found both agents (administered intraperitoneally) to increase skin flap survival significantly compared with controls (no treatment).[158]

Nonsteroidal anti-inflammatory agents have been used widely in patients suffering from myocardial infarctions or cerebral ischemia. Ibuprofen (Motrin) in particular has been shown to reduce the infarct size in myocardial infarctions significantly and to protect the ischemic myocardium in animals.[159, 160] Douglas and associates studied the efficacy of ibuprofen for increasing the safe warm ischemia time of free flaps developed in rats.[161] Control and ibuprofen-treated animals all survived periods of ischemia of from 1 to 8 hours. However, only free flaps in those animals treated with ibuprofen could tolerate ischemia times from 10 to 12 hours. These results suggest that by inhibiting cyclo-oxygenase, nonsteroidal anti-inflammatory agents may block the untoward effects mediated by thromboxane. Although these agents hold promise for allowing increased primary ischemia times for free tissue transfer, as well as for the treatment of secondary ischemia, they remain experimental. Until clinical trials are conducted they cannot be recommended for routine use in microvascular surgery.

Weinberg and associates, using a rat model, showed that the irreversible effects leading to the no-reflow phenomenon could be mitigated by raising a denervated free flap 24 hours prior to transfer. Tolerance to warm ischemia for up to 14 hours was possible in this model. This method, however, is not practical in the clinical setting.

Tsai and coworkers reported an overall vascular complication rate of 15 per cent (182 flaps). One or more explorations and anastomotic revisions were successfully performed on 21 flaps for a salvage rate of 75 per cent. Correctable problems other than vascular thrombosis included vessel kinking in three transfers, compression due to a tight closure in five, hematoma in three, a leaking vein in one, and a hypercoagulable condition in one. Arterial occlusions were more common than venous occlusions. Harii also found that arterial thrombosis was more frequently encountered than venous thrombosis in clinical cases, the most common cause of which was poor intimal continuity.[152] Stenosis or exposure of the adventitia in the vessel lumen was a rarely observed cause for thrombosis. Venous obstruction is less common and may occur later than arterial events. Unlike most arterial occlusions that are usually an all-or-none phenomenon, venous insufficiency may cause only partial flap necro-

sis (see Fig. 27–6). Compensatory bleeding from the flap edges and undersurface may be sufficient to delay irreversible congestion and progressive thrombosis, allowing more time for anastomotic revision.

In general, any sign of ischemia within the first 72 hours after free tissue transfer requires immediate exploration and anastomotic revision. The management of anastomotic failure after the first week following free tissue transfer is controversial. At this point, partial survival of the flap is possible but depends on the degree of recipient site neovascularization. Re-exploration of the anastomosis may not be necessary unless pharmacotherapy fails. It is crucial at the time of re-exploration to attempt to determine the cause of the failure: e.g., vessel kinking, torsion, tension, local trauma, or hematoma. Resection of the anastomotic area, followed by thrombectomy and reanastomosis, should restore flow to the ischemic tissue.

For extensive thrombosis, direct intravascular administration of thrombolytic agents may be beneficial. Lipton and Jupiter reported the first successful free flap salvage utilizing streptokinase to lyse blood clot in a thrombosed vein.[164] Local administration of this drug prevents systemic hemorrhagic problems. Cooley and coworkers compared the efficacy of three thrombolytic agents, including thrombolysin (combination of streptokinase and human plasminogen), streptokinase alone, and urokinase.[165] Urokinase and thrombolysin were both found to be more effective than streptokinase alone. Tissue-type plasminogen activator (t-PA) has the advantage of greater clot-specific thrombolysis and less systemic activation of fibrinolysis than with streptokinase. Hergrueter and coworkers demonstrated that t-PA was 100 per cent effective in lysing fresh clot when infused locally.[166] At the present time, although human recombinant t-PA holds promise as an excellent thrombolytic agent, it is prohibitively expensive for clinical use.

After thrombolytic anastomotic revision, systemic heparinization may be needed to maintain patency. In instances where early exploration of the wound is not possible, systemic heparinization should be considered. During the early stages of venous thrombosis, we found that full heparinization of the patient for one week resulted in flap survival by preventing further thrombus formation (Fig. 27–10). Greenberg and coworkers, using a thrombogenic rabbit inversion graft model, found that systemic administration of heparin could maintain vascular patency for up to one week in 67 per cent of the heparin-treated anastomoses, compared with 19 per cent of the untreated controls.[167] They stress the importance of monitoring the partial thromboplastin time to avoid hemorrhagic complications (3 per cent hematoma rate).

As a last resort, when revision anastomosis is unsuccessful for venous thrombosis, medicinal leeches may be used. Flap salvage using leeches has an estimated success of 60 to 70 per cent (Fig. 27–8).[168] Barnett and coworkers described the "chemical leech" technique that involves blood-letting from the compromised flap, using subcutaneous heparin injections.[169] Continuous bleeding from the wound edge can be titrated by dosage adjustment. Three free tissue transfers were successfully salvaged using this method.

SPECIFIC FLAP AND DONOR SITE COMPLICATIONS

Numerous potential donor sites are available for free tissue transfer. Each site has advantages or disadvantages relative to the specific texture, bulkiness, hair-bearing characteristics, color match, innervation, length and size of the vascular pedicle, difficulty of dissection, and donor site cosmetic and functional disability. Ideal donor sites provide a long vascular pedicle with large diameter vessels (2 to 4 mm), with little morbidity or

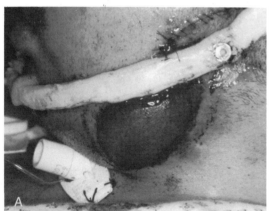
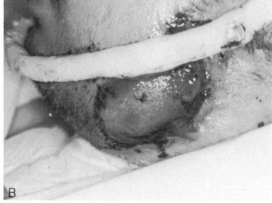
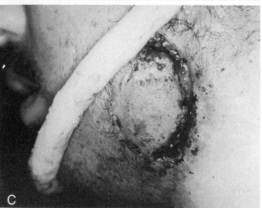

FIGURE 27–10. *A,* Early partial venous thrombosis of free osteomusculocutaneous groin flap marked by cutaneous petechiae. *B,* Full heparinization of the patient produced improvement in venous drainage within 24 hours. *C,* Two weeks after surgery. The entire flap was salvaged with the use of heparinization. (From Baker SR: Microvascular surgery. *In* Johns ME (ed): Complications in Otolaryngology–Head and Neck Surgery. Vol 2: Head and Neck. Toronto, BC Decker, 1986, with permission.)

functional deficit. Several major anatomic areas, including the groin, abdomen, back, and upper extremity, provide fasciocutaneous, musculocutaneous, and osteomusculocutaneous units for transfer. All donor sites are prone to the usual complications associated with soft tissue surgery, including hematoma, infection, wound dehiscence, hemorrhage, and neurovascular injury. Specific problems unique to each of the major donor sites are briefly discussed.

Groin and Thigh Flaps

Flaps harvested from the groin and thigh areas may be based on several branches of the internal and external iliac vessels, including the superficial inferior epigastric, superficial circumflex iliac (cutaneous groin flap), deep circumflex iliac (iliac crest/internal oblique flap), deep inferior epigastric (rectus abdominis flap), and the lateral femoral circumflex [tensor fascia lata musculocutaneous flap (TFLMF)]. The septocutaneous vessels of the profunda femoris system supply the lateral thigh fasciocutaneous flap.

Complications in harvesting the TFLMF and lateral thigh flaps are related to injury of the profunda femoris artery with the potential for vascular compromise of the posterior thigh musculature. The need to incorporate approximately 8 cm of tissue between the vascular pedicle of the TFLMF and the iliac crest may result in an excessively bulky flap for intraoral reconstruction. Redundant tissue often will contribute to oral incompetence. The patient's need to compress the flap against the upper alveolus to control drooling may compromise flap perfusion (Fig. 27–11).

Iliac crest flaps based on the deep iliac system frequently cause a sensory deficit in the lateral aspect of the thigh, due to injury or division of the lateral cutaneous nerve of the thigh that courses through the area of dissection. Detachment of the inguinal ligament during dissection of these flaps may subsequently contribute to inguinal hernia formation. Without the internal oblique modification, the iliac crest osteomusculocutaneous flap may carry excessive immobile soft tissue, thus complicating the reconstruction.

When used for mandibular reconstruction and intraoral defects, this excessive tissue may cause oral incompetence and problems with speech and deglutition.

The inferior rectus abdominis flap is an ideal flap when soft tissue is needed for reconstruction of large defects of the scalp, skull base, or maxilla.[170] Its long vascular pedicle and ease of harvest with the patient supine is advantageous in head and neck reconstruction. A two-team approach can significantly shorten operative time. When used as a myocutaneous flap, excessive bulkiness can be a limiting factor, especially in obese patients. An oblique skin paddle design based on the paraumbilical musculocutaneous perforators requires only a small island of muscle, which can reduce the flap's bulk. Also, the muscle can be harvested alone and skin grafted. This must be done in hirsute males because hair growth may later cause functional and cosmetic problems. Abdominal wall bulging and ventral hernia formation are important complications of this donor site. The incised anterior rectus sheath must be meticulously closed with permanent sutures. In addition, the anterior rectus sheath should not be resected below the arcuate line, and great care should be taken not to injure the transversalis fascia. The amount of rectus muscle sacrificed also should be minimized to maintain the strength of the anterior abdominal wall.[171] Inadvertent entry into the peritoneal cavity may rarely occur during harvest of the rectus abdominis or iliac crest grafts with the internal oblique modification. Late abdominal wall hernias may occur, especially when resecting a portion of the internal oblique muscle. Injury to the nerve supply of the rectus abdominis and transversus muscles may also contribute to abdominal wall weakness.[24] In such situations the use of Marlex mesh is advisable to reinforce the closure.

Flaps Based on the Axillary Vessels

The subscapular artery, a major branch of the axillary artery, supplies the skin overlying the posterior aspect of the scapula (circumflex scapular artery) and the periosteum of the lateral border of the scapular bone. A scapular and parascapular cutaneous or os-

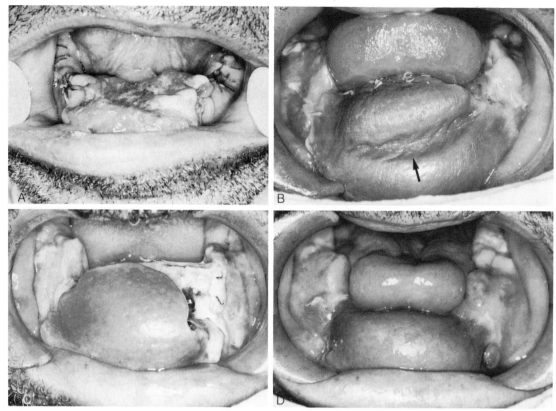

FIGURE 27–11. *A*, Extensive squamous cell carcinoma of the anterior floor of mouth with mandible invasion. *B*, Ten days after transfer of a free tensor fascia lata osteomusculocutaneous flap to reconstruct the floor of mouth and mandible. Note the bulkiness of the flap and depressed area *(arrow)* resulting from compression by the upper mandibular alveolus. *C*, Two weeks after surgery. The distal portion of the flap has undergone necrosis, resulting in exposure of the underlying bone graft. *D*, Three weeks after debridement of necrotic bone and soft tissue. The remaining flap is well healed, resulting in adequate reconstruction of the soft tissues of the floor of the mouth. (From Baker SR: Microvascular surgery. *In* Johns ME (ed): Complications in Otolaryngology–Head and Neck Surgery. Vol 2: Head and Neck. Toronto, BC Decker, 1986, with permission.)

teocutaneous flap may be harvested based on this vessel.[172, 173] The scapular osteocutaneous flap can provide well-vascularized bone up to 14 cm in length for mandibular reconstruction. The excellent mobility of the skin paddle relative to the bone facilitates closure of complex orofacial defects. A skin paddle up to 12 cm wide will allow primary donor site closure. Wider skin islands will cause excessive closing tensions and result in a widened, unsightly scar. A simultaneous two-team approach for flap harvest and preparation of the recipient site is difficult because of patient positioning. This problem is somewhat solved by turning the patient 45° from the supine position to expose the ipsilateral

back, shoulder, entire face, and neck. Positioning is facilitated by use of a vacuum-controlled, beanbag mattress beneath the back and a Mayfield headrest to allow circumferential access to the head and neck region. Harvest of the scapular osteocutaneous free flap necessitates detachment of several upper extremity muscles (long head of triceps, teres major, teres minor, and subscapularis muscles), which may lead to upper extremity weakness. When radical neck dissection is performed, consideration should be given to contralateral flap harvest. Shoulder weakness can be minimized by a rigorous exercise and physical therapy program.[27] During axillary dissection, trauma to the intercostobrachial nerves supplying the medial aspect of the upper arm, and the axillary vessels themselves, can occur but is rare. Excessive arm abduction, causing compression of the brachial plexus between the clavicle and the cervical vertebrae, can cause a temporary neurapraxia.

The thoracodorsal vessels supply the latissimus dorsi muscle and overlying skin along with the serratus anterior muscle.[174] This is an excellent soft tissue flap for reconstruction of orbital-maxillary, craniofacial, and lateral temporal bone defects.[175] It also has been used successfully as an innervated flap (neurorrhaphy between the thoracodorsal and hypoglossal nerves) for reconstruction of glossectomy defects. The donor site is relatively inconspicuous, and denervation and partial resection of the latissimus dorsi muscle usually causes little functional disability.[176] However, when combined with or following an ipsilateral radical neck dissection, shoulder dysfunction may be significant. In this situation, the contralateral side should be chosen as a donor site.

The difficulties encountered with patient positioning during harvest of the scapular free flap also apply to the latissimus dorsi myocutaneous free flap. The bulkiness of this flap is often cited as a major disadvantage. However, this may be overcome by dissecting the vascular pedicle away from the muscle in a caudal direction to the level of the nipple, and division of the muscle close to the point where the thoracodorsal vessels enter.[177] Only muscle that lies directly beneath the skin paddle need be resected. A thin, hairless cutaneous flap up to 10 cm beyond the muscle boundary can be successfully transferred when less tissue bulk is required.[178] Careful handling of the myocutaneous flap and placement of tacking sutures from the skin island to the muscle will prevent shearing of the musculocutaneous perforating vessels. Dissection of the vascular pedicle can be difficult when a large axillary fat pad is present, and extreme arm abduction may cause injury to the brachial plexus. Injury to the long thoracic nerve may rarely cause scapular winging. A 20 per cent incidence of seroma formation has been reported with this flap and dictates the need for prolonged suction drainage.[179] Lumbar herniation and late hematoma formation are rare complications.[180]

Radial Forearm Flap

The radial forearm flap is a fasciocutaneous flap based on the radial artery and its venae comitantes or superficial forearm veins. The lateral antebrachial cutaneous nerve is availabe for reinnervation of the skin island using recipient lingual or glossopharyngeal nerves. When a portion of the radius is harvested with the flap, the arm must be immobilized in a plaster splint for up to 6 weeks. The risk of pathologic fracture resulting in subsequent deformity and difficulty with supination is a significant complication.[181] The skin-grafted defect is unsightly, and problems with graft "take" can occur if the paratenon that nourishes the graft is resected or injured. Both a de-epithelialized forearm flap and the use of tissue expanders prior to harvest have been described to circumvent these problems.[182–184] Injury to the superficial radial nerve will cause numbness in the anatomic snuff box. An Allen test must be performed preoperatively to prevent vascular compromise of the hand. When the test is equivocal, the radial artery may need to be reconstituted with a vein graft.

Lateral Arm Flap

The arterial supply of the lateral arm fasciocutaneous free flap is based on a terminal branch of the profunda brachii artery, the posterior radial collateral artery, and its venae comitantes, which travel with the radial nerve in the spiral groove of the humerus.[185, 186] Arterial branches run through the delicate lateral intermuscular septum dividing the brachialis and brachioradialis muscles to supply the skin of the upper lateral arm between the deltoid insertion and the lateral epicondyle of the humerus.[187] The external diameter of the donor artery ranges from 1.0 mm to 2.4 mm and may make microvascular anastomosis and vessel match difficult. The vascular pedicle is short (4–8 cm). However, additional pedicle length and increased vessel diameters may be obtained by splitting the triceps muscle between its lateral and long heads, and dissecting the pedicle to its origin. When this is done, a mean pedicle length of 11 cm and an artery diameter of 2.45 mm may be achieved.[188] The skin island is innervated by the posterior antebrachial cutaneous nerve of the arm, which can be used to create a sensate flap for oral cavity reconstruction (e.g., neurorrhaphy between the posterior antibrachial cutaneous nerve and the lingual nerve).[189] Sacrifice of this nerve results in a small segmental area of anesthesia along the extensor surface of the forearm and must be discussed with the patient prior to operation. Unlike the radial forearm flap, the donor site usually can be closed primarily when the defect does not exceed 7 to 8 cm in width. Excessive tension potentially could cause a tourniquet effect and compromise forearm perfusion. In this situation, a skin graft should be used.

Harvest of this flap must be done with great care since the intermuscular septum is thin and injury to the vascular pedicle can occur early. The upper portion of the skin incision can be extended cephalad to allow proximal dissection of the vascular pedicle between the brachialis and triceps muscles. This maneuver, facilitated by placement of a self-retaining retractor, will allow dissection of a longer pedicle with larger vessel diameters. Although application of a tourniquet may decrease operative time, excessive pressure may cause a triple nerve palsy of the donor limb.[190] We have not found tourniquet application necessary for rapid dissection. Furthermore, it obviates intraoperative use of the Doppler probe, which is often helpful for initial identification of the major feeding vessels within the intermuscular septum. Injury to the radial nerve, which is exposed throughout the dissection, is a rare complication.

Free Jejunal Graft

The free jejunal autograft has enjoyed much success in pharyngoesophageal reconstruction. Since the operation is extrathoracic the morbidity and mortality associated with mediastinitis are obviated. The jejunum may be used as a free mucosal patch or as a complete bowel segment based on the superior mesenteric vascular arcade. Harvest of the graft is usually performed by a general surgeon, and a simultaneous two-team approach is preferred when possible.

Several technical points are important in harvesting this flap. Identification of the direction of peristalsis by placing a suture at the proximal end of the graft at the time of harvest is important to ensure an isoperistaltic bowel anastomosis. Transilluminating the mesentery will facilitate selection of a bowel segment with sufficient arborization within the vascular arcade to supply the graft. Dissection of the vascular pedicle within the mesentery is considerably less difficult when it is still under stretch in the abdomen. This is especially true in the presence of a fatty mesentery. Generally, 20 cm is the maximum length of a pharyngoesophageal defect that can be bridged with a single loop of jejunum.[191] Longer defects may require an additional loop of jejunum. However, excessive redundancy of the jejunal segment must be avoided to prevent dysphagia. Despite convincing evidence of its necessity, we and others generally cool the bowel to reduce metabolic requirements and allow a greater period of "safe" primary ischemia time. The venous anastomosis can be difficult since the vein wall is thinner than similar diameter veins of other free grafts. The mesenteric artery is very susceptible to vascular spasm, resulting in intimal ruffling and separation from the media, occasionally necessitating placement of a tacking suture.[192]

The bowel must appear pink and show active peristalsis following revascularization. Occasionally more than one artery will supply the bowel segment. The primary vessel may not be correctly identified until revascularization, at which time the second vessel may need to be anastomosed to a second recipient vessel in the neck.

The EEA stapler (United States Surgical Corporation, Stamford, CT) has been used to decrease operative time for bowel anastomoses in the neck. However, accurate alignment of the instrument can be technically difficult, especially when passed through the oral cavity, and may risk avulsion of the microvascular anastomoses. Furthermore, the size discrepancy between the jejunum and the pharynx will not permit its safe use. We prefer a two-layer suture anastomosis with filleting of the proximal jejunum along its antimesenteric border or end-to-side pharyngojejunal anastomosis to compensate for differences in lumen size. The former technique is preferred because deglutition problems associated with diverticulum formation have been reported.[193]

Leakage from the enteric anastomosis in the neck may lead to a salivary fistula. This occurs more commonly at the upper pharyngojejunal anastomosis, presumably due to the greater mismatch in lumen diameters.[194] Small fistulas tend to heal with conservative management. However, infection associated with an early fistula may cause inflammation and edema, resulting in thrombosis of the vascular pedicle.[195] Total flap necrosis, which occurs in up to 15 per cent of jejunal transfers, can be a devastating complication with life-threatening sequelae, including sepsis, carotid artery rupture, hemorrhage, and cerebrovascular accident. Most graft failures are successfully salvaged with a second free jejunal graft, with gastric transposition, or, less frequently, by more complex, staged, pedicled flap reconstructions.

The detection of vascular compromise is especially important for free jejunum, since the graft is buried. Direct postoperative monitoring can be facilitated by exteriorizing an indicator segment based on the vascular arcade.[196, 197] This segment may be observed for peristalsis and evaluated directly with a Doppler probe.

Unlike gastric transposition, regurgitation and reflux following free jejunal flap reconstruction are minimal. However, early postoperative hypersecretion from the revascularized jejunal segment occasionally causes aspiration when laryngectomy is not performed. This factor, combined with uncoordinated peristalsis, also may contribute to dysphagia and failure of tracheojejunal speech rehabilitation.[73] Bates and associates reported successful voice rehabilitation with primary tracheoesophageal puncture in six

of seven patients following resection of hypopharyngeal lesions and free jejunal flap reconstructions.[198]

Extensive dissection required for primary tumor resection or for recipient vessel preparation may devascularize the parathyroid glands, resulting in hypoparathyroidism.[195] Stricture of the upper or lower anastomoses occurs in roughly 12 per cent of free jejunal transfers and responds well to short-term dilatation.[192]

The intra-abdominal portion of the procedure rarely leads to complications. Loss of a tie or clamp on the superior mesenteric artery can be troublesome. Postoperative ileus and problems related to the gastrostomy or jejunostomy may prolong hospitalization.[194] Postoperative adhesions with subsequent bowel obstruction are a late risk, as in any laparotomy. Proximal small bowel surgery rarely causes anastomotic leaks, and peritonitis is seldom encountered.

References

1. Carlson GW, Coleman JJ III: Microvascular free-tissue transfer: The Atlanta Veterans Administration Medical Center experience. Arch Surg 124:438–440, 1989.
2. Hayden RE: Role of microvascular surgery in head and neck reconstruction. In Bloom HJG, et al (eds): Head and Neck Oncology. New York, Raven Press, 1986, pp 65–72.
3. Baker SR: Microsurgical soft tissue augmentation of the head and neck. In Baker SR (ed): Microsurgical Reconstruction of the Head and Neck. New York, Churchill Livingstone, 1989, pp 287–312.
4. Arena S, Fritch M, Hill EY: Free tissue transfer in head and neck reconstruction. Am J Otolaryngol 10:110–123, 1989.
5. Shenaq SM: Reconstruction of complex cranial and craniofacial defects utilizing iliac crest–internal oblique microsurgical free flap. Microsurgery 9:154–158, 1988.
6. Johnson GD, Jackson GC, Fisher J, et al: Management of large dural defects in skull base surgery: An update. Laryngoscope 100:200–202, 1990.
7. Harii K: The free flap in head and neck reconstruction. In Fee WE, Goepfert H, Johns ME, et al (eds): Head and Neck Cancer. Vol 2. Philadelphia, BC Decker, 1990, pp 33–35.
8. Shaw WW: Microvascular free flaps: The first decade. Clin Plast Surg 10:3–20, 1983.
9. Irons GB, Wood MB, Schmitt EH: Experience with one hundred consecutive free flaps. Ann Plast Surg 18:17–23, 1987.
10. Baker SR: Microvascular free flaps in soft-tissue augmentation of the head and neck. Arch Otolaryngol Head Neck Surg 112:733–737, 1986.

11. Jacobson JH, Suarez EL: Microsurgery in the anastomosis of small vessels. Surg Forum 11:243–245, 1960.
12. Malt RA, McKhann J: The classic replantation of severed arms. Clin Orthop 133:3–10, 1978.
13. Seidenberg BS, Rosenak ES, Hurwitt A, Som ML: Immediate reconstruction of the cervical esophagus by a revascularized isolated jejunal segment. Ann Surg 149:162–171, 1959.
14. McGraw JB, Dibbell DG, Carraway JH: Clinical definition of independent myocutaneous vascular territories. Plast Reconstr Surg 60:341–352, 1977.
15. Ariyan S: The pectoralis major myocutaneous flap. A versatile flap for reconstruction in the head and neck. Plast Reconstr Surg 63:73–81, 1979.
16. Baek S, Biller HF, Krespi YP, Lawson W: The pectoralis major myocutaneous flap for reconstruction of the head and neck. Head Neck Surg 1:293–300, 1979.
17. Harii K, Ohmori K, Ohmori S: Hair transplantation with free scalp flaps. Plast Reconstr Surg 53:410–413, 1974.
18. O'Brian BM, Macleod AM, Hayhurst JW, et al: Successful transfer of a large island flap from the groin to the foot by microvascular anastomoses. Plast Reconstr Surg 52:271–278, 1973.
19. Daniel RK, Taylor GI: Distant transfer of an island flap by microvascular anastomoses. Plast Reconstr Surg 52:111–117, 1973.
20. McLean DH, Buncke HJ: Autotransplantation of omentum to a large scalp defect with microsurgical revascularization. Plast Reconstr Surg 49:268–274, 1972.
21. Fujino T, Saito S: Repair of pharyngoesophageal fistula by microvascular transfer of a free skin flap. Plast Reconstr Surg 56:549–553, 1975.
22. Panje WR, Krause CJ, Bardach J, Baker SR: Reconstruction of intraoral defects with the free groin flap. Arch Otolaryngol 103:78–83, 1977.
23. Taylor G, Townsend P, Corlett R: Superiority of the deep circumflex iliac vessels as the supply for free groin flaps: Clinical work. Plast Reconstr Surg 64:745–749, 1979.
24. Urken ML, Vickery C, Weinberg H, et al: The internal oblique–iliac crest osseomyocutaneous microvascular free flap in head and neck reconstruction. J Reconstr Microsurg 5:203–216, 1989.
25. Dos Santos LF: The vascular anatomy and dissection of the free scapular flap. Plast Reconstr Surg 73:599–603, 1984.
26. Swartz WM, Banis JC, Newton ED, et al: The osteocutaneous scapular flap for mandibular and maxillary reconstruction. Plast Reconstr Surg 77:530–545, 1986.
27. Baker SR, Sullivan MJ: Osteocutaneous free scapular flap for one stage mandibular reconstruction. Arch Otolaryngol Head Neck Surg 114:267, 1988.
28. Lukash FN, Sachs SA, Fishman B, Attie JN: Osseointegrated denture in a vascularized bone transfer: Functional jaw reconstruction. Ann Plast Surg 19:538–544, 1987.
29. Urken ML, Buchbinder D, Weinberg H, et al: Primary placement of osseointegrated implants in microvascular mandibular reconstruction. Otolaryngol Head Neck Surg 101:56–73, 1989.
30. Franklin J, Withers E, Madden J: Use of the free dorsalis pedis flap in head and neck repairs. Plast Reconstr Surg 63:195–204, 1979.
31. Urken ML, Weinberg H, Vickery C, Biller HF: The neurofasciocutaneous radial forearm flap in head and neck reconstruction: A preliminary report. Laryngoscope 100:161–173, 1990.
32. Harii K, Ohmori K: Free groin flaps in children. Plast Reconstr Surg 55:588–592, 1975.
33. Peters GE, Grotting JC: Free-flap reconstruction of large head and neck defects in the elderly. Microsurgery 10:325–328, 1989.
34. Ohtsuka H, Kamiishi H, Saito N, et al: Successful free flap transfers with diseased recipient vessels. Br J Plast Surg 29:5–7, 1978.
35. Ohtsuka H, Kamiishi H, Shioya N: Successful free flap transfers in two diabetics. Plast Reconstr Surg 61:715–718, 1978.
36. Van Gelder PA, Klopper PJ: Microvascular surgery and diseased vessels. Surgery 90:860–867, 1981.
37. Kaufman T, Eichenlaub EH, Levin M, et al: Tobacco smoking: Impairment of experimental flap survival. Ann Plast Surg 13:468–472, 1984.
38. Lawrence WT, Murphy RC, Robson MC, Heggers JP: The detrimental effect of cigarette smoking on flap survival: An experimental study in the rat. Br J Plast Surg 37:216–219, 1984.
39. Rao VK, Morrison WA, O'Brien BM: Effect of nicotine on blood flow and patency of experimental microvascular anastomosis. Ann Plast Surg 11:206–209, 1983.
40. Engelberg H, Futterman M: Cigarette smoking and thrombotic coagulation of human blood. Further in vitro studies. Arch Environ Health 14:266–270, 1967.
41. Marchetta FC, Sako KS, Maxwell W: Complications after radical head and neck surgery performed through previously irradiated tissues. Am J Surg 114:835–838, 1967.
42. Murros KE, Toole JF: The effect of radiation on carotid arteries. Arch Neurol 46:449–455, 1989.
43. Butler MJ, Lane RHS, Webster JH: Irradiation injury to large arteries. Br J Surg 67:341–343, 1980.
44. Baker SR, Krause CJ, Panje WR: Radiation effects on microvascular anastomosis. Arch Otolaryngol 104:103–107, 1978.
45. De Wilde RL, Donders G: Scanning electron microscopic study of microvascular anastomoses on irradiated vessels: Long-term effect of irradiation. Microsurgery 7:156–157, 1986.
46. Fried MP: The effects of radiation therapy in microvascular anastomoses. Laryngoscope (Suppl)37:1–33, 1985.
47. Cunningham BL, Shons AR: Free transfers in rats using an irradiated recipient site. Br J Plast Surg 32:137–140, 1979.
48. Watson JS: Experimental microvascular anastomoses in radiated vessels. A study of the patency rate and the histopathology of healing. Plast Reconstr Surg 63:525–533, 1979.
49. Tan E, O'Brian BM, Brennan M: Free flap transfer in rabbits using irradiated recipient vessels. Br J Plast Surg 32:121–123, 1978.
50. Krag C, deRose G, Lyczakowski T: Free flaps and irradiated recipient vessels: An experimental study in rabbits. Br J Plast Surg 35:328–336, 1982.
51. Guelinckx PJ, Boeckx WD, Fossion E, Gruwez JA: Scanning electron microscopy of irradiated recipient blood vessels in head and neck free flaps. Plast Reconstr Surg 74:217–226, 1984.
52. Serafin D, DeLand M, Lesesne CB, et al: Recon-

struction with vascularized composite tissue in patients with excessive injury following surgery and irradiation. Ann Plast Surg 8:35–54, 1982.

53. Black MJM, Chait L, O'Brian BM, et al: How soon may the axial vessels of a surviving free flap be safely ligated: A study in pigs. Br J Plast Surg 31:295–299, 1978.

54. Tsur H, Daniller A, Strauch B: Neo-vascularization of skin flaps: Route and timing. Plast Reconstr Surg 66:85–90, 1980.

55. Serafin D, Shearin JC, Georgiade NG: The vascularization of free flaps: A clinical and experimental correlation. Plast Reconstr Surg 60:233–241, 1977.

56. Rothaus KO, Acland RD: Free flap neo-vascularization: Case report. Br J Plast Surg 36:348–349, 1983.

57. Fisher J, Wood MB: Late necrosis of a latissimus dorsi free flap. Plast Reconstr Surg 74:274–281, 1984.

58. Clark HM, Howard CR, Pynn BR, McKee NH: Delayed neovascularization in free skin flap transfer to irradiated beds in rats. Plast Reconstr Surg 75:560–564, 1985.

59. Franklin JD, Withers EH, Madden JJ Jr, et al: Use of free dorsalis pedis flap in head and neck repairs. Plast Reconstr Surg 63:195–204, 1979.

60. Yaremchuk MJ, Bartlett SP, Sedacca T, May JW Jr: The effect of preoperative angiography on experimental free-flap survival. Plast Reconstr Surg 68:201–207, 1981.

61. Sheppard JE, Dell PC: The effect of preoperative arteriography on vascular endothelium and replant survival in rabbit ears. J Hand Surg 8:145–153, 1983.

62. Hansen EB, Gellett S, Kirkegard L, et al: Tissue oxygen tension in random pattern skin flaps during normovolemic hemodilution. J Surg Res 47:24–29, 1989.

63. Blair WF, Chang L, Pedersen DR, et al: Hemodynamics after autogenous, interpositional grafting in small arteries. Microsurgery 7:84–86, 1986.

64. Melka J, Charbonneau R, Bosse JP: Experimental evaluation of microarterial grafts in rats and rabbits: Long-term histologic studies. Plast Reconstr Surg 63:245–248, 1979.

65. Caffee HH: Venous bypass for decompression of bleeding varices of the pharynx. Head Neck Surg 10:124–128, 1987.

66. Abbott WM, Wieland S, Austen WG: Structural changes during preparation of autogenous venous grafts. Surgery 76:1031–1040, 1974.

67. Osgood CP, Dujovny M, Faille R, et al: Early scanning electron microscopic evaluation of microvascular maneuvers. Angiology 27:96–105, 1976.

68. Roth JH, Urbaniak JR, Boswick JM: Comparison of suture ligation, bipolar cauterization, and hemoclip ligation in the management of small branching vessels in a rat model. J Reconstr Microsurg 1:7–9, 1984.

69. Caffee HH, Ward D: Bipolar coagulation in microvascular surgery. Plast Reconstr Surg 78:374–377, 1986.

70. Zinberg EM, Choo DI, Zotter LA: Effect of heparinized irrigating solutions on patency of experimental microvascular anastomoses. Microsurgery 10:103–107, 1989.

71. Gould JS, Sully L, O'Brian BM, et al: The effects of combined cooling and perfusion on experimental free-flap survival in rabbits. Plast Reconstr Surg 76:104–109, 1985.

72. Chait LA, May JW, O'Brian B, Hurley JV: The effects of perfusion of various solutions on the no-reflow phenomenon in experimental free-flaps. Plast Reconstr Surg 61:421–430, 1978.

73. Panje WR, Moran WJ: Clinical perspectives in microsurgical reconstruction of the head and neck. In Panje WR, Moran WJ (eds): Free Flap Reconstruction of the Head and Neck. New York, Thieme Medical Publishers Inc, 1989, pp 46–56.

74. Shaw WW, Hidalgo DA: Replantation: General considerations. In Microsurgery in Trauma. New York, Futura Publishing Co, 1987, p 61.

75. May JW, Chait LA, O'Brian BM, Hurley JV: The no-reflow phenomenon in experimental free flaps. Plast Reconstr Surg 61:256–267, 1978.

76. Hayhurst JW, O'Brian BM, Ishida H, Baxter TJ: Experimental digital replantation after prolonged cooling. Hand 6:134–141, 1974.

77. Ballantyne DL, Reid CA, Harper AD, Shaw WW: The effects of short-term preservation on microvascular free groin flaps in rats. J Microsurg 2:101–105, 1980.

78. Donski PK, Franklin JD, Hurley JV, O'Brian B: The effects of cooling on experimental free flap survival. Br J Plast Surg 33:353–360, 1980.

79. Anderl H: Storage of a free groin flap. A case report. Chir Plast 4:41, 1979.

80. Urkin ML, Vickery C, Weinberg H, et al: Geometry of the vascular pedicle in free tissue transfers to the head and neck. Arch Otolaryngol Head Neck Surg 115:954–960, 1989.

81. Nam DA, Roberts TL, Ackland RD: An experimental study of end-to-side microvascular anastomosis. Surg Gynecol Obstet 147:339–342, 1978.

82. Frodel JL, Trachy R, Cummings CW: End-to-end and end-to-side microvascular anastomoses: A comparative study. Microsurgery 7:117–123, 1986.

83. Bas L, May JW Jr, Handre J, Fallon J: End-to-end versus end-to-side microvascular anastomosis patency in experimental venous repairs. Plast Reconstr Surg 77:442–450, 1986.

84. Godina M: Preferential use of end-to-side arterial anastomoses in free flap transfers. Plast Reconstr Surg 64:673–682, 1979.

85. Fukui A, Tamai S: Factors influencing the failure of microsurgical composite tissue transplantation. J Reconstr Microsurg 4:285–290, 1988.

86. Sullivan MJ: Microvascular surgical technique. In Baker SR (ed): Microsurgical Reconstruction of the Head and Neck. New York, Churchill Livingstone, 1989, pp 1–25.

87. Mao K, Tang MYM, South JR: A comparison of continuous with interrupted sutures in microvascular anastomosis. Microsurgery 7:158–160, 1986.

88. Siemionow M: Evaluation of long-term patency rates of different techniques of arterial anastomoses in rabbits. Microsurgery 8:25–29, 1987.

89. Kanaujia RR, Hoi KI, Miyamoto Y, et al: Further technical considerations of the sleeve microanastomosis. Plast Reconstr Surg 81:725–734, 1988.

90. Fahmy HWM, Moneim MS: The effect of prolonged blood stasis on a microarterial repair. J Reconstr Microsurg 4:139–143, 1988.

91. Pottie R, Rossouw DJ, Zeeman BJ, Lamont A: Experimental reclamping of free-flap pedicles: The

effect of prolonged stasis on the anastomoses and clamp sites. Plast Reconstr Surg 79:786–795, 1987.

92. Morecraft R, Blair WF, Chang U: Histopathology of microvenous repair. Microsurgery 6:219–228, 1985.

93. Isogai N, Kamiishi H, Chichibu S: Re-endothelialization stages at the microvascular anastomosis. Microsurgery 9:87–92, 1988.

94. Lidman D, Daniel RK: The normal healing process of microvascular anastomoses. Scand J Plast Reconstr Surg 15:103–110, 1981.

95. Tangelder GJ, Egbrink MO, Slaaf DW, Reneman RS: Blood platelets: An overview. J Reconstr Microsurg 5:167–171, 1989.

96. Reichel CA, Croll GH, Puckett CL: A comparison of irrigating solutions for microanastomoses. J Hand Surg 13A:33–36, 1988.

97. Mazer N, Barbieri CH, Goncalves RP: Effect of different irrigating solutions on the endothelium of small arteries: Experimental study in rats. Microsurgery 7:9–28, 1986.

98. Acland RD, Lubbers LL, Grafton RB, Bensimon R: Irrigating solutions for small blood vessel surgery. A histologic comparison. Plast Reconstr Surg 65:460–465, 1980.

99. Acland R: Prevention of thrombosis in microvascular surgery by the use of magnesium sulfate. Br J Plast Surg 25:292–299, 1972.

100. Hoe SM, Seaber AV, Urbaniak JR: Relief of blood-induced arterial vasospasm by pharmacological solutions. J Reconstr Microsurg 3:147–151, 1987.

101. Geter RK, Winters RRW, Puckett CL: Resolution of experimental microvascular spasm and improvement in anastomotic patency by direct topical agent application. Plast Reconstr Surg 77:105–115, 1986.

102. Davies DM: A world survey of anticoagulation practice in clinical microvascular surgery. Br J Plast Surg 35:96–99, 1982.

103. Ketchum LD: Pharmacologic alterations in the clotting mechanism: Use in microvascular surgery. J Hand Surg 3:407–415, 1978.

104. Harris WH, Athanasoulis CA, Waltman AC, Salzman EW: Prophylaxis of deep-vein thrombosis after total hip replacement. J Bone Joint Surg 67A:57–62, 1985.

105. Shoenfeld NA, Eldrup-Jorgensen J, Connolly R, et al: The effect of low molecular weight dextran on platelet deposition onto prosthetic materials. J Vasc Surg 5:76–82, 1987.

106. Weislander JB, Dougan P, Stjernquist U, et al: The influence of dextran and saline solution upon platelet behavior after microarterial anastomosis. Surg Gynecol Obstet 163:256–262, 1986.

107. Aberg M, Heder U, Bergentz S-E: The antithrombotic effect of dextran. Scand J Haematol Suppl 34:61–68, 1979.

108. Aberg M, Arfors KE, Bergentz SE: Effect of dextran on factor VIII and thrombus stability in humans: Significance of varying infusion rates. Acta Chir Scand 143:417–419, 1977.

109. Ljungstrom KG: The antithrombotic efficacy of dextran. Acta Chir Scand Suppl 543:26–30, 1988.

110. Webster AL, Comfort PT, Fisher AJG: Two cases (one fatal) of severe reactions to rheomacrodex. S Afr Med J 47:2421–2422, 1973.

111. Shaw WW: Microvascular free flaps: Survival, donor sites, and applications. In Symposium on Clinical Frontiers in Reconstructive Microsurgery. Vol 24. St. Louis, CV Mosby, 1984, pp 3–10.

112. Irons GB, Wood MB, Schmitt EH: Experience with one hundred consecutive free flaps. Ann Plast Surg 18:17–23, 1987.

113. Harrison DH, Girling M, Mott G: Methods of assessing the viability of free flap transfer during the postoperative period. Clin Plast Surg 10:21–36, 1983.

114. Saeber AV: Experimental vasospasm. Microsurgery 8:234–241, 1987.

115. Luk KDK, Zhou LR, Chow SP: The effect of established infection on microvascular surgery. Plast Reconstr Surg 80:423–427, 1987.

116. Raskin DG, Erk Y, Spira M, Melissinos EG: Tissue pH monitoring in microsurgery: A preliminary evaluation of continuous tissue pH monitoring as an indicator of perfusion disturbances in microvascular free flaps. Ann Plast Surg 11:331–339, 1983.

117. Warner KG, Durham-Smith G, Butler MD, et al: Comparative response of muscle and subcutaneous tissue pH during arterial and venous occlusion in musculocutaneous flaps. Ann Plast Surg 22:108–116, 1989.

118. May JW, Halls MJ: Thermocouple probe monitoring for free tissue transfer, replantation, and revascularization procedures. Clin Plast Surg 12:197–207, 1985.

119. Urken ML, Weinberg H, Vickery C, et al: Free flap design in head and neck reconstruction to achieve an external segment for monitoring. Arch Otolaryngol Head Neck Surg 115:1447–1453, 1989.

120. Fig LM, Shulkin BL, Sullivan MJ, et al: Utility of emission tomography in evaluation of mandibular bone grafts. Arch Otolaryngol Head Neck Surg 116:191–196, 1990.

121. Barron JN, Laing JE, Colbert JG, Veall N: Observations on the circulation of tubed skin pedicles using the local clearance of radioactive sodium. Br J Plast Surg 5:171–180, 1952.

122. Silverman DG, LaRossa DD, Barlow CH, et al: Quantification of tissue fluorescein delivery and prediction of flap viability with the fiberoptic dermofluorometer. Plast Reconstr Surg 66:545–553, 1980.

123. Weisman RA, Silverman DG: Fiberoptic fluorometer for skin flap assessment. Otolaryngol Head Neck Surg 91:377–379, 1983.

124. Glogovac SV, Bitz MD, Whiteside LA: Hydrogen washout technique in monitoring vascular status after replantation surgery. J Hand Surg 7:601–605, 1982.

125. Batchelor A, Kay S, Evans D: A simple and effective method of monitoring free muscle transfers: A preliminary report. Br J Plast Surg 35:343–344, 1982.

126. Fischer JC, Parker PM, Shaw WW, Colen SR: Dynamic computer tomography determining the patency of buried free flaps. Microsurgery 7:190–192, 1986.

127. Harrison DH, Girling M, Mott G: Methods of assessing the viability of free flap transfer during the postoperative period. Clin Plast Surg 10:21–36, 1983.

128. Sloan GM, Sasaki GH: Noninvasive monitoring of tissue viability. Clin Plast Surg 12:185–195, 1985.

129. Jones NF: Postoperative monitoring of microsurgical free tissue transfers for head and neck reconstruction. Microsurgery 9:159–164, 1988.

130. May JW, Halls MJ: Thermocouple probe monitoring for free tissue transfer, replantation, and revascularization procedures. Clin Plast Surg 12:197–207, 1985.

131. Roberts JO, Jones BM, Greenhalgh RM: An experimental investigation into the use of implanted thermocouples and differential thermometry as monitors for microvascular anastomoses. J Reconstr Microsurg 2:51–57, 1985.

132. Marks NJ, Trachy RE, Cummings CW: Dynamic variations in blood flow as measured by laser Doppler velocimetry: A study in rat skin flaps. Plast Reconstr Surg 73:804–810, 1984.

133. Fernando B, Young VL, Logan SE: Miniature implantable laser Doppler probe monitoring of free tissue transfer. Ann Plast Surg 20:434–442, 1988.

134. Walkinshaw M, Holloway A, Bulkley A, Engrav L: Clinical evaluation of laser Doppler blood flow measurements in free flaps. Ann Plast Surg 18:2212–2217, 1987.

135. Rolfe P: Review of chemical sensors for physiological measurement. J Biomed Eng 10:138–145, 1988.

136. Glinz W, Clodius L: Measurement of tissue pH for predicting viability in pedicle flaps: Experimental studies in pigs. Br J Plast Surg 25:111–115, 1972.

137. Dickson MG, Sharpe DT: Continuous subcutaneous tissue pH measurement as a monitor of blood flow in skin flaps: An experimental study. Br J Plast Surg 38:39–42, 1985.

138. Delpy DT: Developments in oxygen monitoring. J Biomed Eng 10:534–540, 1988.

139. Achauer BM, Black KS, Litke DK: Transcutaneous Po$_2$ in flaps: A new method of survival prediction. Plast Reconstr Surg 65:743–745, 1980.

140. Achauer BM, Black KS: Transcutaneous oxygen and flaps. Plast Reconstr Surg 74:721–722, 1984.

141. Matsen I, Bach AW, Wyss CR, Simmons CW: Transcutaneous Po$_2$: A potential monitor of the status of replanted limb parts. Plast Reconstr Surg 65:732–737, 1980.

142. Serafin D, Lesesne CB, Mullen RY, Georgiade NG: Transcutaneous Po$_2$ monitoring for assessing viability and predicting survival of skin flaps: Experimental and clinical correlations. J Microsurg 2:165–178, 1981.

143. Smith AR, Sonneveld GJ, Kort WJ, Van der Meulen JC: Clinical application of transcutaneous oxygen measurements in replantation surgery and free tissue transfer. J Hand Surg 8:139–145, 1983.

144. Eickhoff JH, Jacobsen E: Is transcutaneous oxygen tension independent of variations in blood flow and in arterial blood pressure? Biotel Pat Monitg 9:175–184, 1982.

145. Raskin DJ, Nathan R, Erk Y, Spira M: Critical comparison of transcutaneous Po$_2$ and tissue pH as indices of perfusion. Microsurgery 4:29–33, 1983.

146. Mahoney JL, Lista FR: Variations in flap blood flow and tissue Po$_2$: A new technique for monitoring flap viability. Ann Plast Surg 20:43–47, 1988.

147. Kuriloff DB, Sullivan MS, Berman E, et al: Continuous monitoring of free tissue transfers: Experimental use of an implantable pH/O$_2$ biosensor. Arch Otolaryngol Head Neck Surg, in press.

148. Serafin D, Puckett CL, McCarty G: Successful treatment of acute vascular insufficiency in a hand by intraarterial fibrinolysin, heparin, and reserpine. Plast Reconstr Surg 58:506–509, 1976.

149. Cooly BC, Jones MM, Dellon AL: Comparison of efficacy of thrombolysin, streptokinase and urokinase in a femoral vein clot model in rats. Microsurgery 4:1–4, 1983.

150. Campbell SP, Tattelbaum A, Rosenber M, et al: Fluormetric analysis of an attempt to reclaim ischemic flaps in rats with fluosol. Plast Reconstr Surg 84:484–491, 1989.

151. Biemer E: Salvage operation for complications following replantation and free tissue transfer. Int Surg 66:37–38, 1981.

152. Harii K: Complications. In Microvascular Tissue Transfer: Fundamental Techniques and Clinical Applications. Tokyo, Igaku-Shoin, 1983, pp 205–208.

153. Russell RC: Reperfusion injury and oxygen free radical: A review. J Reconstr Microsurg 5:79–84, 1989.

154. Feller AM, Roth AC, Russell RC, et al: Experimental evaluation of oxygen free radical scavengers in the prevention of reperfusion injury to skeletal muscle. Ann Plast Surg 22:321–331, 1989.

155. Acland RD, Anderson G, Siemionow M, McCabe S: Direct in vivo observations of embolic events in the microcirculation distal to a small-vessel anastomosis. Plast Reconstr Surg 84:280–289, 1989.

156. Angel MF, Narayanan K, Swartz M, et al: Deferoxamine increases skin flap survival: Additional evidence of free radical involvement in ischaemic flap surgery. Br J Plast Surg 39:469–472, 1986.

157. Angel MF, Haddad J, Abramson M: A free radical scavenger reduces hematoma-induced flap necrosis in Fischer rats. Otolaryngol Head Neck Surg 96:96–98, 1987.

158. Pokorny AT, Bright DA, Cummings CW: The effects of allopurinol and superoxide dismutase in a rat model of skin flap necrosis. Arch Otolaryngol Head Neck Surg 115:207–212, 1989.

159. Jugdutt BI, Hutchins GM, Bulkley GH: Salvage of ischemic myocardium by ibuprofen during infarction in the conscious dog. Am J Cardiol 46:74–82, 1980.

160. Lefer AM, Polansky EW: Beneficial effects of ibuprofen in acute myocardial ischemia. Cardiology 64:265–279, 1979.

161. Douglas B, Weinberg H, Song Y, Silverman DG: Beneficial effects of ibuprofen on experimental microvascular free flaps: Pharmacologic alteration of the no-reflow phenomenon. Plast Reconstr Surg 79:366–374, 1987.

162. Weinberg H, Song Y, Douglas B: Enhancement of blood flow in experimental microvascular free flaps. Microsurgery 6:121–124, 1985.

163. Tsai TM, Bennett DL, Pederson WC, Matiko J: Complications and vascular salvage of free-tissue transfers to the extremities. Plast Reconstr Surg 82:1022–1026, 1988.

164. Lipton HA, Jupiter JB: Streptokinase salvage of a free-tissue transfer: Case report and review of the literature. Plast Reconstr Surg 79:977–981, 1987.

165. Cooley BC, Jonel MM, Dellon AL: Comparison of efficacy of thrombolysin, streptokinase, and urokinase in a femoral vein clot model in rats. Microsurgery 4:1–4, 1983.

166. Hergrueter CA, Handren J, Kersh R, May JW: Human recombinant tissue type plasminogen activator and its effects on microvascular thrombosis in the rabbit. Plast Reconstr Surg 81:418–424, 1988.

167. Greenberg BM, Masem M, May JW: Therapeutic

value of intravenous heparin in microvascular surgery: An experimental vascular thrombosis study. Plast Reconstr Surg 82:463–472, 1988.

168. Kraemer BA, Korber KE, Aquino TI, Engleman A: Use of leeches in plastic and reconstructive surgery: A review. J Reconstr Microsurg 4:381–386, 1988.

169. Barnett GR, Taylor GI, Mutimer KL: The "chemical leech": Intra-replant subcutaneous heparin as an alternative to venous anastomosis. Report of three cases. Br J Plast Surg 42:556–558, 1989.

170. Jones NF, Sekhar LN, Schramm VL: Free rectus abdominis muscle flap reconstruction of the middle and posterior cranial base. Plast Reconstr Surg 78:471–479, 1986.

171. Meland NB, Fisher J, Irons GB, et al: Experience with 80 rectus abdominis free-tissue transfers. Plast Reconstr Surg 83:481–487, 1989.

172. Sullivan MJ, Carroll WR, Baker SR: The cutaneous scapular free flap in head and neck reconstruction. Arch Otolaryngol Head Neck Surg 116:600–603, 1990.

173. Sullivan MJ, Baker SR, Cromptom R, Smith-Wheelock M: Free scapular osteocutaneous flap for mandibular reconstruction. Arch Otolaryngol Head Neck Surg 115:1334–1340, 1989.

174. Takayanagi S, Ohtsuka M, Tsukie T: Use of the latissimus dorsi and the serratus anterior muscles as a combined flap. Ann Plast Surg 20:333–339, 1988.

175. Baker SR: Closure of large orbital-maxillary defects with free latissimus dorsi myocutaneous flaps. Head Neck Surg 6:828–835, 1984.

176. Russell RC, Pribaz J, Zook EG, et al: Functional evaluation of the latissimus dorsi donor site. Plast Reconstr Surg 78:336–344, 1986.

177. Godina M: The tailored latissimus dorsi free flap. Plast Reconstr Surg 80:304–306, 1987.

178. Hayashi A, Maruyama Y: The reduced latissimus dorsi musculocutaneous flap. Plast Reconstr Surg 84:290–295, 1989.

179. Colen SR, Shaw WW, McCarthy JG: Review of the morbidity of 300 free-flap donor sites. Plast Reconstr Surg 77:948–953, 1986.

180. Lineaweaver WC, Buncke GM, Buncke HJ: Hematoma in a latissimus dorsi donor site 21 months after surgery. Ann Plast Surg 21:143–144, 1988.

181. Soutar DS, McGregor IA: The radial forearm flap in intraoral reconstruction: The experience of 60 consecutive cases. Plast Reconstr Surg 78:1–8, 1986.

182. Kawashima T, Harii K, Ono I, et al: Intraoral and oropharyngeal reconstruction using a de-epithelial-ized forearm flap. Head Neck Surg 11:358–363, 1989.

183. Hallock GG: Free flap donor site refinement using tissue expansion. Ann Plast Surg 20:566–572, 1988.

184. Hallock GG: Refinement of the radial forearm flap donor site using skin expansion. Plast Reconstr Surg 81:21–25, 1988.

185. Matloub HS, Larson DL, Kuhn JC, et al: Lateral arm free flap in oral cavity reconstruction: A functional evaluation. Head Neck 11:205–211, 1989.

186. Song R, Song Y, Yu Y, et al: The upper arm free flap. Clin Plast Surg 9:27–35, 1982.

187. Katsaros J, Shusterman M, Beppu M, et al: The lateral upper arm flap: Anatomy and clinical applications. Ann Plast Surg 6:489–500, 1984.

188. Moffett T, Madison S, Derr J, et al: An extended approach for the vascular pedicle of the lateral arm free flap. Plast Reconstr Surg 89:259–267, 1992.

189. Sullivan MJ, Carroll WR, Kuriloff DB: The lateral upper arm free flap in head and neck reconstruction. Arch Otolaryngol Head Neck Surg, in press.

190. Waterhouse N, Healy C: The versatility of the lateral arm flap. Br J Plast Surg 43:398–402, 1990.

191. Hynes B, Boyd JB, Gullane PJ, et al: Free jejunal grafts in pharyngoesophageal reconstruction. Can J Surg 30:436–439, 1987.

192. Gluckman JL, McCafferty GJ, Black RJ, et al: Complications associated with free jejunal graft reconstruction of the pharyngoesophagus—A multiinstitutional experience with 52 cases. Head Neck Surg 7:200–205, 1985.

193. Biel MA, Maisel RH: Free jejunal autograft reconstruction of the pharyngoesophagus: Review of a 10-year experience. Otolaryngol Head Neck Surg 97:369–375, 1987.

194. Gluckman J, McDonough JJ: Free jejunal grafts. In Baker SR (ed): Microsurgical Reconstruction of the Head and Neck. New York, Churchill Livingstone, 1989, pp 249–253.

195. Fisher SR, Cameron R, Hoyt DJ, et al: Free jejunal interposition graft for reconstruction of the esophagus. Head Neck 12:126–130, 1990.

196. Bafitis H, Stallings JO, Ban J: A reliable method for monitoring the microvascular patency of free jejunal transfers in reconstructing the pharynx and cervical esophagus. Plast Reconstr Surg 83:896–897, 1988.

197. Katsaros J, Banis JC, Acland RD, Tan E: Monitoring free vascularized jejunum grafts. Br J Plast Surg 38:220–222, 1985.

198. Bates GJ, McFeeter L, Coman W: Pharyngolaryngectomy and voice restoration. Laryngoscope 100:1025–1026, 1990.

CHAPTER 28

Management of Scars

•

FRED J. STUCKER, MD
GARY Y. SHAW, MD

Numerous advances in the surgical treatment of a variety of head and neck disease processes have not altered Gilles' noted comment of the early 20th century, "By your scars you will be judged."[1] While much thought is given to which surgical procedure is best adapted for a particular disease process, frequently incision placement is given insufficient thought. Surgeons will reflexly adopt a "classic" incision, uninfluenced by the fact that the ultimate cosmetic result will be far from ideal. Similarly, when confronted with an unacceptable scar for revision, we are too often willing to blame "poor patient healing" or "inadequate surgical technique," without recognizing which basic principles were violated. Unless there is a fundamental understanding of why unacceptable scars appeared, we are destined to repeat our failures.

The purposes of this chapter are threefold. First, to outline the basic mechanism of wound healing and scar formation. Second, to emphasize principles to be followed when making an elective surgical incision. Finally, to recommend an approach to scar revisions, including hypertrophic scars and keloids.

SCAR FORMATION

A wound that pierces only the epidermis will heal by simple epithelialization. Structural integrity is rapidly restored, and there is rarely any chronic sequela. On the other hand, when a wound penetrates the dermis, repair is characterized by scar formation. The scar itself is the end result of a complex series of biochemical steps, involving a variety of circulating cells (polymorphonuclear cells, mast cells, eosinophils, macrophages, fibroblasts, and so on) and a variety of chemical intermediaries (anaphylaxins, complement, prostaglandins, leukotrienes, lipoperoxidases, and so on), which ultimately result in the deposition of glycosaminoglycan and mature collagen.[2] Although the process is complex, it can be divided conveniently into three phases: substrate phase, proliferative phase, and remodeling phase.

The substrate phase occurs with the initial insult to skin. Polymorphonuclear cells (PMNs) and macrophages aggregate and release a variety of chemotactic messengers for the production and attraction of cells, particularly fibroblasts and myofibroblasts, in addition to more polymorphonucleocytes and macrophages. Relative tissue hypoxia is also a stimulus for macrophages, and they tend to produce growth factors that induce fibroblast proliferation.[3] Additionally, macrophages act as a cellular microdebrider, preparing the wound for subsequent healing. Blood clot fibrin and platelets act as a substrate for the subsequent scar framework. Lipid peroxidases released mostly by the PMNs penetrate cellular membranes within the area of the wound, aiding in debridement. This phase can be delayed by steroid administration, which acts to stabilize the lysozyme membranes, thereby decreasing cellular destruction, and will markedly decrease the number of PMNs and macrophages attracted to the wound. Vitamin A, on the other hand, appears to induce macrophage migration and overcomes the effects of steroids. The first stage of wound healing lasts from 2 to 5 days after insult and consists of leukocyte and macrophage migration, fibrin deposition, and microdebridement.

The proliferative phase of wound healing is characterized by the rapid increase in fibroblasts and myofibroblasts. Fibroblasts are responsible for the synthesis of collagen, the principal component of scar. The critical step in collagen formation occurs at the ribosomal level when proline and lysine are hydroxylated to hydroxyproline and hydroxylysine. This step requires ascorbic acid as a reducing agent. If vitamin C is deficient, inadequate wound healing will result. The myofibroblasts are responsible for early wound contraction. Because of the intense mitotic activity of the cells during this phase, this period of time is quite sensitive to any antimitotic effects, such as chemotherapy or radiation therapy.[4]

The remodeling phase begins approximately 10 days to 2 weeks after injury and continues up to 12 months. Here, the early gel-like collagen matures, with extensive cross-linking and a relative dehydration. A dynamic balance of collagen synthesis and lysis is struck. A defect in this equilibrium is believed to result in hypertrophic scars and keloids.[5]

PLACEMENT OF ELECTIVE INCISIONS

The cosmetic acceptability of scars resulting from elective incisions is directly related to certain principles: the length of an incision, its anatomic location in relation to the direction of the relaxed skin tension lines, the surgical precision and technique, and individual patient variables. All but the last are under the control of the surgeon to a large extent.

Inherent in any surgical procedure is that the incision must be of sufficient length to allow adequate exposure of the underlying structures. There is, however, no redeeming value to excessive length. Typical instances of frustration with inadequate incisions in head and neck surgery are procedures such as tracheostomies and lymphadenectomies. Additionally, it has been well established that, when possible, two or more incisions are preferable to one long incision, particularly in the neck, where a bowstring effect tends to occur. This is one reason why a stair-step incision to deal with such lesions as brachial cleft cysts or the McFee incision for neck dissections is recommended. In practice, many scar revisions occur because a critical incision followed all guidelines but was just too long. Remember the caveat that while an incision can always be lengthened, it can never be shortened; the careful surgeon will proceed accordingly.

The anatomic location of a surgical incision is critical to ultimate cosmesis. Attempts should be made to place incisions inside an orifice when possible, so the healed scar is hidden from view. These are utilitarian incision placements in the head and neck, particularly for exposure of the mandible and maxilla (intraoral), as well as rhinoplasties (endonasal) and most otologic procedures (endaural). When placement of an incision in an orifice is not feasible, another propitious placement is at the patient's hairline; thus, a coronal incision in a patient without alopecia is excellent for the exposure of the frontal sinuses and anterior skull base or indirect brow lift.

Incisions are also well hidden by anatomic

structures, such as the auricle for postauricular incisions, the nose in a lateral rhinotomy or external rhinoplasty, and the mandible in a submental incision for a chin implant or submandibular gland exposure. The head and neck surgeon should have a clear understanding of the aesthetic areas of the face. Incisions placed along the boundaries of these areas, although in the open, usually with proper surgical execution result in barely discernible scars. Among these are the melonasal junction, the melolabial groove, and the labial-mental junction, as well as the preauricular facial sulcus.

Incisions that bisect certain anatomic landmarks, such as the eyebrows, the lips, and the hairline, should be made with care or avoided if possible. These scars tend to be unacceptable if approximation is imprecise. Concave areas tend to scar with a bowstring effect. This is evident in the suprasternal notch or the medial canthus. Similarly, incisions that transect grooves like the nasolabial or postauricular groove also tend to form bowstrings. Conversely, convex surfaces such as the forehead tend to heal incisions well. Some areas, most notably the deltoid and the sternum, tend to produce unacceptable scars and are frequent sites of hypertrophic scars and keloids. This is thought to be due to constant motion and circumferential tension as these areas exert traction on the wound in all directions.[6]

The concept of skin tension lines is deceivingly simple, yet elusive in many applications. This is evidenced by the more than 40 terms used to refer to it.[7] In essence, intact skin is always under tension from all directions, but there is always one direction in which tension is the greatest. An incision made perpendicular to this tension line will gape, whereas one made parallel will tend to remain narrow. This is thought to be the characteristic of skin tension, which is one third greater when perpendicular to relaxed skin tension lines.[8] Relaxed skin tension lines (RSTLs) are frequently confused with wrinkle lines, which are caused by redundant skin overlying muscle fibers at right angles. Thus, the vertical lines at the glabella caused by the corrugator supercilii muscle actually run perpendicular to relaxed skin tension lines. Similarly, the crow's feet of the lateral palpebral commissure, a common site for some upper blepharoplasty incisions, actually run obliquely across RSTLs. However, patients tend to form wrinkles in areas of skin laxity, which by definition have little tension; therefore, surgeons often can "get away" with using these areas to hide scars.

Humans, unlike zebras, do not have obvious markers of their RSTLs; therefore, a method for finding them is necessary. This can sometimes be a challenge. First, some standard facial relaxed skin tension lines are universal and often helpful to know.[9] The *median line* begins at the lateral nasal ala, runs transversely across the floor of the nostril, down a philtral fold, vertically through the upper and lower lip to the mentum, then to an inferior submental point below the mandibular synthesis. The *nasolabial line* originates in the free margin of the nostril, down the nasolabial sulcus inferiorly, down the lateral part of the chin, meeting its opposite below the mental symphysis. The *palpebral line* starts at the medial canthus and runs transversely across the nasal dorsum to meet its opposite. Laterally, it extends from the lateral canthus transversely, then, sloping inferiorly, forms a curve from the cheek, terminating in the submandibular area below the nasolabial line. The *marginal line*, as implied by the name, runs along the lateral margin of the face in the hairline superiorly and then inferiorly extends in a near-vertical fashion in the preauricular area, terminating in the submandibular area inferior to all the other stated lines, where it meets its opposite approximately at the level of the hyoid (Fig. 28–1).

One approach to finding relaxed skin tension lines employs pinching the skin with the thumb and forefinger. The ridges and furrows created are easier to make and extend longer in the direction of relaxed skin tension lines. If one remains uncertain of the direction of relaxed skin tension lines, a 2-mm circular punch of skin may be removed: one actually can observe in which direction the maximum and minimum skin tension exists. A caution about this technique is the

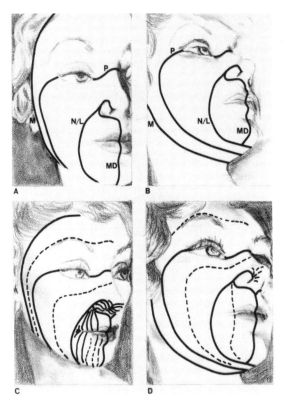

FIGURE 28–1. Four main facial lines. *A*, Anterior, and *B*, oblique views. *M*, Marginal; *P*, palpebral; *N/L*, nasolabial; *MD*, median. *C* and *D* depict other facial lines between the main ones. Note radial configurations at nasal and oral orifices.

a 25-gauge needle. Care should be taken to make the incision perpendicular to the skin. An oblique cut tends to expose a greater area of dermis and lead to subsequent scar formation. This applies to all incisions except those in hair-bearing areas, where the incision should be beveled in the direction of the hair to avoid harm to hair follicles. Wound edges should not be crushed, which occurs with many types of forceps. Rather, small skin hooks or tiny biting forceps such as a Bishop-Harmon should be used to help reflect the skin for both retraction and closure.

The number of sutures and how tightly they are tied has a significant effect on subsequent scar formation. Too many or too-tight sutures tend to cause necrosis of the skin, which leads to greater scar formation. Suture material will be discussed later, but note that all materials cause inflammation, and thus the minimal amount of sutures needed to close deeper dead space and superficial skin will be most beneficial toward alleviating ugly scar formation. Blood and clots accumulate in proportion to the number of sutures and puncture holes, setting up an increased inflammatory process.

effect of patient positioning, such as head extension or lateral rotation, which tends to distort the normal relaxed skin tension line. Distortion of the RSTL also can occur with anesthetic infiltration. Ideally, the surgeon's incision should be planned with the patient in a neutral position prior to any movement or injection.

It is axiomatic that precise surgical execution is mandatory to achieve maximal cosmesis in elective surgical incisions. The alignment of surgical incisions at closure can be aided by making hash marks perpendicular to the demarcated incision prior to cutting. Many surgeons use a knife blade to make these hash marks, but there is risk of penetrating to the dermis and, therefore, creating a scar. When this technique is thought necessary, we recommend small, intradermal, temporary tattooing with gentian violet and

SCAR REVISION

Although ideally incisions could be hidden or placed in accordance to the principles outlined, practically this frequently does not occur. In many instances unacceptable scars are the result of trauma that could not be avoided. Unacceptable scars may result despite excellent plastic techniques in closing these lacerations. In either case, scar revision is in order. Prior to any surgical intervention, both the surgeon and the patient should understand that scars can never be erased and that, at best, one type of scar will be replaced with another more acceptable type. When function is affected, such as an ectropion in eye closure or oral commissure stenosis, the surgeon must explain that new scars will be created to correct the functional deformity. All other psychologic assessment principles that the physician may use in cosmetic surgical procedures must be applied to the scar revision patient. Additionally, the patient (or the parents if the patient is a child) must realize that frequently scar revision may involve several procedures to achieve the desired results. The surgeon who makes the effort to counsel the patient at the onset will find the subsequent dealings to be greatly facilitated.

The revision of scars involves a variety of surgical techniques and understanding of varying principles. The techniques we have most commonly applied have been found satisfactory for most scars. These can be divided into primary and adjunctive techniques. The primary techniques are fusiform excision, Z-plasty, W-plasty, and geometric broken-line closure. The adjunctive techniques include dermabrasion, dermal planing, and steroid injection.

The oldest method of dealing with an unsightly scar is a fusiform excision. While it is clearly not the answer for many scars, it continues to play an important role in revision. We employ this technique generally for two indications: First, when a scar is either in or near a relaxed skin tension line, a groove or furrow, or an aesthetic boundary, we will excise the scar, undermine the surrounding area, and move the scar to the desired area (Fig. 28–2). Second, when the scar is too large to be moved in one step we may employ serial fusiform excisions for the

repositioning. When serial excision is used, care is taken to incise the scar initially from the center where minimal new scar formation would form. Obviously in the last step, one must excise the remaining "border" scar (Fig. 28–3). An alternative recently has been advocated, that of using skin expanders. These are placed under adjacent skin and allowed to expand over a period of time with regular injection of saline. The adjacent expanded skin is used to cover the scar area when the entire scar is removed. We have found a number of drawbacks with this technique and rarely employ it.

The Z-plasty technique was originally described by Denouvilliers in 1856.[10] McCurdy, in 1964, popularized the technique in the United States.[11] The doubly transposed flaps of the Z-plasty lengthen scars, thus freeing contractures. This characteristic of Z-plasties is applied to solve head and neck problems such as ectropion, relief of nasal valve stenosis, and microstomia. If properly designed, the Z-plasty can change an unacceptable scar to an acceptable one by placing it in a relaxed skin tension line. When designing a Z-plasty, the central limb with few exceptions is the scar itself. Ideally, the lateral limbs should run in lines parallel to the relaxed skin tension line. The resulting transposition will place the direction of the scar near or in the relaxed skin tension line. The angles of the limb should not exceed 60 degrees, since

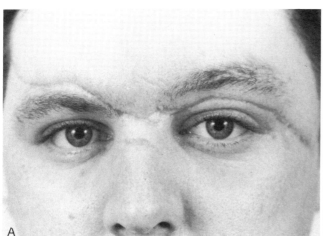
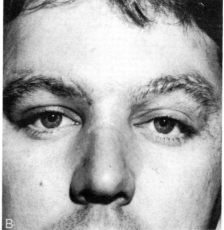

FIGURE 28–2. *A,* A scalping injury resulted in an unsightly scar despite excellent acute management. *B,* The right scar was moved so that it lies in the right eyebrow; the left scar was moved to the palpebral crease.

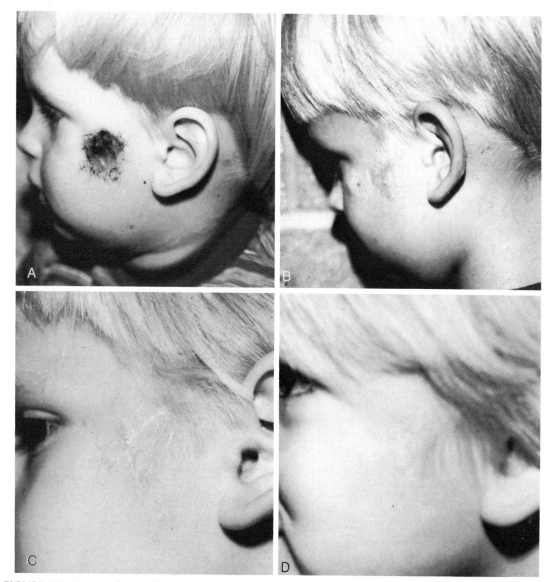

FIGURE 28–3. *A,* Failure of free graft to replace tissue bitten off by a dog. *B,* After first stage of serial resection. *C,* Following second stage of serial resection. *D,* Final result after third stage of serial resection.

larger angles tend to make flap transposition quite difficult. Often, second or multiple Z-plasties are used for superior modification instead of one very large Z-plasty (Fig. 28–4).

In addition to the ability to move scars to relax skin tension lines, it was noted that multiple Z-plasties tended to break a scar, making it hard to follow. This led to the next revision technique, W-plasty. Unlike the Z-plasty, the W-plasty does not involve flap transposition. The negative side of this is that the scar is not lengthened. On the pos-

itive side is that the areas of compression adjacent to skin stretch, which is inevitably produced by the Z-plasty, is not present with the W-plasty. In this technique, small triangles of normal tissue are excised on either side of the scar, along with the scar. The result is a saw-tooth pattern defect. When designing this, the limbs of each triangle are placed as close to relaxed skin tension lines as possible. After adequate undermining of the serrated edges, the margins are advanced and a zigzag closure is produced. Unlike with

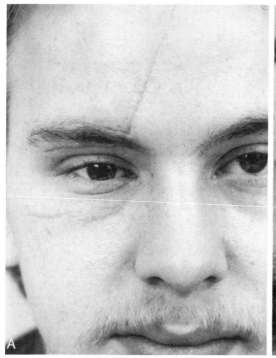

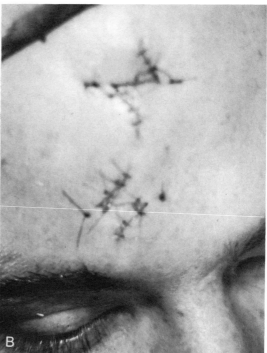

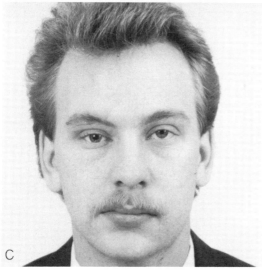

FIGURE 28–4. *A,* Linear scar on forehead secondary to trauma. *B,* Two Z-plasties to bunch up scar. *C,* Final result after abrading Z-plasties.

a linear scar, the healing zigzag can be stretched and compressed like an accordion, yet it does not have the peaks and valleys often characterized by the Z-plasty. We have found this technique useful in long, curved scars, particularly on the cheek (Fig. 28–5). Often, W-plasties can be interrupted with intermittent Z-plasties.

Although the W-plasty smooths out scars, we as well as others[12] note that in longer scars the eye can detect the recurrent pattern of triangles and thus the scar becomes noticeable. Therefore, in longer scars, predominantly of the neck, a broken-line geometric closure is employed. In this technique, the surgeon randomly intersperses squares and rectangles of varying sizes in addition to triangles, though none larger than 6 mm. The advantage of the random unpredictable scar is that the eye has difficulty following

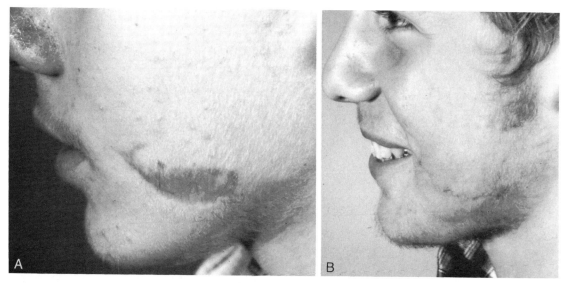

FIGURE 28–5. *A*, Scar on left side of face. *B*, Six months after W-plasty.

it. The disadvantage is that the scar is not as distensible as the W-plasty, with many lines that will run perpendicular to relaxed skin tension lines. Yet, in the proper circumstances, it yields superb results (Fig. 28–6).

We offer some simple surgical guidelines for all these techniques. First, the excision of the scar should be no deeper than the level of the dermis, except when treating contractures. The deeper scar should be left intact where it will act as a type of antitension binder, allowing the resulting wound to be closed easier and under less tension, thus improving the final result. The choice of sutures is important. As previously mentioned, we use as few deep permanent sutures as possible. Those that dissolve will produce a marked inflammation. In all straight line closures, if practical, we employ a pullout subcuticular 5–0 or 6–0 nylon. All epidermal gaps are closed with a fine 5–0 or 6–0 mild Davis and Geck chromic suture, as advocated by Webster and associates.[13] When a zigzag closure is involved, we employ a vertical, half-buried corner mattress suture, often called a Gillies stitch. We take care to orient the extracutaneous portion of the mattress suture in the direction of the relaxed skin tension lines and thus obviate railroad tracks even in sutures left for several weeks. The geometric broken-line closure is closed with a running locking stitch of mild

chromic.[13] Finally, in longer scars, we often keep a small "island" of scar intact. We find that this greatly reduces the amount of gapping of the wound, which will allow a reduced tension closure.

Dermabrasion and dermal planing are adjunctive procedure that will tend to even out raised areas of the scars. A variety of abrasive surfaces are used: wire brush, diamond fraise, and sandpaper. Abrasion is administered by a motorized unit or by hand. The technique is not difficult, but a few principles should be kept in mind. The level of abrasion should not extend deeper than the most superficial dermis. If extended deeper, an unacceptable scar will often follow. The surgeon should abrade in the direction of relaxed skin tension lines and should feather the abrasion where the deepest abrasion occurs in the raised central portion and apply gradually less pressure on the periphery. Adjacent normal tissue should be included. Within hours, epidermal migration begins to occur, which will eventually re-epithelialize the dermabraded segment, resulting in a smoother, cosmetically improved scar. Often it takes up to a year to see the full effect of dermabrasion; nevertheless, we have found often that a second or third procedure may be necessary and can be safely performed after 2 to 3 months.

Dermal planing is similar to dermabrasion

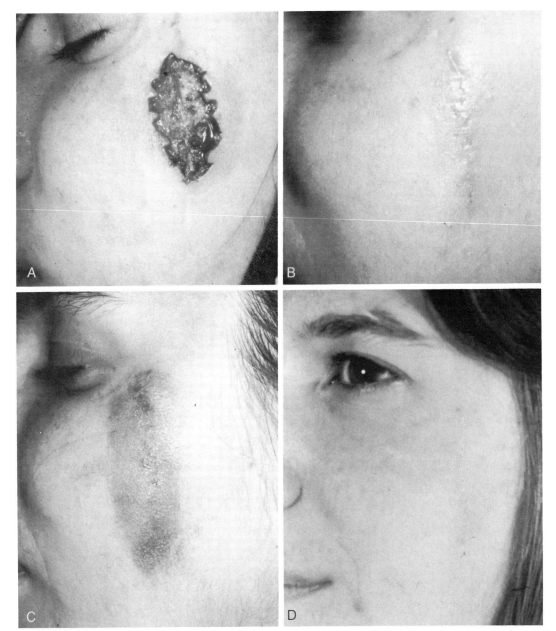

FIGURE 28–6. *A*, Gaping wound with broken-line geometric design. *B*, Two months postoperatively. *C*, Dermabrasion at 6 months. *D*, Photograph at 1 year.

in that the scar and adjacent areas are evened by actually leveling the area with a scalpel blade. Again, care must be taken not to reach the superficial dermis but to include adjacent areas of normal skin to allow a more even result. If a scar is felt to be enlarging or firmer than usual, it is injected with a mixture of triamcinolone acetonide (Kenalog), 40 mg/ml and hyaluronidase (Wydase), 150 units/ml

via a Dermajet or Modajet. This is repeated every 2 weeks until there is palpable softening or visible flattening of the scar.

Unlike normal or hypertrophic scars, keloids invade and expand beyond normal adjacent tissue. Their management has proved most frustrating, which is reflected by the variety of techniques described. Because of the different nature of keloids, our management of these scars differs markedly from that of other scars.[14] We employ the CO_2 laser at 10 watts, using a 0.2 mm spot size with the handpiece to excise the keloid. After the skin is incised, the keloid is resected from its base in the plane beneath the dense collagen of the lesion. This plane is relatively avascular and is found by placing maximal traction on the keloid perpendicular to its base. Most bleeding encountered in this plane can be controlled by a defocused beam. All keloid tissue must be removed.

Once excised, there is no attempt to close the wound since this will tend to initiate a new keloid formation. Rather, the open bed is managed as a full-thickness burn with either silver sulfadiazine (Silvadene) or A&D ointment. The wound is dressed for patient comfort, with the deepest layer being non-adhesive.

Our experience with over 50 keloids of this type demonstrates that the wound will contract significantly so that in 10 days it will approximate the size of the initial keloid base. In the following 3 to 6 weeks, the wound will relentlessly orient itself in the direction of relaxed skin tension until ultimate closure and re-epithelization. The normal contracting forces usually place the final result in a very narrow band and orient it in the direction of RSTLs (Fig. 28–7).

Once the wound is closed, the risk of recurrent keloid is significant. We therefore follow these patients every 2 to 3 weeks initially for the first 3 months and then once a month for 2 years. If a firm collagen bed is palpated beneath the flat atrophic epithelium, we feel that the keloid is attempting to re-establish itself. We then inject with our mixture of Kenalog, 40 mg/ml and Wydase, 150 units/ml via the Dermajet or Modajet every 2 or 3 weeks until the scar has softened. With this technique we have achieved an 80 per cent success rate.

Summary

In summary, scars are an inevitable consequence of any skin incision or traumatic laceration. A knowledgeable surgeon strives to place incisions in areas that will best conceal their presence. When confronted with an unacceptable scar, a variety of revision techniques are available. The surgeon must analyze why a poor scar resulted prior to choosing the techniques with which to revise it. The patient must have a good rapport with the surgeon and understand that no technique is perfect and that often multiple procedures are necessary. Keloids are a difficult management problem characterized by frequent recurrences; we offer a protocol that has been more effective than any other we previously employed.

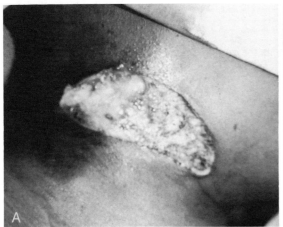 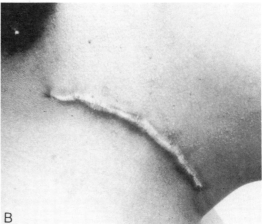

FIGURE 28–7. *A,* Resected bed of a neck keloid. *B,* Six weeks after laser resections, with a narrow scar band oriented in directions of relaxed skin tension lines.

References

1. FitzGibbons GM, Gilles HD: The Commandments of Gilles. Br J Plast Surg 21:226, 1968.
2. Belinger NT: Wound healing. Otolaryngol Clin North Am 15:29–34, 1982.
3. Boucek RJ: Factors affecting wound healing. Otolaryngol Clin North Am 17:243–261, 1984.
4. Ryan GB, Cliff WJ, et al: Myofibroblasts in human granulation tissue. Hum Pathol 5:55–67, 1974.
5. Chuapil M, Koopman CF: Scar formation: Physiology and pathological states. Otolaryngol Clin North Am 17:265–272, 1984.
6. Peacock EE: Keloids and Hypertrophic Scars in Wound Repair. Philadelphia, WB Saunders, 1984, pp 159–166.
7. Borges AF: Major Factors in Scar Prognosis in Elective Incisions and Scar Revision. Boston, Little, Brown, 1972, pp 18–19.
8. Raynell A: The tensability of the skin: An experimental investigation. Plast Reconstr Surg 14:317, 1954.
9. Borges AF, Alexander JG, Block CC: Z-plasty treatment of aesthetic scars. EENT Monthly 44:39, 1965.
10. Denouvilliers CP: Blepharoplastie. Sol Chir Paris 7:243–244, 1856.
11. McCurdy SL: Plastic operations to elongate cicatrical contractions across joints. Cleve Med J 3:123, 1964.
12. Webster RC, Davidson TM, Smith RC: Broken line scar revision. Clin Plast Surg 4:263–274, 1972.
13. Webster RC, Davidson TM, Smith RC: Wound closure with absorbable sutures. Laryngoscope 84:1280–1284, 1976.
14. Stucker FJ, Shaw GY: Management of keloids and hypertrophic scars. In Papel I (ed): Plastic Surgery of the Face. Chicago, Year Book Medical Publishers, 1992.

CHAPTER 29

Stomal Recurrence and Mediastinal Dissection

YOSEF P. KRESPI, MD
GEORGE A. SISSON, MD

STOMAL RECURRENCE

Stomal recurrence following total laryngectomy is associated with poor survival rates. Radical surgery yields the most promising chance of cure. Death following surgical treatment may be related to uncontrolled disease, but in a significant number of patients it is related to surgical complications, including sepsis and large vessel rupture. Diminution of these complications would decrease morbidity and mortality, and therefore enhance ultimate survival.

The incidence of postlaryngectomy stomal recurrence varies from 5 per cent to 15 per cent. Several factors have been implicated in the etiology of stomal recurrence, including the location of the primary tumor, its size, and whether a preliminary tracheotomy was performed before the definitive resection. Stomal recurrence is generally associated with lesions having subglottic extension. However, Myers and Ogura[1] noted increased incidence with bulky transglottic lesions, even in the absence of subglottic involvement. Periostomal recurrence has been reported following tracheostomy that is performed for other primary head and neck tumors, most likely due to implantation of tumor cells around the tracheostoma.

Stomal recurrence is classified into four types and the prognosis can be predicted accordingly. Type I is localized and usually presents as a discrete nodule in the superior aspect of the stoma (Fig. 29–1). The prognosis is very good if the lesion is detected and treated early. Type II indicates an esophageal involvement but no inferior involvement (Fig. 29–2). The prognosis for Type II is fair to good, depending on the amount of esophageal involvement. Type III originates inferior to the laryngostoma and usually has direct extension into the upper mediastinum (Fig. 29–3). Type IV indicates there is an extension laterally and often under the head of the clavicles (Fig. 29–4). We consider all patient with Type IV and some patients with

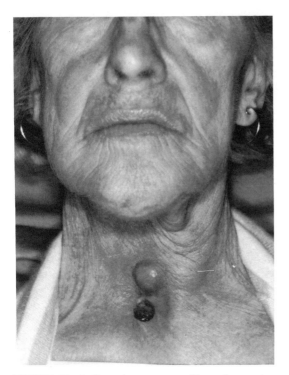

FIGURE 29–1. Stomal recurrence (Type I) superior to the tracheostoma.

Type III stomal recurrences to be nonsurgical candidates. Most often Type III stomal recurrences will undergo mediastinoscopy or mediastinal exploration to determine resectability.

Following Watson's[2] report of the first successful surgical resection for stomal recurrence in 1942, many surgeons explored the feasibility of an operative approach. These early reports stress the difficulties encountered in reconstruction of the surgical defect. The inordinate number of complications and high mortality recorded in the early publications resulted primarily from inadequate protection of the major vessels exposed in the surgical defect. Although radical resection offered the best chance of cure, the technical problems encountered prevented the operation from obtaining wide acceptance as the treatment of choice in the management of stomal recurrences. Various other modalities, including radiotherapy, chemotherapy, and a combination of both, were offered as palliative measures but without predictable results.

Recent reports in the literature have proposed chemotherapy and radiotherapy for the management of stomal recurrence.[3] Data are available on 384 patients with advanced and/or recurrent squamous cell carcinoma treated at Northwestern University Medical School with chemotherapy, surgery, and radiation therapy from 1979 to 1987. Among these patients, 12 with stomal recurrences were treated with *cis*-platinum bolus and 5-fluorouracil infusion. Only one patient survived beyond 12 months. These data support the fact that acceptable palliation in this disease can be expected only from aggressive surgical therapy.

The concept of surgical resection of recurrent stomal carcinoma was stimulated by reports from Sisson,[4, 5] who stressed the importance of protecting the major vessels from postoperative rupture. He employed the medially based pectoral muscle flap to obliterate the operative defect in the mediastinum and to act as a cushion between the trachea and the innominate artery. Sisson[5, 6] later described techniques for staging the removal of the manubrium and clavicles and for preparing the necessary regional cutaneous flaps. He emphasized the importance of proper flap selection to meet the needs of a specific clinical problem. The bipedicle chest visor

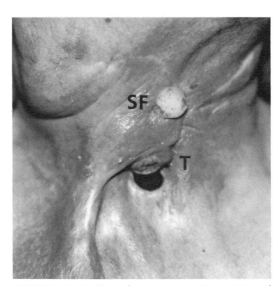

FIGURE 29–2. Stomal recurrence (Type II) with esophageal involvement. Tumor superior to the tracheostoma. T, tumor; SF, salivary fistula.

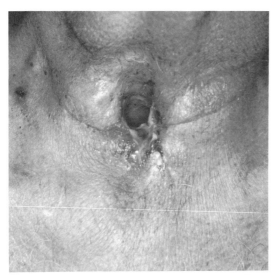

FIGURE 29–3. Stomal recurrence (Type III) inferior to the tracheostoma with mediastinal extension.

flap, the lateral chest flap, and the medial chest flap, along with the pectoralis major muscle flap, were used according to the classification of the type of stomal recurrence. Multiple staged reconstructive procedures for stomal recurrence required flaps with elaborate planning and precise execution. It was mandatory to cover the carotid artery and the innominate artery with dermal grafts. The morbidity associated with multiple staged procedures and the resultant increase in the hospital stay and associated mortality were adequately documented in the literature by Sisson.[7]

The pectoralis major island myocutaneous flap, in our experience, is superior to previously employed staged techniques. Only one operative procedure is necessary. The great vessels are covered by well-vascularized muscle tissue, therefore eliminating the need for dermal grafts. The pectoralis muscle mass also obliterates dead space in the upper mediastinum. The donor defect is closed primarily with minimal deformity, and a skin or dermal graft is not required.

OPERATIVE TECHNIQUE

The procedure is performed with the patient in the supine position. The area of tumor involvement, including the tracheal stoma and a minimum of a 3-cm skin margin, is incised. The sternal ends of the clavicles and the upper portion of the manubrium are removed to obtain an en bloc resection of the involved tracheal stoma and to provide access for the superior mediastinal lymphadenectomy.

Following removal of the manubrium, the internal periosteum is carefully incised. The innominate artery and vein are identified. The node-bearing fat pad of the upper mediastinum is dissected with a combination of sharp and blunt dissection, exposing all the great vessels. The innominate vein may be ligated and transected if necessary for better visualization, and the contents of the superior mediastinum are swept superiorly to connect with the neck dissection specimen. Low paratracheal and tracheoesophageal nodes are also included in the resection and are incorporated into the specimen at this point. When removing these low paratracheal and tracheoesophageal nodes, it is always necessary to include the remaining portion of the thyroid gland. When performing a block dissection in this area, most, if not all, of the patient's parathyroid tissue is removed. This can result in hypoparathyroidism, which must be treated postoperatively.

Reconstruction begins with the design of the skin island of the myocutaneous flap.

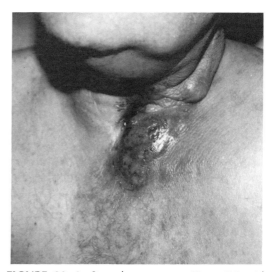

FIGURE 29–4. Stomal recurrence (Type IV) with inferior and lateral extension under the clavicle.

The size and shape of the island depend upon the size of the surgical defect. A circumferential incision is made around the outlined skin island and continued through the subcutaneous tissue to the pectoralis major muscle. The entire muscle is exposed by elevating medial and lateral chest flaps. The pectoralis major muscle with the overlying skin island is elevated. The lateral edge of the muscle is identified and separated from the chest wall. The flap is elevated superiorly, and the lateral thoracic artery and pectoral branch of the thoracoacromial artery are easily identified on the deep surface of the muscle. The tendinous insertion to the humerus is severed. The lateral thoracic artery is usually preserved due to a limited rotation arc. A large subcutaneous tunnel is made through the skin bridge between the neck incision and chest, and the flap is passed beneath the skin bridge into the operative defect.

The skin island is sutured to the cutaneous margins of the cervical defect and to the trachea. Two types of island skin configuration have been used. When the cutaneous defect following stomal resection is primarily superior (Types I or II), the skin island has a semilunar shape. The myocutaneous flap covers the surgical defect above and at both sides of the stoma. The inferior margin of the new stoma is sutured to the upper chest skin. However, with extensive circumferential defects (Type III), the new stoma is placed in the center of the skin island (doughnut shape). A 1.5- to 2-cm skin ellipse is excised from the center of the skin island, and the subcutaneous tissue and muscle are bluntly spread to permit insertion and suturing of the trachea. In either method most of the pectoralis muscle is insinuated between the trachea and the great vessels. The chest donor defect is closed primarily.

Lesions involving the cervical esophagus require immediate reconstruction of the gullet. Following resection of the proximal trachea, the common tracheoesophageal wall is exposed. The posterior tracheal wall is separated from the esophagus by blunt dissection. Tears at the posterior tracheal wall must be avoided by using careful dissection. Once the tumor and the upper esophagus are mo-

bilized and a tumor-free tracheal stump is obtained, the lesion is determined fully resectable and suitable for gastric pull-up reconstruction.

The abdominal surgical team enters the abdomen with a long midline incision. A large, self-retaining retractor (Gomez Retractor, Pilling Company, Philadelphia, PA) is placed after entering the abdominal cavity. The stomach is mobilized, preserving the right gastric and gastroepiploic vessels. The left gastric and left gastroepiploic vessels are ligated. The short gastric arteries are carefully ligated, and the spleen is protected with abdominal pads. A wide Kocher maneuver is performed to mobilize the duodenum. The esophageal hiatus is enlarged, and both vagus nerves are clipped and transected. Pyloroplasty is mandatory to avoid gastric outlet obstruction. Using sharp dissection under direct vision, followed by a blunt dissection, the anterior and posterior walls of the esophagus are mobilized in the posterior mediastinum. The blind simultaneous bimanual mobilization is carried out by two teams— one surgeon working from the neck, the other from the abdomen. After complete mobilization, the specimen is pulled to the neck. The esophagus is divided at the cardioesophageal junction by stapler, and the fundus portion of the stomach is positioned to create a gastropharyngeal anastomosis. This is performed with single layer nonabsorbable sutures. The abdominal team creates a needle jejunostomy. A nasogastric tube is inserted to decompress the stomach. The abdominal cavity is closed in layers in the usual fashion. After completion of the anastomosis, the skin defect is measured and the appropriate sized pectoralis myocutaneous flap is elevated from the chest wall, as described earlier.

REVIEW OF PATIENTS AND RESULTS

Sixty patients operated for stomal recurrence in the last 30 years are reviewed: 53 men (88 per cent) and 7 women (12 per cent) are included in these series. Ages ranged from 31 to 79 years. Owing to major changes in the surgical reconstructive techniques, the statistical analyses are separated into the initial 20 years (1958–1978) and the last 10 years (1979-1988). The turning point in reconstruction represents the development of the pectoralis major myocutaneous flap in 1979.

Thirty-two patients were operated on prior to 1979 and twenty-eight patients were operated on after 1979. Because of complex reconstructive techniques, 57 per cent of the patients (18 of 32) were operated on more than once in the era prior to 1979. Only 14 per cent of the patients were operated on more than once after 1979. The intrasurgical complications were slightly higher in the pre-1979 era. However, this may not be statistically significant. The postoperative complications, on the other hand, were significantly larger in the patients operated on prior to 1979. This is due to multiple reconstructive procedures using only skin flaps. The incidence of postoperative complications has dropped significantly following the development of the pectoralis myocutaneous flap. Survival in the immediate postoperative period has changed significantly because of protection of the large vessels with the myocutaneous flap. Ninety-seven per cent of the patients operated on after 1979 survived 60 days or more, as opposed to 72 per cent with a 60-day survival rate prior to 1979.

The overall survival statistics in the past 10 years are as follows: 61 per cent of patients survived 1 year and 47 per cent of patients survived 2 years or more. The average hospital stay was reduced from 60 days to 20 days after development of the pectoralis major myocutaneous flap.

DISCUSSION

Prior to the development of the transsternal radical neck dissection or mediastinal dissection for the treatment of postlaryngectomy stomal recurrence, patients with low cervical disease or involvement of the upper mediastinum uniformly met a fatal outcome. With application and increased experience with mediastinal dissection, a significant number of patients with stomal recurrence so treated met with a favorable outcome from the standpoint of both palliation and cure.

Since radiotherapy has offered little chance of cure and virtually no potential for palliation, treatment of this disease remains surgical.

Previously, malignant lesions recurring peristomally with esophageal involvement were considered beyond operative intervention. As noted, Sisson,[4] in 1962, popularized the trans-sternal or mediastinal dissection for stomal recurrence. With continued experience, the real danger of great vessel exposure and rupture at the base of the neck was appreciated. Sisson and others solved the arterial exposure problem with a combination of skin flaps, dermal graft, and pectoralis major muscle flap.

The deltopectoral and laterally based chest flap for reconstruction decreased the length of hospitalization and postoperative complications to acceptable levels in the early 1970s. More recently, Biller[8] reported the successful single-stage reconstruction after mediastinal dissection in seven patients, using only the pectoralis major myocutaneous flap. Myocutaneous flap coverage greatly reduced the rate of vessel exposure and rupture after mediastinal dissection. In a recent report the attention was turned to the problematic reconstruction of patients who had cervical esophageal involvement.

Fifteen patients underwent pharyngoesophagectomy and mediastinal dissection for stomal recurrence following previous irradiation and total laryngectomy. Of these 15 patients, 9 are alive after 2 years. Six patients were dead of the disease within 1 year of surgery. This represents a 60 per cent raw survival rate. However, of the nine survivors, four are alive with disease and five have no clinical evidence of disease. Thus, 27 per cent of these patients are alive with disease and 33 per cent are alive and free of disease.

Turning now to the most important aspect of the surgical management of this lesion, survival, we find that it remains essentially unchanged. The previously reported rate for 5-year survival after mediastinal dissection alone is 17 per cent to 33 per cent.

While this new method of immediate reconstruction for patients undergoing pharyngoesophagectomy and mediastinal dissection for recurrent disease may not offer any or very little improvement in survival, it enables the patient to leave the hospital quickly. More importantly, it leaves the patient with the ability to eat a normal diet, which from the palliative standpoint represents a great deal to these individuals.

References

1. Myers EM, Ogura JH: Stomal recurrences: A clinicopathological analysis for future management. Laryngoscope 89:1121–1128, 1979.
2. Watson WL: Cancer of the trachea 15 years after treatment of cancer of the larynx. J Thorac Surg 12:142–150, 1942.
3. Krespi YP, Wurster SF, Sisson GA: Immediate reconstruction after total Laryngopharyngoesophagectomy and mediastinal dissection. Laryngoscope 95:156–161, 1985.
4. Sisson GA, Straehly CJ Jr: Mediastinal dissection for recurrent cancer after laryngectomy. Laryngoscope 72:1069–1077, 1962.
5. Sisson GA: Mediastinal dissection for recurrent cancer after laryngectomy. Trans Am Acad Ophthalmol Otolaryngol 74:767–777, 1970.
6. Sisson GA, Edison BD, Bytell DE: Transsternal radical neck dissection: Postoperative complications and management. Arch Otolaryngol 101:46–49, 1975.
7. Sisson GA, Bytell DE, Edison BD, et al: Transsternal radical neck dissection for control of stomal recurrences–end results. Laryngoscope 85:1504–1510, 1975.
8. Biller HF, Krespi YP, Lawson W, et al: A one-stage reconstruction following resection for stomal recurrence. Otolaryngol Head Neck Surg 88:357–360, 1980.

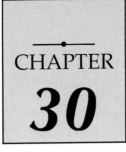

CHAPTER

30

Laser Surgery

ROBERT H. OSSOFF, DMD, MD

Laser is an acronym for **L**ight **A**mplification by the **S**timulated **E**mission of **R**adiation. The development and subsequent addition of laser technology to the existing surgical armamentarium offers new and exciting possibilities for improving conventional surgical approaches and techniques and expanding the scope of modern otolaryngology–head and neck surgery. Lasers are precise, but potentially dangerous, surgical instruments that must be used with caution. Certain distinct and unprecedented advantages have been associated with the use of lasers in performing surgical procedures of the head and neck and upper aerodigestive tract; however, several unique, potentially serious, and sometimes catastrophic complications have occurred in patients undergoing laser surgical procedures in these anatomic sites. Furthermore, reports about many of these unique laser-related complications, complete with conflicting discussions detailing how to avoid these laser-related accidents, appeared to increase as the use of this technology proliferated.[1]

ADMINISTRATIVE CONSIDERATIONS

Because of the risk of laser-related complications, the head and neck surgeon should first determine whether the use of laser technology offers any distinct advantages over conventional surgical techniques. Exposure to some type of formal laser education program, therefore, is essential and must serve as a non-negotiable prerequisite to the use of this technology. For those head and neck surgeons who did not receive adequate instruction in laser surgery during their residency training, mandatory attendance at one of the many excellent hands-on training courses in laser surgery offered in the United States should be considered the minimum necessary exposure to a formal laser education program. The curriculum should include lectures on laser biophysics, tissue interactions, clinical applications, special delivery systems, and safety precautions. Additionally, supervised hands-on laboratory training using living laboratory animals is essential. Following attendance at such a course, it is suggested that the surgeon plan to practice the newly acquired laser surgical skills by working on cadaver or animal specimens before progressing to perform, at first, simple procedures on patients, followed by more difficult procedures.[2]

A laser safety committee should be formed and a laser safety officer appointed by each hospital in which laser surgery is performed. Membership on the committee should consist of the laser safety officer, two or three physicians using lasers, one or two nursing representatives from the operating room, a hospital administrator, a biomedical engineer, and a member of the hospital's quality assurance program. The purpose of this committee is to develop policies and procedures for the safe use of lasers within the hospital. The safety protocols established by this committee will vary with each specialty using lasers, of course. This committee should also make the recommendations regarding the appropriate credential-certifying mechanisms required of each physician and nurse who becomes involved with using the lasers. In other words, the educational policies for surgeons, anesthesiologists, nurses, and other health care personnel working with lasers will be developed by this committee. Two additional responsibilities of this committee include the accumulation of laser-related patient data in cases in which an investigational laser device was used and a periodic review of all laser-related complications.

Because our colleagues in anesthesiology also are concerned with the airway and because potent oxidizing gases frequently pass through the airway via an endotracheal tube in close approximation to the path of the therapeutic laser beam, it is necessary to develop a team approach to the anesthetic management of the patient undergoing laser surgery of the upper aerodigestive tract. Hence, it is highly recommended that anesthesiologists, who will be attending patients upon whom the laser will be used, attend a didactic session that discusses in depth the many anesthetic considerations, precautions, and techniques appropriate for patients

undergoing laser surgery of the head and neck and upper aerodigestive tract.[3] Finally, the operating room staff must receive a formal education with respect to laser surgery. Attendance at an in-service workshop, with exposure to clinical laser biophysics and the fundamental workings of the laser, as well as hands-on orientation to the laser and its delivery systems, should be the minimal requirement for nursing participation in laser surgery cases.[4]

SAFETY PRECAUTIONS

The successful development of an effective laser safety protocol is definitely the single most important reason why this potentially dangerous surgical technology can be used so safely in treating patients with diseases of the head and neck and upper aerodigestive tract. Such a protocol must stress compliance and meticulous attention to detail on the part of the surgeon, anesthesiologist, and operating room nurse (laser surgery team). This protocol must be general enough to include all the major and most of the minor precautions necessary to perform safe and efficacious laser surgery in the anatomic confines of the head and neck (Table 30–1). General considerations include the provision for protection of both the patient's and operating room personnel's eyes and skin and the provision for adequate smoke (laser plume) evacuation from the operative field. Other precautions that must be addressed include the choice of anesthetic techniques and endotracheal tubes, if used, and the selection of proper instruments, including bronchoscopes and laryngoscopes.

Eye Protection

Injury to the eye is certainly possible from an acute exposure to the laser beam. This injury can take the form of either a corneal or lenticular opacity (cataract) or a retinal burn; the actual injury occurs at the area of the eye where the most radiant energy per

TABLE 30–1. Laser Safety Protocol

I. Eye Protection
  A. Patient
    1. Tape patient's eyes shut
    2. Double layer of saline-saturated eye pads placed over the patient's eyes for carbon dioxide laser
    3. Double layer of saline-saturated eye pads placed over the patient's eyes covered by crumpled aluminum foil and wavelength specific protective glasses for Nd:YAG and visible lasers
  B. Operating room personnel
    1. Wear protective glasses with side protectors
    2. Surgeon does not require protective glasses when working with the operating microscope when using carbon dioxide laser
    3. Surgeon does require protective glasses when working with the operating microscope and Nd:YAG and/or visible lasers
  C. Warning signs
    1. Placed outside of all entrances into the operating room when the laser is used
    2. Caution persons entering the room that the laser is in use and that protective glasses are required
  D. Limited access
    1. Limit traffic into the operating room when the laser is in use
    2. Keep doors to the operating room closed when laser is in use
II. Skin Protection
  A. Use a double layer of saline-saturated surgical towels, surgical sponges, or lap pads to cover all exposed skin and mucous membranes of the patient outside of the surgical field
    1. Keep this protective layer wet during the case
    2. Do not forget to protect the teeth, when exposed
  B. When microlaryngeal surgery is performed, the patient's face is completely draped with saline-saturated towels
III. Smoke Evacuation
  A. Aspirate laser-induced smoke from the operative field
  B. Have two separate suction setups available in the operating room
    1. One suction for laser-induced smoke and steam
      a. High-power suction
      b. Disposable filters in suction line
    2. One suction for blood and mucus
IV. Anesthetic Considerations
  A. Use of nonflammable general anesthetic
  B. Limit oxygen concentration to maximum of 40%
    1. Mix oxygen with helium, nitrogen, or air
    2. Do not use nitrous oxide
  C. Use a "laser-safe" endotracheal tube, when available
  D. Use a Rusch red rubber endotracheal tube wrapped with Merocel Laser-Guard or reflective metallic tape when "laser-safe" tube not available
  E. Protection of the endotracheal tube cuff
    1. Use saline-saturated cottonoids to protect the endotracheal tube cuff
      a. Keep the cottonoids moist
      b. Count the cottonoids
    2. Use methylene blue–colored saline to inflate cuff
    3. Use the operating platform
V. Instrument Selection
  A. Use of wide-bore microlaryngoscope
  B. Choose instruments with a nonreflective surface

volume of tissue has been absorbed. When the wavelength of the laser is in the visible and near-infrared range of the electromagnetic spectrum (0.4 to 1.4 μm), retinal injury will occur. Laser radiation in the ultraviolet (less than 0.4 μm) or in the far-infrared range of the spectrum (greater than 1.4 μm) produces effects primarily at the cornea, although certain wavelengths may also reach the lens.[5]

In all laser surgical cases, certain precautions must be adhered to if the risk of ocular injury is to be decreased. First, a sign should be placed on the operating room door warning those persons entering the room that the laser is in use. This sign should specify which laser is in use and that all those entering should wear the proper protective glasses. The doors to the operating room should remain closed, and any windows on the doors should be covered with protective window covers. The protective eyewear for the surgeon and operating room staff will vary according to the wavelength of the laser used.

The mid-infrared wavelength of the carbon dioxide laser requires the patient's eyes to be protected with a double layer of eye pads moistened with saline. Protective glasses with side protectors should be worn by all operating room personnel. Ordinary eyeglasses or contact lenses protect only the areas covered by the lens and do not provide any protection from the possibility of the laser beam entering the eye from the side. The optics of the operating microscope and rod lens telescopes do provide protection for the surgeon when working with the carbon dioxide laser. Here, the surgeon does not need to wear protective glasses.[6]

Use of the Nd:YAG laser requires all operating room personnel to wear wavelength-specific glasses. The patient's eyes should also be protected by a pair of these glasses, when possible. Otherwise, the patient's eyes should be protected by a double layer of saline moistened eye pads covered by a sheet of crumpled aluminum foil. Proper eye protection is always essential when performing Nd:YAG laser surgery, even when it is delivered to the target tissue using a fiber delivery device within an endoscope. It is possible that inadvertent deflection of the beam could occur as a result of a faulty contact, a break in the fiber, or accidental disconnection between the fiber and endoscope.[7]

When working with the argon, KTP, or dye laser, all personnel in the operating room, including the patient, should wear wavelength-specific protective glasses. Use of protective metal eye shields rather than protective glasses works well for patient eye protection when performing photocoagulation procedures for selected cutaneous vascular lesions on the face.[8] Similar precautions are necessary for the newer visible and near-infrared wavelength lasers. The major difference is the type of eye protection that is worn.

Skin Protection

A double layer of saline-saturated surgical towels, surgical sponges, or lap pads should be used to protect all exposed skin and mucous membranes outside the surgical field. When microlaryngeal laser surgery is being performed, there is a possibility that the beam could partially reflect off the proximal rim of the laryngoscope and burn the patient's face or forehead. Therefore, saline-saturated surgical towels are used to drape the patient's face completely, exposing only the proximal lumen of the laryngoscope. During the case it is frequently necessary to resaturate the drapes with saline to prevent them from drying out.

Protection of the teeth in the operative field has proved to be a challenge, especially when performing oral cavity laser surgery. Use of saline-saturated Telfa, surgical sponges, or specially constructed metal dental impression trays will provide protection to the teeth if they are carefully applied over them. Great care is exercised at the beginning of the case to protect the skin and teeth from accidental laser injury; this same compulsion should be displayed for the continued protection of the skin and teeth during the surgical procedure.[6]

Plume Evacuation

When performing laser surgery of the upper aerodigestive tract or head and neck, two separate suction setups should be available; one provides for adequate smoke and steam evacuation from the operative field, and the second is connected to the surgical suction tip for the aspiration of blood and mucus from the operative wound.[4] Constant suctioning is required to remove laser-induced smoke and steam from the operative field when performing laser surgery with a closed anesthetic system. When working with an open anesthetic system or with a jet ventilation system, suctioning should be used only on an intermittent basis to maintain the forced inspiratory oxygen (FIO_2) at a safe level. Laryngoscopes, bronchoscopes, operating platforms, mirrors, and anterior commissure and ventricle retractors with built-in smoke evacuation channels facilitate removal of the laser plume from the operative field.[6] Disposable filters in the suction lines should be used to prevent clogging of the suction lines by the black carbonaceous plume debris created by the laser.[9]

There has been recent concern about the possibility of hazards to health care workers related to laser plume inhalation. Tomita and colleagues suggested that the smoke created by the interaction of the carbon dioxide laser with tissue was probably mutagenic.[10] In another more recent study, Garden and colleagues demonstrated the presence of intact papillomavirus DNA in the smoke plume generated during laser surgery.[11] Although the significance of these findings remains in question, probably the risk of laser plume inhalation injury to health care workers can be reduced significantly by their wearing appropriate surgical masks and using a vacuum evacuation device for the plume.[12]

Anesthetic Considerations

Anesthetic management of the patient undergoing laser surgery of the head and neck or upper aerodigestive tract must include attention to three general areas: the safety of the patient, the requirements of the surgeon, and the hazards of the equipment. General anesthesia with muscle relaxation is usually required for microlaryngeal laser surgical cases, whereas laser surgery of the oral cavity and tracheobronchial tree can sometimes be performed with local anesthesia with or without sedation. General endotracheal anesthesia and jet ventilation with total intravenous anesthesia represent the two most commonly utilized forms of general anesthesia for laser surgery of the upper aerodigestive tract.

Any nonflammable general anesthetic is suitable for general endotracheal anesthesia; halothane and enflurane are most commonly used. The inspired concentration of oxygen, a potent oxidizing gas, is extremely important because of the historical risk of fire associated with microlaryngeal laser surgery cases performed under general endotracheal anesthesia. The oxygen should be diluted with helium, nitrogen, or air to maintain the FIO_2 around but not above 40 per cent and also to ensure that the patient is adequately oxygenated. Nitrous oxide is also a potent oxidizing gas and should not be used in the anesthetic mixture when performing laser surgery of the upper aerodigestive tract. Muscle relaxation is required to prevent movement of the vocal folds when laser surgery is performed in the larynx.

Jet ventilation techniques during laser surgery work well for selected patients.[13] Newer total intravenous anesthetic agents and use of pulse oximeters has facilitated widespread use of jet ventilation by many otolaryngologists–head and neck surgeons when performing microlaryngeal and bronchoscopic laser surgical cases.

At the present time a nonflammable, universally accepted endotracheal tube and cuff system for laser surgery of the upper aerodigestive tract does not exist. However, advances have been made with respect to the endotracheal tube shaft; at least two tubes, Mallinckrodt Laser-Flex and Xomed-Treace Laser Shield II, have shafts that are considered acceptable for both CO_2 and KTP/532 laser surgery of the upper aerodigestive tract.[14, 15] The cuff of both these tubes, however, is readily penetrated by the laser beam and must be protected in a fashion to be described later.

When a special laser-protective endotracheal tube cannot be used, protection of the endotracheal tube from either direct or reflected laser beam irradiation is of primary importance. Should the laser beam strike an unprotected endotracheal tube carrying oxygen, ignition of the tube could result in a catastrophic, intraluminal, blow-torch type of endotracheal tube fire.[16] Polyvinyl endotracheal tubes should not be used, either wrapped or unwrapped, because they offer the least resistance to penetration by the laser beam, their fire breakdown products are the most severe, and their tissue destruction tendencies exceed those of all other tubes tested.[1, 17] Rusch red rubber endotracheal tubes wrapped with Merocel Laser-Guard or circumferentially from the cuff to the top with reflective metallic tape reduce the risk of intraluminal fire. Mylar tape offers no protection and should not be used.[6, 7]

The cuff of the endotracheal tube also needs to be protected. Methylene blue–colored saline should be used to inflate the cuff, and saline-saturated neurosurgical cottonoids should be placed above the cuff in the subglottic larynx to further protect the cuff.[6, 18] These cottonoids will require frequent moistening during the procedure to prevent them from becoming too dry and acting as a wick. Cottonoids should be used only to protect the cuff; it is seductive to attempt to seal off the subglottis with cottonoids when using an uncuffed endotracheal tube. However, in this situation the cottonoids would dry out and act as a fire-causing wick. A cottonoid count prior to and following the procedure is essential and should be documented in both the nursing notes as well as in the operative report. Should the cuff become deflated from an inaccurate hit of the laser beam, the tube should be removed and replaced with a new one. Use of an operating platform is strongly recommended as a further layer of protection against potential danger.[19]

The Nd:YAG laser has a different interaction with endotracheal tubes than the CO_2 or KTP/532 laser. In vitro testing of many different endotracheal tubes with the Nd:YAG laser in our laboratory did not yield any conclusive information about which tube to recommend. Sosis also performed in vitro testing with the Nd:YAG laser and found the Rusch red rubber tube wrapped with reflective metallic tape to be safe for clinical use.[20]

As new laser wavelengths are developed for clinical use, currently acceptable endotracheal tubes will have to be checked with the new laser to make certain that their use will continue to be safe.

Instrument Selection

Instruments used in laser surgery should be prepared with surface characteristics that provide for low specular or direct reflectance and large diffuse or scattered reflectance of the laser beam, should the beam inadvertently strike the instrument. Because plastic instruments melt when irradiated with the laser, their use should be avoided.

When performing laser bronchoscopy with either the CO_2 or Nd:YAG laser, rigid instrumentation represents the preferred endoscopic delivery system. Should active bleeding occur during a case, it would be extremely difficult or impossible to control the airway successfully and evacuate the blood using flexible instrumentation. Additionally, rigid instrumentation allows the surgeon to pass one, two, or three suction cannulas through the bronchoscope to facilitate blood evacuation and airway control.

Bronchoscopic couplers for CO_2 laser surgery must include an optical system that allows the visible helium-neon aiming laser beam to be passed coaxially with the invisible CO_2 laser beam. Furthermore, the surgeon should be able to center the beam within the lumen of the bronchoscope to avoid the hazards associated with beam reflection off the inside wall of the bronchoscope, yielding subsequent loss of power and causing possible heating of the bronchoscope itself. Such a situation could cause burns of the trachea, larynx, pharynx, and oral cavity.[21]

COMPLICATIONS

Serious complications can occur if the laser surgical team deviates from the established laser safety protocol. Therefore, it is appropriate to review several categories of laser-related complications uniquely attributable to the use of the laser. What these complications are, why they occur, and how to avoid them are discussed.

Exposure Hazards to the Patient or Operating Room Personnel

Ocular injury and skin injury represent the two most common potential exposure hazards to the patient or operating room personnel. No cases of ocular injury have been reported in our literature; however, Leibowitz and Peacock discuss this potential in an experimental study they reported in 1969.[22] Most probably, compulsive adherence to the safety protocol has helped prevent this type of injury. Several surgeons have reported laser-induced skin injuries, most of which have occurred secondary to movement of the protective drapes during the case.[1, 6, 22] It follows, then, that the surgical team must check the drapes frequently during the case to prevent such an injury from occurring.

Finger burns suffered by the surgeon also have been reported in association with microlaryngeal laser surgery cases.[1, 6] This injury occurs when the surgeon does not keep the hand out of the line of fire of the laser beam. If the surgeon notices a loss of the brilliance of the red helium-neon aiming laser while performing microlaryngeal laser surgery, he or she should not activate the laser. Instead, the surgeon should look around the binocular tube of the microscope and determine whether the laser beam is reflecting off the shaft of the microlaryngeal instrument, proximal rim of the microlaryngoscope, or the finger. Correcting the alignment of the optical beam path of the microscope and therapeutic beam path of the laser through the lumen of the laryngoscope is frequently necessary to overcome the former two problems, and moving the hand to the extreme side of the operative field is necessary to prevent the latter. It is very helpful to develop surgical skill with both hands when performing microlaryngeal laser surgery. This will allow the surgeon to avoid crossing the hands through the operative field.

Inadvertent Laser Irradiation

Inadvertent laser irradiation of the patient or operating room personnel can lead to several diverse types of complications. Both direct and reflected laser energy can cause burns to the patient or operating room personnel. Chances are greater that this type of complication will occur if the laser in not in proper alignment. Carbon dioxide lasers with their articulated arms are much more prone to go out of alignment than those lasers that use fiber delivery systems. The risk of injury is greatest with a misaligned laser when performing microlaryngeal surgery. Therefore one should test the alignment on a supraglottic area prior to performing the procedure at the level of the vocal folds. A laser shooting to the left could fire through the vocal folds and impact the cottonoids protecting the cuff if the surgeon was working on the right vocal fold. Failure to use cottonoids in this situation would cause the cuff to rupture. Reflected laser energy can occur as the beam passes through the endoscope. This is usually recognized by a characteristic glare of the helium-neon aiming beam as it reflects off the proximal rim or inner lumen of the endoscope. Once again, realignment of the beam path through the endoscope is the corrective action. Using nonreflective instrumentation and taking great care when working in and around the teeth will help reduce reflective laser tissue injuries.

Tracheal perforation, when performing bronchoscopic laser surgery, represents one of the most serious complications from inadvertent laser irradiation. Proper technique is the best preventive measure here. The laser beam should be directed parallel to the long axis of the airway; the surgeon should avoid firing the laser tangentially at the wall of the airway. Knowledge of the airway anatomy beyond the obstruction is essential and can be best determined by careful study of the airway through preoperative radiographic studies and pretreatment flexible bronchoscopy. Finally, the laser should be used in shuttered rather than continuous exposures to help minimize the risk of perforating the airway. In patients in whom either extrinsic compression from a tumor or cartilaginous collapse from a stenosis has been found, bronchoscopic laser surgery should not be performed. These observations represent strong contraindications to performing bronchoscopic laser surgery.

Endotracheal tube ignition can occur from direct or reflected laser beam irradiation. Proper selection of an endotracheal tube in conjunction with using the proper anesthetic gas mixture will help prevent this complication.

Acquired anterior or posterior glottic web secondary to laser surgery for patients with recurrent respiratory papillomatosis has been recently reported.[23, 24] The surgeon must respect the integrity of the anterior and posterior commissures when performing laser surgery for this or any other disease within the larynx. Preservation of a 2- to 3-mm cuff of mucosa on one or the other vocal fold at the anterior or posterior commissure will help prevent this complication.[25, 26] Use of the microspot micromanipulator also will contribute greatly toward reducing this complication.[27]

Subglottic stenosis as a complication secondary to excising a congenital subglottic hemangioma has been reported by Cotton and Tewfik.[28] The best precaution against this complication is to avoid excising mucosa circumferentially in the subglottic larynx.

Vocal fold fibrosis is a complication of inadvertent laser irradiation and may represent the most common complication following laser surgery for benign lesions of the larynx. This complication typically occurs after the vocal ligament has been violated either directly from laser beam penetration or indirectly from thermal injury to the vocal ligament. In either case, the laser had to be applied to the larynx incorrectly. Use of ap-

propriately low power densities and short shuttered exposures rather than continuous exposure will help minimize this complication. The precision afforded by the microspot micromanipulator with low-power application to the larynx also will allow the surgeon to achieve the desired end results without increased risk to the integrity of the vocal ligament. Shapshay and colleagues have performed a study with the microspot that demonstrates the efficacy and safety of laser surgery for benign laryngeal disease when the energy is applied using appropriate power densities with the microspot.[29]

Anesthetic Hazards

Anesthetic hazards represent the greatest concern to the head and neck surgeon with respect to laser surgery of the upper aerodigestive tract. Endotracheal tube ignition is a catastrophic complication and must be avoided; therefore, strict compliance with the safety protocol is imperative. A review of all laser-ignited endotracheal tube fires in the literature through 1988 revealed that these fires occurred because of three reasons.[1] First, there was a controversy in the literature about which tube to use or how to best protect it. Second, there was a deviation in the then-standard of care with respect to protection of the tube or choice of anesthetic gas mixture. Third, a new "laser proof" endotracheal tube was introduced that in fact was not laser proof and caught fire.[30] This latter reason is most distressing and should serve as a warning to both anesthesiologists and otolaryngologists–head and neck surgeons to make certain that the new product is indeed safe for use with the laser that they plan to use. The product insertion package should be carefully reviewed to determine which lasers can be used with the tube and what maximum power density and exposure time the tube will tolerate in a certain oxygen environment.

The polyvinyl chloride endotracheal tube is mentioned here only to condemn its use in upper aerodigestive tract laser surgery. Phosgene and hydrochloride gases are given off from the tube upon impact with the laser. Both these gases are toxic to the airway. Furthermore, this tube is readily penetrated by the laser and causes a fire that deposits black, carbonaceous hydrocarbon debris throughout the airway. The soft tissue effects of a fire with this tube are more extreme than they are with either a Rusch red rubber tube or silicone tube.[17] Although protecting the polyvinyl tube with reflective metallic tape should provide sufficient protection from laser beam penetration, if the beam does find a way through the protective tape the results would be devastating. Thus, the polyvinyl endotracheal tube should not be used when performing laser surgery of the upper aerodigestive tract, either wrapped or unwrapped.

Other anesthetic hazards include inadequate ventilation. Inadequate ventilation can occur from the endotracheal tube's becoming kinked secondary to direct pressure on the tube caused by using the posterior commissure laryngoscope or caused by rupture of the endotracheal tube cuff and intraoperative airway obstruction from foreign bodies in the airway (metallic tape or cottonoids). Other anesthetic hazards are displaced tumor debris, displaced blood clot, or tracheobronchial neoplasm. Should the anesthesiologist inform the surgeon of ventilatory difficulties, these possibilities should be reviewed.

Pneumothorax and several other complications of jet ventilation have been reported in the literature. However, because these complications do not represent unique, laser-related problems, they are not discussed in this chapter.

Suggested Patient Management During and Following an Endotracheal Tube Fire

Compulsive adherence to the laser safety protocol will reduce the risk of laser-induced endotracheal tube fire to as close to 0 per cent as possible.[1] However, it is essential that the proper management of a patient during and following an endotracheal tube fire be discussed.

The first step in the management of the patient during a laser-induced endotracheal tube fire is to immediately extubate the patient. The amount of soft tissue injury to the airway is directly related to the length of time that the fire burns within the airway. Other factors that enter into the equation include the oxygen concentration, the anesthetic gas mixture, the type of endotracheal tube, and the location of the tube within the airway. At the same time that the surgeon extubates the patient he or she should yell to the anesthesiologist to shut off the oxygen and other anesthetic gases.

Following extubation, the anesthesiologist should ventilate the patient by mask while provisions for either endoscopic evaluation or reintubation are made. The ideal step following extubation is for the surgeon to perform direct laryngoscopy to assess the amount of thermal damage at the level of the larynx, followed by rigid bronchoscopy to assess the amount of thermal damage within the tracheobronchial tree. If the bronchoscopic instrumentation is not readily available, then the patient should be reintubated with a small endotracheal tube.

While the surgeon is examining the airway, the anesthesiologist should inspect the burned endotracheal tube to determine whether it is intact. Often, a portion of the tube distal to the cuff separates from the main shaft of the tube and lodges at the carina or within the right main stem bronchus. If the tube had been protected with reflective metallic tape, all the tape must be accounted for. Frequently after a laser-induced endotracheal tube fire, some of the reflective tape dislodges from the tube and remains within the airway. Cottonoids also need to be counted since the possibility of their remaining within the airway as foreign bodies is distinctly possible.

Examination of the airway, then, must not only assess the thermal damage caused from the fire, but also facilitate foreign body removal, if necessary. In addition, gentle debridement of the airway should be performed in appropriate anatomic sites. Tracheotomy should be performed if the degree of thermal injury to the larynx is severe.

Intravenous antibiotics and steroids should be administered and a consultation from the appropriate internist that treats thermal inhalation injuries should be obtained.

Reflective Tape Wrapping of Endotracheal Tubes

Rusch red rubber endotracheal tubes wrapped with reflective metallic tape or Merocel Laser Guard are still commonly used for laser surgery. Retained reflective metallic tape as a cause of acute airway obstruction has been reported by Kaeder and Hirshman.[31] When wrapped tubes are used, the tube must be inspected at extubation to make sure that all the tape that was on the tube at intubation is still there. Should a piece of tape be found to be missing, the oral cavity, oropharynx, hypopharynx, larynx, and trachea must be carefully examined. Vocal fold trauma from the wrapped endotracheal tubes can represent another form of complication from wrapping tubes. Careful wrapping of the tubes to minimize rough edges and careful intubation by the most experienced member of the anesthesia team help reduce this potential complication.

Miscellaneous Complications

Several miscellaneous complications of laser surgery of the upper aerodigestive tract and head and neck can occur. Delayed bleeding is a distinct possibility, especially when performing laser surgery on the floor of the mouth and tongue. The laser is an inefficient specific vessel coagulator; therefore, clamping and tying or cauterizing vessels at these sites represents good surgical technique. Delayed healing following laser surgery has been shown to occur, especially when closing the wound primarily. Choosing suture material that is slower to absorb helps neutralize this potential complication. Postoperative airway obstruction from displaced metallic tape, displaced cottonoids, and excessive coagulum can occur. Counting cottonoids, examining endotracheal tubes on extubation, and

carefully aspirating the operative site and airway following laser surgery will help minimize these complications.

Feder has reported granulomas following laser surgery at the operative site.[32] Because of this possibility, attempts should be made to remove all the black carbonaceous debris from the operative site at the conclusion of the case. Use of the microsuction, irrigation, and gentle rubbing with saline-saturated cottonoids facilitates this removal.

Laser Problems

Laser problems include misuse, malfunctions, and complications of proper use. Misuse of the laser should not occur if the surgeon attended a hands-on course, avoided use of the continuous mode, and used the proper power densities and exposure times. Malfunctions can always occur; however, problems related to laser malfunctions can be minimized if the laser is checked prior to bringing the patient into the operating room. If the laser safety protocol discussed earlier works, then complications of proper use should be minimal.

Effectiveness of a Safety Protocol

Fried published a survey of laser-related complications in the otolaryngology–head and neck surgery literature in 1984.[33] Of the 152 otolaryngologists who reported using the laser in this survey, 49 had experienced a total of 81 complications, including 28 separate incidents of endotracheal tube fires. Healy and associates reviewed 4416 cases of carbon dioxide laser surgery in the upper aerodigestive tract performed at Boston University Medical Center and affiliated hospitals and noted a 0.2 per cent complication rate.[34] Ossoff reported a survey of 218 past registrants in the hands-on laser surgery courses that he had directed; these otolaryngologists had performed over 7200 laser cases since attending the course.[1] Seven physicians reported a total of eight complications (0.1 per cent). No endotracheal tube fires were experienced in this group of physicians. These latter two studies demonstrate the effectiveness of a laser safety protocol.

CONCLUSIONS

The specialty of otolaryngology–head and neck surgery has had over 20 years of experience performing laser surgery in the head and neck and upper aerodigestive tract. Many complications have been experienced, and it is safe to say that as new wavelengths are introduced, new complications unique to this technology will probably arise. Existing safety protocols will have to be updated, and experienced laser surgeons will need to attend additional courses or workshops to become familiar with the new lasers.

The airway remains an area of concern with respect to the risk of a laser-ignited endotracheal tube fire. Newer tubes have reduced the risk of an airway fire but have not eliminated it entirely. Once the danger of a laser-ignited endotracheal tube fire has been put to rest through the introduction of a "laser-safe" endotracheal tube and cuff, more attention can be directed toward identifying and reducing procedure-related soft tissue laser complications.

References

1. Ossoff RH: Laser safety in otolaryngology–head and neck surgery: Anesthetic and educational considerations for laryngeal surgery. Laryngoscope 99:1–26, Suppl 48, 1989.
2. Ossoff RH, Duncavage JA: The CO_2 laser in otolaryngology–head and neck surgery: Advantages, precautions, administrative considerations and complications. In Johnson JT, Blitzer A, Ossoff R, Thomas JD (eds): Instructional Courses. Vol I. St. Louis, CV Mosby, 1988; pp 73–81.
3. Ossoff RH: Laser surgery: Basic principles and safety considerations. In Cummings CW, Fredrickson JM, Harker LA, et al (eds): Otolaryngology–Head and Neck Surgery. St. Louis, CV Mosby, 1986, pp 149–162.
4. Spilman LS: Nursing precautions for CO_2 laser surgery. Symp Proc Laser Inst Am 37:63, 1983.
5. American National Standards for the safe use of lasers, Z136.1. New York, American National Standards Institute, 1981.
6. Ossoff RH, et al: The CO_2 laser in otolaryngology–

head and neck surgery: A retrospective analysis of complications. Laryngoscope 93:1287, 1983.
7. Ossoff RH, Reinisch L: Laser surgery in otolaryngology: Basic principles and safety considerations. In Cummings CW, Fredrickson JM, Harker LA, et al (eds): Otolaryngology–Head and Neck Surgery. 2nd ed. in press.
8. DiBartolomeo JR: The argon and CO_2 lasers in otolaryngology: Which one, when and why? Laryngoscope Suppl 26:91:1–16, 1981.
9. Mohr RM, McDonnel BC, Unger M, Mauer TP: Safety considerations and safety protocol for laser surgery. Surg Clin North Am 64:851–859, 1984.
10. Tomita Y, Mihashi S, Nagata K: Mutagenicity of smoke condensates induced by CO_2 laser irradiation and electrocauterization. Mutat Res 89:145–149, 1981.
11. Garden JM, O'Banion MK, Sheintz LS, et al: Papilloma virus in the vapor of carbon dioxide laser–treated verrucae. JAMA 259:1199–1204, 1988.
12. Wentzell JM, Robinson JK, Schwartz DE, Carlson SE: Physical properties of aerosols produced by dermabrasion. Arch Dermatol 125:1637–1643, 1989.
13. Edelist G, Alberti PW: Anesthesia for CO_2 laser surgery of the larynx. J Otolaryngol 11:107–110, 1982.
14. Fried MP, Mallampati SR, Lui FC, et al: Laser resistant stainless steel endotracheal tube: Experimental and clinical evaluation. Lasers Surg Med 11:301–306, 1991.
15. Ossoff RH, Aly A, Gonzalez D, et al: A new endotracheal tube for carbon dioxide and KTP laser surgery of the aerodigestive tract. Otolaryngol Head Neck Surg, in press.
16. Schramm VL, Mattox DE, Stool SE: Acute management of laser-ignited intratracheal explosion. Laryngoscope 91:1417–1426, 1981.
17. Ossoff RH, Karlan MS: Safe instrumentation in laser surgery. Otolaryngol Head Neck Surg 92:664, 1984.
18. LeJeune FE Jr, LeTard F, Guice C, et al: Heat sink protection against lasering endotracheal cuffs. Ann Otol Rhinol Laryngol 91:606–607, 1982.
19. Ossoff RH, Karlan MS: Instrumentation for CO_2 laser surgery of the larynx and tracheobronchial tree. Surg Clin North Am 64:973–980, 1984.
20. Sosis MB: What is the safest endotracheal tube for Nd:YAG laser surgery? A comparative study. Anesth Analg 69:802–804, 1989.
21. Ossoff RH, Karlan MS: Universal endoscopic coupler for carbon dioxide laser surgery. Ann Otol Rhinol Laryngol 91:608–609, 1982.
22. Leibowitz HM, Peacock GR: Corneal injury produced by carbon dioxide laser radiation. Arch Ophthalmol 81:713–721, 1969.
23. Wetmore SJ, Key JM, Suen JY: Complications of laser surgery for laryngeal papillomatosis. Laryngoscope 95:798–801, 1985.
24. Crockett DM, McCabe BF, Shive CJ: Complications of laser surgery for recurrent respiratory papillomatosis. Ann Otol Rhinol Laryngol 96:639–644, 1987.
25. Benjamin B, Parsons DS: Recurrent respiratory papillomatosis: A ten-year study. J Laryngol Otol 102:1022–1028, 1988.
26. Ossoff RH, Werkhaven JA, Dere H: Soft-tissue complications of laser surgery for recurrent respiratory papillomatosis. Laryngoscope 101:1162–1166, 1991.
27. Ossoff RH, Werkhaven JA, Raif J, Abraham M:

Advanced microspot microslad for the CO_2 laser. Otolaryngol Head Neck Surg 105:411–414, 1991.

28. Cotton RT, Tewfik TL: Laryngeal stenosis following carbon dioxide laser in subglottic hemangioma. Ann Otol Rhinol Laryngol 94:494–497, 1985.

29. Shapshay SM, Rebeiz EE, Bohigian RK, Hybels RL: Benign lesions of the larynx: Should the laser be used? Laryngoscope 100:953–957, 1990.

30. Sosis MB: Airway fire during CO_2 laser surgery using a Xomed laser endotracheal tube. Anesthesiology 72:747–749, 1990.

31. Kaeder CS, Hirshman CA: Acute airway obstruction: A complication of aluminum tape wrapping of tracheal tubes in laser surgery. Can Anaesth Soc J 26:138–139, 1979.

32. Feder RJ: Laryngeal granuloma as a complication of the CO_2 laser. Laryngoscope 93:7, 1983.

33. Fried MP: A survey of the complications of laser laryngoscopy. Arch Otolaryngol 110:31–34, 1984.

34. Healy GB, Strong MS, Shapshay SM, et al: Complications of CO_2 laser surgery of the aerodigestive tract: Experience of 4,416 cases. Otolaryngol Head Neck Surg 92:13–18, 1984.

CHAPTER 31

Acquired Immunodeficiency Syndrome; Precautions for Health Care Workers

RON D. GOTTLIEB, MD
FRANK E. LUCENTE, MD

The acquired immunodeficiency syndrome (AIDS) epidemic that now plagues the country poses specific risks to health care workers who frequently come into contact with infected patients. Much attention has been focused recently on the precautions to be observed by these health care workers. This chapter reviews the currently recommended precautions to be observed in the office and operating room, as well as in other clinical settings, when dealing with all patients.

The first cases of AIDS were recognized in five young homosexual males in Los Angeles in June, 1981. In 1984, human immunodeficiency virus (HIV) was found to be the cause of AIDS. Human immunodeficiency virus is thought to have been present in the United States for over 20 years. Autopsy tissue dating from 20 years before, of a young, sexually active man, was positive for HIV.

AIDS has had a devastating impact on the health care system. At the beginning of 1990, there were thought to be 1.5 million people infected with HIV in this country and up to 10 million people worldwide. The cost of care for AIDS patients will be astronomic, and the disease has an impact on every medical specialty, requiring that all physicians be well educated about this disease.

The definition of AIDS was revised by the Centers for Disease Control in 1987. AIDS may be diagnosed by finding a positive ELISA and western blot blood test for HIV in the presence of certain opportunistic infections or characteristic tumors. The infections may include *Pneumocystis carinii* pneumonia, candidiasis of the esophagus, trachea, bronchi, or lungs, or persistent herpes simplex virus mucocutaneous infections. The diagnosis also may be made without antibody tests (if the test was not performed or was inconclusive) in the presence of opportunistic infections if other causes of immunodeficiency, such as long-term corticosteroid administration or lymphoma, are ruled out.[1] The term *AIDS-related complex* (ARC) has been used for those patients infected with HIV who exhibit fever, nightsweats, fatigue, diarrhea, and weight loss. The frequently used phrase "HIV-positive" implies that the individual described has been exposed to HIV virus and has formed antibodies to the virus.

By January 1, 1989, 82,764 cases of AIDS were diagnosed in the United States. Over 46,000 of these cases have proved to be fatal.[2] Three modes of transmission of AIDS are sexual contact, through blood and blood products, and perinatally.

Of the reported cases of AIDS contracted by sexual contact, most have occurred through sexual contact between men. As of 1989, homosexual men accounted for 62 per cent of all reported cases of AIDS.[3] The proportion of total AIDS cases in adult men who are homosexual has declined from 69 per cent prior to 1985 to 63 per cent in 1988. In contrast, the proportion of AIDS cases made up of intravenous drug abusers (IVDAs) has increased. Thirty per cent of all AIDS cases may be traced to IVDA, with this figure rising to 33 per cent in 1988. Minorities make up a disproportionate number of these cases. Among male heterosexual intravenous drug abusers with AIDS, 48 per cent are black and 32 per cent are Hispanic. Among female IVDAs, or sex partners of IVDAs with AIDS, 55 per cent are black and 23 per cent are Hispanic.[3]

Through 1988, 3069 persons developed AIDS from blood or blood products. Commencing in 1985, blood donations were screened for antibodies to HIV. Since that time, there have been several documented cases of persons acquiring AIDS through screened blood or blood products. People who are at high risk for AIDS are discouraged from donating blood.[3]

Heterosexual contacts account for 4 per cent of all reported AIDS cases. Many of these patients had a prior history of sexually transmitted diseases. There is a record of transmission of the virus through a single contact. However, in some instances hundreds of contacts with an infected person have failed to transmit the virus.[3]

Of the 1346 children below the age of 13 years who have contracted AIDS, 78 per cent contracted it perinatally. Of the perinatal transmissions, 54 per cent of the mothers were IVDAs. The fetus may acquire antibodies transplacentally. Accordingly, the antibody status may not detect true infection until the child is 15 months of age.[3]

Human immunodeficiency virus is the etiologic agent in AIDS. Two subtypes have been identified: HIV-1 and HIV-2. HIV-2 is endemic in Africa and has infrequently been reported elsewhere. Human immunodeficiency virus contains an RNA genome that through a reverse transcriptase becomes incorporated in the infected cell's genome as DNA. This DNA is responsible for the production of the viral proteins.

HIV debilitates the immune system by destroying T lymphocytes expressing the CD4 receptor. The CD4 receptor is most commonly expressed by the T helper cell. All aspects of cell-mediated immune response are altered, including natural killer activity, cytotoxicity, and the production of cytokines. Humoral immunocompetence is also affected, as B cells often fail to produce antibodies to new antigens.

The clinical manifestations of AIDS are varied. As the immune system is significantly impaired, any organ may be the site of opportunistic infections or unusual tumors. In addition, AIDS patients may present with common infections that are seen in a more severe or refractory state.

AIDS patients most commonly develop *Pneumocystis carinii* pneumonia. These patients generally present with dyspnea, fever, and cough. Other pulmonary pathogens include *Mycobacterium avium intracellulare* and now, with increasing frequency, *Mycobacterium tuberculosis*.

Common oral cavity pathogens are *Candida albicans* and herpes simplex virus. *Candida albicans* causes thrush and esophagitis, resulting in symptoms of sore throat with dysphagia. Herpes simplex lesions tend to be persistent and not readily eradicated.

Neuropsychiatric disorders are commonly manifested in AIDS patients. HIV encephalopathy includes findings of impaired cognitive and motor functions in the absence of illness other than HIV infection. *Cryptococcus neoformans* is a common pathogen causing meningitis and progressive dementia. *Toxoplasmosis gondii* frequently presents as an intracranial mass lesion.

Cytomegalovirus (CMV) can have multiple organ involvement. CMV meningitis in an acute or chronic form may be manifested. CMV chorioretinitis results in vision impairment and can lead to blindness. CMV enteritis is a frequent cause of diarrhea.

Among the characteristic tumors, Kaposi's sarcoma is usually manifested by multifocal vascular nodules on the skin or mucosal surfaces. The course may be quite variable. These lesions may cause significant dysphagia, lymphedema, intestinal obstruction, and pulmonary disease. Often these lesions are slowly progressive, causing them to be more of a cosmetic and psychologic issue.

The United States Public Health Service has estimated that between 1.5 and 2 million United States residents are infected with HIV. The seropositivity rate among trauma victims at Johns Hopkins Medical Center in a recent study was 3 per cent.[4] Of 534 patients admitted to Charity Hospital for major trauma, medical emergencies, or in labor, 2 per cent were seropositive for HIV. The authors of the latter study concluded that there is a ". . . substantial risk of exposure to HIV in trauma and medical emergency centers."[5]

The health care worker must protect himself or herself by a physical barrier during likely incidents of exposure to HIV. Universal precautions imply that all patients are potentially infectious for HIV and other bloodborne pathogens. The Centers for Disease Control (CDC) recommends that universal precautions apply to certain body fluids, any body fluid contaminated with blood, and all body fluids in emergency situations, in which the type of body fluid is not easily ascertained. Other body fluids do not necessitate universal precautions. Table 31–1 lists the CDC recommendations.[6] Although HIV has been isolated from nearly all body fluids, trans-

TABLE 31–1. Universal Precautions

Apply to	Do Not Apply Unless Contaminated with Blood
Blood	Feces
Amniotic fluid	Nasal secretions
Pericardial fluid	Sputum
Peritoneal fluid	Sweat
Pleural fluid	Tears
Cerebrospinal fluid	Urine
Semen	Saliva
Vaginal fluid	Cerumen
Synovial fluid	

mission has not been documented from these fluids listed in the righthand column in Table 31–1.

Certain precautions must be observed to minimize health care worker exposure to HIV:

1. All needles and sharp instruments must be disposed of in puncture-proof containers. Needles should never be recapped. Disposal containers must be easily accessible.

2. Although HIV does not penetrate intact skin, hands and skin surfaces should be washed immediately after any exposure to blood or body fluids to prevent transfer of virus to permeable regions. Hands should be washed even if gloves are used. Skin surfaces should be washed with soap and warm water. An antiseptic solution may also be used.

3. Gloves should be worn during exposure to blood and body fluids. Gloves should fit well and allow for manual dexterity. Care should be taken to avoid handling communal objects with soiled gloves.

4. Masks, protective eyewear, and gowns are indicated when droplets of blood and body fluids may be generated. Certain conditions such as major sharp trauma, emergency childbirth, and endotracheal intubation require these protective measures.

5. Health care workers with exudative dermatitis or broken skin should refrain from direct patient contact until the condition

clears. These health care workers lack the natural barrier provided by the skin.

6. All blood and potentially infectious body fluids that are spilled onto inanimate objects must be cleaned appropriately. Gloves must be worn and the spilled material cleaned with either an EPA-approved germicide or a 1:100 household bleach solution. First, all visible spillage should be cleaned with disposable towels, and the surface should be cleansed with an appropriate germicide. A full protective barrier is to be worn if splashing is expected.[6]

7. Sterilization and disinfection protocols should exist for reusable medical instruments. This is necessary to prevent the risk of transmission of HIV between patients as well as to protect health care workers. An ideal protocol would consist of a technique that quickly destroyed all microorganisms while not damaging instruments. The cleansing of the flexible nasopharyngoscope illustrates these principles. After the endoscope is used, it is mechanically cleaned. It is subsequently placed in a 2 per cent glutaraldehyde solution for 10 minutes. It is then rinsed with alcohol or sterile water and dried prior to repeat usage.[7]

8. There is a substantial risk of exposure to HIV in the operating room. Certain precautions may be undertaken to reduce this risk. The scalpel should have minimal usage besides incising skin. Scissors or an electrocautery should be substituted for the scalpel where possible. Blunt retractors should replace sharp ones where possible. The surgical team needs to be aware of the risks of exposure to HIV in the operating room and, consequently, take action in reducing these risks.

Unfortunately, universal precautions are often not adhered to. One recent spot check of a large hospital revealed that 36 per cent of venipunctures in an emergency room were done without gloves. During intubation in emergencies, 50 per cent were done without following the recommendations of mask and glove usage.[5] In a questionnaire mailed to all chief residents in emergency medicine residency programs, the respondents revealed that universal precautions are inconsistently followed. During major resuscitations, only 22 per cent of the respondents stated that protective gear was always used. Eighty-four per cent of the respondents had observed the attending staff not following universal precautions.[8] It is apparent that universal precautions are frequently not followed and need to be further encouraged.

The risk of seroconversion after needle stick exposure from an HIV-positive patient is approximately 0.5 per cent. The CDC, in an ongoing study, tested 1201 health care workers exposed to HIV from either needle sticks or mucous membrane contamination.[6] Four of the workers, all of whom had needle stick exposures, seroconverted. The Morbidity and Mortality Weekly Report of June 23, 1989, listed 25 cases of HIV infection in health care workers who had no nonoccupational risk factors. Fifteen workers seroconverted by needle stick exposure, 4 through nonintact skin, 2 through sharp objects, 2 through mucous membranes, 1 through a puncture wound, and 1 presumably by cutaneous exposure. The latter case involved a mother's numerous contacts with her HIV-infected child's blood and blood products without using proper precautions.

The appropriate management of an exposure to human immunodeficiency virus is essential. All exposures should be clearly documented and reported to Employee Health. The activity of the worker, the type of protection employed, and the nature of the penetration should be provided. Figure 31–1 illustrates the management of health care workers exposed to HIV.[9] Exposed areas should be cleansed appropriately. In the event of a needle stick, the wound should be milked and cleaned with an antiseptic solution such as Betadine. Informed consent should be obtained from the patient. If the patient is HIV-positive or refuses testing, the health care worker should be tested as indicated by Figure 31–1. Presently, many institutions are recommending prophylaxis with zidovudine, 200 mg every 4 hours for 6 weeks, if HIV exposure occurs.

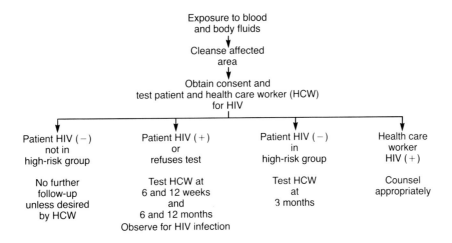

FIGURE 31–1. Management of health care workers exposed to HIV. (Modified from Osguthorpe JD, Patow C: Exposure to AIDS and hepatitis B: Prevention and management. Am Acad Otolaryngol Head Neck Surg Bull Dec 1989, pp 12–13.)

Employers have responsibility in protecting workers against infectious pathogens. The Department of Labor and the Department of Health and Human Services Joint Advisory Notice has made several recommendations about this. Employers need to clarify worker responsibilities, provide a standard operating practice, train and educate employees, and alter working conditions as necessary, in order to reduce risks.

The acquisition of HIV infection or AIDS by a health care worker through an occupational exposure raises multiple issues, including employer responsibility. There is currently a 175 million dollar lawsuit involving a physician who claims she acquired AIDS through her occupation. She is suing two physicians and the New York City Health and Hospitals Corporation. One physician, she claims, was negligent in the actual exposure. The other is accused of breeching the confidentiality of the plaintiff by improperly disclosing that the plaintiff tested positive for HIV. Important issues, such as employer responsibility and maintaining the confidentiality of the HIV-positive health care worker, were raised in the court case.

The management of health care workers with HIV must be individually based. Those with impaired immune responses are susceptible to infectious agents present in the health care environment. The decision to allow health care workers infected with HIV to continue their duties should involve the health care workers, their personal physicians, and the employer's medical advisors.

Treatment and compassion for the AIDS patient should meet the standard of medical care in our society. At the same time, health care workers should take the appropriate steps to ensure their own safety. The universal precautions must be followed with all patients, as any patient is potentially infected with HIV.

There is currently no cure for AIDS. Opportunistic infections are treated medically with impaired assistance from the patient's immune system. AZT has shown promise in prolonging survival, but there are deleterious side effects to this drug. Education of the general public and health care workers is essential in fighting this lethal disease and preventing its transmission.

References

1. Centers for Disease Control: Revision of the CDC Surveillance case definition for acquired immunodeficiency syndrome. MMWR 36:(Suppl 1S), 1987.
2. Centers for Disease Control: AIDS and human immunodeficiency virus infection in the United States: 1988 Update. MMWR 38:(S-4), 1989.

3. Berkelman RL, Heyward WL, Stehr-Green JK, et al: Epidemiology of human immunodeficiency virus infection and acquired immunodeficiency syndrome. Am J Med 86:761–770, 1989.

4. Baker JL, Kelen GD, Sivertson KT, et al: Unsuspected human immunodeficiency virus in critically ill emergency patients. JAMA 257:2609–2611, 1987.

5. Risi, GF Jr, Gaumer RH, Weeks S, et al: Human immunodeficiency virus: Risk of exposure among health care workers at a southern urban hospital. South Med J 82:1079–1082, 1989.

6. Centers for Disease Control: Guidelines for prevention of transmission of human immunodeficiency virus and hepatitis B virus to health care and public safety workers. MMWR 38:(S-6), 1989.

7. Meiteles LZ, Lucente FE: Endoscopic instrument sterilization: Impact of AIDS. Presented at the Eastern Section Meeting of the American Laryngologic, Rhinologic and Otologic Society, New Haven, CT, Jan 26, 1990.

8. Huff JS, Basala M: Universal precautions in emergency medicine residencies: 1989 (letter). Ann Emerg Med 18:798–799, 1989.

9. Osguthorpe JD, Patow L: Exposure to AIDS and hepatitis B: Prevention and management. Am Acad Otolaryngol Head Neck Surg Bull 8:12–13, 1989.

Index

—————•—————